Basic and Clinical Science Course
Section 8

External Disease and Cornea

1999-2000

(Last major revision 1998-1999)

LEO

LIFELONG
EDUCATION FOR THE
OPHTHALMOLOGIST

American Academy of Ophthalmology

The Basic and Clinical Science Course is one component of the Lifelong Education for the Ophthalmologist (LEO) framework, which assists members in planning their continuing medical education. LEO includes an array of clinical education products that members may select to form individualized, self-directed learning plans for updating their clinical knowledge. Active members or fellows who use LEO components may accumulate sufficient CME credits to earn the LEO Award. Contact the Academy's Clinical Education Division for further information on LEO.

This CME activity was planned and produced in accordance with the ACCME Essentials.

Basic and Clinical Science Course

Thomas A. Weingeist, PhD, MD, Iowa City, Iowa
Senior Secretary for Clinical Education

Thomas J. Liesegang, MD, Jacksonville, Florida
Secretary for Instruction

M. Gilbert Grand, MD, St. Louis, Missouri
BCSC Course Chair

Section 8

Faculty Responsible for This Edition

Kirk R. Wilhelmus, MD, MPH, *Chair,* Houston, Texas

Andrew J.W. Huang, MD, Miami, Florida

David G. Hwang, MD, San Francisco, California

Carolyn M. Parrish, MD, Nashville, Tennessee

John E. Sutphin, Jr, MD, Iowa City, Iowa

Jeffrey C. Whitsett, MD, Houston, Texas
Practicing Ophthalmologists Advisory Committee for Education

The authors state the following financial relationships:

Dr. Hwang: research funding from KeraVision, Inc; Nidek Technologies; Tomey Corporation USA.

Dr. Sutphin: research funding from Allergan, Inc; Senju Corporation.

The other authors state that they have no significant financial interest or other relationship with the manufacturer of any commercial product discussed in the chapters that they contributed to this publication or with the manufacturer of any competing commercial product.

Recent Past Faculty

Michael W. Belin, MD

Vincent P. deLuise, MD

Steven P. Dunn, MD

Randy J. Epstein, MD

David J. Harris, Jr, MD

Jeffrey D. Lanier, MD

Priscilla E. Perry, MD

Stephen C. Pflugfelder, MD

Ivan R. Schwab, MD

Paul L. Wright, MD

In addition, the Academy gratefully acknowledges the contributions of numerous past faculty and advisory committee members who have played an important role in the development of previous editions of the Basic and Clinical Science Course.

American Academy of Ophthalmology Staff

Kathryn A. Hecht, EdD
Vice President, Clinical Education

Hal Straus
Director, Publications Department

Margaret Denny
Managing Editor

Fran Taylor
Medical Editor

Maxine Garrett
Administrative Coordinator

American Academy of Ophthalmology
655 Beach Street
Box 7424
San Francisco, CA 94120-7424

CONTENTS

GENERAL INTRODUCTION

The Basic and Clinical Science Course (BCSC) is designed to provide residents and practitioners with a comprehensive yet concise curriculum of the field of ophthalmology. The BCSC has developed from its original brief outline format, which relied heavily on outside readings, to a more convenient and educationally useful self-contained text. The Academy regularly updates and revises the course, with the goals of integrating the basic science and clinical practice of ophthalmology and of keeping current with new developments in the various subspecialties.

The BCSC incorporates the effort and expertise of more than 70 ophthalmologists, organized into 12 section faculties, working with Academy editorial staff. In addition, the course continues to benefit from many lasting contributions made by the faculties of previous editions. Members of the Academy's Practicing Ophthalmologists Advisory Committee for Education serve on each faculty and, as a group, review every volume before and after major revisions.

Organization of the Course

The 12 sections of the Basic and Clinical Science Course are numbered as follows to reflect a logical order of study, proceeding from fundamental subjects to anatomic subdivisions:

1. Update on General Medicine
2. Fundamentals and Principles of Ophthalmology
3. Optics, Refraction, and Contact Lenses
4. Ophthalmic Pathology and Intraocular Tumors
5. Neuro-Ophthalmology
6. Pediatric Ophthalmology and Strabismus
7. Orbit, Eyelids, and Lacrimal System
8. External Disease and Cornea
9. Intraocular Inflammation and Uveitis
10. Glaucoma
11. Lens and Cataract
12. Retina and Vitreous

In addition, a comprehensive Master Index allows the reader to easily locate subjects throughout the entire series.

References

Readers who wish to explore specific topics in greater detail may consult the journal references cited within each chapter and the Basic Texts listed at the back of the book. These references are intended to be selective rather than exhaustive, chosen by the BCSC faculty as being important, current, and readily available to residents and practitioners.

Related Academy educational materials are also listed in the appropriate sections. They include books, audiovisual materials, self-assessment programs, clinical modules, and interactive programs.

Study Questions and CME Credit

Each volume includes multiple-choice study questions designed to be used as a closed-book exercise. The answers are accompanied by explanations to enhance the learning experience. Completing the study questions allows readers both to test their understanding of the material and to demonstrate section completion for the purpose of CME credit, if desired.

The Academy is accredited by the Accreditation Council for Continuing Medical Education to sponsor continuing medical education for physicians. CME credit hours in Category 1 of the Physician's Recognition Award of the AMA may be earned for completing the study of any section of the BCSC. The Academy designates the number of credit hours for each section based upon the scope and complexity of the material covered (see the Credit Reporting Form in each individual section for the maximum number of hours that may be claimed).

Based upon return of the Credit Reporting Form at the back of each book, the Academy will maintain a record, for up to 3 years, of credits earned by Academy members. Upon request, the Academy will send a transcript of credits earned.

Conclusion

The Basic and Clinical Science Course has expanded greatly over the years, with the addition of much new text and numerous illustrations. Recent editions have sought to place a greater emphasis on clinical applicability, while maintaining a solid foundation in basic science. As with any educational program, it reflects the experience of its authors. As its faculties change and as medicine progresses, new viewpoints are always emerging on controversial subjects and techniques. Not all alternate approaches can be included in this series; as with any educational endeavor, the learner should seek additional sources, including such carefully balanced opinions as the Academy's Preferred Practice Patterns.

The BCSC faculty and staff are continuously striving to improve the educational usefulness of the course; you, the reader, can contribute to this ongoing process. If you have any suggestions or questions about the series, please do not hesitate to contact the faculty or the managing editor.

The authors, editors, and reviewers hope that your study of the BCSC will be of lasting value and that each section will serve as a practical resource for quality patient care.

OBJECTIVES FOR BCSC SECTION 8

Upon completion of BCSC Section 8, *External Disease and Cornea,* the reader should be able to:

□ Describe the anatomy and molecular biology of the cornea

□ Explain the pathogenesis of common disorders affecting the eyelid margin, conjunctiva, cornea, and sclera

□ Recognize the distinctive signs of specific diseases of the ocular surface and cornea

□ Describe how the environment can affect the structure and function of the ocular surface

□ Evaluate the diagnostic tests used in ocular microbiology, immunology, and oncology

□ Summarize the developmental and metabolic alterations that lead to structural changes of the cornea

□ Identify topographic changes of the cornea and describe the risks and benefits of corrective measures

□ Assess the indications and techniques of surgical procedures for managing corneal disease, trauma, and refractive error

□ Apply the results of recent clinical research to the management of selected disorders of the conjunctiva and cornea

□ Integrate the discipline of corneal and external eye disease into the practice of ophthalmology

INTRODUCTION TO SECTION 8

The discipline of corneal and external eye disease encompasses a wide variety of ocular and systemic conditions that affect the eyelid skin, eyelid margin, tear film, conjunctiva, cornea, and sclera. This completely revised manual provides an overview of the basic and clinical knowledge needed to understand the disorders and management options pertaining to the outer eye.

Clinical problem-solving involves determining the involved structure and disease process, identifying the distinctive features, and developing a management plan. This manual is organized to facilitate this approach. The authors have sought to provide an introductory curriculum for ophthalmologists in training that can also serve as a review and update for practicing ophthalmologists.

The text begins with chapters on the normal eye, diagnostic techniques, and principles of treatment and prevention. The remainder of the book is organized by specific disease processes and interventions. The principal pathophysiologic responses of the outer eye covered in individual chapters are

- Ocular surface dysfunctions
- Infections
- Immune-mediated diseases
- Neoplasias
- Congenital anomalies
- Dystrophic and metabolic disorders
- Aging and degenerative conditions
- Toxic and traumatic injuries

The manual concludes with chapters on surgery of the conjunctiva and cornea. New sections included in this revision are immunology of the outer eye, genetics and molecular biology of the cornea, diseases and surgery of the ocular surface, corneal topography and biomechanics, and keratorefractive surgery including various laser procedures.

Most parts of the book begin with an overview chapter of the basic science underpinning each major entity. The chapter that follows focuses on diagnostic methods and clinical science. Specific diseases and procedures are ordered and explained, and prevalence is noted. If epidemiologic information is not available, the authors categorize disease frequency by using the following scale based on how often a comprehensive ophthalmologist might typically encounter the problem:

- Very common: one or more cases every month
- Common: more than one per year
- Somewhat common: about one per year
- Somewhat rare: one every several years
- Rare: one or two in a career
- Very rare: heard or read of a case

The length and detail of information devoted to each topic reflect its relative importance in contemporary practice. The pathogenesis, clinical findings, and management are described for ocular disorders, and the indications and complications are given for surgical procedures. Drawings and color photographs show examples of common or important diseases and illustrate the principal surgical techniques. Biologic scientific advances and evidence from randomized clinical trials and other analytic studies are used whenever possible. Much of this manual also relies on general clinical perceptions and consensus of the writing committee and reviewers. Responses from readers are welcomed to correct factual errors before each annual revision.

This section of the Basic and Clinical Science Course is designed to be the basis for understanding corneal and external eye disease and surgery, but it is not a substitute for study or clinical experience. Further reading is essential, and references to key textbooks and atlases and selected chapters and journal articles are interspersed throughout the text. Current materials produced by the American Academy of Ophthalmology are also cited. The Academy's multimedia collection, also entitled *External Disease and Cornea*, contains slides and a photo-CD depicting common corneal and external eye diseases. It is a useful companion to this book.

Study questions are included at the end of the book to encourage review of the text, but the problems that arise in daily practice cannot be answered with this volume alone. BCSC Section 8 is one step in a successful ophthalmologist's lifelong educational program. While ophthalmologists are superfluous for many of nature's afflictions, our goals are to preserve and restore vision by preventing and correcting the various pathophysiologic processes that affect the eye and its adnexa.

PART 1

BASIC AND CLINICAL CONCEPTS OF
CORNEAL AND EXTERNAL EYE DISEASE

CHAPTER I

Structure and Function of the External Eye and Cornea

The Outer Eye and Cornea in Health and Disease

The external eye is the most crucial part of the body exposed to the outside world. The normal structure and function of the healthy eye rely on homeostasis of the entire body for protection against an adverse environment. Genetics and nutrition determine the embryogenesis and growth of the eye. Intact vascular and nervous systems ensure stable metabolism, and the immune system maintains surveillance.

The cushioning effect of the periocular tissues and local barriers like the orbital rim is needed to safeguard the globe. The eyebrows and eyelashes catch small particles, and cilia work like sensors to stimulate reflex eyelid closure. Blinking augments the lacrimal pump to rinse tears over the eye and flush off foreign material. The tear film also dilutes toxins and allergens and contains proteins that control the normal flora. Mucin demarcates our surroundings from the living cells of the ocular surface.

The epidermis and the epithelium of healthy eyelids, conjunctiva, and cornea adhere tightly to their basement membranes. Regulation of cellular growth and metabolism are critical to the maintenance of an intact ocular surface and a transparent cornea. The underlying extracellular matrix of the eye's mucous membrane is rich in blood vessels and conjunctiva-associated lymphoid tissue. The anterior segment of the eye provides a clear, protected exterior for light that is to be seen by the central nervous system to enter.

Understanding the eye's innate defenses requires study of ocular histology and biochemistry and observation of many people, both healthy and ill. The practice of corneal and external eye disease builds on this understanding and extends from clinical examination to clinicopathologic problem-solving, molecular medicine, and microsurgery. The reader is expected to be familiar with the embryology, anatomy, physiology, and biochemistry of the normal eye (see BCSC Section 2, *Fundamentals and Principles of Ophthalmology*).

Development of the Anterior Segment

The eye begins to develop during week 4 of gestation as an evagination from the *neuroectoderm* (Fig I-1). Invagination of the optic vesicle forms the double-layered optic cup of neuroectoderm at week 5. At this time the surface ectoderm forms the lens placode and gives rise to the corneal and conjunctival epithelium and the eyelid epidermis. Also at week 5, the first wave of *mesectoderm (neural crest)* extends under the epithelium from the limbus to begin forming the corneal endothelium. A subsequent wave of mesectoderm at week 6 begins forming the corneal stroma and sclera.

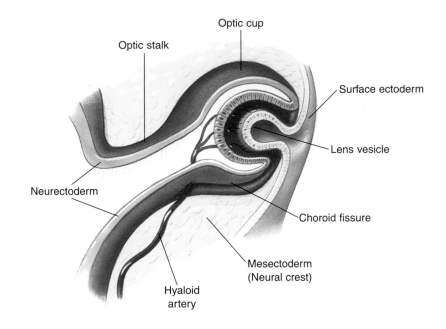

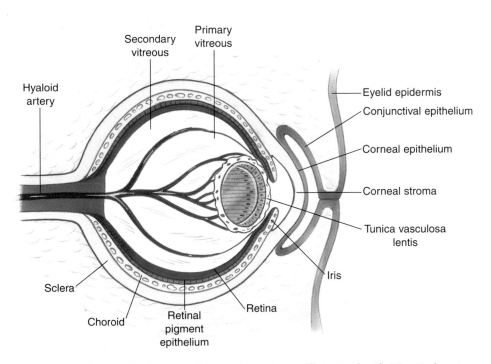

FIG I-1—Embryonic development of the anterior segment. (Illustration by Christine Gralapp.)

At 2 months of gestation the eyelids fuse, and the conjunctiva begins to develop with the eyelid folds. The ocular surface epithelium differentiates shortly afterward. At 3 months all corneal components are present except Bowman's layer, which appears in the fourth month as the scleral spur is also forming. The eyelids begin to open during the sixth month. At birth the globe is 80% of its adult size. The postnatal sclera and cornea are somewhat distensible, gradually becoming more rigid during the first 2 years of life.

Eyelids

Eyelids are unique to vertebrates, and humans have one of the largest interpalpebral fissure width–to–body mass ratios. The eyelid skin blends into the surrounding periorbital skin, varying from 0.5 mm thick at the eyelid margin to 1 mm thick at the orbital rim. Except for fine vellus hairs, the only hairs of the eyelids are the eyelashes, or *cilia*, which are twice as numerous along the upper eyelid margin as the lower. Cilia are replaced every 3–5 months; they will usually regrow in 2 weeks when cut and within 2 months if pulled out.

The epidermis of the eyelids is similar to other facial skin. It abruptly changes to nonkeratinized stratified squamous epithelium at the mucocutaneous junction of the eyelid margin, along the row of *meibomian gland* orifices. Holocrine sebaceous glands and eccrine sweat glands are present in the eyelid skin. Near the eyelid margin are the apocrine sweat glands, the *glands of Moll;* and numerous sebaceous glands, the *glands of Zeis* (Fig I-2).

Sensory nerves from the first division of cranial nerve V (trigeminal) extend to the eyelids through the supraorbital nerve and its lacrimal, supratrochlear, and infratrochlear branches. Innervated by the zygomatic branch of cranial nerve VII (facial), the orbicularis oculi muscle closes the eyelids, whether by volition using its orbital and preseptal portions or by subconscious blinking using the pretarsal portion. Nonstressed, healthy people blink about every 3–4 seconds when not concentrating on a visual task; conscious vision is turned off just before a blink starts. Besides movement toward each other, the eyelids also move medially during a blink, providing a pumping action within the lacrimal drainage system. Eyelid closure during sleep involves active tonus of the orbicularis with sustained inhibition of the levator muscle.

The blood supply of the eyelids comes chiefly from two sources: the external carotid artery through the facial, superficial, temporal, and infraorbital branches of the facial artery; and the internal carotid artery through the dorsal, nasal, frontal, supraorbital, and lacrimal branches of the ophthalmic artery. Venous drainage occurs through the anterior facial and superior temporal veins into the jugular vein and through the ophthalmic vein into the cavernous sinus. Lymphatics drain primarily to the preauricular lymph node, although the medial aspect of the eyelid and conjunctiva drain into the submandibular and submental nodes.

Tarsal plates are situated in the deep upper and lower eyelids, providing a structural foundation for attachment of muscles and the orbital septum. Each tarsus is 0.75 mm thick and measures 10 mm in vertical height in the upper eyelid and 4 mm in the lower. The orbital septum, separating the orbicularis muscle and the orbital fat, extends from the tarsi to the periosteum of the orbital rim. The meibomian glands embedded within each tarsus are composed of several lobules that open in a common secretory duct.

Krachmer JH, Mannis MJ, Holland EJ, eds. *Cornea.* St Louis: Mosby; 1997;1:61–67.

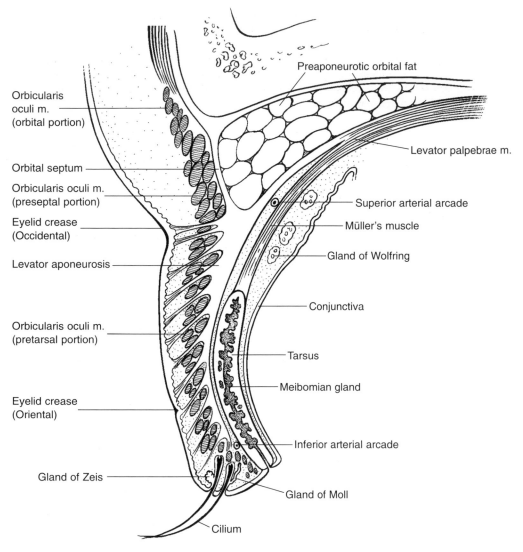

Orbicularis
oculi m.
(orbital portion)

Orbital septum

Orbicularis oculi m.
(preseptal portion)

Eyelid crease
(Occidental)

Levator aponeurosis

Orbicularis oculi m.
(pretarsal portion)

Eyelid crease
(Oriental)

Gland of Zeis

Preaponeurotic orbital fat

Levator palpebrae m.

Superior arterial arcade

Müller's muscle

Gland of Wolfring

Conjunctiva

Tarsus

Meibomian gland

Inferior arterial arcade

Gland of Moll

Cilium

FIG I-2—Cross-section of the upper eyelid. (Illustration by Christine Gralapp.)

Conjunctiva

The conjunctival sac includes the *bulbar conjunctiva,* a *fornix* on three sides and a
medial *semilunar fold,* and the *palpebral conjunctiva.* Smooth-muscle fibers from
the levator muscle maintain the superior fornix, and fibrous slips extend from the
horizontal rectus tendons into the temporal conjunctiva and plica to form cul-de-
sacs during horizontal gaze. The *caruncle* is a fleshy tissue mass containing hairs and
sebaceous glands. The *tarsal conjunctiva* is tightly adherent to the underlying tarsus,

and the bulbar conjunctiva is loosely adherent to Tenon's capsule. These tissues blend at the limbus, where a series of radiating ridges called the *palisades of Vogt* appear.

The conjunctival epithelium varies from stratified cuboidal over the tarsus to columnar in the fornices to squamous on the globe. Multiple surface folds are present. Goblet cells account for up to 10% of basal cells of the conjunctival epithelium; they are most numerous in the tarsal conjunctiva and the inferonasal bulbar conjunctiva.

The *substantia propria* of the conjunctiva consists of loose connective tissue. Lymphocytes and other leukocytes are present, especially in the fornices. Lymphocytes interact with mucosal epithelial cells through reciprocal regulatory signals mediated by growth factors, cytokines, and neuropeptides.

The palpebral conjunctiva shares its blood supply with the eyelids. The bulbar conjunctiva is supplied by the anterior ciliary arteries, branches of the ophthalmic artery. These capillaries are fenestrated and leak fluorescein just like the choriocapillaris. Sensory innervation is controlled by the lacrimal, supraorbital, supratrochlear, and infraorbital branches of the ophthalmic division of cranial nerve V.

Krachmer JH, Mannis MJ, Holland EJ, eds. *Cornea.* St Louis: Mosby; 1997;1:41–47.

Cornea

The cornea is a transparent, avascular tissue that measures 11–12 mm horizontally and 9–11 mm vertically. Its refractive index is 1.376, although an index of refraction of 1.3375 is used in calibrating the keratometer to account for the combined optical power of the anterior and posterior curvatures of the cornea. The cornea is aspheric, although its radius of curvature is often recorded as a spherocylindrical convex mirror representing the central anterior corneal surface, also called the *corneal cap.*

The average radius of curvature of the central cornea is 7.8 mm (6.7–9.4 mm). The cornea thus contributes 74%, or 43.25 diopters (D), of the total 58.60 dioptric power of a normal human eye, and it is the major source of astigmatism. Most of the total corneal power occurs at the air–tear surface. Some refraction occurs at the tear–cornea and cornea–aqueous interfaces because of slight differences in refractive index between the cornea (1.376) and the tear film and aqueous humor (1.336).

Nutrition of the cornea is dependent on glucose diffusing from the aqueous humor and oxygen diffusing through the tear film. In addition, the peripheral cornea is supplied with oxygen from the limbal circulation.

The cornea has one of the body's highest densities of nerve endings, and corneal sensation is 100 times that of the conjunctiva. Sensory nerve fibers extend from the long ciliary nerves and form a subepithelial plexus. Neurotransmitters in the cornea include acetylcholine, catecholamines, substance P, and calcitonin gene–related peptide.

Epithelium

The corneal *epithelium* is composed of stratified squamous epithelial cells and makes up about 5% (0.05 mm) of the total corneal thickness (Fig I-3). The epithelium and tear film form an optically smooth surface. Tight junctions between superficial epithelial cells prevent penetration of tear fluid into the stroma. Continuous proliferation of basal epithelial cells gives rise to the other layers that differentiate subsequently into superficial cells. With maturation these cells become coated with

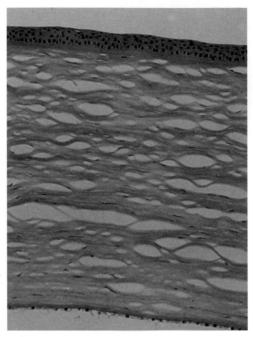

FIG I-3—Normal cornea. The epithelium, normally five cell layers, will thicken to maintain a smooth surface (H&E ×32).

microvilli on their outermost surface, thus appearing dark by scanning electron microscopy and bright by specular microscopy, and then desquamate into the tears. This process of differentiation takes about 7–14 days. Basal epithelial cells secrete a continuous, 50-nm-thick basement membrane, composed of type IV collagen, laminin, and other proteins.

Stroma

Optimal corneal optics requires a smooth surface with a healthy tear film and epithelium. A clear cornea needs tight packing of epithelial cells to produce a layer with a nearly uniform refractive index and minimal light scattering. The regular arrangement of stromal cells and macromolecules is also necessary for a clear cornea. Keratocytes form a three-dimensional network throughout the cornea, and these corneal fibroblasts continually digest and manufacture stromal molecules.

Beneath the acellular *Bowman's layer* the corneal *stroma* is composed of an extracellular matrix formed of collagens and proteoglycans. Type I and type V fibrillar collagens are intertwined by filaments of type VI collagen. The major corneal proteoglycans are decorin associated with dermatan sulfate and lumican associated with keratan sulfate. The lamellae of the anterior stroma are short, narrow sheets with extensive interweaving between layers, while the posterior stroma have long, wide, thick lamellae with minimal interlamellar connections. The human cornea has little elasticity and stretches only 0.25% at normal intraocular pressures.

The lattice arrangement of collagen fibrils embedded in the extracellular matrix is partly responsible for corneal transparency. This pattern acts like a diffraction grating to reduce light scattering by destructive interference. The cornea is transparent because the size of the lattice elements is smaller than the wavelength of visible light.

Transparency also depends on keeping the water content of the corneal stroma at 78%. Corneal hydration is largely controlled by intact epithelial and endothelial barriers and the functioning of the endothelial pump, which is linked to an ion-transport system controlled by temperature-dependent enzymes such as Na^+,K^+-ATPase. In addition, negatively charged stromal glycosaminoglycans tend to repel each other, producing a swelling pressure (SP). Because the intraocular pressure (IOP) tends to compress the cornea, the overall imbibition pressure of the corneal stroma is given as IOP − SP. The total transendothelial osmotic force is calculated by adding the imbibition pressure and the various electrolyte gradients produced by the endothelial transport channels.

Endothelium

The *endothelium* is made up of closely interdigitated cells arranged in a mosaic pattern of mostly hexagonal shapes. Human endothelial cells do not proliferate in vivo. Cell loss results in enlargement and spread of neighboring cells to cover the defective area.

Descemet's membrane is the basement membrane of the corneal endothelium. It increases in thickness from 3 µm at birth to 10–12 µm in adults as the endothelium gradually lays down a posterior amorphous nonbanded zone.

Krachmer JH, Mannis MJ, Holland FJ, eds. *Cornea.* St Louis: Mosby; 1997;1:3–27.

Smolin G, Thoft RA, eds. *The Cornea: Scientific Foundations and Clinical Practice.* 3rd ed. Boston: Little, Brown; 1994:3–67.

Sclera

The sclera is composed primarily of type I collagen and proteoglycans (decorin, biglycan, and aggrecan). Other components include elastin and glycoproteins such as fibronectin. Fibroblasts lie along collagen bundles. The long posterior ciliary nerves supply the anterior sclera. An intrascleral loop from a branch of one of these nerves sometimes forms a visible nodule over the ciliary body.

Normally a densely white tissue, sclera becomes more translucent when thinning occurs or the water content changes, falling below 40% or rising above 80%. For example, senile scleral plaques are areas of calcium phosphate deposits just anterior to the insertions of the medial and lateral rectus muscles that become dehydrated and reveal the blue color of the underlying uvea.

Krachmer JH, Mannis MJ, Holland EJ, eds. *Cornea.* St Louis: Mosby; 1997;1:29–40.

CHAPTER II

Examination Techniques of the External Eye and Cornea

Examination of the patient begins the moment the examiner enters the room. Since the reader should have already become familiar with the basic techniques of the complete eye examination, this chapter will describe how to recognize abnormalities produced by disorders of the external eye and cornea. *Practical Ophthalmology: A Manual for Beginning Residents,* published by the American Academy of Ophthalmology, offers a concise review of examination techniques.

Vision

Visual acuity testing is an essential part of the examination, and the refraction of a patient with an abnormal cornea requires special attention. Occasionally, it is necessary to use a rigid gas-permeable (RGP) contact lens with overrefraction when visual acuity is reduced because of surface irregularity. One method is to obtain keratometry readings and select a large-diameter hard contact lens with a base curve halfway between the two powers and with a power near the patient's spherical equivalent. Topical anesthesia helps reduce tearing as the spherical overrefraction is performed. The potential acuity meter is another way to assess visual acuity potential in a patient with focal corneal opacification or surface irregularity, but this instrument can give misleading results. BCSC Section 3, *Optics, Refraction, and Contact Lenses,* discusses these difficulties in detail in its appendix on prescribing cylinders.

External Examination

Physical examination of the eye begins with inspection, palpation, and occasionally auscultation. The examiner observes the patient's appearance and notes the condition of the skin, the position and action of the eyelids, the presence of preauricular lymph nodes, and the placement of the globes. Eversion of the eyelids permits examination of the palpebral conjunctiva. Infants and frightened patients may need to have their eyelids gently pried open with the thumbs or a retractor.

Common measurements include interpalpebral fissure height and levator function. The examiner should measure each visible or palpable mass by the longest dimension and its perpendicular. Tear production is measured with sterile filter-paper strips and may be done without anesthetic (Schirmer test) or with anesthetic (basic secretion test).

External examination of the outer eye and adnexa begins by looking at the patient, preferably in daylight or bright room light, then proceeds to magnification with focal illumination. The simplest magnifying instruments are loupes and condensing lenses like those used for indirect ophthalmoscopy. Many handheld penlights and transilluminators are also available, and these tools are helpful at the bedside and for external surgical procedures.

Krachmer JH, Mannis MJ, Holland EJ, eds. *Cornea.* St Louis: Mosby; 1997;1:237–242.

Slit-Lamp Biomicroscopy

The slit-lamp biomicroscope has two rotating arms—one for the slit illuminator and the other for the biomicroscope—mounted on a common axis. The illumination unit is essentially a projector with a light beam that is adjustable in width, height, direction, intensity, and color. The biomicroscope is a binocular Galilean telescope with multiple magnifications. A headrest immobilizes the patient, and a joystick lever and adjustable eyepieces allow the examiner to focus the stereoscopic image.

The illumination and microscope arms are parfocal, arranged so both focus on the same spot, with the slit beam centered in the field of view. This setup provides direct illumination, and purposeful shifting of alignment allows for indirect illumination. Variations of these illumination techniques, using both dark-field and brightfield contrast, are used to examine the anterior segment of the eye.

Leibowitz HM, Waring GO III, eds. *Corneal Disorders: Clinical Diagnosis and Management.* 2nd ed. Philadelphia: Saunders; 1998:34–81.

Direct Illumination Methods

Diffuse illumination   The light beam is broadened, reduced in intensity, and directed at the eye from an oblique angle. Diffuse illumination is usually used at low magnification to give an overview of the eyelids, conjunctiva, sclera, and cornea. Swinging the illuminator arm to produce highlights and shadows can enhance the visibility of surface changes.

Slit illumination   The light and the microscope are focused on the same spot, and the slit aperture is adjusted from wide to narrow. Broad-beam illumination, using a slit width of around 3 mm, can help the examiner visualize opaque lesions. Slit-beam illumination, using a beam width of about 1 mm or less, gives an optical section of the cornea (Fig II-1). A very narrow slit beam helps identify refractive index differences in transparent structures as light rays pass through the cornea, anterior chamber, and lens. The examiner can reduce the height of a narrow beam to determine the presence and amount of cells and flare in the anterior chamber.

Specular reflection   Specular reflections are normal light reflexes bouncing off a surface. An example is the bright round or oval spot seen reflected from the ocular surface in a typical flash photograph of an eye. These mirror images of the light source can be annoying, and it is tempting to subliminally ignore them during slit-lamp examination. However, the clarity and sharpness of these shiny reflections from the tear film give clues to the condition of the underlying tissue.

A faint reflection also comes from the posterior corneal surface. The examiner can enhance this specular reflection by using a light beam at an appropriate angle,

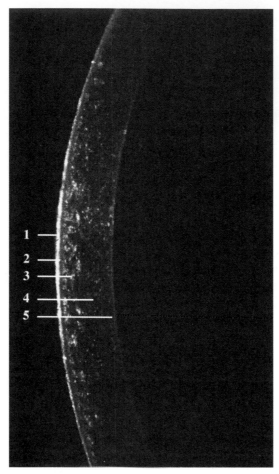

FIG II-1—Slit section of normal cornea. *1,* Tear film. *2,* Epithelium. *3,* Anterior stroma with high density of keratocytes. *4,* Posterior stroma with lower density of keratocytes. *5,* Descemet's membrane and endothelium. (Reproduced with permission from Krachmer JH, Mannis MJ, Holland EJ, eds. *Cornea.* St Louis: Mosby; 1997;1:249. ©CL Mártonyi, WK Kellogg Eye Center, University of Michigan.)

revealing the corneal endothelium (Fig II-2). To examine the corneal endothelium using specular reflection the examiner performs the following steps:

☐ Begin with setting the slit-beam arm at an angle of 60° from the viewing arm and using a short slit or 0.2-mm spot

☐ Identify the very bright mirror image of the light bulb's filament and the paired epithelial and endothelial Purkinje light reflexes

☐ Superimpose the corneal endothelial light reflex onto the filament's mirror image, giving a bright glare

☐ Use the joystick to move the biomicroscope slightly forward in order to focus the endothelial reflex

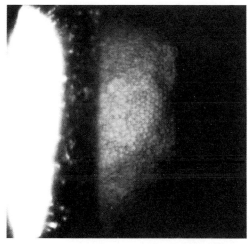

FIG II-2—Corneal endothelium seen with specular reflection using the slit-lamp biomicroscope at ×40 magnification. (Reproduced with permission from Krachmer JH, Mannis MJ, Holland EJ, eds. *Cornea.* St Louis: Mosby; 1997;1:255. ©CL Mártonyi, WK Kellogg Eye Center, University of Michigan.)

Specular microscopy is monocular, and one eyepiece may require focusing. A setting of ×25 to ×40 is usually needed to obtain a clear view of the endothelial mosaic. Cell density and morphology are noted; guttatae and keratic precipitates appear as dark areas of nonreflectivity.

Indirect Illumination Methods

Proximal illumination Turning a knob on the illumination arm slightly decenters the light beam from its isocentric position, causing the light beam and the microscope to be focused at different but adjacent spots. This technique highlights an opacity against deeper tissue layers and allows the examiner to see small irregularities that have a refractive index similar to their surroundings. Moving the light beam back and forth in small oscillations can help the examiner detect small three-dimensional lesions.

Sclerotic scatter Total internal reflection in the cornea makes another form of indirect illumination possible. Decentering the isocentric light beam so that an intense beam shines on the limbus and scatters off the sclera causes a very faint glow of the cornea. Reflective opacities stand out against the dark field, while areas of reduced light transmission in the cornea are seen as shades of gray.

Retroillumination This technique can be used to examine more than one area. Retroillumination from the iris is performed by displacing the beam tangentially while examining the cornea. The examiner observing the zone between the light and dark backgrounds can detect subtle corneal abnormalities. Retroillumination from the fundus is performed by aligning the light beam nearly parallel with the examiner's visual axis and rotating the light so it shines through the edge of the pupil.

Opacities in the cornea or lens are highlighted against the red reflex, and iris defects are transilluminated. Retroillumination from light reflected off the retinal pigment epithelium is used with the Hruby lens or an indirect condensing lens to reveal vitreous floaters.

Farrell TA, Alward WLM, Verdick RE. *Fundamentals of Slit-Lamp Biomicroscopy.* Videotape. San Francisco: American Academy of Ophthalmology; 1993.

Clinical Use

Slit-lamp examination is performed in a coordinated sequence:

- Eyelids
- Eyelid margins
- Tear film
- Conjunctiva
- Cornea
- Aqueous humor
- Iris
- Lens
- Vitreous

After adjusting the focus of the eyepieces, the clinician usually begins the examination with direct illumination of the conjunctiva and sclera. A broad beam illuminates the cornea and overlying tear film in optical section. Details are examined with a narrow beam. The clinician can estimate the height of the tear meniscus and measure discrete lesions using a slit-beam micrometer or an eyepiece reticle. Retroillumination and indirect illumination accentuate fine changes. The examiner then uses specular reflection to inspect the endothelium and has the patient shift gaze in different directions so that each corneal quadrant can be surveyed. A slit beam is used to judge the corneal thickness and the depth of the anterior chamber. A short beam or spot will show flare or cells in the aqueous humor. Direct, slit, and retroillumination techniques are used to identify abnormalities of the iris and lens.

The experienced examiner actively uses the light beam with multiple illumination methods to sweep across the eye, using shadows and reflections to bring out details. Having the patient blink can also help the examiner to distinguish changes of the ocular surface from tiny opacities floating in the tear film. After initial low-power screening, much of the slit-lamp examination is performed using higher magnifications.

Except for the anterior vitreous humor, other intraocular structures require special lenses. A contact lens permits examination of the medial and posterior portions of the eye and is often combined with angled mirrors and prisms for gonioscopy and peripheral fundus examination. A concave Hruby lens or a convex condensing lens allows diffuse and focal illumination of the posterior segment.

Stains

Hydroxyxanthene dyes such as fluorescein have been in clinical use for more than a century. They are commonly used to detect corneal epithelial lesions, to aid in applanation tonometry, and to evaluate lacrimal drainage. In clinical practice, fluorescein is used to detect disruption of intercellular junctions, and rose bengal staining is used to evaluate abnormal epithelial cells and ocular surface changes associated with insufficient tear film protection. Other dyes such as lissamine green are available but not in widespread use.

Fluorescein Topical fluorescein is a nontoxic, water-soluble dye that is available as a 0.25% solution with an anesthetic (benoxinate or proparacaine), an antiseptic (povidone-iodine), and a preservative; as a 2% nonpreserved unit-dose eyedrop; and in impregnated paper strips. Fluorexon is a related compound available as a 0.35% nonpreserved solution that will not stain most contact lenses. Fluorescence is easily detected with a cobalt blue filter.

Fluorescein is most commonly used for applanation tonometry and evaluation of the tear film. Tear breakup time is measured by instilling fluorescein, asking the patient to hold the eyelids open after one or two blinks, and counting the seconds until a dry spot appears. Fluorescein will pool in punctate and macroulcerative epithelial defects *(positive staining),* and it can highlight nonstaining lesions that project through the tear film *(negative staining).* Different disease states can produce various punctate staining patterns (Fig II-3). Fluorescein that pools in an epithelial defect will diffuse into the corneal stroma and then cause a green flare in the anterior chamber.

The Seidel test is used to detect seepage of aqueous humor through a corneal perforation. The examiner applies fluorescein using a moistened strip or concentrated drop to the site of suspected leakage and looks for a flow of clear fluid streaming through the orange dye.

Rose bengal Rose bengal is a halide derivative of fluorescein that is available as a 1% solution and in impregnated paper strips. This dye is routinely used for evaluation of tear deficiency states and detection of various epithelial lesions. Rose bengal stains devitalized cells and cells that have lost their normal mucin surface (e.g., punctate epithelial keratitis). The red-free light filter accentuates its visibility. The compound is a photosensitizer and has antiviral and other toxic effects.

Krachmer JH, Mannis MJ, Holland EJ, eds. *Cornea.* St Louis: Mosby; 1997;1:243–273.

Clinical Evaluation of Ocular Inflammation

Classification of disease becomes easy when the cause is known, but this situation is unlikely. It is often preferable in clinical practice to use key distinctive features to categorize a patient's problem. The major disease mechanisms of the outer eye that the clinician should recognize by the history and examination are the following:

- Infection
- Immune alteration
- Neoplasia
- Maldevelopment
- Degeneration
- Trauma

These pathogenic categories are discussed in greater detail in individual chapters that follow. Since redness is often a feature of infection, allergy, neoplasia, injury, and other conditions, this introduction offers a summary of the various signs of ocular inflammation (Table II-1).

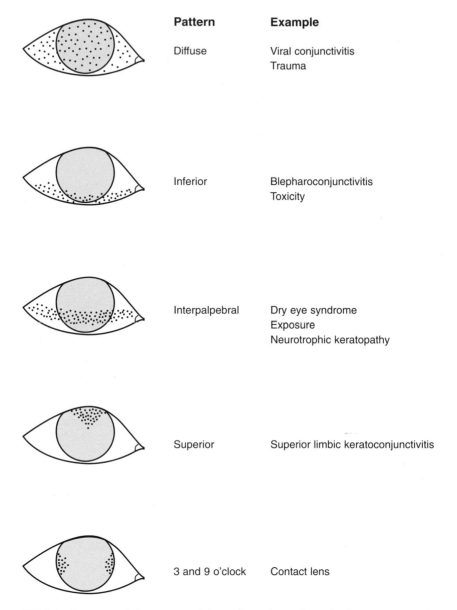

Pattern	Example
Diffuse	Viral conjunctivitis Trauma
Inferior	Blepharoconjunctivitis Toxicity
Interpalpebral	Dry eye syndrome Exposure Neurotrophic keratopathy
Superior	Superior limbic keratoconjunctivitis
3 and 9 o'clock	Contact lens

FIG II-3—Punctate staining patterns of the ocular surface. (Illustration by Joyce Zavarro.)

Leibowitz HM, Waring GO III, eds. *Corneal Disorders: Clinical Diagnosis and Management.* 2nd ed. Philadelphia: Saunders; 1998:502–542.

TABLE II-1

COMMON CLINICAL CHANGES OF THE EXTERNAL EYE AND CORNEA

TISSUE	FINDING	DESCRIPTION
Eyelid	Macule	Spot of skin color change
	Papule	Solid, raised spot
	Vesicle	Blister filled with serous fluid
	Bulla	Large blister
	Pustule	Pus-filled blister
	Keratosis	Scaling from accumulated keratinizing cells
	Eczema	Scaly crust on a red base
	Erosion	Excoriated epidermal defect
	Ulcer	Epidermal erosion with deeper tissue loss
Conjunctiva	Hyperemia	Focal or diffuse dilation of the subepithelial plexus of conjunctival blood vessels, usually with increased blood flow; other changes include fusiform vascular dilations, saccular aneurysms, petechiae, and intra-conjunctival hemorrhage
	Chemosis	Conjunctival edema caused by a transudate leaking through fenestrated conjunctival capillaries as a result of altered vascular integrity (e.g., inflammation and vasomotor changes) or hemodynamic changes (e.g., impaired venous drainage or intravascular hyposmolarity)
	Tearing	Excess tears from increased lacrimation or impaired lacrimal outflow
	Mucous excess	Increased amount of mucin relative to aqueous component of tears
	Discharge	Exudate on the conjunctival surface, varying from proteinaceous (serous) to cellular (purulent)
	Papilla	Dilated, telangiectatic conjunctival blood vessels, varying from dotlike changes to enlarged tufts surrounded by edema and inflammatory cells
	Follicle	Focal lymphoid nodule with accessory vascularization
	Pseudomembrane	Inflammatory coagulum on the conjunctival surface that does not bleed during removal
	Membrane	Inflammatory coagulum suffusing the conjunctival epithelium that bleeds when stripped
	Granuloma	Nodule of chronic inflammatory cells with fibrovascular proliferation
	Phlyctenule	Nodule of chronic inflammatory cells, often at or near the limbus
	Punctate epithelial erosion	Loss of individual epithelial cells in a stippled pattern
	Epithelial defect	Focal area of epithelial loss

TABLE II-1 (Continued)

COMMON CLINICAL CHANGES OF THE EXTERNAL EYE AND CORNEA

TISSUE	FINDING	DESCRIPTION
Cornea	Punctate epithelial erosion	Fine, slightly depressed stippling caused by altered or desquamated superficial epithelium
	Punctate epithelial keratitis	Swollen, slightly raised epithelial cells that can be finely scattered, coarsely grouped, or arranged in an arborescent pattern
	Epithelial edema	Swollen epithelial cells (intraepithelial edema) or intercellular vacuoles (microcystic edema)
	Bulla	Fluid pocket within or under the epithelium
	Epithelial defect	Focal area of epithelial loss, caused by trauma (abrasion) or other condition
	Ulcer	Epithelial defect, stromal loss, stromal inflammation, or any combination of these changes
	Filament	Strand (filament) or clump (mucous plaque) of mucus and degenerating epithelial cells attached to an altered ocular surface
	Subepithelial infiltrate	Coin-shaped inflammatory opacity in the anterior portion of Bowman's layer
	Suppurative stromal keratitis	Focal yellow-white infiltrate composed of neutrophils
	Nonsuppurative stromal keratitis	Focal gray-white infiltrate of lymphocytes and other mononuclear cells; also called interstitial keratitis, especially when accompanied by stromal neovascularization
Sclera	Episcleritis	Focal or diffuse dilation of radial superficial episcleral vessels
	Nonnecrotizing scleritis	Dilated deep episcleral vessels with scleral edema
	Necrotizing scleritis	Area of avascular sclera

Eyelid Signs of Inflammation

Individual skin changes should be described by their size, shape, and borders. Multiple lesions or a generalized skin eruption should be characterized by arrangement and distribution, using such terms as *disseminated, grouped,* or *confluent.* Several commonly encountered cutaneous lesions and their accompanying characteristics are described in Table II-1.

Cellular infiltration and edema of the upper eyelid can cause eyelid drooping, called *mechanical blepharoptosis.* Protective ptosis is a result of ocular surface discomfort.

TABLE II-2

COMMON CAUSES OF CONJUNCTIVAL INFLAMMATION

FINDING	EXAMPLES
Papillary conjunctivitis	Allergic conjunctivitis Bacterial conjunctivitis
Follicular conjunctivitis	Adenovirus conjunctivitis Herpes simplex virus conjunctivitis Molluscum contagiosum blepharoconjunctivitis Chlamydial conjunctivitis Drug induced (e.g., dipivetrin) conjunctivitis
Conjunctival pseudomembrane or membrane	Severe viral or bacterial conjunctivitis Stevens-Johnson syndrome Chemical burn
Conjunctival granuloma	Cat-scratch disease Sarcoidosis Foreign-body reaction
Conjunctival ulceration	Stevens-Johnson syndrome Ocular cicatricial pemphigoid Factitious conjunctivitis

Conjunctival Signs of Inflammation

Many forms of conjunctivitis heal without complications, but permanent changes may occur with severe or chronic inflammation. Keratinization of the ocular surface epithelium may occur over a chronically inflamed, indurated lesion. Conjunctival scarring can range from subepithelial reticular or lacy fibrosis to extensive symblepharon formation with eyelid distortion and secondary dry eye changes. Identification of the principal clinical feature of ocular inflammation can help in the differential diagnosis of common causes of conjunctivitis. Characteristics of different forms of conjunctivitis are described in Table II-2. Two common changes are papillae and follicles.

Papillae Papillae are vascular changes that are most easily visible in the palpebral conjunctiva where fibrous septa anchor the conjunctiva to the tarsus (Fig II-4). With progression these dilated vessels sprout spokelike capillaries that become surrounded by edema and a mixed inflammatory cell infiltrate, producing raised elevations under the conjunctival epithelium.

A mild papillary reaction produces a smooth, velvety appearance (Fig II-5A). Chronic or progressive changes result in enlarged vascular tufts that obscure the underlying blood vessels (Fig II-5B). Connective tissue septa restrict inflammatory changes to the fibrovascular core, producing the appearance of elevated, polygonal, hyperemic mounds. Each papilla has a central red dot that represents a dilated capillary viewed end-on. Because the anchoring septa become sparser toward the fornix

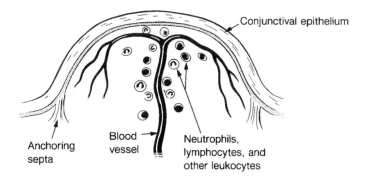

Conjunctival epithelium

Anchoring septa

Blood vessel

Neutrophils, lymphocytes, and other leukocytes

FIG II-4—Cross-sectional diagram of conjunctival papilla with a central vascular tuft surrounded by acute and chronic leukocytes.

and permit undulation of less adherent tissue, the palpebral and forniceal conjunctiva beyond the tarsus is less helpful to the examiner hoping to determine the nature of an inflammatory reaction. With prolonged, recurrent, or severe conjunctival inflammation the anchoring fibers of the tarsal conjunctiva stretch and weaken, leading to confluent papillary hypertrophy (Fig II-5C). The furrows between these enlarged fibrovascular structures collect mucus and pus.

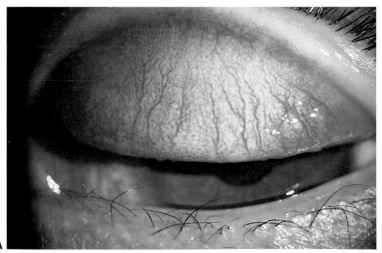

A

FIG II-5—Papillary conjunctivitis. *A,* Mild papillae. *B (facing page),* Moderate papillae. *C,* Marked (giant) papillae.

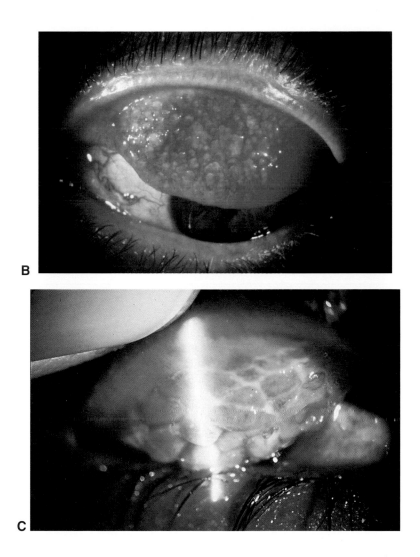

B

C

Follicles Except in neonates, conjunctival lymphoid tissue is normally present within the substantia propria. Conjunctival follicles are clusters of lymphocytes with an active germinal center surrounded by plasma cells and some mast cells (Fig II-6). Small follicles are often found in the normal lower fornix. Clusters of enlarged, non-inflamed follicles are occasionally found in the inferotemporal palpebral and forniceal conjunctiva of children and adolescents, a condition known as *benign lymphoid folliculosis* (Fig II-7).

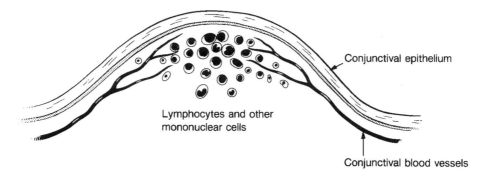

Conjunctival epithelium

Lymphocytes and other
mononuclear cells

Conjunctival blood vessels

FIG II-6—Cross-sectional diagram of conjunctival follicle with mononuclear cells obscuring conjunctival blood vessels.

Follicular conjunctivitis involves redness and new or enlarged follicles. Vessels surround and encroach on the raised surface of follicles but are not prominently visible within the follicle (Fig II-8). Follicles can be seen in the inferior and superior tarsal conjunctiva and, less often, on the bulbar or limbal conjunctiva. They must be differentiated from cysts produced by tubular epithelial infoldings during chronic inflammation and from distended meibomian glands.

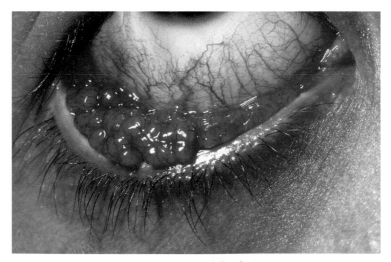

FIG II-7—Benign folliculosis.

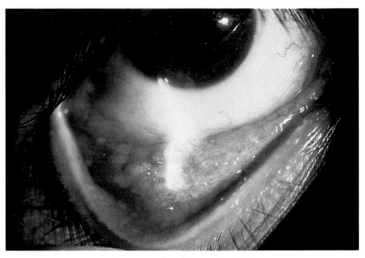

FIG II-8—Follicular conjunctivitis.

Corneal Signs of Inflammation

Inflammation can affect any layer of the cornea. The pattern of corneal inflammation, or *keratitis*, can be described according to the following:

- Distribution: diffuse, focal, or multifocal
- Depth: epithelial, subepithelial, stromal, or endothelial
- Location: central or peripheral
- Shape: dendritic, disciform, etc.

An accurate description of keratitis also notes any structural or physiologic changes such as ulceration or endothelial dysfunction.

Punctate epithelial keratopathy is a nonspecific term that includes a spectrum of biomicroscopic changes from punctate epithelial granularity to erosive and inflammatory changes (Fig II-9).

Key features of *stromal inflammation* are the type of inflammatory infiltrate (e.g., suppurative, nonsuppurative, or necrotizing) and presence of new blood vessels. Active corneal stromal inflammation is identified by interlamellar infiltration of leukocytes. Inflammatory cells most commonly come from the limbal vascular arcades and migrate into the peripheral cornea. Cells can also enter the stroma from the tear film through an epithelial defect or, less often, from inflamed aqueous humor in the presence of endothelial injury. In a vascularized cornea, inflammatory cells can emanate directly from infiltrating blood and lymphatic vessels.

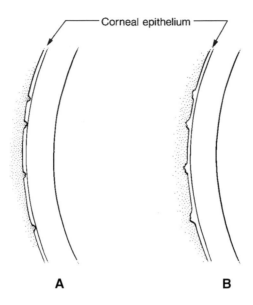

Corneal epithelium

A   B

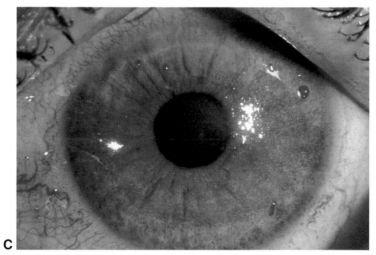

C

FIG II-9—Punctate lesions of the corneal epithelium. *A,* Punctate epithelial erosions. *B,* Punctate epithelial keratitis. *C,* Punctate epithelial erosions. *D (facing page),* Punctate epithelial keratitis.

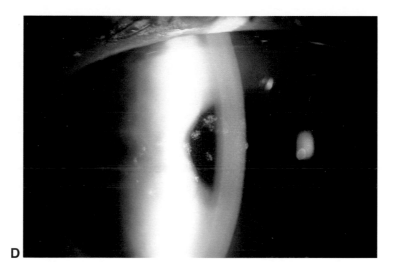

D

Stromal inflammation is characterized as *suppurative* or *nonsuppurative* (Fig II-10). It is further described by its distribution into focal or multifocal infiltrates and by its location, either central (or paracentral) or peripheral. The various morphological changes of corneal inflammation, categorized by the principal clinical features, aid in differential diagnosis (Table II-3).

TABLE II-3

COMMON CAUSES OF CORNEAL INFLAMMATION

FINDING	EXAMPLES
Punctate epithelial erosions	Dry eye syndrome Toxicity Atopic keratoconjunctivitis
Punctate epithelial keratitis	Adenovirus keratoconjunctivitis Herpes simplex virus epithelial keratitis Thygeson superficial punctate keratitis
Stromal keratitis, suppurative	Bacterial keratitis Fungal keratitis
Stromal keratitis, nonsuppurative	Herpes simplex virus stromal keratitis Varicella-zoster virus stromal keratitis Syphilitic interstitial keratitis
Peripheral keratitis	Blepharitis-associated marginal infiltrates Peripheral ulcerative keratitis caused by connective tissue diseases Mooren ulcer

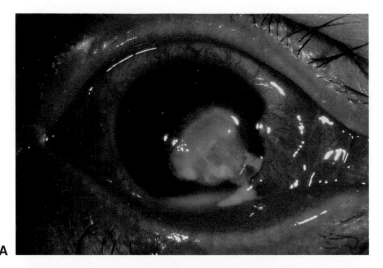

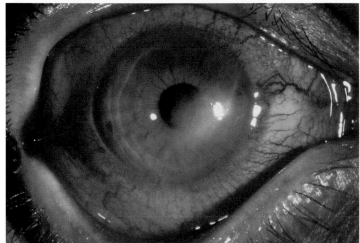

FIG II-10—Inflammation of the corneal stroma. *A,* Suppurative keratitis. *B,* Nonsuppurative, nonnecrotizing (disciform) stromal keratitis.

Endothelial dysfunction often accompanies corneal stromal inflammation and contributes to epithelial and stromal edema. Swollen endothelial cells called *inflammatory pseudoguttatae* are visible by specular reflection as dark areas of the normal mosaic pattern. *Keratic precipitates (KPs)* are clumps of inflammatory cells on the back of the cornea that come from the anterior uvea during the course of keratitis and/or uveitis. The clinical appearance of KP depends on the composition:

- ☐ Fibrin and other proteins coagulate into small dots and strands
- ☐ Neutrophils and lymphocytes aggregate into punctate opacities
- ☐ Macrophages form larger "mutton-fat" clumps

Inflammation can lead to corneal opacification. Altered stromal keratocytes produce new collagen fibers that are disarrayed and scatter light to form a nontransparent scar. Scarring can also incorporate calcium complexes, lipids, and proteinaceous material. Dark pigmentation of a residual corneal opacity is often a result of incorporated melanin or iron salts.

Corneal inflammation can also lead to neovascularization. Superficial stromal blood vessels begin as capillary buds of limbal vascular arcades in the palisades of Vogt. New lymphatic vessels may also form but cannot be distinguished clinically. Subepithelial fibrovascular ingrowth into the peripheral cornea is called a *pannus* (Fig II-11). Neovascularization may invade the cornea at deeper levels depending on the nature and location of the inflammatory stimulus. Any vessel tends to remain at a single lamellar plane as it grows unless stromal disorganization has occurred.

Leibowitz HM, Waring GO III, eds. *Corneal Disorders: Clinical Diagnosis and Management.* 2nd ed. Philadelphia: Saunders; 1998:432–479.

Scleral Signs of Inflammation

Episcleritis and scleritis may be nodular or diffuse. The red-free light filter is used to see which level of blood vessels is dilated. Areas of increased translucency are detected by direct observation and by transillumination.

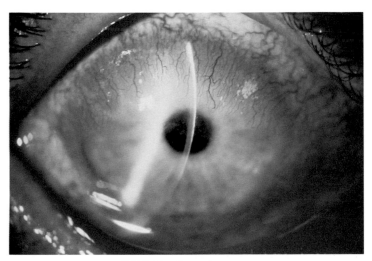

FIG II-11—Corneal pannus.

Corneal Pachymetry

A corneal pachymeter measures corneal thickness, which is a sensitive indicator of endothelial physiology that correlates well with functional measurements such as aqueous fluorophotometry. The normal cornea has a central thickness of about 0.52 mm and becomes thicker in the paracentral zone (from about 0.52 inferiorly to 0.57 mm superiorly) and peripheral zone (from 0.63 inferiorly to 0.67 superiorly). The thinnest zone is about 1.50 mm temporal to the geographic center.

Optical pachymetry can be performed using a device that attaches to the slit-lamp biomicroscope, but it is somewhat imprecise. Ultrasonic pachymetry is both easier and more accurate. Instrumentation is based on the speed of sound in the normal cornea (1640 m/sec). The applanating tip must be perpendicular to the surface since errors are induced by tilting. Improved signal processing and other methods such as laser interferometry allow the examiner to map the corneal thickness very precisely.

Corneal pachymetry can aid in the diagnosis of corneal thinning disorders and can also be used to assess the function of the corneal endothelium. Folds in Descemet's membrane begin when corneal thickness is increased by 10% or more; epithelial edema occurs when the corneal thickness exceeds 0.70 mm. A central corneal thickness greater than 0.62 mm suggests a higher risk for symptomatic corneal edema after intraocular surgery.

Corneal Edema

The corneal endothelium maintains corneal clarity through two functions: acting as a barrier to the aqueous humor and providing a metabolic pump. Alteration of either function by damage or maldevelopment leads to corneal edema. Increased permeability and insufficient pump sites occur with an endothelial cell density lower than 500 cells/mm^2.

Corneal edema is a condition of abnormal homeostasis resulting in excess fluid within the corneal stroma and/or epithelium. *Acute corneal edema* is often the result of an altered barrier effect of the endothelium or epithelium. *Chronic corneal edema* is usually the result of an inadequate endothelial pump. The normally functioning endothelial pump balances the leak rate, keeping the corneal stromal water content at 78% and the central corneal thickness at 0.52 mm. *Stromal edema* alters corneal transparency, but visual loss is most severe when epithelial microcysts or bullae occur. A *posterior collagenous layer,* or retrocorneal membrane, can arise after endothelial cell damage.

Various traumatic, inflammatory, and dystrophic mechanisms can produce corneal edema (Table II-4). The examiner can consider duration, laterality, and the presence of associated ocular disease in identifying the underlying etiology. Clinical examination should use the various illumination techniques of slit-lamp biomicroscopy. Early signs include a patchy or diffuse haze of the epithelium, mild stromal thickening, faint deep stromal wrinkles (Waite-Beetham lines), Descemet's membrane folds, and a patchy or diffuse posterior collagenous layer. Endothelial alterations include reversible changes such as pseudoguttata and permanent alterations such as corneal guttae *(cornea guttatae).*

TABLE II-4

CAUSES OF CORNEAL EDEMA

TYPE	CAUSE
Acute	Trauma (e.g., epithelial defect, intraocular surgery)
	Inflammation (e.g., infectious or immune-mediated keratitis, corneal graft rejection)
	Hypoxia (e.g., contact lens overwear)
	Hydrops from ruptured Descemet's membrane (e.g., keratoconus)
	Increased intraocular pressure
Chronic	Trauma or toxins (e.g., intraocular surgery)
	Fuchs dystrophy
	Posterior polymorphous dystrophy
	Iridocorneal endothelial syndrome

Esthesiometry

Esthesiometry is the measurement of corneal sensation, a function of the ophthalmic branch of cranial nerve V. Its primary use is in the evaluation of neurotrophic keratopathy. In most clinical circumstances reduced corneal sensitivity can be diagnosed qualitatively without special instruments, but quantitative esthesiometry is useful in unusual cases and for research. Obviously, the examiner does not apply topical anesthesia (or any other topical agent, preferably) to the patient if corneal sensation is to be evaluated. The patient should be advised as well not to apply topical medications before the examination.

Corneal sensation is most easily tested in comparison to a normal fellow eye. A rolled wisp of cotton from a cotton-tipped applicator is touched lightly to corresponding quadrants of each cornea. The patient is asked to report the degree of sensation in the first eye relative to that of the fellow eye, and sensation is recorded as normal, reduced, or absent for each quadrant. This method can be used to detect most clinically relevant cases of reduced corneal sensation.

The handheld esthesiometer gives quantitative information about corneal sensation. This device contains a thin, flexible, retractable filament. The patient's cornea is touched with the filament extended to the full 6 cm. The filament is then retracted incrementally in 0.5-cm steps until it becomes rigid enough to allow the patient to feel its contact. This length is then recorded. Esthesiometry readings may vary with user technique, but in general a lower number, or shorter filament, indicates reduced corneal sensation. After the central cornea's sensitivity is measured, a map is produced of the cornea (and sometimes of the bulbar conjunctiva) by testing the superior, temporal, inferior, and nasal quadrants sequentially.

Krachmer JH, Mannis MJ, Holland EJ, eds. *Cornea*. St Louis: Mosby; 1997;1:275–281.

Anterior Segment Photography

External and Slit-Lamp Photography

External eye photography is usually performed with a single-lens reflex camera. Magnification up to 1:1 (life-size) can be obtained with a bellows, extension ring, or close-focusing lens. A 35-mm camera can also be attached with an adapter to a slit lamp, but the low light level and long exposure time make it challenging to get a good picture.

Slit-lamp photography and videophotography allow a permanent record of most anterior segment conditions. A photo slit-lamp biomicroscope is an instrument with a fill light and an electronic flash.

Krachmer JH, Mannis MJ, Holland EJ, eds. *Cornea.* St Louis: Mosby; 1997;1:283–304.

Specular Photomicroscopy

Because slit-lamp illumination techniques are only semiquantitative and slit-lamp photography is difficult, specular photomicroscopes are available to photograph the endothelium for closer evaluation. Specular reflection permits visualization of the corneal endothelial mosaic. Wide-field specular microscopy can be performed throughout the entire cornea, permitting the study of regional variability. Posterior corneal rings function as fingerprint lines on the back of the cornea to help the examiner relocate a specific area.

Most specular microscopy techniques involve the use of a photomicroscope attached to an applanating cone and a coupling fluid. They are best performed following the application of a topical anesthetic, although noncontact techniques have been employed. A relatively clear cornea is generally required in order to obtain a good specular image. As fine focus is obtained, the endothelial mosaic comes into view (Fig II-12). The stroma and epithelium can also be examined and photographed. Most instruments have a pachymeter attached to the focusing apparatus so that corneal thickness can be measured. The parameters that can be calculated from the image include the following:

☐ *Density.* The normal endothelial cell density decreases with age. Endothelial cell density normally exceeds 3500 cells/mm^2 in children and gradually declines with age to about 2000 cells/mm^2 in older eyes. An average value for adults is 2400 cells/mm^2 (1500–3500), with a mean cell size of 150–350 μm^2 (i.e., 10^6/cell density). Other morphometric parameters that can be calculated by analyzing the specular photograph can be used to evaluate polymegethism and pleomorphism.

☐ *Coefficient of variation.* The mean cell area divided by the standard deviation of the mean cell area gives the coefficient of variation of mean cell area, a unitless number normally less than 0.30. *Polymegethism* is increased variation in individual cell areas.

☐ *Percentage of hexagonal cells.* The percentage of cells with six apices should ideally approach 100%. Lower percentages indicate a diminishing state of health of the endothelium. *Pleomorphism* is increased variability in cell shape.

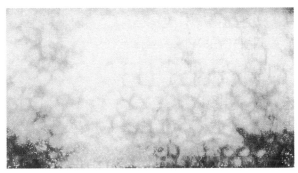

FIG II-12—Specular photomicrograph of normal corneal endothelium, with cell density of 3300 cells/mm^2.

Specular microscopy can be an important diagnostic tool, especially for differentiating between difficult or overlapping diagnostic entities, such as the iridocorneal endothelial (ICE) syndrome and posterior polymorphous corneal dystrophy. The following parameters indicate that a cornea may not tolerate intraocular surgery:

☐ A low cell density (e.g., less than 1000 cells/mm^2); donor corneas for transplantation should have at least 2000 cells/mm^2

☐ High polymegethism (coefficient of variation greater than 0.40)

☐ High pleomorphism (proportion of nonhexagonal cells greater than 50%)

American Academy of Ophthalmology. Ophthalmic procedures assessment. Corneal endothelial photography. *Ophthalmology.* 1991;98:1464–1468.

Krachmer JH, Mannis MJ, Holland EJ, eds. *Cornea.* St Louis: Mosby; 1997;1:313–334.

Leibowitz HM, Waring GO III, eds. *Corneal Disorders: Clinical Diagnosis and Management.* 2nd ed. Philadelphia: Saunders; 1998:83–122.

Anterior Segment Fluorescein Angiography

Anterior segment fluorescein angiography has been used to study the circulatory dynamics of normal and pathologic bulbar conjunctival, episcleral, scleral, and iris blood vessels. This technique is performed using a slit-lamp camera equipped with a power supply for high-speed serial fluorescein fundus photography. This technique is rarely used clinically and appears to be most valuable for evaluating patients who might have areas of vascular nonperfusion as in necrotizing scleritis and some forms of iritis.

Anterior Segment Echography

Echography of the anterior segment is occasionally required to detect foreign bodies, evaluate iris and ciliary body tumors, evaluate the extent of trauma, and determine the position of the crystalline lens or intraocular lens. Anterior segment echography may use an immersion technique, which involves inserting a small scleral shell between the eyelids and filling the shell with methylcellulose. This technique can be used to examine the cornea, anterior chamber, iris, lens, retrolental or retroiridal spaces, and ciliary body by B- and A-scan methods. A B-scan method called *ultrasound biomicroscopy* provides high resolution for examining anterior segment structures (see Figures VII-3 and VIII-2 in BCSC Section 10, *Glaucoma*).

Confocal Microscopy

The scanning confocal microscope can be used to study cell layers of the cornea even in cases with edema and scarring.

Krachmer JH, Mannis MJ, Holland EJ, eds. *Cornea.* St Louis: Mosby; 1997;1:335–359.

Leibowitz HM, Waring GO III, eds. *Corneal Disorders: Clinical Diagnosis and Management.* 2nd ed. Philadelphia: Saunders; 1998:123–127.

Measurement of Corneal Topography

Retinoscopy

Retinoscopy can detect irregular astigmatism by showing nonlinear or multiple reflexes that cannot be completely neutralized with a spherocylindrical lens. The retinoscopic finding of a multifocal cornea is that of multiple regular reflexes that move in different directions. Irregular astigmatism and a multifocal cornea can occur with keratoconus and after keratorefractive surgery. Abnormalities found with retinoscopy can help explain why a patient with a clear cornea cannot see well.

Retinoscopy can also disclose disrupted light reflexes caused by disturbances of the corneal surface. In cases where retinoscopic findings exceed the corresponding slit-lamp findings, retinoscopy can help gauge the relative impact on vision of changes at the corneal surface.

Krachmer JH, Mannis MJ, Holland EJ, eds. *Cornea.* St Louis: Mosby; 1997;1:215–221.

Keratometry

Keratometry determines corneal curvature by use of an image-doubling device that measures the greater and lesser radii of the virtual oval image generated by a circular keratometric target reflected from the spherocylindrical corneal surface. The longer axis of the elliptical image is produced by the flattest portion of the cornea (i.e., that part of the central cornea that has the longest radius of curvature and the lowest dioptric power). The average corneal curvature at two sets of diametrically opposed points about 3 mm apart on the central cornea is deduced from these measurements. Results are reported as *radius of curvature* in millimeters or *refracting power* in diopters.

For most normal corneas keratometry allows the curvature of the cornea to be inferred with enough accuracy for contact lens fitting or intraocular lens power calculation. Keratometry has limited usefulness in irregular astigmatism, since keratometric images cannot be superimposed or are not regular ovals. In other circumstances, such as with keratoconus or after radial keratotomy, optical properties of the cornea may arise from zones other than those measured by keratometry. Topographic keratometry can be performed with a special attachment to the instrument. See also BCSC Section 3, *Optics, Refraction, and Contact Lenses.*

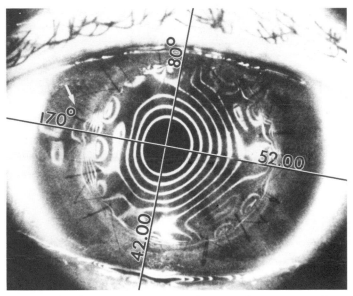

FIG II-13—Photokeratoscopic mires are closer together in a zone of steep curvature (arrow) induced by a tight suture after penetrating keratoplasty. Keratometric values and meridians are superimposed.

Keratoscopy

Information about corneal curvature can be obtained with a variety of instruments that reflect the images of multiple concentric circles from the corneal surface. These devices allow analysis of corneal curvature in zones both central and peripheral to those measured by keratometry. In general, the reflected mires appear closer together on steeper parts of the cornea (Fig II-13). The handheld Placido disk is a keratoscope with a flat target. Collimating keratoscopes use rings inside a column or a curve to maximize the area of the ocular surface that can reflect the target mires. Photokeratoscopy preserves the virtual image of concentric circles on film, and videokeratoscopy stores the images on video.

Computerized keratoscopes produce a dioptric map of the corneal surface. The instrument digitizes the reflected circles by creating 256–360 individual points along the mires and then assigns each point a location, mapped by polar coordinates, and a shape measurement. The shape measurement can be calculated to give *corneal slope* (also called *axial power*) or *local curvature* (also called *instantaneous power*). A central fixation point that gives a reproducible reference for the statistical analysis of the points on the keratoscopic rings is displayed as a small dot or cross on the corneal map. Calculations of corneal power change depending on where the target mires are positioned on the cornea.

The computer interpolates corneal shape between the calculated points and presents this information as a color-coded topographic map where blues identify lower diopters and reds, higher ones (Fig II-14). The scale, and hence the color that corresponds to a given power, can be altered. The position of the pupillary margin is often shown as well.

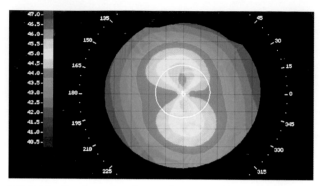

FIG II-14—Keratography of normal cornea with regular astigmatism. White circle indicates pupil.

Clinical use Qualitative analysis of a keratoscope photograph begins with examining for artifacts such as nose and eyelash shadows and tear film breakup. Three aspects of the image are then inspected:

□ The shape of the central mire is examined to determine whether a regular central cornea or nonorthogonal astigmatism is present. A round or oval shape indicates a spherical or spherocylindrical surface; an egg shape or other distortion is a sign of central irregular astigmatism.

□ The size of the central mires is determined. The larger the central mire, the lower the power.

□ The spacing between mires is examined, proceeding from the central cornea to the periphery. Mires that are closer together suggest steepening of the corneal contour; wider separation of adjacent mires indicates flattening.

The examiner can use qualitative assessment of a keratograph to categorize patients as having a particular topographic pattern. About two thirds of patients with normal corneas have a symmetric pattern that is round, oval, or bowtie-shaped, as in Figure II-14. The other patients are classified as having an asymmetric pattern: inferior steepening, superior steepening, asymmetric bowtie patterns, or nonspecific irregularity.

Many corneas are found to have a complex shape that would be oversimplified by using the qualitative pattern descriptions. To calculate several topographic parameters the examiner can use a computer-assisted topographic instrument such as simulated keratometry (Sim K), which uses mires close to the position of the standard keratometric mire. Different values obtained at different examinations can signal a change in corneal contour if the alignment of the eye and the instrument is the same. Computer-assisted topographic modeling systems allow the clinician to detect subtle and minor variations in power distribution of the anterior corneal surface.

Krachmer JH, Mannis MJ, Holland EJ, eds. *Cornea.* St Louis: Mosby; 1997;1:223–235.

Maguire LJ. Computerized corneal analysis. In: *Focal Points: Clinical Modules for Ophthalmologists.* San Francisco: American Academy of Ophthalmology. 1996;14:5.

CHAPTER III

Principles of Corneal Pharmacology and Surgery

Medical Treatment

Drug Delivery

Topical routes   Many medications can be delivered as topical dermatologic preparations or as topical ophthalmic solutions, suspensions, or ointments. Liposomes, collagen shields, and other drug-delivery modalities have potential use in the management of certain corneal diseases.

Periocular routes   Subcutaneous administration is most often used around the eye for delivering local anesthetics. Subconjunctival, sub-Tenon, or retrobulbar injection can achieve therapeutic intracorneal and intraocular levels of antibiotics, corticosteroids, and other agents. Care must be taken to avoid accidental perforation of the globe.

Systemic routes   Intravenous, intramuscular, and oral administration usually produce relatively low levels in tears but can sometimes help attain therapeutic concentrations in ocular and periocular tissues. The nature and site of disease and the possible adverse effects and drug interactions that may occur affect the use of parenteral and oral therapy.

Pharmacokinetics

Most pharmacologic studies in ophthalmology pertain to topically applied drugs. Drugs penetrating the eyelids and the conjunctiva are absorbed into the bloodstream. Closing the eyelids or pressing on the lacrimal sac can decrease systemic absorption from the ocular surface. To reach the inner eye, topically applied drugs must penetrate the cornea. Because the cornea has a lipophilic epithelium and a hydrophilic stroma, drugs that possess both lipid and water solubility, such as weak bases, penetrate more easily. Penetration is also affected by the concentration of a drug and the contact time. A *corneal permeability coefficient,* generally from 10×10^{-6} to 80×10^{-6} cm/sec, can be determined for any topical ophthalmic drug.

   The proportion of a drug that reaches an ocular compartment is known as its *ocular bioavailability.* A topical ophthalmic drug must be absorbed quickly because most of it will be diluted and washed away by the tears within 5 minutes. Studies relating the amount of administered to absorbed drug show that pharmacokinetics involves several individual variables. Most ophthalmic drugs follow first-order kinetics, but protein binding, melanin binding, and other factors alter the drug-delivery rate. Generally, only 1%–10% of a topically instilled drug reaches the aqueous humor compartment. BCSC Section 2, *Fundamentals and Principles of Ophthalmology,* discusses these and related issues in greater detail in Part 5 of that volume, Ocular Pharmacology.

Ocular Surface Agents

A *lubricant* is an aqueous solution of electrolytes and buffers that usually contains a viscous agent such as hydroxypropyl methylcellulose or polyvinyl alcohol, which prolongs contact time, and a polymer demulcent, which forms an adsorptive film and increases surface tension. The efficacy of different tear substitutes also depends on the osmolarity, pH, and preservatives of the agents and the wettability of the patient's ocular surface.

Preservatives are surface-active agents that are microbicidal by disruption of cellular membranes. Benzalkonium chloride, thimerosal, and chlorbutol are popular additives in many eyedrops, but they can cause allergic reactions and produce epithelial cytotoxicity. Povidone-iodine is a germicide used as an antiseptic.

Anti-Inflammatory Agents

The anti-inflammatory medications listed in Table III-1 can accomplish control of the anti inflammatory response, but host defenses and wound healing can be impaired. BCSC Section 4, *Ophthalmic Pathology and Intraocular Tumors,* discusses wound healing in depth. If available, specific treatment designed to eliminate or neutralize the agent causing ocular inflammation should be used before nonspecific measures are employed.

Vasoconstrictors   Topical vasoconstrictors are used to control the symptoms and signs of conjunctival inflammation, but they may not shorten its course. These $alpha_1$-adrenergic vasoconstrictors are generally restricted to short-term use for self-limited causes of conjunctival hyperemia that cannot be treated with more specific measures.

Antihistamines   Antihistamines are available in topical and oral forms. All topical antihistamines are selective H_1-receptor blockers that inhibit ocular itching. Some H_1 antihistamines (antazoline and pheniramine) are only available in combination with a vasoconstrictor. Levocabastine is a topical H_1 antihistamine with rapid onset and prolonged duration. Several oral antihistamines, including non-sedating forms, are available.

Mast-cell stabilizers   Mast-cell inhibitors block the release of histamine and other vasoactive substances. In conditions such as vernal conjunctivitis and seasonal allergic conjunctivitis, where mast-cell degranulation plays a major pathogenetic role, a topical mast-cell inhibitor can be used effectively as a prophylactic agent prior to allergen exposure and as a maintenance drug for chronic control.

Nonsteroidal anti-inflammatory agents   By inhibiting the cyclooxygenase pathway that controls prostaglandin biosynthesis, nonsteroidal agents can inhibit pupillary miosis during intraocular surgery. Anticyclooxygenase and, possibly, antilipoxygenase properties account for the anti-inflammatory effects of these agents.

TABLE III-1

ANTI-INFLAMMATORY OPHTHALMIC PREPARATIONS
COMMERCIALLY AVAILABLE IN THE UNITED STATES

CATEGORY	SOLUTIONS	SUSPENSIONS	OINTMENTS
Vasoconstrictors*	Naphazoline 0.012%, 0.02%, 0.03%, 0.1% Oxymetazoline 0.025% Phenylephrine 0.12% Tetrahydrozoline 0.05%		
Vasoconstrictor- antihistamine combinations	Naphazoline 0.05%– antazoline 0.5% Naphazoline 0.025%– pheniramine 0.3%		
Antihistamines	Emedastine 0.05% Levocabastine 0.05% Olopatadine 0.1%		
Mast-cell stabilizers	Cromolyn 4% Lodoxamide 0.1% Olopatadine 0.1%		
Nonsteroidal anti-inflammatory agents	Diclofenac 0.1% Flurbiprofen 0.03% Ketorolac 0.5% Suprofen 1%		
Corticosteroids	Dexamethasone sodium phosphate 0.1% Prednisolone sodium phosphate 0.125%, 1%	Dexamethasone alcohol 0.1% Prednisolone acetate 0.12%, 0.125%, 1% Rimexolone alcohol 1% Loteprednol etabonate 0.2%, 0.5% Fluorometholone alcohol 0.1%, 0.25% Fluorometholone acetate 0.1% Medrysone 1%	Dexamethasone sodium phosphate 0.05% Fluorometholone 0.1%

* Some vasoconstrictors are available in combination with zinc sulfate 0.25%, an astringent agent that aggregates and precipitates many proteins. Phenylephrine 0.12% is available in combination with sulfac-etamide 15%. Homeopathic preparations are also marketed.

Corticosteroids   While experimental data show variable and sometimes conflict-ing effects, clinical observations suggest that the anti-inflammatory efficacy and pressure-elevating potency of commonly used topical corticosteroids can be ranked approximately as follows:

prednisolone, dexamethasone > rimexolone, loteprednol, fluorometholone
> medrysone

The bioeffectiveness of different corticosteroid preparations is influenced by the base compound, its derivative, and the vehicle of the agent as well as the status of the patient's epithelium.

Phosphate preparations are water soluble and available as solutions. Acetate and alcohol preparations marketed as suspensions are biphasic in solubility and thus better able to penetrate the cornea with an intact epithelial surface than are the phosphate compounds. With an intact epithelium, dexamethasone alcohol 0.1% penetrates more than dexamethasone sodium phosphate 0.1%, and prednisolone acetate 1% more than prednisolone sodium phosphate 1%. These differences are less marked with an altered or missing epithelium.

The choice of an appropriate corticosteroid agent and concentration is also based on the location and severity of the ocular inflammation and the risk of adverse effects such as steroid-induced glaucoma, cataract, and retardation of wound healing. Topical application is generally superior to periocular injection for corneal inflammation, but administration by both routes has a potential additive effect for severe intraocular inflammation.

Dosage adjustment in response to the severity of ocular inflammation and the occurrence of side effects is essential in judicious corticosteroid use. Abrupt discontinuation should be avoided for many forms of ocular disease in order to minimize rebound of inflammation.

Combined corticosteroid-antibiotic preparations are commercially available (Table III-2). Because of the fixed ratio in these two-, three-, and four-drug combinations, careful observation is needed to ensure treatment efficacy and to minimize allergic and toxic reactions.

Immunosuppressives Dapsone and related sulfones interfere with the function of polymorphonuclear leukocytes and can be used for some autoimmune disorders, but hemolytic anemia and other adverse reactions can occur.

Alkylating agents such as chlorambucil and cyclophosphamide cross-link DNA and inhibit the division of leukocytes and other cells. Antifibrotic agents, or antimetabolites, such as azathioprine and methotrexate inhibit nucleotide metabolism needed for nucleic acid synthesis. Bone-marrow suppression, teratogenicity, and other severe side effects are potential risks with the use of these cytotoxic agents.

TABLE III-2

COMBINED CORTICOSTEROID-ANTIBIOTIC OPHTHALMIC PREPARATIONS
COMMERCIALLY AVAILABLE IN THE UNITED STATES

EYEDROPS	OINTMENTS
Dexamethasone/Neomycin	Dexamethasone/Neomycin
Dexamethasone/Neomycin/Polymyxin B	Dexamethasone/Neomycin/Polymyxin B
Dexamethasone/Tobramycin	Dexamethasone/Tobramycin
Hydrocortisone/Neomycin/Polymyxin B	Hydrocortisone/Neomycin/Polymyxin B/Bacitracin
Hydrocortisone/Chloramphenicol	Hydrocortisone/Chloramphenicol/Polymyxin B
Prednisolone/Sulfacetamide	Prednisolone/Sulfacetamide
Prednisolone/Gentamicin	Prednisolone/Gentamicin
Prednisolone/Neomycin/Polymyxin B	
Fluorometholone/Sulfacetamide	

Systemic administration is reserved for progressive inflammatory eye conditions such as pemphigoid and necrotizing scleritis. Local cytotoxic therapy to the eye is currently limited to the use of antifibrotics such as 5-fluorouracil and mitomycin-C that affect wound healing after surgery.

Cyclosporine and tacrolimus are lipophilic peptides that reduce T-cell activation and recruitment through effects on interleukins. Oral use of cyclosporine is limited by renal toxicity and other adverse effects. Topical use may be beneficial for some immune-mediated diseases.

Anti-Infective Agents

Several commercially available antibiotics are useful for superficial infections (Table III-3). Some anti-infective agents can be fortified to a higher concentration by the addition of a corresponding intravenous or intrathecal preparation to the eyedropper vial. Others can be freshly prepared from medications marketed for systemic use by using appropriate pharmaceutical methods.

TABLE III-3

ANTI-INFECTIVE OPHTHALMIC PREPARATIONS
COMMERCIALLY AVAILABLE IN THE UNITED STATES

CATEGORY	EYEDROPS	OINTMENTS
Single antibacterial agents	Sulfacetamide 10%, 15%, 30%	Sulfacetamide 10%
	Sulfisoxazole 4%	Sulfisoxazole 4%
	Chloramphenicol 0.5%	Chloramphenicol 1%
	Gentamicin 0.3%	Gentamicin 0.3%
	Tobramycin 0.3%	Tobramycin 0.3%
	Ciprofloxacin 0.3%	Ciprofloxacin 0.3%
	Norfloxacin 0.3%	Bacitracin 0.5%
	Ofloxacin 0.3%	Erythromycin 0.5%
	Tetracycline 1%	Tetracycline 1%
		Chlortetracycline 1%
		Oxytetracycline 1%
Combination antibacterial agents	Neomycin/Polymyxin B	Neomycin/Polymyxin B
	Neomycin/Polymyxin B/ Gramicidin	Neomycin/Polymyxin B/ Bacitracin
	Polymyxin B/Trimethoprim	Polymyxin B/Bacitracin
		Polymyxin B/ Oxytetracycline
Antifungal agents	Natamycin 5%	
Antiviral agents	Trifluridine 1%	Vidarabine 3%

Agents effective against Chlamydia   Sulfonamides inhibit a wide variety of bacteria including *C trachomatis* by interfering with utilization of para-aminobenzoic acid, but because of increasing resistance these agents are used selectively. Tetracycline, doxycycline, minocycline, and related agents inhibit bacterial protein synthesis, are bacteriostatic against many bacterial species, and are effective in adult chlamydial conjunctivitis. Erythromycin is used in the treatment of neonatal and adult chlamydial eye disease. Azithromycin is another macrolide antibiotic useful for chlamydial infection.

Agents effective against spirochetes   The penicillins and cephalosporins are β-lactam antibiotics that interfere with bacterial cell-wall peptidoglycan synthesis. Penicillin G remains the preferred agent for syphilis. Penicillin G or ceftriaxone is used in the treatment of Lyme borreliosis.

Agents effective against gram-negative cocci   Penicillin G has previously been the preferred treatment of gonococcal eye disease. Because of the increasing occurrence of penicillinase-producing *N gonorrhoeae* (PPNG), ceftriaxone or cefotaxime is now used in many communities. Alternative therapy includes bacteriostatic agents that inhibit protein synthesis by binding to ribosomal proteins: erythromycin, tetracycline, and chloramphenicol.

Agents effective against gram-negative rods   Aminoglycoside antibiotics such as gentamicin and tobramycin have a broad range of bactericidal activity against many bacterial species, particularly gram-negative rods. Topical allergic reactions of the eyelids and conjunctiva can occur, and frequent or chronic use can cause epithelial toxicity. Extended-spectrum cephalosporins such as ceftazidime have a broad spectrum of activity, including *Haemophilus* spp. Extended-spectrum penicillins such as piperacillin have shown efficacy against many gram-negative bacilli. Because of the risk of bone-marrow suppression, chloramphenicol is generally reserved for specific infections, such as those caused by *H influenzae*. Polymyxin B–containing preparations have a broad spectrum of antibacterial activity. Ciprofloxacin, norfloxacin, ofloxacin, and other fluoroquinolones inhibit bacterial nucleic acid synthesis and exhibit bactericidal activity against most gram-negative rods.

Agents effective against gram-positive cocci   Agents that are effective in inhibiting cell-wall function in gram-positive cocci include bacitracin, gramicidin, β-lactam antibiotics (penicillins and cephalosporins), streptomycin, and vancomycin. Because of the common occurrence of penicillin resistance, penicillinase-resistant penicillins such as methicillin and first-generation cephalosporins such as cefazolin are used against susceptible staphylococci and streptococci. Vancomycin is useful against methicillin-resistant strains. Neomycin, contained in several combinations, is effective against many staphylococci but not streptococci. Bacteriostatic agents such as erythromycin and tetracycline can suppress the growth of susceptible gram-positive cocci.

Agents effective against gram-positive rods   Most penicillins and aminoglycosides are useful for many gram-positive bacilli.

Agents effective against gram-positive filaments   Of the acid-fast filamentous bacteria, amikacin is generally preferred for atypical mycobacterial infections and a sulfonamide for disease caused by *Nocardia* spp. The anaerobic actinomycetes are susceptible to the penicillins.

Agents effective against yeasts Amphotericin B is a polyene antifungal agent that is effective against most *Candida* spp by altering fungal cell membrane permeability. Amphotericin B can be reconstituted as a diluted topical eyedrop from the intravenous formulation. Management of fungal eye infections is limited by poor tissue penetration and ocular surface toxicity when medications are administered topically. An oral pyrimidine derivative, flucytosine, has been used as an adjunctive agent. Ketoconazole, fluconazole, and itraconazole are imidazoles that are marketed as oral preparations.

Agents effective against hyphal fungi Natamycin is a lipophilic polyene compound commercially available as a 5% suspension that is useful as topical treatment against several filamentous fungi such as *Fusarium* spp. While none of the imidazole antifungal agents are available as an ophthalmic preparation, IV formulations such as miconazole and fluconazole have been used undiluted as eyedrops, and oral preparations such as ketoconazole and itraconazole can be dissolved in an ophthalmic vehicle. Clotrimazole and econazole are available as dermatologic creams that are not recommended for topical ocular use. The relative aqueous insolubility of these agents generally restricts their use to a relatively low concentration in water or to an oil-based solvent. The susceptibility of filamentous fungi to different imidazoles varies markedly among the genera causing ocular fungal infection.

Agents effective against protozoa Some of the antibacterial and antifungal agents show activity against some protozoa. For example, two aminoglycosides (neomycin and paramomycin) and several imidazoles have been sucessfully used in the management of *Acanthamoeba* keratitis. Other agents that have been used against *Acanthamoeba* are propamidine, hexamidine, polyhexamethylene, biguanide (polyhexanide), and chlorhexidine.

Agents effective against nematodes Oral ivermectin is widely used in the management of onchocerciasis.

Agents effective against herpesviruses Nucleoside analogues can inhibit viral DNA polymerase. Topical preparations currently available are vidarabine and trifluridine. Topical antivirals can cause adverse effects on the ocular surface, particularly with chronic administration, including follicular conjunctivitis, conjunctival scarring, punctal occlusion, punctate epithelial erosions, and retardation of wound healing. Oral antiviral agents include acyclovir (available in 200 mg, 400 mg, and 800 mg capsules), famciclovir (500 mg tablets), and valacyclovir (500 mg tablets). α-interferon is commercially available as a systemic agent, and β- and γ-interferons are under development.

Agents effective against retroviruses Nucleoside reverse transcriptase inhibitors include zidovudine (AZT), didanosine (ddl), zalcitabine (ddC), stavudine (d4T), lamivudine (3TC), and abacavir. Non-nucleoside reverse transcriptase inhibitors are nevirapine, delavirdine, and efavirenz. Protease inhibitors include saquinavir, ritonavir, indinavir, nelfinavir, and vertex-141. The therapeutic and preventive roles of HIV vaccines, including antigens derived from the envelope (gp-120 and gp-160) and the core (p17 and p24), are under investigation.

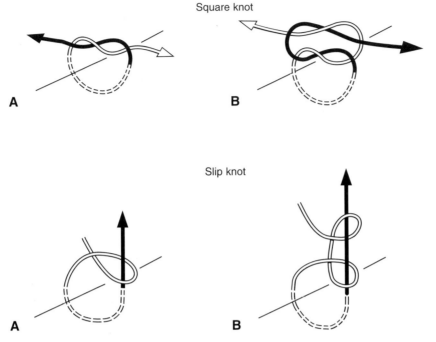

Square knot

A   B

Slip knot

A   B

FIG III-1—Surgical knots. Square and slip knots are tied differently, but both end up with a similar loop configuration. (Illustration by Joyce Zavarro.)

Hodge WG, Hwang DG. Antibiotic use in corneal and external eye infections. In: *Focal Points: Clinical Modules for Ophthalmologists.* San Francisco: American Academy of Ophthalmology; 1997;15:10.

Surgical Management

The techniques of anterior segment microsurgery include accurate needle placement, optimal tissue union, and tying of square and slip knots (Fig III-1). A familiarity with the instruments and materials used in microsurgery is essential.

Needles and Sutures

Hollow-bore needles for injection and aspiration come in a range of lengths and diameters (Table III-4). Besides the typical pointed tip, needles and cannulas are available with rounded tips (e.g., Atkinson needle for retrobulbar injection), blunted ends (e.g., Ashey needle for intraocular irrigation), olive-tipped ends, and other configurations.

Microsurgical needles are made of stainless steel directly swaged onto suture ends. Needles are assessed by their curvature, including radius and chord length, length, and diameter (Fig III-2). The needle tip may be taper point, conventional cutting, reverse cutting, and spatula or side cutting.

TABLE III-4

NEEDLE SIZES

GAUGE #	OUTER DIAMETER
30	0.3 mm
25	0.5 mm
20	0.9 mm
18	1.2 mm

Suture threads may be almost nonabsorbable or absorbable, and they can be made from either natural or synthetic materials. Natural sources include silk obtained from the silkworm cocoon, surgical gut from the mucosal tissue of the small intestine of sheep or cattle, and collagen from cattle tendon. Gut and collagen are available plain or chromicized to delay slightly the absorption time. Synthetic materials are polymers that are usually less flexible, more elastic, and more easily buried than silk. Virgin silk (multifilament) and nylon (monofilament) are both nonabsorbable, while surgical gut, collagen, and polyglycolic acid are all absorbable (Table III-5). A 10-0 suture has a diameter of 13–25 μm, and an 8-0 suture measures 38–51 μm, with some variation among manufacturers.

Eisner G. *Eye Surgery: An Introduction to Operative Technique.* 2nd ed. New York: Springer-Verlag; 1990:1–48.

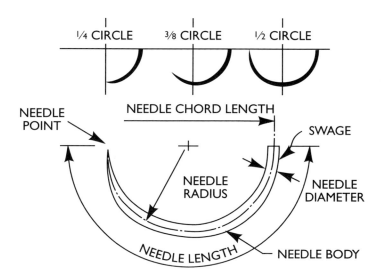

FIG III-2—Parts and terminology of a surgical needle. (Illustration courtesy of Ethicon, Inc.)

TABLE III-5

OPHTHALMIC SUTURES

TYPE	NONABSORBABLE	ABSORBABLE
Natural	Virgin silk	Surgical gut
	Braided silk	Collagen
Synthetic	Nylon (Ethilon, Dermalon, Supramid, Perlon)	Polyglycolic acid (Dexon)
	Polyester fiber (Dacron, Mersilene)	Polyglactin 910 (Vicryl)
		Polydioxanone (PDS)
	Polypropylene (Prolene)	

Surgical Instruments

Floor- and ceiling-mounted operating microscopes have variable magnification and illumination settings and are typically focused 15–20 cm from the operative field. A ×10 magnification gives a binocular field about 20 mm in diameter; higher settings reduce the size and depth of field. Diffuse oblique and coaxial illuminations use halogen lamps or fiberoptics, and a slit-beam attachment is available. Zoom, horizontal (X–Y) excursion, and focus are controlled by the foot pedal. A camera and a keratometer can be attached to the instrument.

Ophthalmic microsurgical instruments are available from several manufacturers with various designs. Some common instruments are listed in Table III-6. Other materials and instruments include a waterproof drape, utility scissors, hemostats to fixate traction sutures, a muscle hook to move the globe, and sponges to absorb blood and fluid.

Surgical Fluids

An ophthalmic irrigant such as balanced salt solution (BSS) is saline with other salts at a pH of 7.4 and osmolality of 305 mOsm. Viscoelastic agents are polysaccharides such as sodium hyaluronate, chondroitin sulfate, or hydroxypropyl methylcellulose. BCSC Section 11, *Lens and Cataract,* describes the viscoelastic substances used in ophthalmic surgery in more detail.

Prevention Practices

Some corneal and external eye diseases can be prevented. Strategies for prevention include adequate hygiene and nutrition, aseptic surgical techniques, protective spectacles that minimize ocular trauma, and prophylactic antibiotics. Prevention begins with immunization. Practicing ophthalmologists should provide an opportunity for hepatitis B vaccination for their office staff and follow other regulations of the Occupational Safety and Health Administration. Universal precautions that safeguard the health of patients' eyes as well as the ophthalmologist and staff should be a part of daily practice.

TABLE III-6

INSTRUMENTS USED IN CORNEAL AND ANTERIOR SEGMENT SURGERY

INSTRUMENT	USE
Eyelid speculum	Separate the eyelids without compressing the globe
Ring	Prevent collapse of the open globe
Toothed forceps	Grasp tissue; tying platforms aid in suture placement; knurled handle gives a firm grip; tips come in different sizes (e.g., 0.12 mm, 0.3 mm) and designs (e.g., open-cup, splay-tooth, dog-tooth)
Smooth forceps	Grasp suture using platforms
Westcott type scissors	Cut tissues (e.g., conjunctiva) and sutures
Vannas type scissors	Cut tissues or small sutures
Corneal/corneoscleral scissors	Follow the curvature of the globe while cutting; a slightly longer innermost blade keeps tip inside eye; rounded handle permits rotational positioning
Iris scissors	Perform iridectomy or iridotomy and cut vitreous strands
Knife	Incise tissue by using a blade holder with a disposable blade, a disposable knife, or a permanent (e.g., diamond) knife
Trephine	Incise cornea; an obturator limits the depth of penetration and, when extended, protects blade
Caliper	Measure chord length on the globe
Spatula	Perform blunt dissection
Iris retractor	Open pupil
Cannula	Attach to syringe or bottle for wetting surface or injecting fluid or air into the eye
Wet-field cautery	Provide hemostasis; bipolar cautery electrocoagulates only tissue between tips
Needle holder	Grasp needle; spring action releases needle; locking and nonlocking types available

Universal Precautions

Optimal infection control is based on the assumption that all specified human body fluids are potentially infectious. Many transmissible diseases of the external eye, such as adenovirus conjunctivitis, cause redness that immediately indicates infection. Other infectious agents, however, can be present on the ocular surface without causing inflammation. Human immunodeficiency virus (HIV), hepatitis B virus, hepatitis C virus, rabies virus, and the agent of Creutzfeldt-Jakob disease are not immediately obvious without systemic clues or laboratory testing. Every patient must be approached as potentially contagious. Guidelines for routine ophthalmic examinations include the following:

- *Wash hands between patient examinations.* Use disposable gloves if an open sore, blood, or blood-contaminated fluid is present. Using cotton-tipped applicators to manipulate the eyelids can also minimize direct contact.

- *Avoid unnecessary contact.* Eyedropper bottles used in the office should not directly touch the ocular surface of any patient.

- *Disinfect all contact instruments after each use.* Tonometer tips and pachymeter tips should be soaked in diluted bleach or hydrogen peroxide or cleansed with isopropyl alcohol after every use. Trial contact lenses must be disinfected between patients. BCSC Section 10, *Glaucoma,* discusses infection control in clinical tonometry in greater detail.

- *Handle sharp devices carefully.* Needles must always be discarded into puncture-resistant (sharps) containers.

> Updated recommendations for ophthalmic practice in relation to the human immunodeficiency virus and other infectious agents. *Information Statement.* San Francisco: American Academy of Ophthalmology; 1992.

Public Health Campaigns

Worldwide, the major infectious causes of visual loss are the following:

- Trachoma
- Onchocerciasis
- Herpes simplex virus keratitis
- Microbial keratitis
- Hansen disease (leprosy)

In the absence of an available vaccine for these conditions, specific programs are designed to reduce the risk of communicable diseases. Examples of such efforts are the following:

- Improved hygiene and mass distribution of antibiotics to interrupt hyperendemic trachoma
- Eradication of the insect vector to control onchocerciasis
- Vitamin A supplementation in communities with childhood xerophthalmia
- Education about contact lens disinfection in industrialized countries

These preventive strategies seek to reduce the global burden of blindness caused by diseases of the outer eye.

> Schwab L. *Eye Care in Developing Nations.* 3rd ed. San Francisco: American Academy of Ophthalmology; 1999.

PART 2

OCULAR SURFACE DISORDERS

CHAPTER IV

Normal Physiology of the Ocular Surface

Problems of the ocular surface are diverse with respect to etiology, symptoms, and prognosis. They range from relatively minor irritations of recurrent corneal epithelial erosions with excellent preservation of vision to devastating and potentially blinding chemical injuries with persistent epithelial defects and stromal ulceration. The discussion in Part 2 of the maintenance of ocular surface integrity begins with a review of normal physiology of the external eye.

Eyelids

The ocular surface encompasses the entire epithelial surface of the cornea, limbus, and conjunctiva. It is physically contiguous with the adjacent eyelids and adnexa and shares important functional relationships with the external eye. The eyelids have important protective functions for the globe, both voluntary and involuntary. The involuntary fright blink reflex in response to external stimuli without physical contact is mediated by the optic nerve or cranial nerve VIII (auditory) as the afferent arc and by primarily cranial nerve VII (facial) as the efferent arc. A neuronally controlled eyelid blinking, which occurs approximately every 5–10 seconds, mechanically spreads the tear film to lubricate the ocular surface. This subconscious blink reflex is mediated by the ophthalmic division of cranial nerve V (trigeminal) as afferent arc and CN VII as efferent arc.

The blinking movement protects the ocular surface from untoward stimuli and allows the upper eyelid to drag the tear meniscus upward over the ocular surface. Impairment of this protective reflex mechanism may render the ocular surface susceptible to pathologic insults, as may be seen in neuroparalytic keratopathy. Through blinking and contraction of eyelid muscles, the old used tears are removed from the ocular surface and drained through the puncta and nasolacrimal ducts into the nose. BCSC Section 7, *Orbit, Eyelids, and Lacrimal System,* discusses and illustrates the functions of the eyelids and lacrimal system in depth. Ocular surface integrity can also be compromised by malfunctioning or malpositioning of the eyelid apparatus, as in entropion, ectropion, or imbrication of eyelids.

Precorneal Tear Film

The normal ocular surface is covered by a layer of tear film. Because the precorneal tear film–air interface is the initial refractive surface of the eye, the maintenance of a stable, healthy tear film is of paramount importance with regard to vision. Tears provide a moist environment for epithelial cells, lubricating the ocular surface while they dilute and remove noxious stimuli. Tear film provides the cornea with essential

Epithelial cell

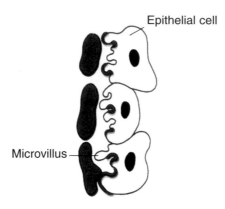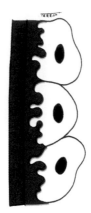

FIG IV-1—Function of the mucin layer. *Left,* With mucin deficiency the aqueous layer (blue) does not wet the corneal epithelium. *Right,* A normal amount of mucin (red) allows proper wetting of the corneal epithelium by the aqueous layer. (Reproduced with permission from Kanski JJ. *Clinical Ophthalmology: A Systematic Approach.* 3rd ed. Oxford: Butterworth-Heinemann; 1994:93.)

nutrients and oxygen, and leukocytes gain access to the cornea through the tear film. The solutes contained within the tear film, including lactoferrin, immunoglobulins, lysozyme, and β-lysin, render it bactericidal. Lack of this physiologic lubricating fluid, as in tear deficiency states, may predispose the eye to microbial infections.

Until recently, the tear film was believed to be tripartite, with a lipid superficial layer about 0.1 μm in thickness (with the eyelids open), an aqueous midphase 7 μm thick, and a mucin basal layer 20–50 nm thick. Recent evidence, however, indicates that the tear film may be as thick as 40 μm and is largely made up of a mucin gel or partial mucin layer, with an increase in mucin content basally and without discrete separation of the aqueous and mucin layers (Fig IV-1).

The most superficial layer of the tear film is the *lipid layer* produced by the meibomian glands. Its principal function is to retard tear evaporation and enhance stability, while maintaining the tear meniscus. Meibomian gland dysfunction (MGD) can lead to unstable tear film and associated ocular surface disorders. The *aqueous component* is produced by the main lacrimal glands, as well as the accessory lacrimal glands of Krause and Wolfring. The aqueous layer transports all of the water-soluble nutrients, and aqueous tear deficiency (ATD) is the most common cause of dry eye. The layer coating the cornea is the *mucin layer,* which is produced by both conjunctival goblet cells and ocular surface epithelium. The mucin is hydrophilic, and this quality enhances the ability of the aqueous layer to spread over the corneal epithelium. The loss of conjunctival goblet cells, which occurs for example in chemical burns, leads to xerosis of the ocular surface.

Normal tear film has a pH of about 7.2, an osmolarity of 302 mOsm per liter, and a volume of 7.0 μl in the precorneal film. It is produced at a rate of 1.2 μl per minute and has a refractive index of 1.336. BCSC Section 2, *Fundamentals and Principles of Ophthalmology,* discusses the tear film in detail in Part 4, Biochemistry and Metabolism.

Lipid Tear Secretion

The meibomian glands are richly innervated. The nerve fibers surrounding them are probably cholinergic since they contain cholinesterase, and cholinergic agonists such as pilocarpine stimulate release of meibomian oil. However, no evidence has yet been produced to show that meibomian gland secretion in humans is controlled by either parasympathetic or sympathetic innervation. Hormones may influence meibomian secretion. Androgens, such as testosterone, increase production of these lipids, while antiandrogens and estrogens depress secretion of all sebaceous glands. Bacteria colonizing the eyelids also modify the lipid secretion in meibomian gland dysfunction.

Blinking is thought to be important in the release of meibomian gland lipid. It has been estimated that a gravitational force of 50–70 g is applied to the globe during a blink, and the globe is retroplaced on average 1.5 mm. When the eye is open, the muscle of Riolan surrounding the meibomian gland ducts contracts and compresses the ducts, thereby preventing outflow. The palpebral portion of the orbicularis may possibly act as an opponent by milking the glands on contraction. Blinking would lead to expression or jetting of the oil onto the precorneal tear film; between blinks, with the muscle of Riolan contracted and the orbicularis relaxed, secretion would be prevented. Cells in the acinar wall may act as valves to control lipid flow.

Aqueous Tear Secretion

Aqueous tear secretion is largely a reflex mechanism. Cranial nerve V is the afferent pathway in the reflex tear arc. Stimulation of receptors in the fifth nerve distribution in the cornea or nasal mucosa induces tear secretion from the lacrimal gland. The efferent pathway is more roundabout. Parasympathetic fibers leave cranial nerve VII in the greater superficial petrosal nerve and pass to the sphenopalatine ganglion. From there the lacrimal secretory nerve fibers travel with the zygomaticotemporal nerve of the maxillary division (V_2) and join the lacrimal (sensory) nerve of the ophthalmic division (V_1) of CN V before entering the lacrimal gland. Sympathetic efferent pathways may also be involved. Reduction of tear secretions and associated dry eye syndrome can be caused by diseases such as familial dysautonomia or by medications affecting the autonomic system.

Mucin Tear Secretion

Mucin secreted by conjunctival goblet cells, which makes up the inner portion of the precorneal tear film, is essential for proper ocular surface wetting. When mucin production is deficient, as with Stevens-Johnson syndrome or following severe chemical injury, poor wetting of the corneal surface with subsequent desiccation and epithelial damage may occur, even in the setting of sufficient aqueous tear production. However, the controlling mechanism of mucin secretion by the conjunctival goblet cells and ocular surface epithelium is not known. The mucin of the preocular tear film represents a hydrophilic layer that overlies the hydrophobic ocular surface, conferring hydrophilia to the solid surface. This property is important because aqueous films of less than 200–300 μm in thickness spontaneously rupture over hydrophobic surfaces. A continuous aqueous tear of 7–40 μm thickness can exist only on a hydrophilic surface.

Tear Breakup

Meibomian lipids cannot spread over mucin or an aqueous film surface containing surfactants, as the lipid will disperse and emulsify. Tear film breakup has been attributed to lipid contamination of the hydrophilic supporting solid, or mucin layer, rendering it hydrophobic. Polar lipids could diffuse to the mucin layer and cause focal disruption in the open eye, especially over areas of thinning, such as irregularities in the surface epithelium, or during conditions of increased evaporation. This model has been questioned, however, and it is postulated that the key step in tear film breakup is instability and rupture of the mucin layer caused by van der Waals forces acting on the mucin layer. Precise biomechanical and biophysical structures of the tear film await further investigation.

Decreased tear breakup time rapidly returns to normal once the meibomian glands are expressed. A decrease in secretion of the meibomian glands as a result of plugging or decreased blinking and the consequent absence of milking of the glands could result in a compromised lipid layer and increased evaporation of the aqueous layer with thinning of the tear film and increased contamination. Blinking can remove the lipid-contaminated mucin, and a decrease in blinking can also result in evaporative loss of the aqueous layer with increased hydrophobicity of the mucin layer. Blinking increases to compensate for conditions, as in blepharitis, associated with decreased tear breakup time secondary to increased tear evaporation. Incomplete blinking and abnormalities in eyelid congruity have similar effects.

The Ocular Surface

Epithelium

Corneal epithelium Under the precorneal tear film lies the anterior surface of the cornea, which is made up of nonkeratinized, stratified squamous epithelium. This highly organized epithelium is rich in desmosomes and tight junctions, thereby providing paracellular permeability barriers to limit the nonionic solutes and maintaining the homeostasis of the intraocular milieu. Disruption of this physiologic barrier by preservatives in ocular medications or topical anesthetics may lead to punctate epitheliopathy and compromised epithelial wound healing. Since corneal epithelium is highly differentiated with rapid self-renewal, it depends on its stem cells for continual migration and replacement. Cumulative research and clinical evidence have indicated that the stem cells of the corneal epithelium are located at the limbal basal epithelium.

The *limbus* is a unique structure that acts as a junctional barrier to separate the cornea and conjunctiva. Phenotypical and biochemical characteristics of limbal epithelium have been shown to be intermediate between corneal and conjunctival epithelium. In humans the limbal palisades of Vogt, representing specialized regions of epithelial structure, are the location of the limbal stem cells. Similar to the rete ridges of the epidermal stem cells, the limbal palisades of Vogt are also rich in melanin to protect the corneal stem cells. The palisades are tightly attached to the underlying basement membrane and have a rich limbal vascular network to nourish the metabolically active stem cells. In the absence of these limbal stem cells, epithelial wound healing becomes compromised. Persistent epithelial defects or abnormal wound healing associated with the invasion of conjunctival goblet cells is often observed in the conditions associated with limbal stem-cell deficiency.

Tseng SC, Tsubota K. Important concepts for treating ocular surface and tear disorders. *Am J Ophthalmol.* 1997;124:825 835.

Conjunctival epithelium In contrast to the corneal structure, conjunctival epithelium is a stratified columnar epithelium with numerous mucin-secreting goblet cells. The junctional structures of conjunctival epithelium are less developed than those of corneal epithelium, and increased epithelial permeability has been observed in conjunctiva. Healthy conjunctival epithelium can be an alternative source for corneal epithelial wound healing, and, in the absence of corneal vascularization, it may transform into a corneal phenotype, a process known as *conjunctival transdifferentiation*. However, such a transformation does not occur in vascularized corneas associated with limbal stem-cell deficiency. The conjunctiva-derived epithelium on the cornea is less competent than the normal corneal epithelium. The locations of stem cells of conjunctival epithelium remain unclear. Research suggests that the proliferative potential and the density of goblet cells are higher in the conjunctival epithelium of the fornix than in the bulbar or tarsal conjunctiva.

Near the eyelid margins the stratified columnar epithelium of the conjunctiva merges with the keratinized, stratified squamous epithelium of the eyelid skin. Similar to the palpebral eyelid margin, the transition at the limbus is gradual from the stratified columnar epithelium of the conjunctiva to the stratified squamous epithelium of the cornea. The areas of stratified squamous epithelium at the eyelid margin and limbus correspond to the areas of most frequent contact and greatest pressure between the palpebral and bulbar surfaces. These mechanical factors of eyelid movement and appositional pressure have been suggested as the greatest stimulus for the formation of stratified squamous epithelium about the eyelid margin and the limbus. Such mechanical forces may be crucial in stimulating the limbal stem cells to maintain corneal epithelial proliferation and differentiation. Through such a mechanism, the eyelids also play a proactive role in regulating the surface epithelial turnover, in addition to their passive role in protecting the ocular surface.

Unlike the normal cornea, the conjunctival epithelium lacks an organized basement membrane and rests loosely on the fibrovascular tissue of the substantia propria. Because of the various immunocompetent and parenchymal cells such as T cells, mast cells, dendritic cells, and fibroblasts in the subconjunctival layer, as well as its lymphatic and vascular pathways, the conjunctiva is a complex element of the mucosal immune defense system. Specialized lymphoid follicles located in the substantia propria, known as the *conjunctiva-associated lymphoid tissue (CALT),* have a modified overlying epithelium. These M cells have elongated microvilli and are thought to increase the antigen-capturing capacity of the mucosa and to confer immune tolerance, rather than sensitization, upon the mucosal surface.

Blood Supply

Conjunctival blood vessels derived from anterior ciliary arteries maintain their superficial position, and a deeper circulation furnishes blood to the peripheral corneal arcades, iris, and ciliary body. Inflammatory processes of the conjunctiva result in prominence of the superficial vessels, which increases away from limbus. In contrast, inflammatory processes of the cornea, iris, or ciliary body result in prominence of the deep vessels, which increases toward the limbus. Clinically, this process manifests as ciliary flush at the limbus. Conjunctival blood vessels near the limbus provide nourishment for the peripheral cornea and limbus, the location of the corneal epithelial stem cells. In pathologic circumstances these vessels transport inflammatory cells for combating infection (e.g., infectious keratitis) or serum proteases for preventing stromal degradation (e.g., peripheral ulcerative keratitis). When the conjunctiva in the involved eye is relatively normal (e.g., neurotrophic keratopathy or after microbial keratitis), a conjunctival flap may supply the necessary corneal vascularity to prevent further stromal degradation and support repair. In situations of ischemia-induced sterile stromal ulceration related to a severe chemical burn involving the cornea, limbus, and conjunctiva, advancement of the conjunctiva or Tenon's tissue or autologous limbal transplantations may restore the limbal vascular supply, reversing ischemia-related complications.

Normal cornea is avascular and angiostatic. A healthy cornea has an intact Bowman's layer and compact stroma. Inflammatory reactions or degenerative processes of the peripheral cornea often lead to breakdown of the basement membrane and perturbation of limbal barrier functions (limbal deficiency), and they can result in corneal vascularization and conjunctival ingrowth such as pterygium, which is discussed in detail in chapters XVIII and XXII.

Mechanical Functions

In addition to their physiologic functions, the conjunctiva and especially the limbus also contribute mechanically to the maintainance of corneal epithelial integrity. For example, a smooth palpebral conjunctiva permits the eyelid to move atraumatically over the cornea, thereby affording protection, distribution of the tear film, and debridement of foreign matter. Diseases that produce keratinization of the palpebral conjunctiva (e.g., Stevens-Johnson syndrome) can induce significant corneal epithelial damage mechanically. Flexible conjunctival folds are essential for the proper movements of the globe and maintenance of the normal eyelid-globe relationship. Thus conditions that produce conjunctival scarring (e.g., ocular cicatricial pemphigoid) can obliterate the normal forniceal anatomy, creating cicatricial entropion, trichiasis, and secondary corneal erosion and scarring.

CHAPTER V

Diagnostic Approach to Ocular Surface Disease

Tear Film Evaluation

Tests for dry eye lend some degree of objectivity to what is essentially a clinical diagnosis. Some of these tests may help persuade a skeptical patient that the diagnosis is indeed correct. No one test is sufficiently specific to permit an absolute diagnosis of dry eye. The diagnosis is made by combining information from the history and examination with the results of one or more of the following diagnostic tests. The tests described may be performed in the following sequence to minimize the potential for alteration of subsequent test results by preceding procedures. However, any of the tests may affect the outcome of subsequent ones.

Inspection

Inspection of the tear meniscus between the globe and the lower eyelid (normally 1.0 mm and convex) is a common starting point. *Tear breakup time* is determined by instilling fluorescein in the inferior cul-de-sac and then evaluating the stability of the precorneal tear film. Tear breakup time should be measured prior to the instillation of any eyedrops and before the eyelids are manipulated in any way. The examiner moistens a fluorescein strip with sterile saline and applies it to the tarsal conjunctiva. (Fluorescein-anesthetic combination drops are not suitable for this purpose.) After several blinks, the tear film is examined using a broad beam of the slit lamp with a blue filter. The time lapse between instillation of fluorescein and the appearance of the first randomly distributed dry spot is the tear breakup time. Dry spots appearing in less than 10 seconds are considered abnormal.

The ocular surface can then be evaluated with rose bengal staining. A drop of 1% rose bengal solution is instilled in the inferior cul-de-sac. Some ophthalmologists prefer to drop the solution directly onto the superior bulbar conjunctiva. At present, ophthalmic rose bengal solution is not available commercially and a thorough wetting of the rose bengal strips may be a viable alternative. The specific pattern of corneal and bulbar conjunctival staining can be very helpful in establishing the diagnosis. Diffuse corneal and bulbar conjunctival staining is commonly seen in the early stages of viral keratoconjunctivitis and medicamentosus. Staining of the inferior cornea and bulbar conjunctiva is often associated with staphylococcal blepharitis, while staining that occurs superiorly is more likely to be caused by superior limbic keratoconjunctivitis. Interpalpebral staining of the cornea and adjacent bulbar conjunctiva is commonly associated with keratoconjunctivitis sicca or exposure.

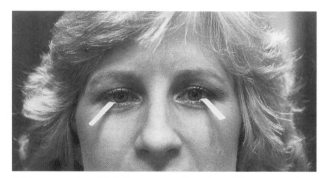

FIG V-1—The Schirmer test, in which the amount of wetting of the paper strips is a measure of tear flow. (Reproduced with permission from Stamper RL, Wasson PJ, eds. *Ophthalmic Medical Assisting.* San Francisco: American Academy of Ophthalmology; 1994:92.)

Tests of Tear Production

Aqueous tear production can be assessed in a variety of ways. *Schirmer testing* is performed by placing a thin strip of filter paper in the inferior cul-de-sac (Fig V-1). The amount of wetting can be measured to quantify aqueous tear production. The *basic secretion test* is performed following the instillation of a topical anesthetic, followed by drying out of the inferior fornix with a cotton-tipped applicator. Whatman #41 filter paper, 5 mm wide and 35 mm long, is placed at the junction of the middle and lateral thirds of the lower eyelids to minimize irritation to the cornea during the test. The eyes are then closed to limit the effect of blinking. Although normal measurements are quite variable, repetitive measurements of less than 5 mm of wetting, with anesthesia, can be highly suggestive of aqueous tear deficiency, while 5–10 mm is equivocal. The *Schirmer I test,* which consists of this same test without the use of topical anesthesia, measures both basic and reflex tearing combined. Less than 10 mm of wetting after 5 minutes is diagnostic of ATD. While this test is relatively specific, the level of sensitivity is poor. Using lower cutoff measurements increases the specificity of these tests but decreases their sensitivity. The *Schirmer II test* measures reflex secretion and is performed in a manner similar to the basic secretion test. However, after the filter paper strips have been inserted into the inferior fornices, a cotton-tipped applicator is used to irritate the nasal mucosa. Wetting of less than 15 mm after 5 minutes is consistent with a defect in reflex secretion. While an isolated abnormal result for any of these tests can be misleading, serially consistent results are highly suggestive. Schirmer testing is also useful in demonstrating to patients the presence of an aqueous tear deficiency.

Tear Composition Assays

Other procedures may be useful in supporting the diagnosis of ATD. Cultures of the eyelid margins are infrequently helpful, but they may provide useful information in selected cases. Additional tests include tear film osmolarity, tear lysozyme, and tear lactoferrin. In lacrimal gland dysfunction states, the normal production of proteins by the lacrimal gland is diminished. A decreased tear lysozyme or lactoferrin level is highly suggestive of dry eye. A commercial assay is available for the measurement of lactoferrin in tears. Tear film osmolarity has been shown to be increased in patients with ATD as well as those with MGD. At the present time no consensus has formed as to which of these tests is most sensitive and/or specific for the diagnosis of ATD, and some are not readily available.

Ocular Cytology

An important step in the diagnosis of many infectious and inflammatory conditions is the examination by light microscopy of conjunctival or corneal specimens. Standard staining procedures are widely used to facilitate the detection of microbial and human cells. This chapter discusses the procedures used in these investigations and the implications that can be drawn from their results. See also BCSC Section 4, *Ophthalmic Pathology and Intraocular Tumors.*

Specimen Collection

Conjunctival scrapings are generally preferred to swabbings that harvest surface exudate. To obtain a conjunctival specimen for cytological examination, the clinician applies a topical anesthetic and everts the upper eyelid. The tarsal conjunctiva is lightly scraped with a sterile spatula. When epithelial cells are removed, the conjunctival surface should blanch slightly during scrapings, avoiding excessive bleeding. An alternative method of gathering conjunctival cells involves a cytobrush. After the conjunctiva is rubbed, the brush is dipped into buffer solution, and the floated cells are concentrated on a Millipore filter. Rapid immersion into fixative avoids excessive air drying of material on a glass slide or filter paper.

Ideally, swabbings of the conjunctiva for culture are obtained prior to the instillation of a topical anesthetic. Calcium alginate, cotton, or polyester swabs are available for collecting specimens of epithelial cells and microflora from the conjunctival or corneal surface. Specimens can also be obtained from the contralateral conjunctiva for comparison.

Impression cytology uses a piece of filter paper pressed onto a specific area of the conjunctival or corneal surface to lift off superficial cells. This procedure can be considered a noninvasive superficial biopsy that provides a means to map specific cell changes topographically and to quantify surface abnormalities.

Preferred Practice Patterns Committee, Cornea Panel. *Conjunctivitis.* San Francisco: American Academy of Ophthalmology; 1998.

Tseng SC. Staging of conjunctival squamous metaplasia by impression cytology. *Ophthalmology.* 1985;92:728–733.

TABLE V-1

CLINICAL INTERPRETATION OF OCULAR SURFACE CYTOLOGY

FINDING	EXAMPLES
Predominance of neutrophils	Bacterial conjunctivitis Early stage of severe viral conjunctivitis Severe allergic or atopic conjunctivitis
Predominance of lymphocytes and monocytes	Viral conjunctivitis Chronic toxic or allergic conjunctivitis
Eosinophils	Acute allergic conjunctivitis Parasitic conjunctivitis
Basophils or mast cells	Vernal conjunctivitis
Plasma cells and macrophages	Chlamydial conjunctivitis
Multinucleated cells	Herpes simplex blepharoconjunctivitis
Keratinized epithelial cells	Tear dysfunction states Pemphigoid Stevens-Johnson syndrome
Cytoplasmic inclusions	Chlamydial conjunctivitis

Interpretation of Ocular Cytology

Microscopic examination of material collected from the ocular surface can reveal cells, cellular elements, and microorganisms that can be helpful in diagnostic evaluation (Table V-1). The staining procedures used in ocular cytology are described in Table V-2.

Microbes The Gram stain helps to identify microorganisms and aids in bacterial classification. The Giemsa stain is used to evaluate cytologic features, and it shows chlamydial inclusions within epithelial cells and most bacteria and fungi. Acridine orange and calcofluor white are chemofluorescent stains that are examined with a fluorescent microscope. Acridine orange will stain most bacteria orange against a dark background, and calcofluor white results in green fluorescence of fungi and amoebic cysts. Acid-fast staining aids in the differentiation of filamentous bacteria. All smears should be fixed in methanol or other fixative before staining.

> Brinser JH, Burd EM. Principles of diagnostic ocular microbiology. In: Tabbara KV, Hyndiuk RA, eds. *Infections of the Eye.* 2nd ed. Boston: Little, Brown & Co; 1996.

Human cells A methylene blue–based dye such as the Giemsa or Wright's stain is useful to highlight specific morphologic characteristics that aid in identifying the following cell types:

□ *Normal conjunctival and corneal epithelial cells:* Slightly larger than leukocytes, epithelial cells have a central round nucleus (sometimes with a prominent nucleolus) and homogeneous cytoplasm (Fig V-2). The usually flat, squamous epithelial cells can appear cuboidal when smeared onto a glass slide, and they tend to clump together in sheets.

TABLE V-2

STAINING PROCEDURES IN OCULAR CYTOLOGY

Gram staining
1. Flood the slide with crystal violet for 1 minute. Rinse gently with tap water.
2. Apply Gram's iodine for 1 minute. Rinse.
3. Tilt slide, and allow the decolorizing solvent to run over the slide until the purple color ceases to be washed off. Rinse.
4. Apply safranin solution for 1 minute. Rinse and blot dry.
5. Examine with oil-immersion light microscopy. Gram-positive cocci and rods stain blue purple, and gram-negative bacteria stain pink-red.

Giemsa staining
1. Immerse slide in freshly prepared Giemsa stain solution for 1 hour.
2. Rinse briefly in ethanol and blot dry.
3. Examine by light microscopy. Leukocytes have lavender cytoplasm with purple nuclei. Neutrophilic granules stain pink-purple, and eosinophilic granules stain bright purple-red. Chlamydial inclusions, as well as bacteria and fungi, stain blue-purple.

Acridine orange staining
1. Apply acidic acridine orange dye to slide for 2 minutes.
2. Rinse and blot dry.
3. Examine by fluorescent microscopy. Bacteria and amoebae generally stain orange, and tissue cells and fungi stain green.

Calcofluor white staining
1. Apply several drops of calcofluor white–Evans blue solution, and apply a coverslip.
2. Examine by fluorescent microscopy. Fungi and amoebic cysts stain green against a dark red background.

Acid-fast staining
1. Apply carbolfuchsin solution for 5 minutes. Rinse with tap water.
2. Decolorize with acid-alcohol.
3. Apply malachite green solution for 5 minutes. Rinse.
4. Examine by light microscopy. Most mycobacteria and nocardioforms stain red.

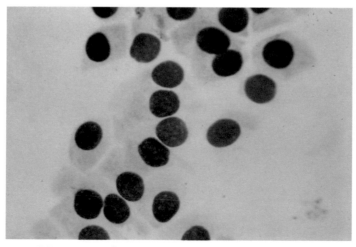

FIG V-2—Normal conjunctival epithelial cells (Giemsa ×400).

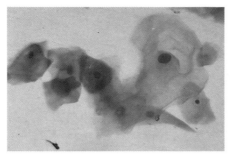 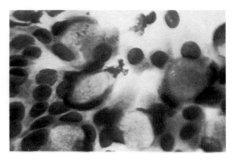

FIG V-3—Degenerated epithelial cells (Giemsa ×1000).

FIG V-4—Conjunctival goblet cells (Giemsa ×1000).

- *Degenerated or keratinized epithelial cells:* Degenerating epithelial cells have a faint, ghostlike appearance with faded or no nuclei (Fig V-3). Keratinization is visualized as eosinophilic cytoplasmic granularity. Keratinized epidermal cells of the normal eyelid margin can also be seen, occasionally with adherent bacteria.

- *Goblet cells:* Conjunctival goblet cells contain a clump of pale staining mucus that displaces the cytoplasm and nucleus toward the edge of the cell membrane. Goblet cells may be found singly or in clusters. The cell can be identified by its mucin contents stained magenta by periodic acid–Schiff reagent (PAS) (Fig V-4).

- *Neutrophils:* Like other granulocytes that are derived from promyelocytes of the bone marrow, neutrophils are polymorphonuclear; that is, the nucleus is usually separated into definite lobes connected by narrow strands (Fig V-5). Less mature neutrophils (band cells) have an indented nucleus. About twice the size of erythrocytes, neutrophils have a fairly homogeneous cytoplasm that contains pale or nonstaining granules. Dark intracytoplasmic granules are sometimes visible in certain toxic and infectious conditions, and intracellular bacteria can be identified within phagolysosomes.

- *Eosinophils:* About the same size as neutrophils, eosinophils usually have a bilobed nucleus and eosinophilic, uniformly spherical granules that fill the cytoplasm (Fig V-6). In chronic allergy, intact eosinophils may be less prominent than ruptured cells, extracellular granules, and Charcot-Leyden crystals.

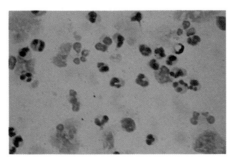

FIG V 5—Neutrophils (Giemsa ×100).

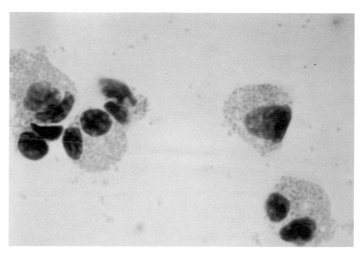
FIG V-6—Eosinophils (Giemsa ×1000).

□ *Basophils and mast cells:* Basophilic leukocytes have banded or lobulated nuclei and dark, basophilic intracytoplasmic granules that are unevenly distributed and vary in size and shape.

□ *Lymphocytes:* Lymphocytes vary in size. Larger, more mature cells resemble other mononuclear cells such as monocytes. The cell contains a single large nucleus and scant, faintly staining cytoplasm that sometimes has scattered granules or vacuoles. Lymphocytes that are usually round and larger can be compressed or ruptured.

□ *Monocytes and macrophages:* These large mononuclear cells can be difficult to distinguish from neutrophils and lymphocytes (Fig V-7). Characteristic features of monocytes include dull coloration of the cytoplasm, blunt pseudopods, and a brainlike convolution of the nucleus. Histiocytes contain phagocytized particles and have pseudopods or shaggy cytoplasmic margins. Large engorged macrophages are sometimes referred to as *Leber* or *epithelioid cells.*

□ *Plasma cells:* These large oval cells have eccentric nuclei and a velvety cytoplasm that is paler adjacent to the nucleus (Fig V-8).

□ *Erythrocytes:* Red blood cells are doughnut-shaped cells without nuclei that measure 7 μm across.

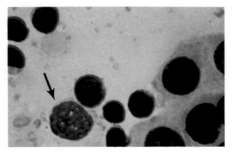

FIG V-7—Mononuclear inflammatory response. Cells with large deeply basophilic nuclei and scant, barely noticeable cytoplasm are lymphocytes. The cell with the larger, violet nucleus and moderate amount of light blue cytoplasm is a monocyte (arrow). Large, clustered cells at lower right are normal epithelial cells (Giemsa ×1000).

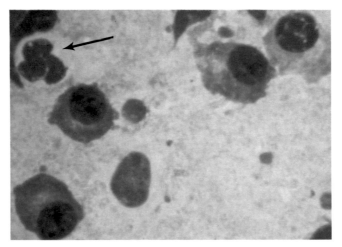

FIG V-8—Plasma cells (arrow) (Giemsa ×1000).

□ *Multinucleated cells:* Multinucleated epithelial cells usually result from failure of the nucleus to divide during mitosis, but they can also arise from a syncytium of coalescent cells. Staining characteristics of these polykaryocytes resemble those of normal conjunctival epithelial cells (Fig V-9). Giant cells produced by a granulomatous reaction can be identified in histopathologic sections but are rarely seen on conjunctival scrapings.

□ *Cytoplasmic inclusions:* A basophilic inclusion within epithelial cells, typically capping the nucleus, is formed by a mass of *C trachomatis* elementary bodies. These Halberstaedter-Prowazek inclusion bodies are more likely to be found in neonatal chlamydial conjunctivitis than in adult infection. At least 1000 epithelial

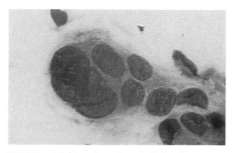

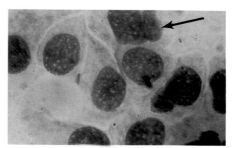

FIG V-9—Multinucleated epithelial cell (Giemsa ×1000).

FIG V-10—Chlamydial inclusion within conjunctival epithelial cell (arrow) (Giemsa ×1000). (Photograph courtesy of Francis I. Proctor Foundation, San Francisco.)

cells should be present on the smear to permit adequate search for chlamydial inclusions (Fig V-10). Extracellular elementary bodies are usually too small to be identified with cytologic stains but can be visualized by immunofluorescence.

□ *Nuclear inclusions:* Eosinophilic, intranuclear inclusions are more easily detectable by Papanicolaou's stain than by the Giemsa stain. A pale halo surrounds the clump, the nucleolus is displaced, and nuclear chromatin is usually clumped or rimmed along the nuclear margins. Lipschütz bodies, classified as Cowdry type I inclusion bodies, are sometimes seen in herpes simplex and varicella-zoster viral blepharoconjunctivitis. Viral inclusions are difficult to identify without electron microscopy.

□ *Pigment and other material:* Small pigment granules are sometimes visible within phagocytic inflammatory cells or scattered extracellularly (Fig V-11). Melanin granules of the uvea are uniformly spherical, and pigment granules from the retinal pigment epithelium are ellipsoid. Mascara, carbon from the collecting device, and precipitated stain particles vary in size and shape. Remnants of extruded nuclei can clump into basophilic fragments. Basophilic mucin and eosinophilic fibrin strands are sometimes visible in the background.

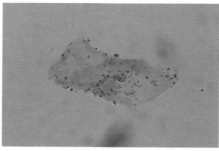

FIG V-11—Melanin pigment granules on degenerated epithelial cell (Giemsa ×1000).

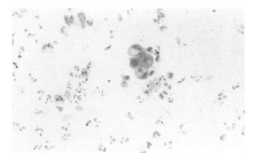

FIG V-12—Sebaceous cell carcinoma (conjunctival impression cytology).

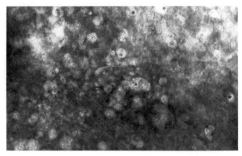

FIG V-13—*Acanthamoeba* in the corneal epithelial cells (corneal impression cytology).

- □ *Tumor cells:* Neoplastic cells can exhibit several features, including aberrant or multiple nuclei, variable cell shapes and sizes, and mitotic figures (Fig V-12).

- □ *Microorganisms:* Bacterial cocci and bacilli, fungi, and protozoa can be visualized with cytologic methods. Gram and acridine orange stains are used to facilitate detection and to highlight the morphology of these microorganisms (Fig V-13).

CHAPTER VI

Clinical Aspects of Ocular Surface Disorders

External diseases are best addressed in a unified manner, as they affect the eyelids, conjunctiva, and cornea. Collectively, these structures constitute what has come to be known as the *ocular surface*. This chapter discusses the diseases of the ocular surface as they affect each of its component parts as well as the ocular surface as a whole.

Dermatoses Affecting the Ocular Surface

Meibomian Gland Dysfunction

PATHOGENESIS. Meibomian gland dysfunction is now recognized as a very common yet frequently overlooked cause of ocular irritation. Patients with meibomian gland dysfunction develop lipid tear deficiency, which results in tear film instability, an increased tear film evaporation rate, and elevated tear osmolarity. Risk factors for meibomian gland disease include rosacea and oral retinoid therapy.

CLINICAL PRESENTATION. Symptoms consist of burning, foreign body sensation, redness of the eyelids and conjunctiva, filmy vision, and recurrent chalazia. The inflammation in this condition is confined predominantly to the posterior eyelid margins, conjunctiva, and cornea, although patients may occasionally have associated seborrheic changes on the anterior eyelid margin (Fig VI-1). The posterior eyelid margins are often irregular and have prominent blood vessel "brush marks" coursing from the posterior to anterior eyelid margins. The meibomian gland orifices may pout or show metaplasia with a white plug of keratin protein extending through the glandular orifice. The meibomian secretions in active disease may be turbid and have increased viscosity. Following years of meibomian gland inflammation, extensive atrophy of the meibomian gland acini may develop, and eyelid compression can no longer express the meibomian secretions. The atrophy of meibomian gland acini and derangement of glandular architecture can be demonstrated by infrared photography.

Patients may have foam in the tear meniscus along the lower eyelid. Frequently, they have an unstable tear film with abnormally rapid tear breakup times, particularly in long-standing disease with meibomian gland atrophy and reduced lipid production. Mild to severe ocular surface inflammation may accompany meibomian gland dysfunction, which includes the following manifestions:

☐ Bulbar and tarsal conjunctival injection

☐ Papillary reaction on the inferior tarsus

☐ Episcleritis

☐ Punctate epithelial erosions in the inferior cornea that stain with fluorescein and rose bengal

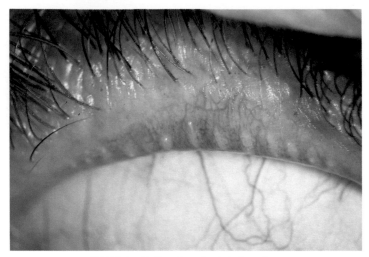

FIG VI-1—Meibomian gland dysfunction.

- Inferior marginal epithelial and subepithelial infiltrates
- Pannus
- Corneal thinning, occasionally

In 60% of cases of meibomian gland dysfunction one or more manifestations of rosacea are observed in the facial flush areas, including telangiectasia, persistent erythema, papules, pustules, hypertrophic sebaceous glands, and rhinophyma.

MANAGEMENT. Systemic antibiotics are the mainstay of treatment in meibomian gland dysfunction. The most commonly used antibiotic is tetracycline, but doxycycline is being used with increasing frequency because it has fewer gastrointestinal side effects and because food does not interfere with its absorption. In addition, doxycycline requires less frequent dosage than tetracycline and does not accumulate in patients with renal failure. Minocycline is also effective in the treatment of meibomian gland dysfunction, but it may induce vestibular dysfunction (vertigo). Erythromycin is sometimes used as an alternative, but its efficacy in treating meibomian gland dysfunction is not well established. Therapeutic regimens include a 3–6 week course of systemic tetracycline 250 mg qid (or 500 mg bid), doxycycline 50–100 mg/day, or minocycline 100 mg/day. If patients experience symptomatic improvement on these medications, the dosage can be slowly tapered to the lowest possible daily dose that controls their symptoms.

Patients with meibomian gland dysfunction should be informed that therapy may control but not eliminate their condition. Warm eyelid compresses and scrubbing of the eyelid margins with a gentle shampoo to remove lipid and inflammatory debris may reduce burning symptoms. Patients rarely observe improvement of meibomian gland dysfunctions before 2–3 weeks after the systemic treatment begins. They should be informed about the side effects of tetracycline, such as gastrointestinal upset and photosensitization, before therapy is started. Tetracyclines are contraindicated in pregnant women and children under 10 years of age and in patients with candidiasis. Topical corticosteroids may be required for short periods in cases with moderate to severe inflammation, particularly those with corneal infiltrates and vascularization. Patients treated with topical steroids should be warned about the complications of chronic use, because this stubborn condition may prompt patients to become dependent.

Bowman RW, Miller KN, McCulley JP. Diagnosis and treatment of chronic blepharitis. In: *Focal Points: Clinical Modules for Ophthalmologists.* San Francisco: American Academy of Ophthalmology; 1989;7:10.

Driver PJ, Lemp MA. Meibomian gland dysfunction. *Surv Ophthalmol* 1996;40: 343–368.

Seborrheic Blepharitis

CLINICAL PRESENTATION. Seborrheic blepharitis may occur alone or in combination with staphylococcal blepharitis or meibomian gland dysfunction. Inflammation is located predominantly at the anterior eyelid margin. A variable amount of crusting, typically of an oily or greasy nature, may be found on the eyelids and lashes. Patients with seborrheic blepharitis experience chronic eyelid redness, burning, and occasionally foreign body sensation. A small percentage of patients (approximately 15%) have been found to have an associated keratitis or conjunctivitis. The keratitis is characterized by punctate epithelial erosions on the lower third of the cornea. Conjunctival inflammation may consist of bulbar and/or tarsal injection with either a follicular or papillary reaction on the inferior tarsal conjunctiva. Approximately one third of patients with seborrheic blepharitis have aqueous tear deficiency.

MANAGEMENT. Eyelid hygiene is the primary treatment in patients with blepharitis. This hygiene includes the following:

- Use of warm compresses
- Expression of meibomian gland secretions
- Cleaning of the eyelid margins to remove keratinized cells and debris

The cleaning process may be enhanced by using a mild, well-diluted detergent such as baby shampoo or a commercially available eyelid scrub.

In cases of blepharitis where inflammation is a prominent component a brief course of topical steroid applied to the eyelid margins may be helpful. When blepharitis involves primarily the posterior eyelid margin (i.e., meibomian gland dysfunction), systemic antibiotics such as doxycycline are the mainstay of treatment. Blepharitis caused by bacteria (e.g., staphylococcus) often responds to the use of a topical antibiotic ointment such as bacitracin or erythromycin. A topical steroid/antibiotic mixture may also be useful. Because topical steroids are associated with a number of well-known complications such as glaucoma, cataract, and aggravation of undiagnosed herpes simplex virus infection, they should be used with caution.

Chalazion

CLINICAL PRESENTATION. A chalazion is a chronic granuloma that develops when a Zeis or meibomian gland becomes plugged. The nodules frequently arise in and around the meibomian glands and may be more prominent on either the skin or the conjunctiva (Fig VI-2). The lesion disappears in weeks to months when the extruded

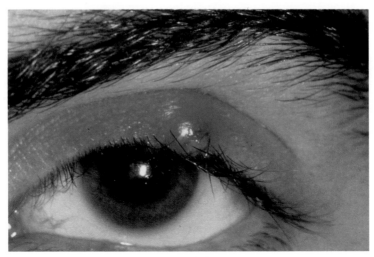

FIG VI-2—Chalazion.

lipid is phagocytosed and the granuloma dissipates. A small amount of scar tissue can remain. Occasionally, patients with a chalazion may experience blurred vision secondary to astigmatism induced by the chalazion pressing on the globe.

PATHOGENESIS AND LABORATORY EVALUATION. Sebaceous material trapped by the plugging of a Zeis or meibomian gland extrudes into adjacent tissues where it elicits a chronic granulomatous inflammation. A zonal granulomatous inflammation centered around lipid is seen histologically. As is typical of all granulomas, epithelioid cells are prominent. Also present are admixtures of other cells, including lymphocytes, macrophages, neutrophils, plasma cells, and giant cells. It must be emphasized that basal cell or sebaceous carcinoma can be misdiagnosed as chalazion, a serious misidentification. The histopathologic examination for persistent, recurrent, or atypical chalazia is therefore quite important.

MANAGEMENT. Because most chalazia are sterile, antibiotic therapy is of no value. Chalazia may be treated with hot compresses and attempted expression of the inflamed meibomian gland. Lesions that fail to respond to conservative therapy may be treated with intralesional injection of steroid (0.1–0.2 ml of triamcinolone 10 mg/ml), incision and drainage, or a combination of both. Surgical incisions can be performed under topical or perilesional anesthesia. Internal chalazia require vertical incisions on the tarsal conjunctiva along the meibomian gland to facilitate the drainage and avoid horizontal scarring of the tarsal plates. Topical anesthesia may also be required for intralesional steroid injection.

    The reported cure rate of chalazia after intralesional steroid injection varies widely from 9% to 90%. In some cases intralesional steroid injection may cause the lesion to shrink to a small, firm nodule that can persist for some time. Intralesional steroid injection in darkly pigmented patients may lead to depigmentation of the overlying eyelid skin.

Epstein GA, Putterman AM. Combined excision and drainage with intralesional corticosteroid injection in the treatment of chronic chalazia. *Arch Ophthalmol.* 1988; 106:514–516.

Hordeolum

This acute, suppurative, nodular inflammation of the eyelid is associated with pain, redness, and a localized purulent abscess. Hordeola occurring on the anterior eyelid (in the glands of Zeis or lash follicles) are called *external hordeola,* or *styes,* and they are usually caused by staphylococcus infection. Hordeola occurring in the meibomian glands are termed *internal hordeola,* which can be either infectious or sterile. Sterile hordeola represent acute inflammatory reactions to lipids in and around obstructed meibomian glands and may be called *acute chalazia.* External hordeola can also be called acute chalazia when they originate in sebaceous (Zeis) glands, but this origin is generally impossible to determine clinically. Thus, all acute pustules of the anterior lamella of the eyelid are referred to as external hordeola or styes.

Hordeola frequently show spontaneous improvement, although warm compresses may relieve symptoms. Topically applied antibiotics are usually not effective, and systemic antibiotics are indicated only for secondary eyelid cellulitis. Incision and drainage may occasionally be required for large or particularly bothersome lesions. See also p 160.

Rosacea

PATHOGENESIS. Rosacea is a common disease that has no proven cause. It is associated with cutaneous sebaceous gland dysfunction of the face, neck, and shoulders. Although this condition has generally been thought to be more common in fair-skinned individuals, it may simply be more difficult to diagnose in persons with dark skin. It is infrequently diagnosed by ophthalmologists, in spite of its relatively frequent association with blepharitis and/or aqueous tear deficiency. Although alcohol can contribute to a worsening of this disorder, because of its effect on vasomotor instability, not all patients with rosacea have a history of excessive alcohol intake. Recently, experimental studies based on immunohistochemical staining of inflammatory cell infiltrates have shown this disease to represent a delayed hypersensitivity reaction. Dysfunction of the meibomian and other lipid-producing glands of the eyelids and skin of the face is believed to be responsible for these infiltrates.

CLINICAL PRESENTATION. A skin condition that frequently involves the eyes, rosacea is characterized by excessive sebum secretion with a frequently recalcitrant chronic blepharitis. Eyelid margin telangiectasia is very common, as are meibomian gland distortion, disruption, and dysfunction, which lead to recurrent chalazia. Ocular involvement can also progress, leading to chronic conjunctivitis, marginal corneal infiltrates, sterile ulceration, episcleritis, or iridocyclitis (Fig VI-3). If properly treated, these lesions can resolve with few sequelae. Repeated bouts of ocular surface inflammation can bring about corneal neovascularization and scarring, often in a characteristic triangular configuration (Fig VI-4).

This disorder is generally found in patients aged 30–50 with a slight female preponderance. However, ocular rosacea can be encountered in younger patients and is often underdiagnosed. Facial lesions consist of telangiectasias, recurrent papules and pustules, and midfacial erythema (Fig VI-5). Rosacea is characterized by a malar

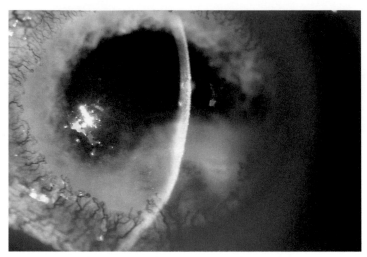

FIG VI-3—Marginal keratitis associated with rosacea.

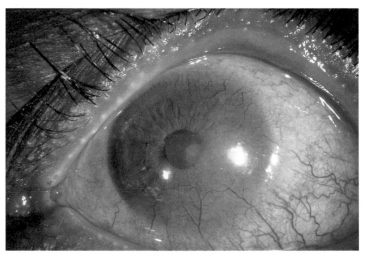

FIG VI-4—Rosacea with chronic superficial keratopathy and corneal neovascularization.

rash with unpredictable flushing episodes, sometimes associated with the consumption of alcohol, coffee, or other foods. Rhinophyma, thickening of the skin and connective tissue of the nose, is a characteristic and obvious sign associated with this disorder, but such hypertrophic cutaneous changes occur relatively late in the disease process.

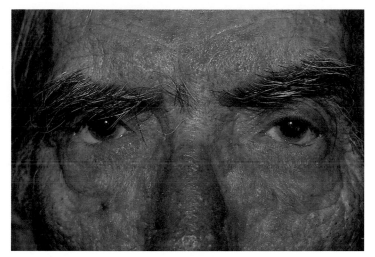

FIG VI-5—Facial changes of rosacea.

MANAGEMENT. Management of the ocular and systemic disease takes place simultaneously. The mainstay of therapy is oral tetracycline, which affects the production of lipids by the sebaceous glands or the interaction between these glands and the resident bacteria by mechanisms that are still unclear. Alternatively, oral doxycycline, 100 mg sid, or oral minocycline, 100 mg bid, can be administered. Using these compounds circumvents the interaction between tetracyclines and many foods, which can be useful in patients who are intolerant of tetracycline because of gastrointestinal side effects or photosensitivity.

With time oral therapy with teracycline or doxycycline can be tapered, although it is recommended that a low dose be continued indefinitely. In addition to oral therapy, application of topical metronidazole 0.75% gel (Metrogel) to the affected facial areas can lead to a significant reduction in facial erythema. A clinical trial using topical 0.5% metronidazole solution for ocular rosacea is currently under way. Topical dermatologic therapy should also be continued indefinitely at a low dose.

Ulcerative keratitis can be associated with infectious agents in rosacea, or it may have a sterile, inflammatory etiology. Once it is ascertained that ulceration is noninfectious, topical corticosteroids used judiciously can play a significant role in reducing sterile inflammation and enhancing epithelialization of the cornea. In advanced cases with scarring and neovascularization, conservative therapy is generally recommended. Penetrating keratoplasty in rosacea patients is a high-risk procedure that may have a poor prognosis if the ocular surface is severely compromised.

Browning DJ, Proia AD. Ocular rosacea. *Surv Ophthalmol.* 1986;31:145–158.

Sarcoidosis

A multisystem disorder of uncertain etiology, sarcoidosis is characterized by noncaseating granulomas in affected tissues. After pulmonary involvement, ocular involvement is the most common manifestation, seen in up to 50% of affected patients. Nontender small (millet seed) or large nodules may be seen in the eyelid skin and in the canthal region. Lacrimal gland involvement occurs in up to 25% of patients with ocular involvement, resulting in keratoconjunctivitis sicca. With the additional involvement of salivary glands the clinical presentation may resemble that of typical Sjögren syndrome.

Visible granulomas may be present in the conjunctiva. The follicles of conjunctival sarcoidosis are often small and easily overlooked, and they may be difficult to distinguish from normal conjunctival follicles. The most common corneal finding is calcific band keratopathy with elevated serum calcium level. Nummular keratitis, thickening of Descemet's membrane, and deep stromal vessels as a result of chronic intraocular inflammation can be seen. Granulomatous uveitis with mutton-fat keratic precipitates and iris nodules occurs in up to two thirds of patients with ocular involvement. Periphlebitis is the most common fundus finding. Chronic cystoid macular edema and exudative retinal detachment are related to intense and longstanding inflammation. Granulomatous involvement of the optic nerve is also seen.

Desquamating Skin Conditions

Ichthyosis   This spectrum of diverse skin disorders is characterized by excessively dry skin and the accumulation of scale. Ichthyosis vulgaris, an autosomal dominant trait, is the most common hereditary scaling disorder, affecting 1 in 250–300 persons. Ocular involvement varies with the form of ichthyosis. Eyelid scaling, ectropion, and conjunctival thickening are common. Primary corneal opacities are seen in 50% of patients with X-linked ichthyosis but are rarely seen in ichthyosis vulgaris. Dots or filament-shaped opacities appear diffusely located in pre–Descemet's membrane or in deep stroma and become more apparent with age without affecting vision. Nodular corneal degeneration and band keratopathy have been described. Secondary corneal changes such as vascularization and scarring from severe ectropion-related exposure can develop.

Ichthyosis is a prominent feature in several genetic disorders, including Sjögren-Larsson, Rud, and Conradi syndromes, congenital keratitis-ichthyosiform-deafness (KID) syndrome, Refsum disease, and congenital hemidysplasia with ichthyosiform erythroderma and limb defects (CHILD). Vascularizing keratitis is a prominent feature of KID syndrome that may worsen with isotretinoin therapy. Treatment for the ichthyosis spectrum is aimed at hydrating the skin and eyelids, removing scale, and slowing the turnover of epidermis when appropriate. These disorders are not responsive to corticosteroids.

Darier disease (keratosis follicularis)   PATHOGENESIS. Darier disease is an autosomal dominant disorder that affects vitamin A metabolism. Histopathologic skin findings are hyperkeratosis, parakeratosis, acanthosis, formation of suprabasal lacunae, and upward proliferation of villi into the lacunae. Distinctive dyskeratotic cells are present in the lacunae. Electron microscopic studies have shown a defect in the tonofilament-desmosomal complex. Histopathology of the peripheral corneal opacities has shown basal epithelial cell edema and decreased desmosomes.

CLINICAL PRESENTATION. Darier disease is characterized by firm brown papular excrescences that tend to coalesce into patches on symmetric areas of the scalp, face, trunk, and flexures of the extremities. The nails and mucous membrane may be involved. The usual onset is in childhood, and all races and genders are affected equally. Ocular manifestations are common, including keratotic eyelid plaques, blepharoconjunctivitis, corneal opacities, and pannus. The corneal lesions seen in 75% of patients in one study were distinctive waxy, intraepithelial, variously shaped opacities combined with a central corneal whorling epithelial irregularity. The corneal changes are asymptomatic and may be helpful in diagnosing the disease.

MANAGEMENT. Treatment can include systemic vitamin A, isotretinoin, and etretinate and topical tretinoin. Corticosteroids are also administered. Treatment does not affect the corneal lesions.

Ectodermal Dysplasia

This heterogeneous group of conditions is characterized by the following:

□ Presence of abnormalities at birth

□ Nonprogressive course

□ Diffuse involvement of the epidermis plus at least one of its appendages (hair, nails, teeth, sweat glands)

□ Various inheritance patterns

Many ocular abnormalities have been described in the ectodermal dysplasias, including sparse lashes and brows, blepharitis, ankyloblepharon, hypoplastic lacrimal ducts, diminished tear production, abnormal meibomian glands, dry conjunctivae, pterygia, corneal scarring and neovascularization, cataract and glaucoma.

Anhidrotic ectodermal dysplasia is usually an X-linked disorder consisting of hypotrichosis, anodontia, and anhidrosis. Sweating is almost completely lacking, and hyperpyrexia is a common problem in childhood. Atopic disease is often an associated finding. The *ectrodactyly–ectodermal dysplasial–clefting (EEC) syndrome* is an association of ectodermal dysplasia, cleft lip and/or palate, and a clefting deformity of the hands and/or feet ("lobster claw deformity").

Xeroderma Pigmentosum

This recessively transmitted disease is characterized by an impaired ability to repair sunlight-induced damage to DNA. During the first or second decade of life the patient's exposed skin develops areas of focal hyperpigmentation, atrophy, actinic keratosis, and telangiectasia as if the patient had received a heavy dose of radiation. Many cutaneous neoplasms appear later, including squamous cell carcinoma, basal cell carcinoma, and melanoma.

Ophthalmic manifestations include photophobia, tearing, blepharospasm, and signs and symptoms of keratoconjunctivitis sicca, or dry eye. The conjunctiva is dry and inflamed with telangiectasia and hyperpigmentation. Pingueculae and pterygia often occur. Corneal complications include exposure keratitis, ulceration, neovascularization, scarring, and even perforation. Keratoconus, band-shaped nodular corneal dystrophy, and gelatinous dystrophy have also been reported. Ocular neoplasms occur in 11% of patients, most frequently at the limbus. Squamous cell carcinoma is the most frequent histologic type seen, followed by basal cell carcinoma and melanoma, similar to the cutaneous tumors. The eyelids can be involved with progressive atrophy, madarosis, trichiasis, scarring, symblepharon, entropion, ectropion, and sometimes even loss of the entire lower eyelid.

Mannis MJ, Macsai MS, Huntley AC, eds. *Eye and Skin Disease*. Philadelphia: Lippincott-Raven; 1996;3–12, 39–44, 131–145.

Noninflammatory Vascular Anomalies of the Conjunctiva

Causes of conjunctival hyperemia include the following:

☐ Inflammation: infection, allergy, toxicity, neoplasia

☐ Direct irritation: foreign body, eyelash

☐ Reflex response: eyestrain, emotional weeping

☐ Systemic or topical vasodilator: alcohol, oxygen, carcinoid tumor

☐ Autonomic dysfunction: sympathetic paresis, sphenopalatine ganglion syndrome

☐ Vascular engorgement: venous obstruction, hyperviscosity

Conjunctival vascular tortuosities may follow trauma or be a result of disorders causing chronic conjunctival vascular dilation, such as rosacea. Systemic disorders that cause sludging and segmentation of blood flow in conjunctival vessels, as well as conjunctival varicosities and aneurysms, include

☐ Hypertension

☐ Diabetes mellitus

☐ Sickle cell disease

☐ Multiple myeloma

☐ Polycythemia vera

☐ Old age

Causes of intraconjunctival hemorrhage, and less commonly of bloody tears, are listed in Table VI-1. Hereditary causes of conjunctival telangiectasia and hemorrhage are hereditary hemorrhagic telangiectasia and ataxia-telangiectasia.

Hereditary Hemorrhagic Telangiectasia

Spontaneous hemorrhage from telangiectatic vessels of the palpebral and bulbar conjunctiva may occur in individuals with hereditary hemorrhagic telangiectasia (Rendu-Osler-Weber disease), a vascular disorder that also involves the skin, nasal and oral mucous membranes, gastrointestinal tract, lungs, and brain. This dominantly inherited (but occasionally sporadic) disease usually is not apparent in early childhood, and its onset during early adult life may be subtle. Initial manifestations may be intermittent, painless gastrointestinal bleeding leading to iron deficiency anemia or recurrent epistaxis following a minor trauma or occurring spontaneously.

TABLE VI-1

CAUSES OF SUBCONJUNCTIVAL HEMORRHAGE

OCULAR	SYSTEMIC
Conjunctival, orbital, or cranial trauma	Sudden venous congestion (Valsalva maneuver)
Acute viral or bacterial conjunctivitis	Vascular fragility
	Thrombocytopenia and impaired clotting
	Systemic febrile illness

Conjunctival hemorrhage may be associated with foreign body sensation, and it usually occurs spontaneously or after minor trauma, such as rubbing of the eyelids. The hemorrhage may extend into the subepithelial connective tissues or may be external (bloody tears). Conjunctival bleeding can be copious, but in most instances it can be controlled with local pressure. The conjunctival telangiectasias appear sharply circumscribed, are slightly elevated, and are composed of arborizing dilated channels. Typically, they involve the palpebral region, although lesions of the bulbar conjunctiva have been reported.

Histologic study has shown superficial, dilated, thin-walled vascular channels. Similar findings have been noted in telangiectatic lesions of the skin and nasal and oral mucous membranes. It is likely that hemorrhage results from minor trauma to these superficial vessels; however, intravascular factors affecting bleeding time also may play a role.

Lymphangiectasia

This condition may be a developmental anomaly or may occur in association with trauma or inflammation. Unlike lymphangiomas, which are cellular proliferations of lymphatic channel elements, lymphangiectasias are irregularly dilated, periodically hemorrhage-filled, lymphatic channels of the bulbar conjunctiva. Surrounding conjunctival edema or subconjunctival hemorrhage may also be present, especially upon crying or exertion. Treatment is local excision or diathermy.

Lymphangiectasia must be distinguished from *ataxia-telangiectasia (Louis-Bar syndrome),* in which the epibulbar and interpalpebral telangiectasia of the arteries lacks an associated lymphatic component. The conjunctival lesions of Louis-Bar syndrome are a marker for associated cerebellar and immunologic abnormalities (e.g., hypogammaglobulinemia), which are conducive to sinopulmonary infection and lymphoreticular proliferations, particularly T-cell leukemias. The epibulbar vascular lesions do not acquire a tumefactive characteristic (hamartia) because they are simple telangiectasia that grow with the patient and the eyeball. No episodic events of hemorrhage or swelling are encountered. Ataxia-telangiectasia is discussed in greater detail in BCSC Section 6, *Pediatric Ophthalmology and Strabismus.*

Tear Deficiency States

Dry Eye (Keratoconjunctivitis Sicca)

Dry eye is a very common disorder of tear film that results from either decreased tear production or excessive tear evaporation. The tear film becomes unstable with the loss of water, and a progressive deterioration of the ocular surface ensues. Interpretation of studies investigating risk factors, pathogenesis, and therapy of dry eye conditions has been complicated in the past by a lack of accepted diagnostic criteria and a lack of standardized, specific diagnostic tests. A diagnostic classification scheme for dry eye disorders has now been established along with uniform guidelines for the evaluation of both the disorder and its response to therapy. The major subclassification in this scheme separates dry eye patients into those with aqueous tear deficiency and those with evaporative loss, predominantly patients with meibomian gland dysfunction (Table VI-2).

TABLE VI-2

CLASSIFICATION OF DRY EYE

Tear-deficient dry eye

 Non–Sjögren syndrome
  Lacrimal disease (primary or secondary)
  Lacrimal obstructive disease
  Decreased corneal sensation
  Other (e.g., multiple neuromatosis)

 Sjögren syndrome

Evaporative dry eye

 Blepharitis-associated
  Obstructive meibomian gland disease

 Blink disorders

 Disorders of eyelid aperture and eyelid/globe congruity

CLINICAL PRESENTATION. The spectrum of aqueous tear deficiency ranges from mild irritation with minimal ocular surface disease to severe and disabling irritation, occasionally associated with sight-threatening corneal complications. Symptoms tend to be worse toward the end of the day, with prolonged use of the eyes, or with exposure to environmental extremes. Patients who live in temperate climates and are exposed to the lower levels of humidity associated with indoor heating systems during the winter tend to become particularly symptomatic. Foreign body sensation is a symptom frequently associated with punctate keratopathy. Associated complaints include burning, a dry sensation, photophobia, and blurred vision.

The signs of a dry eye include bulbar conjunctival vascular dilation, conjunctival pleating (redundancy of the bulbar conjunctiva), a decreased tear meniscus, irregular corneal surface, and increased debris in the tear film. Epithelial keratopathy, which can be fine and granular, coarse, or confluent, is best demonstrated following the instillation of rose bengal or fluorescein. Particularly useful in the evaluation of the dry eye patient is staining with 1% rose bengal. Previously, rose bengal was thought to stain only dead and devitalized cells and mucus. It has recently been demonstrated that it may be staining those epithelial cells that are inadequately protected by a mucin tear coating. Rose bengal staining can be a more sensitive indicator than fluorescein of early or mild cases of keratoconjunctivitis sicca; it may be seen at the nasal and temporal limbus and/or inferior paracentral cornea (exposure staining) (Fig VI-6). Alternatively, it can be most prominent along the inferior cornea and inferior conjunctiva (linear staining), as seen in MGD.

Fluorescein pools in epithelial erosions and stains exposed basement membrane, and it can appear as fine or coarse granular staining of the inferior or central cornea. Lissamine green B and sulforhodamine B have also been used as vital dyes; neither stains healthy conjunctival epithelium. Although these two agents are reportedly less irritating than rose bengal, they are not commercially available.

In more advanced states filaments and mucous plaques can be seen. Filaments represent strands of epithelial cells attached to the surface of the cornea over a core

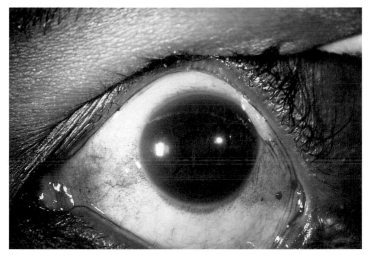

FIG VI-6—Keratoconjunctivitis sicca with punctate epithelial erosions, shown by rose bengal stain.

of mucus. Filamentary keratopathy can be quite painful, as these strands are firmly attached to the richly innervated surface epithelium (Fig VI-7). Marginal or paracentral thinning and even perforation can occur in more advanced states. Inadequate or insufficient blinking is frequently noted. Associated local eye disease, such as blepharitis, MGD, and eyelid abnormalities, can contribute significantly to the patient's level of discomfort.

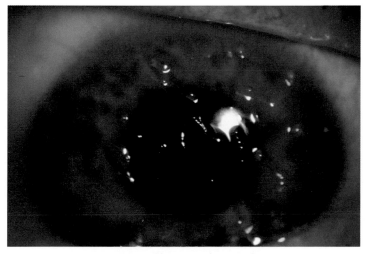

FIG VI-7—Filamentary keratopathy.

Aqueous Tear Deficiency

Findings that are particularly indicative of ATD include, by definition, decreased aqueous tear production as measured by Schirmer testing. In addition, the characteristic exposure pattern of conjunctival and/or corneal staining with rose bengal, corneal staining by fluorescein, and filamentary keratitis support a diagnosis of ATD. There is increasing recognition that lacrimal gland secretory dysfunction results in the ocular surface condition known as *keratoconjunctivitis sicca (KCS),* and that the severity of aqueous tear deficiency is positively correlated with the severity of KCS. ATD can be congenital, as in Riley-Day syndrome (familial dysautonomia); congenital alacrimia, or absence of the lacrimal gland; anhidrotic ectodermal dysplasia; Adie syndrome; and idiopathic autonomic dysfunction (Shy-Drager syndrome). Contact lens wear has also been associated with decreased tear production, possibly as a result of decreased corneal sensation. However, acquired ATD secondary to dysfunction of the lacrimal gland is the more frequently encountered clinical problem. Most commonly seen in association with inflammatory diseases of the main lacrimal gland, it can also be caused by trauma to the lacrimal glands, numerous anticholinergic medications (Table VI-3), and neuroparalytic hyposecretion. Sarcoidosis and mumps can cause significant inflammation and dysfunction of the main lacrimal gland. Severe ATD is frequently associated with Sjögren syndrome, a systemic immune dysfunction.

Patients with ATD are considered to have Sjögren syndrome (SS) if they have an associated xerostomia and/or a connective tissue disorder. Patients with primary SS include a homogeneous group of young to middle-aged women with evidence of systemic immune dysfunction and very severe ATD and ocular surface disease. These patients do not have any connective tissue disease that has currently been defined, and 90% have the HLA-B8 haplotype. Patients with primary SS are very likely to have anti-La (SS-B) autoantibodies. Another group of women have a similar clinical presentation but do not have serum autoantibodies detectable using current techniques. Patients with secondary SS are those who have a defined connective tissue disease. The Sjögren syndrome usually represents a multisystem autoimmune connective tissue disease and is most often seen in middle-aged women. Secondary SS is most commonly associated with rheumatoid arthritis, although numerous other autoimmune and systemic vasculitic diseases are also frequently encountered. Additional associations can include monocular exocrine gland dysfunction, atrophy of the gastric and vaginal mucosa, and lymphocytic infiltration of the kidney, lung, muscle, or visceral organs. Associated symptoms include fever, fatigue, Raynaud's phenomenon, arthralgias, and myalgias. With regard to the pathogenesis of Sjögren syndrome, these patients have been noted to have immunologic abnormalities, including hypergammaglobulinemia, autoantibodies, impaired lymphocytic function, and lymphoreticular neoplasms.

The precise cause of KCS in SS is unknown, although it is probably related to autoimmune infiltration of the lacrimal glands and salivary glands by lymphocytes. Viral infections such as Epstein-Barr virus and human immunodeficiency virus (HIV) have been implicated as the potential etiology since ATD has been observed to develop in patients after mononucleosis or HIV infection. Lacrimal gland histology provides many insights into the pathogenesis of Sjögren syndrome. The histologic changes are usually identical to those noted in the salivary glands, with focal areas of glandular degeneration associated with infiltration by lymphocytes and plasma cells in the earliest stages. As the disease advances, fibrosis and replacement of

TABLE VI-3

MEDICATIONS WITH ANTICHOLINERGIC SIDE EFFECTS THAT DECREASE TEAR PRODUCTION

Antihypertensives
    Clonidine (alpha₁ blocker)
    Prazosin (alpha₂ blocker)
    Propranolol (beta blocker)
    Reserpine
    Methyldopa, guanethidine

Antidepressants and psychotropics
    Amitriptyline, nortriptyline
    Imipramine, desipramine, clomipramine
    Doxepin
    Phenelzine, tranylcypromine
    Amoxapine, trimipramine
    Phenothiazines
    Nitrazepam, diazepam

Cardiac antiarrhythmia drugs
    Disopyramide
    Mexiletine

Parkinson disease medications
    Trihexyphenidyl
    Benztropine
    Biperiden
    Procyclidine

Antiulcer agents
    Atropine-like agents
    Metoclopramide, other drugs that decrease gastric motility

Muscle spasm medications
    Cyclobenzaprine
    Methocarbamol

Decongestants (nonprescription cold remedies)
    Ephedrine
    Pseudoephedrine

Antihistamines

Anesthetics
    Enflurane
    Halothane
    Nitrous oxide

the glandular tissue with connective tissue may occur. Immunoglobulin and complement are rarely detected within the glandular tissue. The lymphocytes are predominantly helper T cells, and the overall histology suggests a cell-mediated pathogenesis.

LABORATORY EVALUATION. A lacrimal gland biopsy can be performed to aid the diagnosis, but it may actually aggravate dry eye conditions, so judicious use is recommended. Minor (labial) salivary gland biopsy is occasionally performed by oral surgeons to confirm the diagnosis of Sjögren syndrome. Finally, conjunctival impression cytology can be used to monitor the progression of ocular surface changes, beginning with decreased goblet cell density, followed by squamous metaplasia, and in later stages, keratinization.

Many patients with ATD have either circulating autoantibodies, including anti-nuclear antibody (ANA), or SS antibodies (SS-A and SS-B). The presence of these antibodies has been correlated with the severity of symptoms and ocular surface changes, including a higher incidence of sterile and bacterial keratitis, suggesting that a component of immune dysregulation may play a role in pathogenesis. As discussed, many systemic diseases have been associated with ATD (Table VI-4). Mikulicz syndrome consists of enlargement of the salivary or lacrimal glands, or both, as a result of underlying systemic diseases such as leukemia, lymphoma, and sarcoidosis.

The psychological problems associated with a highly symptomatic, incurable, chronic disease can require considerable support. Organizations such as the Sjögren's Syndrome Foundation (http://www.sjogrens.com) and the National Sjögren's Syndrome Association (http://www.sjogrens.org) are groups that can provide valuable resources to these patients.

TABLE VI-4

SYSTEMIC DISEASES ASSOCIATED WITH DRY EYE

Autoimmune disorders

    Primary Sjögren syndrome

    Secondary Sjögren syndrome associated with
        Rheumatoid arthritis
        Systemic lupus erythematosus
        Progressive systemic sclerosis (scleroderma)
        Polymyositis and dermatomyositis
        Primary biliary cirrhosis

    Graft-versus-host disease

    Immune reactions after radiation to head and neck

Infiltrative processes

    Lymphoma

    Amyloidosis

    Hemochromatosis

    Sarcoidosis

Infectious processes

    HIV-diffuse infiltrative lymphadenopathy syndrome

    Trachoma

Neuropathic dysfunction of the glands

    Multiple sclerosis

    Cranial neuropathies (Bell palsy, vasculitis)

MEDICAL MANAGEMENT. The selection of treatment modalities for patients with dry eye depends largely on the severity of their disease (Table VI-5). The most effective treatments for dry eye disorders act on the earliest and most crucial milestones in dry eye surface disease. Mild cases of dry eye may require no more than the use of topical solutions. Altering or stopping any topical or systemic medications contributing to the condition should also be considered. Hot compresses with eyelid massage can also help by bolstering the lipid layer. If the condition is not sufficiently managed with artificial tears, the use of sustained-release ocular lubricants may be considered. It may also be appropriate to modify the patient's environment in an effort to reduce evaporation of the tear film; a humidifier and/or moisture shields on glasses can be helpful. Therapy for patients with severe dry eye syndrome includes all of the above measures as well as punctal occlusion in addition to overnight patching or eyelid taping and daily part-time taping.

The mainstay of treatment for dry eye syndrome is the use of topical tear substitutes (eyedrops and, less frequently, ointments). Preservative-free tear substitutes are recommended to avoid toxicity in patients who use these agents frequently. Demulcents are polymers added to artificial tear solutions to improve their lubricant properties. Demulcent solutions are mucomimetic agents that can briefly substitute for glycoproteins lost late in the disease process. Demulcents alone, however, are unable to restore lost glycoproteins or conjunctival goblet cells, reduce corneal cell desquamation, or decrease osmolarity. Until relatively recently, all demulcent solutions contained preservatives. Preservative-free demulcent solutions were introduced after it was recognized that preservatives increased corneal desquamation. The elimination of preservatives from traditional demulcent solutions has led to improved corneal barrier function, and subsequent attempts have been made to improve the effect of preservative-free solutions on corneal barrier function by adding various ions to the solutions.

Pharmacologic stimulation of tear secretion has been attempted with many compounds, with varying degrees of success. Topical cyclosporine has been shown to stimulate tear secretion in dogs and in humans, and oral bromhexine has been

TABLE VI-5

RECOMMENDED TREATMENT FOR DRY EYE

SEVERITY	THERAPEUTIC OPTIONS
Mild	Artificial tears with preservatives up to 4× daily Lubricating ointment at bedtime Hot compresses and eyelid massage
Moderate	Artificial tears without preservatives 4× daily to hourly Lubricating ointment at bedtime Reversible occlusion, lower puncta (plugs)
Severe	All of the above Punctal occlusion (lower and upper) Sustained-release tear inserts Moist environment (humidifier, moisture shields) Tarsorrhaphy Bandage lenses (rarely)

used with some success in studies performed outside the United States. Filamentary keratopathy is best treated by controlling the underlying condition, particularly if ATD is responsible. Acetylcysteine 10%, dispensed in an eyedrop container, can be used as a mucolytic agent and is helpful in alleviating these symptoms. Wearing goggles, shields, or moisture bubbles can decrease the evaporation of tears, although these strategies are generally unacceptable to the patient. The surface area available for evaporation can also be decreased simply by fitting the patient with spectacles, which can be further augmented with plastic side shields fitted to the glasses. Soft contact lenses are used with a high degree of risk in dry eye patients, although gas-permeable lenses are frequently well tolerated. Keratorefractive surgery is an increasingly popular option for many contact lens–intolerant dry eye patients.

A subgroup of patients with dry eye disorders also have glaucoma, and certain topical glaucoma medications can decrease conjunctival goblet cell density. Non-cardioselective beta blockers used to manage glaucoma (e.g., timolol and levobunolol) have been associated with an increased incidence of systemic and ocular side effects including dry eye. Corneal sensitivity may decrease with the use of these topical agents. Compared with beta blockers that do not have intrinsic sympathomimetic activity, topical beta blockers with intrinsic sympathomimetic agents (e.g., carteolol) have fewer systemic side effects, less effect on corneal sensitivity (no local anesthetic effect), decreased stinging and red eye, and better local tolerability. Although selective beta blockers (e.g., betaxolol) have fewer systemic side effects, ocular tolerability is another issue; many patients complain of stinging with the use of selective beta blockers. Oral administration of drugs such as carbonic anhydrase inhibitors (e.g., acetazolamide and methazolamide) can decrease tear production. Topical agents (e.g., dorzolamide) commonly cause burning and stinging but have fewer systemic side effects. See also BCSC Section 10, *Glaucoma.*

Many systemic medications decrease aqueous tear production, producing increased symptoms of dry eye. These drugs include diuretics, antihistamines, anticholinergics, and psychotropics, and they should be avoided, if possible, in patients who are symptomatic from ATD. Advanced stages can see the development of corneal calcification, particularly in association with certain topical medications (especially antiglaucoma medications); band keratopathy; and keratinization of the cornea and conjunctiva.

SURGICAL MANAGEMENT. Surgical treatment is generally reserved for patients with severe disease for whom medical treatment is either inadequate or impractical. Patients with moderately dry eyes may be helped by punctal occlusion, although it occasionally results in chronic epiphora. Tear drainage may be decreased with either temporary or permanent punctal occlusion. Temporary punctal occlusion may be performed in a number of ways, with varying degrees of effectiveness, using collagen implants or silicone punctal plugs (Fig VI-8). The collagen plugs may dissolve within days and can be used as diagnostic adjuncts prior to permanent occlusion of the puncta. Silicone plugs are continuously visible at the slit lamp, making it obvious when they have fallen out. Recently, these plugs have become available in a variety of sizes and shapes, facilitating their insertion and removal. The subcutaneous injection of a small amount of local anesthetic makes insertion considerably less stressful to the patient and physician. One disadvantage of punctal plugs is that they can be inadvertently forced into the nasolacrimal system, requiring surgical removal. Occasionally, patients find the plugs irritating.

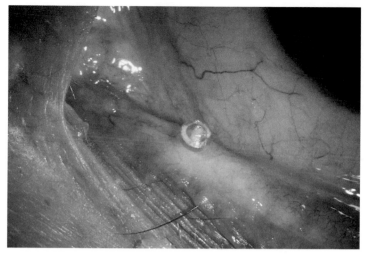

FIG VI-8—Nonabsorbable punctal plug.

When patients have successfully tolerated temporary punctal plugs, permanent punctal occlusion can be performed in the most cost-effective manner with either a hyfrecator tip or disposable cautery (Fig VI 9). The value of punctal occlusion for ocular surface disease other than dry eye is unproven. This procedure Is recommended primarily for those patients in whom basal tear secretion is minimal and

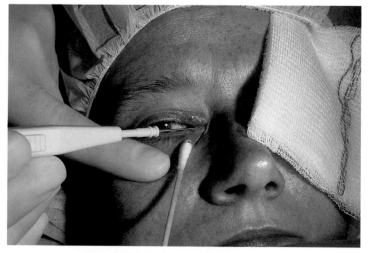

FIG VI-9—Cautery of punctum.

without significant ocular surface inflammation, especially in elderly patients, where risk of iatrogenically induced epiphora is minimal. Correction of eyelid malpositions such as entropion and ectropion may also be useful in managing patients with dry eye.

Mucin Tear Deficiency

Systemic vitamin A deficiency is the most common cause of mucin deficiency, if areas outside the United States are also considered. Conditions associated with goblet cell dysfunction can also cause mucin deficiency, including severe dry eye, alkali burns, cicatricial pemphigoid, Stevens-Johnson syndrome, and trachoma. Signs indicative of mucin deficiency include an increased tear breakup time, which is also indicative of lipid tear deficiency, as well as conjunctival and eyelid changes associated with cicatricial conditions. The treatment of patients with mucin or lipid (see below) deficiency states requires that the underlying condition responsible for the deficiency (i.e., blepharitis or other forms of ocular surface disease) be brought under control. The measures described for treatment of aqueous tear deficiency are also used.

Lipid Tear Deficiency

Lipid tear deficiency states can be manifested by an increased tear breakup time, meibomian gland dysfunction, normal aqueous tear production, and a characteristic linear pattern of rose bengal staining of the inferior conjunctiva and/or cornea. Abnormalities of the lipid layer can also be caused by the conditions causing MGD, as with rosacea or following oral isotretinoin therapy.

de Luise VP. Management of dry eyes. In: *Focal Points: Clinical Modules for Ophthalmologists.* San Francisco: American Academy of Ophthalmology; 1985;3:3.

Farris RL, Stuchell RN, Nisengard R. Sjögren's syndrome and keratoconjunctivitis sicca. *Cornea.* 1991;10:207–209.

Fox RI, Robinson CA, Curd JG, et al. Sjögren's syndrome. Proposed criteria for classification. *Arthritis Rheum.* 1986;29:577–585.

Friedlaender MH. Ocular manifestations of Sjögren's syndrome: keratoconjunctivitis sicca. *Rheum Dis Clin North Am.* 1992;18:591–608.

Pflugfelder W, Whitcher JP, Daniels TG. Sjögren syndrome. In: Pepose JS, Holland GN, Wilhelmus KR, eds. *Ocular Infection and Immunity.* St Louis: Mosby; 1996:313–333.

Preferred Practice Patterns Committee, Cornea Panel. *Blepharitis.* San Francisco: American Academy of Ophthalmology; 1998.

Preferred Practice Patterns Committee, Cornea Panel. *Dry Eye Syndrome.* San Francisco: American Academy of Ophthalmology; 1998.

Nutritional and Physiologic Disorders

Vitamin A Deficiency

PATHOGENESIS. Vitamin A is an essential fat-soluble vitamin. Human disease can be caused by too little or too much vitamin A intake. Table VI-6 presents an overview of vitamin A metabolism.

Vitamin A–induced xerosis is found in epithelial cells of the gastrointestinal, genitourinary, and respiratory tracts. Xerosis is associated with loss of mucus production by the goblet cells. The ocular consequence is Bitôt's spot, a superficial, foamy, gray triangular area on the bulbar conjunctiva that appears in the palpebral aperture (Fig VI-10). This spot consists of keratinized epithelium, inflammatory cells, debris, and also *Corynebacterium xerosis*. These bacilli metabolize the debris and produce a foamy appearance.

Vitamin A deficiency leads to *xerophthalmia,* which is responsible for at least 20,000–100,000 new cases of blindness worldwide each year. At greatest risk of xerophthalmia are the malnourished infant and the baby born to a vitamin A–deficient mother, especially if the infant has another biological stress such as measles or diarrhea. Superficial concurrent infections with herpes simplex, measles, or bacterial agents probably further predispose the child to keratomalacia and blindness. While xerophthalmia usually represents a dietary deficiency as a result of low intake, decreased absorption of vitamin A may also be responsible. Most instances of vitamin A deficiency and xerophthalmia in countries with a low rate of malnutrition are the result of unusual self-imposed dietary practices, chronic alcoholism, or lipid malabsorption (particularly cystic fibrosis, biliary cirrhosis, and bowel resection).

CLINICAL PRESENTATION. *Nyctalopia* is often the earliest symptom of hypovitaminosis A, but retinal function does not always correlate with anterior segment findings. Xerophthalmia fundus, a rare associated abnormality, features yellow-white spots in the peripheral retina.

Prolonged vitamin A deficiency leads to external involvement, including xerosis (dryness of the conjunctiva and cornea), metaplastic keratinization of areas of the conjunctiva (Bitôt spots), corneal ulcers and scars, and eventually diffuse corneal

TABLE VI-6

METABOLISM OF VITAMIN A

LEVEL	METABOLITE
Diet	Plant (carotenoids) and animal (retinyl-palmitate and retinol) foods
Intestine	Retinol-micelle
Portal circulation	Retinyl-palmitate
Liver	Retinol–retinol-binding protein
Target tissues	Retinoic acid (epithelium, epidermis, and lymphocytes)
	Retinal (rod photoreceptors)

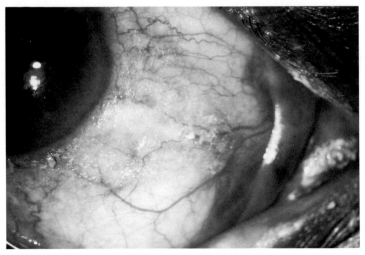

FIG VI-10—Conjunctival xerosis with focal keratinization (Bitôt spot) as a result of vitamin A deficiency.

necrosis (*keratomalacia*). The World Health Organization classifies the ocular surface changes into three stages:

□ Conjunctival xerosis, without (X1A) or with (X1B) Bitôt spots

□ Corneal xerosis (X2)

□ Corneal ulceration, with keratomalacia involving less than one third (X3A) or more than one third (X3B) of the corneal surface

Patients with chronic alcoholism may present with persistent epithelial defect and corneal ulceration unresponsive to antimicrobial therapy. Night blindness with an abnormal electroretinogram and conjunctival xerosis or Bitôt spots may be the presenting manifestation of the chronic malabsorption syndromes mentioned above. Laboratory diagnosis of low serum level of vitamin A or retinol-binding proteins is usually used to confirm the clinical suspicion.

MANAGEMENT. Systemic vitamin A deficiency, best characterized by keratomalacia, is a medical emergency with an untreated mortality rate of 50%. While the administration of oral or parenteral vitamin A will address the acute manifestations of keratomalacia, these patients are usually affected by a much larger protein-energy malnutrition and should be treated with both vitamin and protein-calorie supplements. Problems with malabsorption may prevent oral administration from being effective in patients with acute vitamin A deficiency. Maintenance of adequate corneal lubrication and prevention of secondary infection and corneal melting are essential steps in treating keratomalacia, but identification and proper treatment of the underlying causes are vital to successful clinical management of the ocular complications.

As a result of the beneficial effects of retinoids in xerophthalmia, studies were undertaken to determine if topical retinoids would be useful in reversing the squamous metaplasia and symptoms associated with dry eye syndromes. Although double-blind, placebo-controlled studies failed to demonstrate the efficacy of topical therapy for patients with keratoconjunctivitis sicca alone, subsequent studies revealed that topical retinoids were primarily useful in conditions with severe squamous metaplasia and keratinization, such as Stevens-Johnson syndrome, cicatricial pemphigoid, radiation-induced dry eye, drug-induced pseudopemphigoid, and toxic epidermal necrolysis (see pp 201–207 for discussion of these conditions). At the present time, an effective ophthalmic preparation of topical retinoids is not readily available for general clinical use.

Harris EW, Loewenstein JI, Azar D. Vitamin A deficiency and its effects on the eye. *Int Ophthalmol Clin.* 1998;38:155–162.

Sommer A, West KP. *Vitamin A Deficiency: Health, Survival, and Vision.* New York: Oxford University Press; 1996.

Soong HK, Martin NF, Wagoner MD, et al. Topical retinoid therapy for squamous metaplasia of various ocular surface disorders. A multicenter, placebo-controlled double-masked study. *Ophthalmology.* 1988;95:1442–1446.

Vitamin C Deficiency

Ascorbic acid, or vitamin C, is an essential vitamin in humans because they lack its synthetic enzyme, L-gulonolactone oxidase. A major action mechanism of ascorbic acid is its effect as a cofactor on the hydroxylation of lysine and proline in ribosomal collagen synthesis. Impairment of hydroxylation secondary to ascorbic acid deficiency results in unstable collagen fiber formation.

Following transport through the ciliary epithelium, ascorbic acid is about 15–20 times more concentrated in aqueous humor than in plasma. In a vitamin C deprivation trial extending over approximately 3 months some subjects developed xerosis. In animal studies scorbutic guinea pig corneas subjected to injury showed impaired wound healing. Animal studies also suggest that the alkali-burned cornea represents a localized scorbutic state that is unable to synthesize adequate collagen to repair the stromal wound. Topical and subcutaneous ascorbate can restore the ascorbate level in aqueous humor after alkali burn and significantly reduce the incidence of corneal ulcer and perforation in rabbit eyes.

Neurotrophic Keratopathy

PATHOGENESIS. Neurotrophic keratopathy results from damage to cranial nerve V, causing corneal hypoesthesia or anesthesia. This damage may result from surgical trauma (ablation of the trigeminal ganglion), cerebrovascular accidents, aneurysms, multiple sclerosis, tumors (such as neurofibroma or angioma), herpes zoster ophthalmicus, herpes simplex keratitis, Hansen disease (leprosy), or topical anesthetic abuse. Another cause is hereditary sensory neuropathy, an autosomal recessive disorder with reduction of small myelinated nerve fibers. This condition can result in dramatic, persistent, nonhealing epithelial defects in infants in association with other defects of sensory nerves.

A recently reported animal model demonstrated that, following corneal denervation, tear film osmolarity increased. This study showed that, in addition to the ocular surface findings associated with ATD as a result of depressed tearing reflex, an additional mechanism for corneal disease, related to the trophic influence of cranial nerve V, was operational. Tarsorrhaphy decreased tear film evaporation and effectively decreased tear film osmolarity. Presumably, decreasing the surface area of corneal exposure is the mechanistic explanation for the efficacy of this procedure.

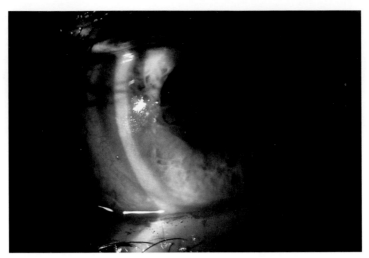

FIG VI-11—Neurotrophic ulcer.

CLINICAL PRESENTATION. Neurotrophic keratopathy is characterized by a keratopathy that generally involves the central or inferior paracentral cornea as a result of corneal denervation or damage to cranial nerve V. Herpes zoster ophthalmicus can lead to a severe neurotrophic keratopathy. A patient showing other signs of herpes zoster ophthalmicus should undergo an assessment of corneal sensation in order to determine the relative level of risk. Vesicles at the side of the tip of the nose, indicative of the involvement of nasociliary branch of the ophthalmic division of cranial nerve V (V_1), are known as *Hutchinson's sign* and are indicative of future ocular involvement. Sensation may return to some extent during healing but is usually permanently depressed. Neurotrophic keratopathy resulting from herpes simplex keratitis can result in persistent epithelial defects in the absence of replicating virus or active corneal inflammation. These epithelial defects stain intensely with fluorescein and are surrounded by raised, rolled-up gray edges (Fig VI-11). Progressive sterile ulceration or superinfection can result in perforation.

Familial dysautonomia (Riley-Day syndrome) This condition is inherited in an autosomal recessive manner, predominantly but not exclusively in Jewish families of eastern European origin (Ashkenazi). Patients usually present with emotional instability, skin blotching, transient but marked hypertension, excessive sweating and salivation, insensitivity to pain, failure to thrive, postural hypotension, and recurrent respiratory tract infection. Constantly diminished production of tears while crying and corneal hypoesthesia are the most consistent ophthalmic findings. The autonomic dysfunction affects the tear production of the lacrimal gland and leads to secondary conjunctival xerosis. Affected individuals frequently develop keratitis ranging in severity from mild punctuate stippling of the lower portion of the corneal epithelium to frank neurotrophic ulcerations.

MANAGEMENT. Management of neurotrophic keratopathy includes treatment of the underlying disease and use of the full spectrum of approaches outlined above and below for dry eyes and exposure keratopathy. The choice of nonpreserved ointments or eyedrops lacking potentially toxic preservatives such as benzalkonium chloride (BAK) is particularly important in these cases. Management of toxic ulcerative keratopathy includes discontinuation of the offending agent, patching, and the use of nonpreserved medications. Rarely, therapeutic contact lenses or collagen shields are used.

Tarsorrhaphy, either lateral or medial or, occasionally, both, is frequently required in order to prevent surface desiccation. Penetrating keratoplasty, although generally hazardous in cases of neurotrophic keratopathy, has recently been used with increasing success in patients with residual scarring from clinically inactive herpes zoster keratopathy. It is essential that this surgery be performed in association with a temporary or permanent tarsorrhaphy.

Donaghy M, Hakin RN, Bamford JM, et al. Hereditary sensory neuropathy with neurotrophic keratitis. Description of an autosomal recessive disorder with a selective reduction of small myelinated nerve fibers and a discussion of the classification of the hereditary sensory neuropathies. *Brain.* 1987;110:563–583.

Structural and Exogenous Disorders

Exposure Keratopathy

PATHOGENESIS. Exposure keratopathy can result from any disease process that limits eyelid closure. Lagophthalmos can be caused by the following:

- Neurogenic diseases such as seventh nerve palsy (neuroparalytic keratopathy) or acoustic neuroma
- Inattentive mental states such as coma, parkinsonism, or thalamic infarct or nocturnal exposure
- Cicatricial or restrictive eyelid diseases such as ectropion
- Following blepharoplasty
- Skin disorders such as Stevens-Johnson syndrome or xeroderma pigmentosum

Proptosis caused by thyroid orbitopathy or other inflammatory or infiltrative orbital diseases can also result in exposure keratopathy.

CLINICAL PRESENTATION. Exposure keratopathy is characterized by a punctate epithelial keratopathy that usually involves the inferior third of the cornea. In more severe cases the entire corneal surface can be involved. Large, coalescent epithelial defects may result, which may lead to ulceration, melting, and perforation. Symptoms are similar to those associated with dry eye, including foreign body sensation, photophobia, and tearing, unless there is an associated neurotrophic component with resultant corneal anesthesia.

MANAGEMENT. Therapy is similar to that described for severe dry eyes. In the earliest stages nonpreserved artificial tears during the day and ointment at bedtime may suffice. Taping the eyelid shut at bedtime can be helpful if the problem is primarily one of nocturnal exposure. The use of bandage contact lenses can be hazardous in these patients with high incidence of desiccation and infection. In cases where the problem is likely to be temporary or self-limited, a temporary tarsorrhaphy using tissue adhesive and Frost sutures should be performed. However, when the problem is likely to be long-standing, definitive surgical therapy to correct the eyelid position is mandated. Correction of any associated eyelid abnormalities, such as ectropion and/or trichiasis, is also indicated.

Most commonly, surgical management consists of permanent lateral and/or medial tarsorrhaphy. Insertion of gold weights into the upper tarsus that mechanically closes the eyelids is also an effective technique to promote eyelid closure. The weights are fabricated from 99.99% pure gold and are available in sizes ranging from 0.6 g to 1.6 g in 0.2 g increments. Implantation of a gold weight does not alter the dimension of the horizontal eyelid fissure and thus creates a less obvious cosmetic change than does a lateral tarsorrhaphy.

A horizontal tightening procedure is also beneficial in correcting the flaccid lower eyelid. Occasionally, a hard palate mucosal graft is needed to augment eyelid elevation, as horizontal tightening alone may be insufficient. Reported complications of gold weight implants include infection, position shifting, implant extrusion, induced astigmatism, unacceptable ptosis, and noninfectious inflammatory response to the gold. The weights remain stable when exposed to MRI.

Donzis PB, Mondino BJ. Management of noninfectious corneal ulcers. *Surv Ophthalmol.* 1987;32:94–110.

Involutional lower eyelid malposition   The lower eyelid retractors are the *capsulopalpebral fascia* and the sympathetic *inferior tarsal muscle.* Detailed histologic study has shown that the capsulopalpebral fascia originates as the capsulopalpebral head, with delicate attachments to the inferior rectus muscle and tendon. Appreciation of this lower eyelid anatomy has allowed a better understanding of involutional entropion and ectropion. These two common lower eyelid malposition problems share some similar pathophysiologic mechanisms. Both conditions may feature horizontal eyelid laxity and retractor disinsertion, causing instability of the eyelid margin and punctal malposition. Differential vector forces between the anterior and posterior lamella often determine which condition—ectropion or entropion—will manifest.

Ectropion is caused by horizontal eyelid laxity resulting from elongation of the lateral tendon. For *entropion* it is well recognized that three basic anatomic defects may be contributory:

□ Horizontal lower eyelid laxity

□ Disinsertion or attenuation of the retractors

□ Preseptal orbicularis muscle overriding the pretarsal orbicularis muscle

Newer surgical repair techniques reflect the anatomic etiology of involutional eyelid malposition in many cases. For horizontal eyelid laxity a lateral tarsal strip procedure and retractor disinsertion reattachment may be performed using an anterior skin approach or a posterior transconjunctival incision. See also BCSC Section 7, *Orbit, Eyelids, and Lacrimal System.*

Floppy Eyelid Syndrome

This syndrome of chronic ocular irritation and inflammation typically occurs in obese individuals. Patients have a flimsy, lax upper tarsus that everts with minimal upward force applied to the upper eyelid. Clinical findings include small to large papillae on the upper palpebral conjunctiva, mucous discharge, and corneal involvement ranging from mild punctate epitheliopathy to superficial vascularization (Fig VI-12). Keratoconus has also been reported in patients with floppy eyelid syndrome. The problem may result from spontaneous eversion of the upper eyelid when it contacts the pillow or other bedclothes during sleep. Direct contact of the upper

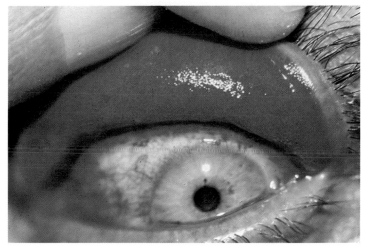

FIG VI-12—Floppy eyelid syndrome with papillary response on superior tarsus.

eyelid with bed linens may traumatize the upper tarsal conjunctiva and induce inflammation and chronic irritation. The disease may be unilateral if the patient always sleeps in the same position. Treatment consists of covering the affected eye(s) with a metal shield or taping eyelids closed at night or performing surgical eyelid-tightening procedures. Differential diagnosis includes vernal conjunctivitis, giant papillary conjunctivitis, atopic keratoconjunctivitis, bacterial conjunctivitis, and toxic keratopathy.

> Culbertson WW, Ostler HB. The floppy eyelid syndrome. *Am J Ophthalmol.* 1981; 92:568–575.

Superior Limbic Keratoconjunctivitis (SLK)

PATHOGENESIS. The pathogenesis of superior limbic keratoconjunctivitis has not been established, although it is thought to result from mechanical trauma to the superior bulbar and tarsal conjunctiva. Some patients have a history of thyroid dysfunction and associated bulbar conjunctival edema that may increase friction between the superior eyelid and the globe.

CLINICAL PRESENTATION. SLK is a chronic, recurrent condition of ocular irritation and redness. The condition typically develops in adult women, 20–70 years of age. SLK may recur over a period of 1–10 years. Usually the condition resolves spontaneously. It is often bilateral, although one eye may be more severely affected than the other. Ocular findings may include the following:

- A fine papillary reaction on the superior tarsal conjunctiva
- Injection and thickening of the superior bulbar conjunctiva (Fig VI-13)
- Hypertrophy of the superior limbus

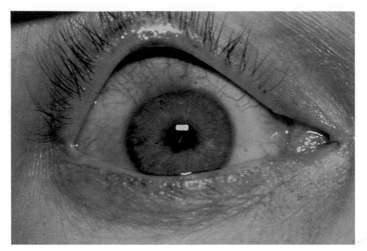

FIG VI-13—Superior limbic keratoconjunctivitis.

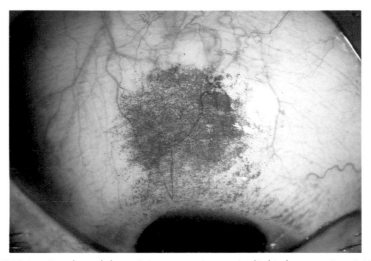

FIG VI-14—Rose bengal dye staining pattern in superior limbic keratoconjunctivitis.

▫ Fine punctate fluorescein and rose bengal staining of the superior bulbar conjunctiva above the limbus and superior cornea just below the limbus (Fig VI-14)

▫ Superior corneal filamentary keratitis

SLK can be associated with aqueous tear deficiency or blepharospasm.

LABORATORY EVALUATION. Hyperproliferation, acanthosis, loss of goblet cells, and keratinization are seen in histologic sections of the superior bulbar conjunctiva. Diagnosis of the condition can often be based on clinical signs, although scrapings or impression cytology of the superior bulbar conjunctiva showing characteristic features of nuclear pyknosis with "snake nuclei," increased epithelial cytoplasm–to–nucleus ratio, loss of goblet cells, and keratinization may be a helpful diagnostic test in mild or confusing cases. Patients with SLK should have thyroid function tests including T_3, T_4, and TSH.

MANAGEMENT. A variety of therapies have been reported to provide temporary or permanent relief of symptoms. These include chemical cauterization of superior bulbar conjunctiva and superior tarsal conjunctiva with 0.5%–1.0% silver nitrate solution (silver nitrate solution in wax ampoules, not silver nitrate cauterization sticks), large-diameter bandage contact lenses, topical vitamin A ointment (0.1% transretinoic acid), thermocauterization of the superior bulbar conjunctiva, and resection of the bulbar conjunctiva superior to the limbus.

Theodore FH, Ferry AP. Superior limbic keratoconjunctivitis. Clinical and pathological correlations. *Arch Ophthalmol.* 1970;84:481 484.

Udell IJ, Kenyon KR, Sawa M, et al. Treatment of superior limbic keratoconjunctivitis by thermocauterization of the superior bulbar conjunctiva. *Ophthalmology.* 1986;93: 162–166.

Recurrent Corneal Erosion

PATHOGENESIS. Recurrent erosions typically occur in eyes that have suffered a sudden, sharp, abrading injury as from a fingernail or paper edge. The superficial injury produces an epithelial abrasion that heals rapidly, frequently leaving no clinical evidence of damage. Some patients even fail to recall encountering this antecedent injury. After an interval varying from days to years, symptoms suddenly recur without any obvious precipitating event. Symptoms subside spontaneously in most cases, only to recur periodically. In contrast to shearing injuries, small and partially penetrating foreign bodies that strike the cornea directly and become embedded in the epithelium or superficial stroma rarely produce recurrent erosions. Defective basement membrane and deficient hemidesmosomal attachments of epithelium to subjacent basement membrane and Bowman's layer have been demonstrated in traumatic recurrent erosions. Epithelial basement membrane dystrophy can predispose a cornea to developing posttraumatic erosions, or it can itself be the cause of spontaneously occurring, nontraumatic erosions.

CLINICAL PRESENTATION. Recurrent corneal erosions are characterized by acute attacks of ocular pain that frequently have their onset in the early morning hours or at the time of awakening. These episodes are also characterized by photophobia and lacrimation. Objective signs vary from a localized roughening or edema of the epithelium to true abrasions. The less severe corneal signs resolve rapidly; often when the patient is examined within hours of an acute recurrence, no abnormality is discernible on slit-lamp examination. Many patients seem to suffer from ocular discomfort that is out of proportion to the amount of observable pathology. However, slit-lamp examination using retroillumination can frequently reveal subtle corneal abnormalities. The corneal epithelium is loosely attached to its basement membrane and Bowman's layer, both at the time of a recurrent attack and between attacks when the cornea appears to be entirely healed. During the acute attack, the epithelium in the involved area frequently appears heaped up, and while no frank epithelial staining defect may be present, significant pooling of fluorescein over this area is easily visible.

LABORATORY EVALUATION. The key to making the distinction between a posttraumatic erosion and a dystrophic erosion in a patient who has no clear-cut history of superficial trauma lies in careful examination of the contralateral eye, following maximal pupillary dilation. Occasionally, subtle areas of loosely adherent epithelium can be identified by gentle pressure with a cotton-tipped applicator following the instillation of topical anesthetics. The presence of basement membrane changes in the *unaffected* eye implicates a primary basement membrane defect in the pathogenesis, while the absence of such findings strongly suggests a posttraumatic etiology. (See also discussion in chapter XVI on corneal dystrophies.)

The prevalence of epithelial basement membrane dystrophy has been found to be as high as 76% in populations over the age of 50. Electron microscopic autopsy studies have established that basement membrane abnormalities are almost ubiquitous in the general population, leading some to suggest that epithelial basement membrane dystrophy should actually be classified as a corneal degeneration. Animal studies have shown that defective hemidesmosome production is the underlying pathologic abnormality in posttraumatic recurrent erosions. In addition to trauma, secondary basement membrane abnormalities can have diabetes mellitus, corneal stromal dystrophies such as lattice dystrophy, and postinfectious etiologies.

MANAGEMENT. Conservative therapy for this condition in the acute phase consists of frequent lubrication with antibiotic ointments with or without pressure patching, followed by use of nonpreserved lubricants or hypertonic saline solution (5% NaCl) during the day and ointment at bedtime for 6–12 months to promote proper regeneration of hemidesmosomes and epithelial attachment. More severe cases may require 40% glucose ointment as a hypertonic agent. Hypertonic agents provide lubrication and may transiently produce an osmotic gradient, drawing fluid from the epithelium and theoretically promoting the adherence of epithelial cells to the underlying tissue. Some patients find hypertonic medications unacceptably irritating, although many patients do quite well with this therapy indefinitely.

Although use of a therapeutic bandage contact lens may be of value, proper patient education and judicious monitoring are crucial. Tight lens syndrome caused by lens desiccation and corneal hypoxia can occur, especially during sleep, resulting in severe pain and the need for emergent removal of the lens. Cycloplegics should be used in eyes that have a significant anterior chamber reaction. Occasionally, judicious use of topical corticosteroids is necessary to treat associated secondary keratitis or uveitis.

It is best to approach the management of patients with recalcitrant disease using a stepwise, rational sequence of interventions. When consistent conservative management fails to control the symptoms, invasive therapy may be indicated. In patients with posttraumatic recurrent erosions *anterior stromal micropuncture* can be very effective (Fig VI-15). Using a specially designed prebent 25-gauge needle (see Rubinfeld reference below), the clinician produces numerous superficial puncture wounds in the involved area, creating a firm adhesion between the epithelium and the underlying stroma. This procedure should be used with caution in the visual axis. Rarely is a significant scar visible for more than a few months after this procedure. The treatment may have to be repeated if patients who are adequately controlled initially subsequently become symptomatic, usually because the area of treatment is

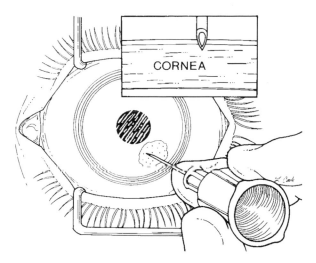

FIG VI-15—Anterior stromal puncture. A No. 20 hypodermic needle is used to encourage microcicatrization between epithelium, Bowman's layer, and stroma. (Reproduced with permission from Kenyon KR, Wagoner MD. Therapy of recurrent erosion and persistent defects of the corneal epithelium. In: *Focal Points: Clinical Modules for Ophthalmologists.* San Francisco: American Academy of Ophthalmology; 1991;9:9. Illustration by Laurel Cook.)

inadequate. Pressure patching for 24–48 hours following treatment is advisable. Histologic studies have revealed that the lesions produced by this procedure do create subepithelial scars. Use of diathermy to create similar lesions in experimental animals has shown that the efficacy of these procedures is related to their ability to stimulate the formation of new basement membrane complexes.

In patients with dystrophic, degenerative, or other severe secondary basement membrane disorder–related recurrent erosions, the procedure of choice is *epithelial debridement,* which can easily be performed at the slit lamp, even in the most uncomfortable patients. Following adequate applications of topical anesthetics and topical nonsteroidal anti-inflammatory agents for analgesia, the epithelium is usually debrided easily using sterile cotton-tipped applicators or a surgical cellulose sponge. An ophthalmic diamond burr sometimes can be used to remove the loose epithelial sheets. It is important to debride the entire epithelium, as this disease is diffuse, rather than limiting the area of debridement to the erosion itself. Care should be taken to avoid damaging the underlying Bowman's layer.

Because a significant amount of discomfort can be expected for 3–4 days following this procedure, the patient will likely be more tolerant if debridement is performed at the time of a painful recurrent episode. Pressure patching, topical antibiotics, and in some cases bandage contact lenses are used until epithelialization is complete (generally 5–7 days). While patients are warned that debridement may need to be repeated at some point in the future, most patients will be symptom-free for at least 1–2 years following a properly performed procedure.

Excimer laser phototherapeutic keratectomy has recently emerged as an alternative modality for the treatment of patients with recalcitrant recurrent erosions, particularly the dystrophic variant. By using a large, shallow zone of ablation, this procedure can minimize the refractive effects, or it can be used to correct an associated myopic refractive error as well. The mechanism of action of this procedure for this condition has yet to be established. See Part 12 for further discussion.

Kenyon KR, Wagoner MD. Therapy of recurrent erosion and persistent defects of the corneal epithelium. In: *Focal Points: Clinical Modules for Ophthalmologists.* San Francisco: American Academy of Ophthalmology; 1991;9:9.

McLean EN, MacRae SM, Rich LF. Recurrent erosion. Treatment by anterior stromal puncture. *Ophthalmology.* 1986;93:784–788.

Payant JA, Eggenberger LR, Wood TO. Electron microscopic findings in corneal epithelial basement membrane degeneration. *Cornea.* 1991;10:390–394.

Rubinfeld RS, Laibson PR, Cohen EJ, et al. Anterior stromal puncture for recurrent erosion: further experience and new instrumentation. *Ophthalmic Surg.* 1990;21:318–326.

Persistent Corneal Epithelial Defect

PATHOGENESIS. Persistent corneal epithelial defects are generally related to some underlying disease process. In a large series the most common causes of these defects were, in order of frequency:

□ Herpetic corneal disease

□ Delayed postsurgical epithelial healing

□ Chemical burns

□ Recurrent corneal erosions

□ Dry eye syndromes

□ Anterior segment necrosis

□ Infections

□ Neuroparalytic keratopathy

In many cases the drugs used to treat some of these conditions impair epithelial wound healing and cause a perpetuation of the epithelial defect. A study has highlighted the drugs most frequently implicated and the characteristic clinical appearance of the affected defects. The authors called this condition *toxic ulcerative keratopathy*. It usually occurs secondary to administration of ocular medications and/or their preservatives. This clinical problem, which is commonly encountered and frequently unrecognized, can begin as a diffuse punctate keratopathy. Nonhealing pseudogeographic defects may result that can be misinterpreted as a worsening of the underlying disease and thus may lead to still heavier doses of the offending medication. Not infrequently, topical anesthetic abuse has been implicated. Frank ulceration can result as sterile inflammation ensues.

CLINICAL PRESENTATION. Persistent corneal epithelial defects are characterized by central or paracentral areas of chronic nonhealing epithelium that resist maximal therapeutic endeavors. They frequently have elevated, rounded edges and may be associated with significant underlying stromal inflammation. Corneal anesthesia is frequently an accompanying sign, and it should always be evaluated. Left untreated, this condition can progress to vascularization and corneal opacification or scarring. Alternatively, progressive inflammation can lead to necrosis and thinning of the stroma, occasionally resulting in perforation.

LABORATORY EVALUATION. The diagnosis is based upon careful history taking, paying particular attention to the preservatives present in any ophthalmic medications being administered. These lesions are frequently round and oval epithelial defects with grayish edges that are rolled under without heaped margins. The defects tend to be inferior or inferonasal and can be associated with an intense, coarse superficial keratitis. The inferonasal predilection of these lesions may be a result of the area's easy access and the protective effect of Bell's phenomenon on the superior cornea. Keratoconjunctivitis sicca is a frequently accompanying disease. Other associated conditions include corneal hypoethesia as a result of previous cataract extraction or keratoplasty and prior herpes zoster or herpes simplex infections.

MANAGEMENT. Aside from removing the offending stimulus or aggravating drugs or treating the underlying condition, a number of strategies have been employed in the treatment of persistent epithelial defects. Pharmacologic therapies have included systemic tetracycline, which has been used for its anticollagenolytic effect, unrelated to the drug's antimicrobial properties. Topical fibronectin, a plasma and extracellular matrix glycoprotein that functions as a cellular attachment factor, has been reported in preliminary clinical trials to facilitate epithelial healing. However, a multicentered, prospective, randomized clinical trial failed to show that this therapy had a significantly positive effect when compared with nonpreserved artificial tears and the elimination of any potentially offending medications.

Other therapies, including use of recombinant epidermal growth factor (EGF), have met with some success. Generally, conventional therapies can be effective in promoting a closure of the epithelial defect. These include the frequent lubrication with nonpreserved ointments and, if necessary, temporary tarsorrhaphy or permanent lateral canthoplasty to encourage the epithelial migration and minimize mechanical trauma from exposure and desiccation.

Persistent epithelial defects often occur in patients with diabetic retinopathy following epithelial debridement during vitreoretinal procedures. In addition to diabetic neuropathy potentially resulting in neurotrophic keratopathy and nonhealing epithelial defects, abnormal metabolism of aldose reductase has been implicated in the pathogenesis of persistent epithelial defects in these patients. A clinical trial is currently investigating the efficacy of a topical aldose reductase inhibitor for persistent epithelial defects in patients with diabetes.

For more extensive insults, such as alkali injuries or other causes of devastating ocular surface trauma, damage to limbal stem cells cannot be overcome by conventional conservative therapies. Various strategies using healthy conjunctiva or limbal stem cells have been employed in ocular surface reconstruction with success. (Limbal stem-cell dysfunction is discussed at the end of this chapter; surgery of the ocular surface is covered in chapters XXI–XXIII.)

Cavanagh HD, Pihlaja D, Thoft RA, et al. The pathogenesis and treatment of persistent epithelial defects. *Trans Am Acad Ophthalmol Otolaryngol.* 1976;81:754–769.

Phan TM, Foster CS, Boruchoff SA, et al. Topical fibronectin in the treatment of persistent corneal epithelial defects and trophic ulcers. *Am J Ophthalmol.* 1987;104:494–501.

Trichiasis and Distichiasis

Trichiasis refers to an acquired condition in which lashes emerging from their normal anterior origin are curved backward toward the cornea. Most cases are probably the result of subtle cicatricial entropion of the eyelid margin. Trichiasis can be idiopathic or secondary to chronic inflammatory conditions such as trachoma, ocular cicatricial pemphigoid, Stevens-Johnson syndrome, blepharitis, or chemical burns.

Distichiasis is a congenital (often autosomal dominant) or acquired condition in which an extra row of lashes is seen emerging from the ducts of meibomian glands. These lashes can be fine and well tolerated or coarser and a threat to corneal integrity. Chronic inflammatory conditions of the eyelids and conjunctiva and trauma are frequent causes of the acquired type of distichiasis.

Careful clinical examination for abnormalities of the lashes, eyelids, and ocular surface is mandatory. Aberrant lashes and poor eyelid position and movement should be corrected. Aberrant lashes may be removed by epilation, electrolysis, or cryotherapy. Epilation is temporary because the lashes will normally regrow within 2–3 weeks. Electrolysis works well only for removing a few lashes, although it can be preferred for cosmetic reasons in younger patients. Cryotherapy is still a common treatment for aberrant eyelashes, but freezing can result in eyelid margin thinning, loss of adjacent normal lashes, and persistent lanugo hairs that may continue to abrade the cornea. Treatment at −20°C should be limited to less than 30 seconds to minimize complications. The preferred surgical technique for aberrant eyelashes is a tarsotomy with eyelid margin rotation.

Factitious Conjunctivitis

Factitious disorders include a spectrum of self-induced injuries with symptoms or physical findings intentionally produced by the patient in order to assume the sick role. Factitious conjunctivitis usually shows evidence of mechanical injury to the inferior and nasal quadrants of the cornea and conjunctiva. The areas of involvement show sharply delineated borders: linear or square. Patients often have medical training or work in a medical setting, and they generally show an attitude of serene indifference. The detached conjunctival tissues usually show no evidence of inflammation by pathologic examination. Other types of noncorneal factitious ocular disorders include self-induced solar retinopathy, eyelid ulceration, and anisocoria.

Mucus fishing syndrome This condition is typified by a well-circumscribed pattern of rose bengal staining on the nasal and inferior bulbar conjunctiva. All patients have a history of increased mucus production as a nonspecific response to ocular surface damage. The inciting event is typically keratoconjunctivitis sicca. However, allergic conjunctivitis, atopic conjunctivitis, corneal foreign body, and conjunctival squamous carcinoma have all been found. Patients usually demonstrate vigorous eye rubbing and compulsive removal of the mucus strands from the fornix (mucus fishing). The epithelial injury created by mucus fishing heightens the ocular surface irritation, which results in further mucus production, creating a vicious cycle. The nasal and inferior bulbar conjunctiva are the most frequently involved, as these seem to be the most accessible areas.

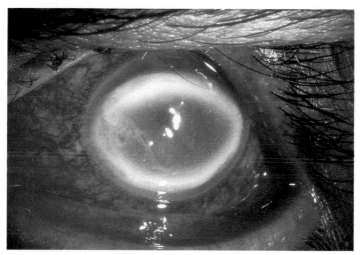

FIG VI-16—Topical anesthetic overuse with persistent corneal epithelial defect and necrotic ring opacity.

Topical anesthetic abuse   Clinical application of topical anesthetics has become an integral part of the modern practice of ophthalmology. However, indiscriminate use of topical anesthetics can cause serious ocular toxicities and complications. Local anesthetics are known to inhibit epithelial migration and division. Loss of microvilli, reduction of desmosomes and other intercellular contacts, and swelling of mitochondria and lysosomes have been reported by ultrastructure studies. The clinical features of anesthetic abuse are characterized by the failure of the presenting conditions, such as corneal abrasions or infectious keratitis, to respond to appropriate therapy.

Initially a punctate keratopathy is seen. As the abuse continues, the eye becomes more injected and epithelial defects appear or transform to a neurotrophic-like appearance. As the process perpetuates, keratic precipitates and hypopyon can be observed, thus mimicking an infectious course. Diffuse stromal edema, dense stromal infiltrates, and a large ring opacity are common presenting signs (Fig VI-16). Stromal vascularization may take place in chronic abuse, and secondary infection may ensue. Because of the presence of corneal infiltrates and anterior segment inflammation, infectious keratitis must be ruled out with corneal scraping, culture, or biopsy.

Differential diagnosis includes bacterial, fungal, herpetic, and amoebic keratitis. Suspicion should be maintained in the face of negative cultures in any patient who is not responding to appropriate therapy. Many times the diagnosis is made only when the patient is discovered concealing the anesthetic drops. Once the diagnosis is made and infectious keratitis is ruled out, corneal healing usually occurs if all exposure to anesthetics is removed. In advanced cases permanent corneal scarring or perforation may occur. Occasionally, anesthetic abuse may continue after surgery. Psychiatric counseling is sometimes helpful.

Delle

Desiccation of the epithelium and subepithelial tissues occurs at or near the limbus adjacent to surface elevations such as those produced by pterygia or dermoids. The tear film is interrupted by these surface elevations, and normal blinking does not wet the involved area properly. Clinically, dellen are saucerlike depressions in the corneal surface. The epithelium exhibits punctate irregularities overlying a thinned area of dehydrated corneal stroma, resulting in depression of the surface. Treatment with frequent ocular lubrication or pressure patching will accelerate the healing process and restore stromal hydration.

The orbital and conjunctival tissues surrounding the sclera also play a role in maintaining scleral hydration. This function becomes especially evident during surgical procedures, when the conjunctiva and extraocular muscles are removed from the scleral surface. The exposed sclera becomes thinner and partially translucent unless it is continually remoistened. Removal of the perilimbal conjunctiva and interference with the wetting effect of the tear film (as after excision of a pterygium by the bare sclera technique) can cause the underlying sclera to become markedly thinned and translucent, forming a scleral delle.

Ocular Surface Problems Secondary to Contact Lens Wear

Metabolic epithelial damage   Contact lens overwear syndromes can be manifested in several forms. *Central epithelial edema* (Sattler's veil) is found after many hours of wear, more commonly with hard contact lenses. This epithelial edema creates blurred vision that may persist for many hours or even progress to acute epithelial necrosis. Although acute epithelial necrosis is rarely seen, central epithelial edema can create epithelial erosions or frank ulceration. Physiologic stress as a result of hypoxia with lactate accumulation and impaired carbon dioxide efflux is responsible for these complications.

Another condition that is caused by impaired metabolic activities in epithelium, *microcystic epitheliopathy* shows fine epithelial cysts best seen with retroillumination. These cysts are common, and they may be either asymptomatic or cause recurrent brief episodes of pain and epiphora.

Toxic conjunctivitis   Conjunctival injection, epithelial staining, punctate epithelial keratopathy, erosions, and microcysts are all potential signs of conjunctival or corneal toxicity from contact lens–wear solutions. Any of the proteolytic enzymes or chemicals used for cleaning contact lenses, or the preservative-containing soaking solution, can be the culprit. Cleaning agents such as benzalkonium chloride, chlorhexidine, hydrogen peroxide, and other substances used for chemical sterilization, if not properly removed from contact lenses, can cause an immediate, severe epitheliopathy with accompanying pain.

Allergic reactions   The preservative thimerosal can produce a delayed hypersensitivity response, resulting in conjunctivitis, keratitis with epithelial involvement, and even coarse epithelial and subepithelial opacities. Thimerosal may be also implicated in contact lens–induced superior limbic keratoconjunctivitis. The ocular signs of this disorder include injection of superior bulbar conjunctiva, epitheliopathy of cornea and conjunctiva, papillary conjunctivitis, and some superficial pannus (Fig VI-17). This condition has declined in prevalence, probably as a result of substitution of thimerosal with other preservatives in the contact lens solutions

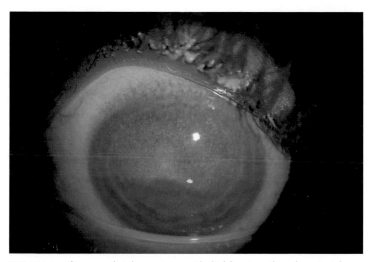

FIG VI-17—The superficial punctate epithelial keratopathy of contact lens–induced superior limbic keratoconjunctivitis often extends over the superior and middle thirds of the cornea.

Neovascularization Neovascular ingrowth into the peripheral cornea is common in soft contact lens wear. Less than 2 mm of such growth is believed to be acceptable, but once the neovascularization extends farther than 2 mm into the cornea, contact lens wear should be discontinued. Superficial pannus is rarely associated with hard or rigid gas-permeable (RGP) contact lens wear but is encountered more frequently in patients using soft lenses. This type of neovascularization is probably caused by hypoxia and chronic trauma to the limbus, which leads to the release of angiogenic mediators. Other causes of pannus such as staphylococcal or chlamydial keratoconjunctivitis should be considered in the presence of appropriate accompanying signs.

Deep stromal neovascularization has been associated with extended-wear contact lenses, especially in aphakia. This condition is not usually symptomatic unless there is associated circinate lipid deposition, *interstitial keratopathy*. Deep neovascularization of the cornea is often irreversible and is best managed by discontinuing contact lens wear and resorting to other alternatives such as secondary intraocular lens implantation.

Stapleton F, Dart J, Minassian D. Nonulcerative complications of contact lens wear. Relative risks for different lens types. *Arch Ophthalmol.* 1992;110:1601–1606.

Stein RM, Stein HA. Corneal complications of contact lenses. In: *Focal Points: Clinical Modules for Ophthalmologists.* San Francisco: American Academy of Ophthalmology; 1993;11:2.

Limbal Stem-Cell Dysfunction

PATHOGENESIS. Corneal epithelium can be regenerated efficiently by limbal epithelium. In the absence of limbal epithelium, as with a total corneal epithelial defect extending beyond the limbus, the denuded corneal surface can only be healed by the surrounding conjunctival epithelium. During this healing process, the fate of the migrating conjunctival epithelium is determined by the presence or absence of corneal vascularization. In the absence of vascularization, the healing conjunctival epithelium will undergo a process of morphologic and physiologic transformation into a cornea-like epithelium with the loss of goblet cells. This process is known as *conjunctival transdifferentiation.* In contrast, if corneal vascularization is present during the wound healing, the conjunctival characteristics are preserved in the healing epithelium, as shown by the persistence of goblet cells on the corneal surface. The absence of limbal stem cells reduces the effectiveness of epithelial wound healing, as evidenced by compromised ocular surface integrity with irregular ocular surface and recurrent epithelial breakdown.

CLINICAL PRESENTATION. Clinically, the conjunctivalization of the cornea can be observed in several ocular surface disorders (Table VI-7). Patients usually suffer from recurrent erosions and decreased vision as a result of irregular corneal surface. Corneal pannus is invariably present in the involved cornea. Increased epithelial permeability can be observed clinically by diffuse permeation of topical fluorescein into the anterior stroma. Related to either primary or secondary limbal stem-cell deficiency, the diseases listed in Table VI-6 are characterized by invasion of the corneal surface by conjunctival epithelium, disruption of epithelial basement membrane, corneal vascularization, and infiltration of inflammatory cells.

LABORATORY EVALUATION. Impression cytology of the involved corneal surface usually shows the presence of goblet cells and conjunctival epithelium. Aniridia might be accompanied by a deficiency in the development or maintenance of limbal stem cells associated with the absence of the iris and the abnormal angle structure of the anterior chamber. In multiple endocrine neoplasia (MEN IIb or MFN III) prominent perilimbal blood vessels are frequently observed in addition to prominent corneal nerves. Neuromas are common in mucosas such as conjunctiva or intestine. MEN

TABLE VI-7

OCULAR SURFACE DISORDERS CHARACTERIZED BY
THE ABSENCE (APLASIA) OF LIMBAL STEM CELLS

HEREDITARY	ACQUIRED
Aniridia (bilateral)	**Diffuse**
Keratitis associated with multiple endocrine deficiency (bilateral)	Stevens-Johnson syndrome (bilateral)
	Chemical injuries (unilateral/bilateral)
	Contact lens–induced keratopathy (unilateral/bilateral)
	Focal
	Pterygium

IIb is thought to originate as a genetic defect leading to abnormalities in tissues of neural crest origin, including the limbus.

In chemical burns or some cases of Stevens-Johnson syndrome the limbal stem-cell deficiency is caused by severe trauma or intense inflammation. The extent of limbal destruction and associated limbal ischemia is an important prognostic factor in determining the clinical outcome. The contact lens–induced keratopathy is a rare occurrence compared to other types of lens-related complications. The fact that it is associated more with soft lenses suggests that limbal stem cells might be more susceptible to such insults as constant mechanical trauma, hypoxia, or toxicity of lens care solution. In pterygium conjunctival invasion may be caused by focal disruption of the limbal barrier by ultraviolet phototoxicity in the interpalpebral exposure zone of bulbar conjunctiva.

MANAGEMENT. For diseases associated with limbal stem-cell deficiency, replacement of stem cells by limbal transplantation seems to the logical choice for ocular surface reconstruction. When the limbus is focally affected in one eye, as with a pterygium, a healthy limbal or conjunctival autograft can be obtained from the ipsilateral eye. For unilateral moderate or severe chemical injuries, a limbal autograft can be obtained from the healthy fellow eye. For bilateral limbal deficiency, as with Stevens-Johnson syndrome or bilateral chemical burns, limbal allograft from a living relative or eye bank donor eye can be considered. Dramatic restoration of the ocular surface with limbal reconstruction has been reported in selected cases with desperate clinical situations. (See the discussion of ocular surface surgery in chapters XXI–XXII.)

PART 3

INFECTIOUS DISEASES OF THE EYELID, CONJUNCTIVA, CORNEA, AND SCLERA

CHAPTER VII

Basic Concepts of Ocular Infection

Defense Mechanisms of the Outer Eye

The surface of the eye is exposed to a hostile environment. An array of anatomic adaptations and immunologic defenses have evolved to protect the human eye from physical trauma, noxious stimuli, and microorganisms, while also maintaining the integrity of an optical interface. Chapter IX, Ocular Immunity, discusses the immunologic aspect of these defenses in depth.

Orbit, Eyelids, and Tear Film

The bony orbital rim protects the globe from blunt trauma delivered by large objects, while the elastic properties of the globe and the cushioning ability of the orbital fat help diffuse the impact of a direct compressive blow. The eyelids serve as a specialized, retractable skin covering, providing physical protection during sleep, reflexive blink closure in response to noxious stimuli, and periodic rewetting and pumping of the tear layer.

Part 2 has also discussed the role of the tear film in combating ocular surface disorders. The tear film provides a measure of physical defense by flushing away and diluting microbes, toxins, and allergens. In addition, a number of soluble macromolecules in the tear film exert antimicrobial properties. Lactoferrin binds free iron ions, which are essential for the function of enzymes involved in bacterial metabolism. Lysozyme, which degrades the mucopeptides of bacterial cell walls, works in concert with β-lysin, which disrupts the integrity of bacterial plasma membranes. Immunoglobulins (predominantly secretory IgA) and complement components in the tear film mediate antigen-specific humoral immunity. Immediately overlying the epithelial microvilli is a layer of mucin, which inhibits the ability of many pathogens to attach to the corneal epithelium. BCSC Section 2, *Fundamentals and Principles of Ophthalmology,* discusses the biochemistry and metabolism of the tear film (and cornea) in detail.

Conjunctiva and Cornea

The epithelium of the cornea and conjunctiva guards against microbial invasion. The stratified cell layers of the epithelium are tightly adherent to each other and to the underlying basement membrane, forming a substantial physical barrier against the penetration of noxious agents and the invasion of pathogens. If disrupted, the epithelium rapidly heals, thus protecting the vulnerable underlying stroma from prolonged exposure. In the human cornea, the condensed collagen that forms Bowman's layer forms an additional barrier to the entry of microbes.

Besides acting as a physical barrier, the epithelium can also resist bacteria through phagocytosis, trapping and digesting bacteria within intracellular phagosomes. Cytokine-stimulated epithelial cells can facilitate humoral immunity and delayed (Type IV) hypersensitivity by presenting endocytosed antigen to CD4+ (T-helper) lymphocytes (see chapter IX). The rapid cycling of the corneal epithelium creates periodic sloughing of the surface squamous cells, a process that may aid in the removal of microbes that have attached to or invaded the superficial cell layer. In response to direct viral invasion or a variety of inflammatory mediators, corneal and conjunctival epithelium secretes interleukin-1 and other inflammatory cytokines. These cytokines can further boost the localized immune response through the enhancement of immune-cell migration, adhesion, and activation. BCSC Section 9, *Intraocular Inflammation and Uveitis,* discusses the immune response in depth.

The vascular and lymphatic channels of the conjunctiva form afferent and efferent conduits for humoral and cellular immune components. During bouts of infection, the flow through these channels is augmented by the action of inflammatory mediators that promote vascular dilation, permeability, and diapedesis. Inflammatory cells that participate in the immune response include circulating cells that are recruited into tissues during active inflammation and native inflammatory cells that reside in uninflamed tissue. The conjunctival epithelium and substantia propria contain lymphocytes, plasma cells, mast cells, Langerhans' cells, and polymorphonuclear leukocytes. Aggregates of lymphocytes and other immune cells are found within the substantia propria in the form of conjunctiva-associated lymphoid tissue, a loosely demarcated structure analogous to Peyer patches of the gut.

The cornea is devoid of immune cells, except for a few lymphocytes and Langerhans' cells. These dendritic cells reside in the epithelium and peripheral corneal stroma and present antigen to CD4+ T cells. Many cells of the cornea, including epithelial cells, stromal keratocytes, and endothelial cells, are capable of secreting interleukins and other pro-inflammatory cytokines that can stimulate and potentiate the inflammatory cascade. During active inflammation, lymphocytes and neutrophils are recruited into the cornea from the tear film, the limbal vascular arcades, and the anterior chamber.

The Normal Ocular Flora

Colonization of the eyelids and the conjunctiva by normal microbial flora contributes to the defense of the ocular surface. Indigenous bacterial flora inhibit the establishment of foreign, potentially pathogenic bacteria by elaborating antibacterial substances and by competing for space and nutrients. The predominant isolates recovered from the eyelids and conjunctiva are *Staphylococcus epidermidis, Staphylococcus aureus, Corynebacterium* spp, and *Propionibacterium acnes* (Table VII-1). The topical use of antimicrobials, local immunosuppression caused by topical corticosteroids, or the presence of ocular surface diseases can alter the normal resident flora and promote the growth of strains with increased antimicrobial resistance or pathogenicity.

Osato MS. Normal ocular flora. In: Pepose JS, Holland GN, Wilhelmus KR, eds. *Ocular Infection and Immunity.* St Louis: Mosby; 1996:191–199.

TABLE VII-1

RELATIVE PREVALENCE OF THE NORMAL FLORA OF THE OUTER EYE

MICROORGANISMS	NORMAL CONJUNCTIVA	NORMAL EYELID MARGIN
Staphylococcus epidermidis	+ + +	+ + +
Staphylococcus aureus	+ +	+ +
Micrococcus spp	+	+ +
Corynebacterium spp (diphtheroids)	+ +	+ +
Propionibacterium acnes	+ +	+ +
Streptococcus spp*	+	±
*Haemophilus influenzae**	±	–
Moraxella spp	±	–
Enteric gram-negative bacilli	±	–
Bacillus spp	±	–
Anaerobic bacteria	+	±
Yeasts (*Malassezia furfur, Candida* spp, etc)	–	+
Filamentous fungi	±	–
Demodex spp	–	+ +

*More common in children.

Pathogenesis of Ocular Infections

The establishment and severity of infection are influenced by the interplay between the following factors:

- Virulence of the pathogen
- Size and route of the inoculum
- Presence or absence of risk factors that compromise host defenses
- Nature of the host's immune and inflammatory response

Virulence Factors

Successful infection of ocular surface tissues requires the microorganism to attach, penetrate, invade, persist, and replicate in the face of many protective mechanisms in the host. Virulence factors are microbial evolutionary adaptations that help the organism carry out one or more of these steps, usually increasing the likelihood and severity of the infection. Virulence factors are as varied and numerous as the types of pathogens that can cause ocular infectious disease.

Attachment   Examples of virulence factors that enhance adherence to the epithelium include herpes simplex virus glycoprotein C, which binds to heparan sulfate of the cell surface; the pili of *Pseudomonas aeruginosa,* which bind to epithelial glycoproteins; and candidal proteins, which mimic mammalian integrins (transmembrane proteins that mediate adhesive cell-cell and cell-matrix interactions).

Penetration Another key step in the pathogenesis of infection is penetration. The intact epithelial layer presents a formidable barrier that few pathogens can overcome. The ability to directly penetrate intact epithelium is limited to a minority of bacterial species, such as *Neisseria gonorrhoeae*. Other pathogens, including *P aeruginosa*, require disruption of the epithelium for adherence and penetration. Experimental evidence suggests that large inocula of bacteria placed on an intact conjunctival or corneal surface rarely result in infection, whereas mechanical disruption of the ocular surface predisposes to infection with small inocula.

Invasion Virulence factors that facilitate tissue invasion include microbial exotoxins and proteases that destroy tissue cells, inflammatory cells, and tissue matrix. Exotoxins important in the pathogenesis of bacterial infections include those elaborated by certain strains of streptococci, staphylococci, and *P aeruginosa*. These enzymes can lead to localized cell death and in some cases cause systemic effects.

Proteases include streptolysin, produced by *Streptococcus pyogenes*, and collagenases secreted by *Acanthamoeba* spp and certain fungi. *Pseudomonas* elastase and alkaline protease not only destroy collagen and proteoglycan components of the cornea but can also affect host immunity by degrading immunoglobulins, complement, interleukins, and other inflammatory cytokines. Endotoxin, the lipopolysaccharide cell-wall component of gram-negative bacteria, is liberated upon death of the microorganism and elicits a severe inflammatory response.

Persistence and replication A number of virulence factors facilitate persistence and evasion of host defense mechanisms. Herpes simplex virus and varicella-zoster virus enter a latent phase in infected trigeminal ganglion cells. Reactivation, which can occur in response to fever, trauma, or ultraviolet radiation, can stimulate the virus to enter a lytic, disease-associated phase. Chlamydia are able to survive within intracellular phagosomes, protected from circulating antibodies and immune cells. The polysaccharide capsules of streptococci, *Haemophilus*, and *Neisseria* inhibit phagocytosis. Proteases released by certain strains of *P aeruginosa*, *Neisseria* spp, and *Haemophilus* spp can cleave and inactivate immunoglobulins and other immune factors.

A number of bacterial species can secrete a protective, extracellular polysaccharide glycocalyx that can encase and shield a bacterial colony, creating a biofilm that is resistant to immune clearance and antimicrobial drug effects. Biofilm formation is believed to play an important role in the pathogenesis of contact lens–associated keratitis and infectious crystalline keratopathy.

Inoculum Size and Route

Organisms differ in their infective ability. For example, experimental bacterial keratitis can be established with *P aeruginosa* using an inoculum size that is several orders of magnitude smaller than that required with *S aureus*. For a given microorganism, however, the larger the inoculum, the greater the likelihood of infection. The capability of the host's defenses determines the threshold of inoculum size at which infection is inevitable.

The route of infection is an important factor in the pathogenesis of infection. The most common route of entry is a break in the epithelium. Microorganisms that enter along a transepithelial route can originate from the eyelids or the nasolacrimal duct or from the environment through trauma, surgery, contact lens wear, or exposure to foreign matter or fluids. Uncommonly, contiguous infection of the ocular surface can occur from superficial spread of a primary orbital or intraocular infection to the sclera or by lateral spread from the conjunctiva to the cornea. The least common mechanism of transmission of infection to the ocular surface involves the hematogenous or lymphatic route.

Host Risk Factors

Risk factors are mechanisms that increase the host's likelihood of infection.

Microbial transmission   The transmission of communicable infections is enhanced by behaviors or circumstances that facilitate the exposure to the pathogen. The risk of contiguously spread infections of the ocular surface and adnexa is increased in the presence of severe and/or chronic infection in adjacent tissues, such as the sinuses, eyelids, or orbit. Epidemic adenovirus conjunctivitis, which develops after exogenous contact with infected secretions, can be spread by eye-to-hand contact or by intermediary contact with a contaminated surface, or fomite, such as a tonometer tip. Sexually transmitted ocular infections such as gonococcal conjunctivitis and chlamydial conjunctivitis are spread through ocular contact with infected genital secretions during sexual activity or, in the case of neonatal infections, during passage through the birth canal. Zoonotic infections such as cat-scratch disease or Lyme disease are transmitted by contact with an infected animal host or vector.

Bacteria, fungi, and protozoa that can exist in a free-living state in the soil or water can cause opportunistic ocular infections. These infections are often difficult to eradicate because of natural defenses that have evolved to help the pathogen withstand harsh environmental conditions. Exposure to these environmental pathogens may occur by a variety of means, including use of chemically disinfected but not fully sterilized surgical instruments *(Mycobacterium chelonae)*, exposure to homemade saline or freshwater *(Acanthamoeba)*, and trauma involving soil or vegetable matter (various fungi).

Compromised physical defenses   Disruption of the eye's physical defenses can occur by several mechanisms. Lagophthalmos or keratoconjunctivitis sicca can lead to desiccation of the tear film. Microtrauma to the epithelium can occur from trichiasis, contact lens wear, use of an ocular prosthesis, or exposure to a surgical suture. A traumatic abrasion or retained foreign body can predispose the ocular surface to infection. Chronic exposure caused by lagophthalmos or ectropion and decreased blink reflex caused by neurotrophic or neuroparalytic processes can also compromise physical defenses.

Compromised immunity   Local or systemic immunocompromise predisposes to ocular infection. The use of topical corticosteroids is frequently a contributing factor in the pathogenesis of postoperative infections. Preexisting corneal or conjunctival pathology may cause structural and functional alterations that affect normal tissue responses to injury, inflammation, or infection. The propensity for development of ocular infection also increases with systemic immunocompromise in hosts with naturally depressed immune function (e.g., neonates) or acquired immunodeficiency (e.g., AIDS patients, patients on systemic immunosuppression regimens, and patients with debilitating chronic illnesses).

O'Brien TP, Hazlett LD. Pathogenesis of ocular infection. In: Pepose JS, Holland GN, Wilhelmus KR, eds. *Ocular Infection and Immunity.* St Louis: Mosby; 1996:200–214.

Ocular Microbiology

The microbial flora of the normal eyelids and conjunctiva is similar to that of the skin and the upper respiratory tract. Occasionally, gastrointestinal flora are found, and airborne contaminants can be transiently recovered. Asymptomatic shedding of viruses, such as herpes simplex virus, can occur intermittently. Postmortem, the microorganisms that normally colonize the ocular surface can proliferate, and an increased diversity of species is sometimes found. Of the many potentially pathogenic microorganisms capable of causing infectious eye disease, those encountered most often are listed in Table VII-2.

Virology

Human viruses contain a single- or double-stranded nucleic acid surrounded by an isometric or tubular protein capsid. Some viruses (such as adenovirus and enterovirus) are naked nucleocapsids, whereas others (such as herpes simplex virus and human immunodeficiency virus) are enclosed within a lipoprotein envelope.

DNA viruses *Herpes simplex virus.* Human herpesviruses that affect the eye include herpes simplex virus (HSV) types 1 and 2, varicella-zoster virus, Epstein-Barr virus, cytomegalovirus, and human herpes virus 8. Neurotropic viruses include HSV types 1 and 2 and varicella-zoster. Herpes simplex virus contains double-stranded DNA in an icosahedral capsid within a lipid envelope. Of the two HSV serotypes, type 1 causes the majority of HSV eye infections. After initial exposure HSV may cause a subclinical infection or an overt primary disease. Transport to the trigeminal ganglion results in latency. Reactivation with asymptomatic viral shedding may subsequently occur, possibly leading to recurrent ocular disease.

HSV blepharitis and conjunctivitis, with or without punctate epithelial keratitis, are occasionally manifestations of primary infection, but they may also be signs of recurrent disease. Recurrent HSV epithelial keratitis typically forms a dendrite that can progress to geographic epithelial keratitis, particularly if the patient has been inappropriately treated with corticosteroids (Fig VII-1).

Stromal keratitis and iridocyclitis may either follow epithelial keratitis or appear as the first apparent ocular involvement. Possibly related to an inflammatory or an immunogenic response to intrastromal and/or intraocular viral antigens, stromal inflammation can take on various manifestations ranging from disciform keratitis to necrotizing keratitis. It can be associated with iridocyclitis, frequently called *stromal keratouveitis.* Other manifestations include trabeculitis and endotheliitis.

Demonstration of HSV is possible during epidermal or epithelial infection using antigen- or DNA-detection methods or culture isolation. Laboratory testing is not available to prove the etiology of herpes simplex stromal keratitis. Serologic tests for neutralizing or complement-fixing immunoglobulins can be used to show a rising antibody titer during primary infection. Antibody titers do not show diagnostic

TABLE VII-2

PRINCIPAL CAUSES OF OCULAR INFECTIONS

CONDITION	VIRUSES	BACTERIA	FUNGI	PARASITES
Dermatoblepharitis	Herpes simplex	Staphylococcus aureus		
	Varicella-zoster	Streptococcus spp		
Blepharitis	Herpes simplex Molluscum contagiosum	Staphylococcus spp Moraxella spp		Phthirus pubis
Conjunctivitis	Adenovirus	Chlamydia trachomatis		
	Herpes simplex	Staphylococcus aureus Steptococcus spp Neisseria gonorrhoeae Haemophilus influenzae Moraxella spp		
Keratitis	Herpes simplex	Pseudomonas aeruginosa Staphylococcus aureus Staphylococcus epidermidis Streptococcus pneumoniae Moraxella spp	Fusarium spp Aspergillus spp Candida albicans	Acanthamoeba spp
Dacryoadenitis	Epstein-Barr virus Mumps	Staphylococcus aureus Streptococcus pneumoniae		
Canaliculitis		Actinomycetes		
Dacryocystitis		Staphylococcus spp Streptococcus spp		

changes during recurrent episodes but can confirm prior exposure. However, since the vast majority of adults have had prior HSV exposure and are thus antibody positive, serologic testing is generally helpful only if it yields a negative result.

> Parrish CM. Herpes simplex virus eye disease. In: *Focal Points: Clinical Modules for Ophthalmologists.* San Francisco: American Academy of Ophthalmology; 1997;15:2.

Varicella-zoster virus. Varicella-zoster virus (VZV) is an enveloped DNA virus that looks identical to herpes simplex virus by electron microscopy. As with other herpesviruses, infection involves a primary infection (varicella) with subsequent latency, which is sometimes followed by recurrent disease (zoster) many years later. Except for an eyelid skin rash and mild conjunctivitis during chickenpox, ocular

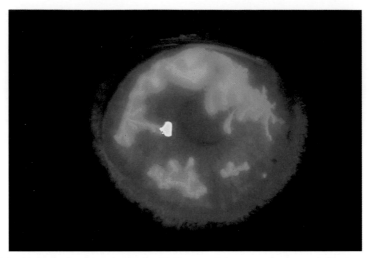

FIG VII-1—Multiple dendrites (stained with fluorescein) occurred when a follicular conjunctivitis was misdiagnosed as adenovirus and treated with topical corticosteroid. (Reproduced with permission from Parrish CM. Herpes simplex virus eye disease. In: *Focal Points: Clinical Modules for Ophthalmologists.* San Francisco: American Academy of Ophthalmology; 1997;15:2.)

involvement is uncommon during primary infection. Approximately 20% of affected individuals subsequently develop zoster, often in later life.

Of all cases with zoster dermatitis, 15% involve the ophthalmic division of cranial nerve V (trigeminal) to cause herpes zoster ophthalmicus. Common ocular complications of trigeminal zoster are epithelial keratitis, marginal corneal infiltrates, stromal keratitis, and neurotrophic keratopathy. Laboratory demonstration of acute VZV infection is possible by immunodiagnostic methods, viral culture, and serologic testing.

Epstein-Barr virus. Interpersonal spread of Epstein-Barr virus (EBV) is common and can result in infectious mononucleosis. The virus remains latent in B lymphocytes and mucosal epithelial cells throughout life, and ocular disease is uncommon. Because of difficulties in culture isolation, diagnosis depends on the detection of various antibodies to viral components. During acute infection, IgM and IgG antibodies to viral capsid antigens appear, and IgG may persist at a low level. Antibodies to early antigens also rise during the acute phases of the disease and subsequently decrease to low or undetectable levels in most individuals. Antibodies to EBV nuclear antigens appear weeks to months later, providing serologic evidence of past infection.

Cytomegalovirus. Cytomegalovirus (CMV) usually produces subclinical infection except in immunocompromised hosts. In acquired immunodeficiency syndrome (AIDS) CMV retinitis becomes more likely as the CD4+ lymphocyte level falls to levels below 50/μl.

Human herpes virus 8 (HHV8). Kaposi sarcoma, the most frequent malignancy in AIDS patients, is caused by HHV8. Its mode of transmission and management are under investigation.

Adenovirus. Each adenovirus (ADV) is a nonenveloped virion composed of double-stranded DNA and two types of capsomers, one of which elicits a type-specific antibody. Serotypes 3, 4, 7, 8, 19, 37, and several others can cause acute conjunctivitis, with or without upper respiratory tract involvement. Some serotypes appear more likely to produce punctate epithelial keratitis and subepithelial infiltrates, often referred to as *epidemic keratoconjunctivitis* (EKC). ADV can be demonstrated by immunodiagnostic methods, culture isolation, and a rise in antibody titer.

Poxviruses. Now that smallpox (variola) is nearly extinct, vaccinia keratitis is relegated to a historical curiosity. Another poxvirus that causes eye disease is molluscum contagiosum, an obligate human virus that produces an umbilicated, wartlike lesion of the eyelid skin as a result of intradermal viral proliferation. Incomplete virogenesis in conjunctival epithelial cells can produce a toxic follicular reaction. Histopathologic examination of an expressed or excised nodule shows eosinophilic, intracytoplasmic inclusions (Henderson-Patterson bodies) within epidermal cells.

Papovaviruses. Human papillomaviruses (HPV) cause warts (verrucae) and have been implicated in mucocutaneous neoplasia. Certain serotypes (including 6, 11, and 16) have been found in association with conjunctival tumors ranging from benign papillomas to squamous dysplasia and carcinoma. Whether HPV initiates epithelial metaplasia or acts in concert with ultraviolet light or another cofactor remains to be determined.

RNA viruses   *Picornaviruses.* These nonenveloped viruses include *rhinoviruses* and *enteroviruses.* Enterovirus type 70 and coxsackievirus type A24 are enteroviruses that cause acute hemorrhagic conjunctivitis.

Orthomyxoviruses and paramyxoviruses. Influenza and parainfluenza viruses are orthomyxoviruses, single-stranded RNA viruses that cause respiratory infection, sometimes with mild conjunctivitis. Paramyxoviruses of ocular importance include those causing mumps, measles, and Newcastle disease.

Like other paramyxoviruses, the *mumps virus* has an outer lipid envelope containing a hemolysin that mediates viral fusion with the host cell membrane and hemagglutinin-neuraminidase protein spikes. Epidemic spread is limited by widespread vaccination. Besides parotitis, mumps can cause dacryoadenitis, conjunctivitis, and, less commonly, stromal keratitis and episcleritis. Serologic tests are limited by cross-reactivity with related viruses, but high or rising titers can indicate recent infection.

The *measles (rubeola) virus* often causes a mild conjunctivitis with punctate epithelial keratitis that is self-limited in affected patients. Severe cases of measles keratitis can produce stromal keratitis with subsequent vascularization (interstitial keratitis). Malnourished children with vitamin A deficiency appear susceptible to progressive keratomalacia with corneal perforation.

Usually a disease of chickens, the *Newcastle disease virus* can cause a follicular conjunctivitis in people likely to be exposed, such as veterinarians and poultry handlers.

Retroviruses. The most important retrovirus is *human immunodeficiency virus type 1 (HIV-1),* the etiologic agent of AIDS. HIV contains double-stranded RNA in a protein core with an outer envelope. The virus enters through mucosa or directly into the circulation, resulting in a viremia that seeds multiple lymph nodes and produces generalized lymphadenopathy. Humoral and cellular responses ensue. Circulating antibodies are detected by enzyme immunoassays that are then confirmed by two-dimensional electrophoresis with immunoblotting (Western blot testing).

In infected cells, including cells of the conjunctiva, cornea, and retina, viral reverse transcriptase translates viral RNA into DNA that is incorporated into the cell genome. Infected patients remain asymptomatic for several years, but CD4+ T lymphocytes are progressively depleted by immunopathogenic mechanisms. Kaposi sarcoma, HIV-directed neurologic disease, and autoimmune disorders such as dry eye syndrome can occur before severe immunosuppression has taken place. When the CD4+ T-cell count falls below a critical level, opportunistic diseases become more likely.

The current AIDS surveillance case definition includes all HIV-infected persons whose CD4+ T-lymphocyte count is <200/µl (or <14% total lymphocytes) or who have an indicator condition such as CMV retinitis or toxoplasmosis of the central nervous system. Associated or opportunistic infections that affect the eye include CMV retinopathy, ophthalmic zoster, syphilitic uveitis, toxoplasmic retinochoroiditis, microsporidial keratoconjunctivitis, cryptococcal optic neuritis, pneumocystis choroiditis, and Kaposi sarcoma of the conjunctiva or orbit.

Anti–HIV antibody testing by ELISA, with confirmation by Western blot, is used for diagnostic screening. The following tests can provide quantitative markers to assess viral burden and to monitor antiretroviral therapy in patients with a low CD4+ count:

- HIV-1 p24 antigen (both free and immune-complexed)
- Proviral DNA and viral RNA amplified by polymerase chain reaction (PCR)
- Viral isolation from plasma and from peripheral blood mononuclear cells

Bacteriology

Bacteria are prokaryotes whose DNA is dispersed in the cytoplasm and in plasmids rather than confined within a membrane-bound nucleus. A rigid cell wall is responsible for the shape and gram reaction of bacteria. Classification is based on morphology, biochemical reactions, DNA composition, and other tests. The discussion below groups bacteria according to the following categories:

- Chlamydia and rickettsia
- Gram-negative cocci
- Gram-negative rods
- Gram-positive cocci
- Gram-positive filaments
- Spirochetes

Chlamydia and rickettsia   *Chlamydia trachomatis.* This bacterium lacks respiratory enzymes and is an intracellular parasite with an affinity for mucosal epithelium. The developmental cycle evolves from an elementary body that is taken up into a mucosal epithelial cell. Chlamydial DNA reorganization produces reticulate bodies within an endosomal vacuole. The organisms multiply, then form an inclusion body containing elementary bodies. Related species are *C pneumoniae* and *C psittaci.*

C trachomatis is classified by the major outer membrane protein antigens. Serotypes A through C are epidemiologically associated with trachoma, and types E through K cause genital infection and keratoconjunctivitis in sexually active adults and in neonates. The pattern of disease relates to the mode of spread and the occurrence of sequential infections.

Intracytoplasmic inclusions are visible by light microscopy. Extracellular elementary bodies are detectable by immunofluorescence. *C trachomatis* can be demonstrated by several immunodiagnostic methods and by culture isolation using McCoy or other cells. Serologic testing can be unreliable because of prior exposure. Certain serotypes have been associated with lymphogranuloma venereum and Reiter syndrome.

Rickettsia. Bartonella henselae and, less often, *Afipia felis* are causes of cat-scratch disease. Both domesticated and feral cats frequently harbor *Bartonella* on an endemic basis. Biopsy material from granulomatous conjunctivitis can show these small pleomorphic organisms with special stains, but culture isolation is often not possible.

Gram-negative cocci   *Neisseria species*. The family Neisseriaceae includes both *Moraxella* and *Acinetobacter*, which are discussed below, as well as *Neisseria. N gonorrhoeae* can cause acute purulent conjunctivitis in newborns and adults and can apparently adhere to and penetrate intact corneal epithelium to produce acute corneal suppuration and ulceration. *N meningitidis* can cause ocular infection without meningitis. On smears of ocular specimens, neisserial organisms typically appear as gram-negative diplococci with a characteristic kidney bean shape. They are usually identified not only extracellularly but also within neutrophils (Fig VII-2).

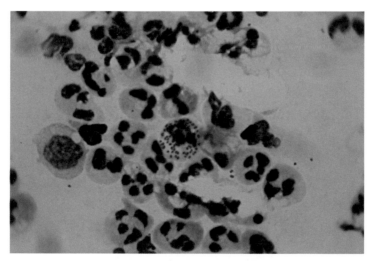

FIG VII-2—Gram-negative cocci (*Neisseria gonorrhoeae*, Gram ×1000).

These strict aerobes have complex growth requirements. While culture is possible on blood agar, optimal isolation is achieved with chocolate agar or similar media incubated under 5%–10% CO_2 with adequate humidity. Species identification is based on differential carbohydrate (e.g., dextrose, maltose, and sucrose) fermentation.

Gram-negative rods   *Moraxella species. Moraxella* can vary from coccobacilli to large dumbbell-shaped diplobacilli arranged in boxcarlike chains. Common ocular isolates include *M lacunata* (formerly *M liquefaciens), M nonliquefaciens,* and *M catarrhalis* (formerly *Branhamella).* On the eyelid margin or conjunctiva *Moraxella* may produce an exoenzyme that contributes to excoriation of the mucocutaneous junction. A chronically damaged corneal epithelial surface is susceptible to adherence and colonization by *Moraxella* species that can lead to stromal infection.

Acinetobacter species. In contrast to *Neisseria* and *Moraxella* species, these pleomorphic gram-negative bacteria are oxidase-negative. *Acinetobacter* species are infrequently encountered as a cause of bacterial conjunctivitis or keratitis.

Pseudomonas species. The family Pseudomonadaceae includes *Pseudomonas aeruginosa* (Fig VII-3) and many other species (e.g., *P fluorescens, P cepacia).* These slender rods with polar flagella are common contaminants of many aqueous solutions and grow on most common microbiological media. *Stenotrophomonas maltophilia* is a related organism that is occasionally a cause of ocular infection.

Azotobacter species. The family Azotobacteraceae includes *Azotobacter* and *Azomonas* species, but these are uncommon causes of corneal infection.

Enterobacteriaceae. This family includes multiple genera of enteric gram-negative rods such as *Escherichia coli, Klebsiella* spp, *Enterobacter* spp, *Citrobacter* spp, *Serratia* spp, *Proteus* spp, and *Morganella* spp. Colony morphology and various biochemical tests are used to differentiate this group of related bacteria.

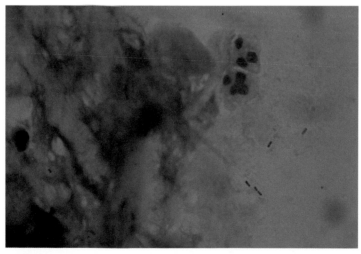

FIG VII-3—Gram-negative rods (*Pseudomonas aeruginosa,* Gram ×1000).

Haemophilus species. Haemophilus species vary in morphology from cocco-bacilli to short rods. Culture isolation requires enriched media such as chocolate agar. *H influenzae* can be divided into biotypes based on biochemical reactions such as indole production, urease activity, and ornithine decarboxylase activity and serotypes based on their capsular polysaccharides. The former *H aegyptius* is now classified as *H influenzae* biotype III.

H influenzae is a cause of purulent conjunctivitis and preseptal cellulitis in unvaccinated children, often distinguished by the purplish discoloration of skin involvement. *Haemophilus* species occasionally cause bacterial keratitis and bleb-associated endophthalmitis. Other species besides *H influenzae* are also occasion-ally encountered as a cause of ocular infection as well (e.g., *H aphrophilus, H haemolyticus*).

Pasteurella species. Pasteurella multocida is a member of the Pasteurellaceae family that is a common cause of respiratory infection and conjunctivitis in experi-mental animals. Clinical infection in human beings usually results from animal bites or scratches and may manifest as preseptal cellulitis and keratitis.

Other genera. Capnocytophaga species, *Alcaligenes* species, and *Eikenella corrodens* are diverse, unrelated bacilli that are uncommon causes of corneal infec-tion. Unlike most other gram-negative rods, these bacteria are usually resistant to most aminoglycosides.

Gram-positive cocci   *Staphylococcus and Micrococcus species.* The family Micro-coccaceae includes gram-positive cocci that grow in short chains and clumps. Staphylococci are arranged in grapelike clusters, but they are frequently seen singly, in pairs, or in short chains on smears of ocular specimens (Fig VII-4). *S aureus* is coagulase-positive (as are *S intermedius* and *S hyicus*) and is differentiated from other staphylococcal species by aerobic fermentation of mannitol. Coagulase-negative, mannitol-negative species include *S epidermidis, S hominis,* and *S auricularis.*

Penicillinase production is common among staphylococcal strains, and some are resistant to synthetic β-lactam agents, such as methicillin and first-generation

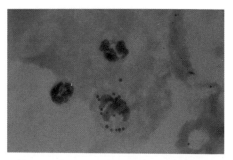

FIG VII-4—Gram-positive cocci (*Staphylococcus aureus,* Gram ×1000).

cephalosporins. *S aureus* and some strains of *S epidermidis* produce a dermato-necrotoxin that may account for the erythema and other clinical changes seen during staphylococcal blepharitis. Hypersensitivity reactions to staphylococcal components can produce ocular surface inflammation such as marginal corneal infiltrates. *S epidermidis* is difficult to establish as an etiologic agent in acute conjunctivitis because it is a normal component of the ocular surface flora. However, it is commonly recognized as a cause of bacterial keratitis and endophthalmitis.

Micrococcus species are gram-positive cocci that usually grow more slowly than staphylococci. One species is the basis for the lysozyme bioassay. *Micrococcus* species are occasionally a component of polymicrobial infection.

Streptococcus species and Enterococcus species. These gram-positive cocci grow in pairs and chains. Streptococci are classified according to their ability to hemolyze erythrocytes during growth on blood agar and by their carbohydrate composition (Lancefield groups):

□ α-hemolysis: a visible green discoloration around colonies

□ β-hemolysis: a clear zone surrounding colonies

□ γ-hemolysis: no hemolysis

With aerobic incubation, oxygen can neutralize the activity of a streptolysin and may make the detection of hemolysis difficult.

Several streptococcal exotoxins can stimulate an inflammatory reaction. Formerly the leading cause of bacterial keratitis, streptococci still account for many cases of suppurative keratitis, acute conjunctivitis, and endophthalmitis (especially bleb-associated and postkeratoplasty infections). Streptococci and enterococci are frequently resistant to aminoglycosides and fluoroquinolones.

α-hemolytic streptococci include *S pneumoniae,* which can be differentiated by its resistance to optochin and to bile solubility, and the viridans streptococci (*S anginosus, S mitis, S mutans, S salivarius,* and *S sanguis*). Pneumococci are lancet-shaped diplococci arranged with their flattened ends together and surrounded by a polysaccharide capsule. β-hemolytic streptococci are often classified according to their specific carbohydrate composition; for example, group A includes *S pyogenes.* *Enterococcus* species, formerly classified among group D streptococci, show variable hemolysis on blood agar.

Other genera. Other gram-positive cocci that are infrequently associated with ocular infections are *Aerococcus* spp and *Pediococcus* spp. Anaerobic gram-positive cocci include *Peptococcus* spp and *Peptostreptococcus* spp.

Gram-positive rods   *Corynebacterium species.* These pleomorphic bacilli are seen in palisading or Chinese-character configurations on stained smears. Besides *C diphtheriae,* a toxin-producing, highly pathogenic cause of membranous conjunctivitis, many other species (e.g., *C haemolyticum, C xerosis*) are described, often referred to as diphtheroids. These other species form part of the normal flora of the outer eye. Occasionally, they can be isolated with other microorganisms during external ocular infections but usually not as the single pathogen.

Propionibacterium acnes. *P acnes* and related species are usually considered anaerobic bacilli, but they do grow under microaerophilic conditions. These slender, slightly curved gram-positive rods sometimes have a beaded appearance (Fig VII-5). They form a normal part of the skin flora. They are known to cause delayed-onset,

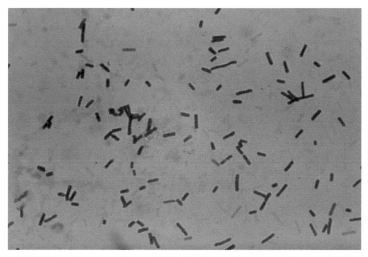

FIG VII-5—Gram-positive rods (*Propionibacterium acnes*, Gram ×1000).

chronic endophthalmitis following intraocular surgery but have rarely been isolated from cases of corneal or external ocular infections.

Bacillus species. These gram-positive bacteria produce endospores. Several species are reported causes of bacterial keratitis, and *Bacillus cereus* is an important cause of posttraumatic endophthalmitis, particularly in the setting of a retained intraocular foreign body. *Clostridium* species are anaerobic spore-forming bacteria.

Gram-positive filaments *Mycobacterium species.* M tuberculosis and other mycobacterial species are aerobic, pleomorphic, gram-positive, acid-fast bacilli that show various growth patterns on blood agar and special media such as Löwenstein-Jensen culture medium. *M leprae* cannot be isolated on artificial media. Atypical (nontuberculous) mycobacteria are classified by growth rate and pigment production into four groups that are further differentiated by biochemical and susceptibility profiles. *M fortuitum* and *M chelonei* are the mycobacteria most commonly isolated from cases of corneal infection. These rapidly growing atypical mycobacteria can be isolated on blood agar as well as Löwenstein-Jensen culture medium.

Nocardia species. N asteroides and related filamentous bacilli are weakly acid-fast. They are infrequent causes of keratitis and endophthalmitis.

Actinomyces species. Actinomyces species (e.g., A israelii) are anaerobic bacteria that grow in reduced media such as thioglycollate broth and on agar plates incubated anaerobically. Several actinomycetes can cause canaliculitis. *Propionibacterium propionicus* (formerly *Arachnia propionica*) is a closely related organism that probably accounts for many of these cases of lacrimal infection.

Spirochetes *Treponema species.* Treponema pallidum is the cause of venereal syphilis, and *T pallidum* subsp *endemicum* is the cause of endemic syphilis, or bejel. Treponemes are so slender they fall below the resolution of light microscopy, but they can be visualized using dark-field illumination from a fresh, infectious muco-cutaneous lesion. Direct demonstration of *T pallidum* or isolation on artificial medium or in experimental animals is usually not feasible in clinical ophthalmic practice. The serologic diagnosis of secondary or tertiary syphilis is based on

□ *Nontreponemal tests:* rapid plasma reagin (RPR) or venereal disease research laboratory (VDRL) assays

□ *Treponemal tests:* fluorescent treponemal antibody absorption (FTA-ABS) test or microhemagglutination assay–*T pallidum* (MHA-TP)

In clinical practice the serum MHA-TP or FTA-ABS test is used to confirm the clinical suspicion of ocular or neuro-ophthalmic syphilis, and the quantitative RPR test is performed to determine disease activity and to compare with subsequent testing following treatment.

Borrelia burgdorferi. This spirochete causing Lyme disease is transmitted to humans by ticks from wildlife hosts in endemic areas. An erythematous skin rash begins at the bite site. Disseminated infection can cause cardiac disease, meningoencephalitis with papilledema and cranial nerve palsies, and conjunctivitis. An immunologic component contributes to the pathogenesis of arthritis, stromal keratitis, and posterior uveitis. The diagnosis of borreliosis is determined by serologic assays and relevant clinical findings.

Mycology

Fungi are nucleated eukaryotes with rigid cell walls composed of polysaccharides such as chitin. The principal morphologic forms in infected human tissues are yeasts and molds. Molds are threadlike hyphae that are either septate or nonseptate. Some fungi are dimorphic, existing in either a yeast or hyphal form depending on environmental factors.

Yeasts   *Candida species.* Unicellular yeasts, also known as *blastoconidia,* grow by budding. Concatenation of elongated budding cells forms pseudohyphae. *Candida* spp produce pseudohyphae during tissue penetration, and these yeasts frequently show gram-positive budding forms on smears (Fig VII-6). Identification of *C albicans* is usually based on the formation of germ tubes in vitro, and further speciation is based on sugar fermentation. Classification of noncandidal yeasts is based on biochemical testing. *C albicans* and other species (e.g., *C parapsilosis, C tropicalis*) are rarely implicated in infections of the eyelid or conjunctiva, except in the mucocutaneous candidiasis syndrome and other immunocompromised states. *Candida* keratitis typically occurs in patients with a preexisting corneal disease or in the setting of altered host defenses, such as comatose patients with exposure or postkeratoplasty patients being treated with topical corticosteroids. *Candida* fungemia can give rise to retinochoroiditis and endogenous endophthalmitis.

Other genera. Yeasts that do not produce pseudohyphae occasionally colonize the outer eye. *Malassezia furfur* (formerly referred to as *Pityrosporum ovale* and *P orbiculare)* is a yeast that digests lipids and is frequently present along the normal eyelid margins. *Cryptococcus neoformans* can involve the posterior segment during meningoencephalitis.

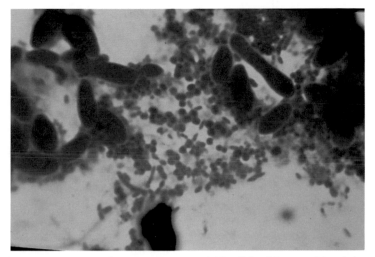

FIG VII-6—Yeasts with gram-positive cocci (*Candida albicans* and *Staphylococcus aureus,* Gram ×1000).

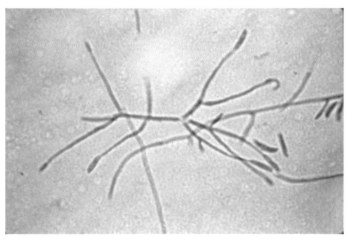

FIG VII-7—Septate hyphae of filamentous fungus (*Fusarium solani,* Gram ×1000).

Septate filamentous fungi Multiple genera of molds, including colorless and dematiaceous (pigmented) fungi, have been isolated from patients with corneal infection. These multicellular fungi have filamentous projections called *hyphae* that branch, forming a tangled colony known as a *mycelium.* Septate fungi are distinguished by crosswalls dividing the filaments into separate cells, each containing one or more nuclei (Fig VII-7).

Isolation is often achieved on blood agar and other standard media, but Sabouraud dextrose agar (without cycloheximide) and brain-heart infusion broth incubated at room temperature under controlled humidity are useful adjuncts. Many fungal cultures show visible colonies within a few days, but growth can take weeks. Classification is based on microscopic features of conidia that form on specialized hyphae called *conidiophores*. Microbiology laboratories must be aware that all ocular fungal isolates, including those formerly considered nonpathogenic saprophytes, should be reported.

Fusarium species (e.g., *F solani*), often encountered in tropical climates, can produce acute suppurative keratitis. Most other filamentous fungal corneal infections present in a more indolent course. Among the many other genera that have been isolated are *Aspergillus* spp, *Bipolaris* spp, *Curvularia* spp, *Drechslera* spp, *Paecilomyces* spp, and *Penicillium* spp. Many cases of oculomycosis follow trauma, especially when vegetative and other organic matter is involved.

Nonseptate filamentous fungi   Nonseptate fungi, which are sometimes referred to as Phycomycetes, include *Mucor* species and *Rhizopus* species, members of the family Mucoraceae and class Zygomycetes. Hyphae are nonseptate and branch at right angles. Rhinoorbitocerebral infection is more common in patients with diabetes mellitus or immunosuppression. Orbital mucormycosis can invade arterioles and cause ischemic necrosis of the eye.

Dimorphic fungi   These fungi grow in two distinct forms: a yeast phase that is usually present in infected tissues and a mycelial phase that occurs during active growth on artificial media. *Blastomyces dermatitidis* and *Sporothrix schenckii* are rare causes of granulomatous blepharoconjunctivitis. *Histoplasma capsulatum* and *Coccidioides immitis* can cause inflammation of the posterior segment.

Parasitology

Parasites of ophthalmic importance include protozoa, helminths (roundworms and flatworms), and arthropods. Many parasites pass through various morphological stages, and their life cycles may involve not only a definitive host that permits development into adult stages but also an intermediate host that allows only larval existence.

Protozoa   *Acanthamoeba species.* Classified on the basis of their cyst morphology and antigenic composition, several species of *Acanthamoeba* have been encountered. Their life cycle includes both a motile trophozoite form and a dormant cystic stage (Fig VII-8). Cysts can be found in water, soil, and air samples, and they are able to survive under adverse conditions.

Laboratory demonstration is possible by stained smears and culture isolation. Acanthamoebae grow on many standard media, and isolation can sometimes be facilitated by the use of nonnutrient agar with an overlay of live or dead gram-negative bacilli (usually *E coli*). Magnification shows lucent trails of motile trophozoites produced by phagocytosis of the bacterial overlay at the edges of inoculation sites. These trails must be differentiated from the short tracks made by wandering leukocytes.

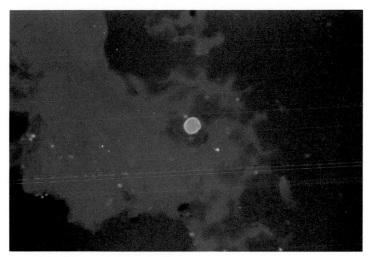

FIG VII-8—Amoebic cyst (*Acanthamoeba polyphaga,* calcofluor white
×1000).

Microsporida. Microsporida are intracellular parasites that can cause corneal
and conjunctival infection. Two clinical forms of microsporidal ocular infection are
described:

□ Focal stromal keratitis in otherwise healthy individuals

□ Superficial keratoconjunctivitis in patients with AIDS

Spores, sporoblasts, meronts, and sporonts can be found in scrapings and in biopsy
material from affected patients. Spores are gram-positive and acid-fast and stain with
other cytopathologic stains. Speciation is aided by use of electron microscopy to
evaluate spore size, nuclear arrangement, and polar filament spirals. Tissue-culture
isolation of *Nosema corneum, Enterocytozoon hellem,* and other microsporidia is
problematic.

Toxoplasma gondii. Sexual reproduction of *Toxoplasma* protozoa in the feline
intestine results in fecal oocysts that subsequently release infective sporozoites.
Many mammals, including humans, can acquire toxoplasmosis by ingesting oocysts
or, more commonly, by eating meat with viable toxoplasmic cysts. Asexual reproduction in these intermediate hosts involves the rapid proliferation of crescentic
tachyzoites in acute infection and encysted bradyzoites during persistent disease.
Transplacental spread during maternal primary disease can result in fetal infection.
See BCSC Section 6, *Pediatric Ophthalmology and Strabismus,* for discussion of the
consequences of maternal transmission.

Pneumocystis carinii. Trophozoites and cysts of *P carinii* develop slowly in the
pulmonary alveoli, causing pneumonia and, rarely, retinochoroiditis in patients with
AIDS and other immunosuppressed states.

Leishmania species. Cutaneous leishmaniasis begins at the bite site of the sand-
fly vector in endemic areas of tropical Asia, Africa, and Latin America. An infected
eyelid ulcer leads to granulomatous conjunctivitis and subcutaneous lymphangitis as
macrophages carry amastigotes away from the lesion. Scrapings or biopsy material

can show intracellular parasites by histopathologic immunofluorescent stains. Flagellated promastigotes can sometimes be isolated on special media.

Helminths *Onchocerca volvulus.* In endemic areas of sub-Saharan Africa, the Middle East, and Latin America, onchocercal filariae penetrate the skin at the bite site of the blackfly vector. Gradual development into adult worms subsequently results in mating of these nematodes, leading to the release of microfilariae that migrate subcutaneously. Microfilariae of *Onchocerca volvulus* enter the peripheral cornea and can reach the inner eye but do not usually cause much inflammation while they are alive. Dead microfilariae cause stromal keratitis and intraocular inflammation. Skin snips can be examined microscopically to demonstrate microfilariae in patients with onchocerciasis.

Loa loa. Filarial larvae enter the skin after the bite of an infected fly and slowly mature into adult worms that migrate subcutaneously. *Loa loa* occasionally appear under the conjunctiva.

Toxocara species. Larvae of *T canis* nematodes develop and mate in the intestines of their canine natural host. Human ingestion of fertilized eggs results in larvae in the intestine that then migrate, sometimes reaching the posterior segment of the eye.

Taenia solium. An adult *T solium* tapeworm can survive in the intestines of humans and other intermediate hosts. Eggs of these cestodes that hatch in the stomach release larvae that can then disseminate. A hydatid cyst can subsequently form in various tissues, including the eye and orbit, to cause cysticercosis.

Arthropods *Phthirus pubis.* Adult lice (Fig VII-9) and the immature nits of *Phthirus pubis* may infest the eyelashes and cause eyelid margin inflammation with mild keratoconjunctivitis.

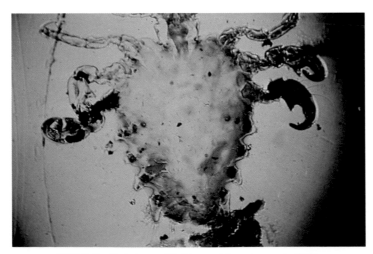

FIG VII-9—Crab louse (*Phthirus pubis,* wet mount ×200).

Demodex species. Demodex folliculorum and *D brevis* normally inhabit hair and eyelash follicles and sebaceous glands. These normal, commensal parasites are found more often in older people. Cylindrical sleeves can collect around the eyelash bases during extensive mite infestation.

Fly larvae. If deposited on the eyelid or conjunctiva, the larva of a botfly or fly of *Calliphoria* genus can cause a granulomatous reaction. Ocular myiasis may involve any of the ocular or adnexal structures.

Insect hairs and stings. The hairs of caterpillars, insects, and arachnids can cause a focal conjunctival granuloma called *ophthalmia nodosa.* Hairs can also migrate into the cornea. *Hymenoptera* (wasp) stings and venomous or toxic substances from beetles and other insects can cause necrotizing ocular inflammation.

Diagnostic Laboratory Techniques

Decisions about when and which laboratory studies should be performed must be based on a knowledgeable clinical assessment. The next chapter discusses the clinical aspects of conditions mentioned in this chapter. Interpretation of diagnostic specimens requires an understanding of the normal flora and cytologic pattern of the ocular surface. Appropriate materials should be available for optimal specimen collection (Table VII-3).

TABLE VII-3

MATERIALS FOR COLLECTING EYELID,
CONJUNCTIVAL, AND CORNEAL SPECIMENS FOR OCULAR MICROBIOLOGY

VIRAL INFECTIONS	CHLAMYDIAL INFECTIONS	MICROBIAL INFECTIONS
Topical anesthetic	Topical anesthetic	Topical anesthetic
Dacron or cotton swabs	Calcium alginate swabs	Calcium alginate swabs
Spatula	Spatula	Spatula
Glass slides	Glass slides	Glass slides
Acetone fixative	Methanol or acetone fixative	Methanol fixative
Viral transport medium	Chlamydial transport medium	Blood agar plate
Ice	Ice	Chocolate agar plate
		Thioglycollate or chopped-meat broth
		Sabouraud's dextrose agar plate
		Special media: Anaerobic plate Brain-heart infusion broth Mycobacterial medium Nonnutrient agar plate

Specimen Collection

Eyelid specimens   Eyelid vesicles are opened by gentle scraping or aspirated with a small-gauge needle and syringe. Material is smeared onto a glass slide that is fixed in methanol for cytologic staining and in cold acetone or methanol for immuno-fluorescent processing. Collected vesicular fluid is inoculated into a viral transport medium that is sent on ice to the laboratory for culture isolation.

Microbial culture specimens are obtained by swabbing the skin ulceration or eyelid margins with a moistened pledget that is used to inoculate culture media. Material expressed from an infected lacrimal sac or other soft tissue is collected and inoculated in a similar way.

Conjunctival specimens   Chapter V, Diagnostic Approach to Ocular Surface Disease, describes the steps of obtaining conjunctival specimens (see p 61). A conjunctival biopsy can be helpful in the evaluation of chronic conjunctivitis, including conditions such as Parinaud oculoglandular syndrome and pemphigoid. Forceps and scissors are used to snip a conjunctival specimen under local anesthesia, avoiding tissue crushing. The sample is placed on a carrier template and inserted into appropriate fixative, such as formalin or glutaraldehyde (for electron microscopy), or sent for immunopathologic processing in saline.

Corneal specimens   After removing adherent mucopurulent material, the clinician swabs the margins of the corneal lesion with a calcium alginate microswab and scrapes with a platinum Kimura spatula. Specimens are smeared onto glass slides and inoculated on prewarmed culture or transport media. Material from viral epithelial keratitis should be sent on ice immediately to the virology laboratory. For microbial keratitis multiple scrapings are obtained to inoculate culture media, using rows of small C-streak inoculation marks and avoiding the perimeter of agar plates. The spatula or swab that is used to collect material should be resterilized or discarded after each sampling. Liquid media are inoculated by transferring the specimen onto a moistened swab.

Corneal material can also be collected by a superficial keratectomy or corneal biopsy. A surgical blade is used to excise corneal fragments, or a small 2–3 mm trephine can be used to partially incise the cornea that is then excised with a microsurgical knife or scissors. One specimen is transported in a liquid medium to the microbiology laboratory for tissue grinding and inoculation, and another is sent for histopathologic examination.

Staining Methods

Chapter V, Diagnostic Approach to Ocular Surface Disease, describes commonly used stains on p 62 and in Table V-2, p 63.

Wilhelmus KR, Liesegang TJ, Osato MS, et al. *Laboratory Diagnosis of Ocular Infections.* Washington, DC: American Society for Microbiology; 1994.

Isolation Techniques

Viral and chlamydial diseases   An appropriate tissue-culture cell line is selected for inoculation and examined for the development of cytopathic effects (CPE) and inclusions based on clinical assessment of likely viral disease. *C trachomatis* can be isolated on cell culture if inoculated soon after the specimen is collected. Because of expense and technical difficulties, viral and chlamydial cultures are not routine diagnostic steps in the evaluation of corneal and external eye diseases.

Bacterial and fungal infections   Artificial media are inoculated and examined daily to detect visible colonies on the inoculation marks. After the number of identical colonies is counted and their morphology described, a sample is transferred to differential media for further growth and testing. Finding organisms compatible with the initial smears that are isolated on multiple media helps to substantiate a definitive etiology. Antimicrobial susceptibility testing is performed by disc-diffusion and broth-dilution procedures.

Parasites   Acanthamoebae are identified as meandering trails of trophozoites on the surface of an agar plate. Other protozoa and parasites are difficult to isolate.

CHAPTER VIII

Clinical Aspects of Infectious Diseases of the Eyelids, Conjunctiva, Cornea, and Sclera

Proper management of patients with external ocular inflammation must be guided by a specific diagnosis. Evaluation of patients with external ocular disease should begin with a detailed history of the patient's condition, which includes prior ocular inflammation, the nature of the patient's symptoms, risk factors such as contact lens wear in patients with corneal ulcers, and previous therapy. A careful and systematic examination of the patient's skin, face, and external eye—including the eyelids, meibomian glands, lacrimal puncta, tarsal and bulbar conjunctiva, sclera, cornea, and anterior chamber—should be performed next (see chapter II). Relevant diagnostic tests may then be performed to confirm a clinical impression (e.g., herpes simplex virus as a cause of dendritic epithelial keratitis) or to assist in therapy (e.g., antimicrobial sensitivity testing for microbial keratitis). After the inflammation has been localized to one or more external ocular tissues, clinical history and specific inflammatory signs can be used to classify the condition so that specific therapy can be instituted. A precise diagnosis may be difficult at the time of the initial evaluation in certain cases:

- Patients who present early in the course of the disease, when specific clinical signs may not yet have evolved
- Patients who have already received treatment (antibiotics or anti-inflammatory agents) that masks specific diagnostic features of their condition

In these cases, if the disease is not severe, it may be justifiable to withhold treatment until specific signs have evolved and/or diagnostic tests have shown results.

Viral Infections

Molluscum Contagiosum

PATHOGENESIS. Molluscum contagiosum is a DNA poxvirus that is spread by direct contact with infected individuals and possibly by fomites. The virus produces one or more asymptomatic umbilicated lesions that release poxvirus particles into the tear film. This release can result in an associated toxic keratoconjunctivitis, which is the major cause of symptoms and clinical pathology.

CLINICAL PRESENTATION. A molluscum is a smooth nodule that develops an umbilicated central core. It is smaller and associated with less inflammation than a keratoacanthoma. Molluscum contagiosum may produce elevated, pearly, umbilicated nodules on the eyelids (Fig VIII-1). These lesions are usually easily visualized on the

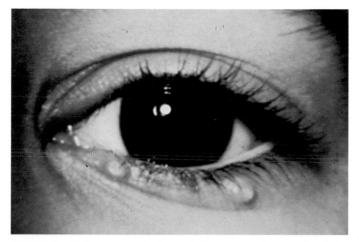

FIG VIII-1—Molluscum contagiosum lesions along the margin of the lower eyelid.

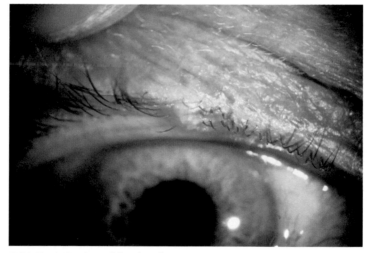

FIG VIII-2—Single nodule of molluscum contagiosum at the eyelid margin.

eyelid margin, but occasionally lesions are small and can be missed during a casual examination (Fig VIII-2). Chronic follicular conjunctivitis is often present, and punctate epithelial erosions and/or a superficial vascular pannus on the cornea may occur. Severe cases of molluscum contagiosum–associated keratitis mimic chlamydial keratoconjunctivitis.

LABORATORY EVALUATION AND MANAGEMENT. The poxvirus responsible for mollus-cum lesions cannot be cultured using standard techniques. Diagnosis is therefore based on careful clinical examination and the detection of the characteristic skin lesions.

Molluscum contagiosum is a self-limited disease, but spontaneous resolution may take months to years. Treatment can involve completely excising the nodule, freezing the lesion, or curetting the central portion of the lesion (production of bleeding within the lesion is felt to speed resolution). Extensive facial and eyelid molluscum lesions have been reported in patients with AIDS. Complete resolution in these cases is often difficult to effect.

Other Neoplastic Infections of the Eyelid and Conjunctiva

Verruca and *papillomas* are caused, in part, by papillomavirus infection of the epi-dermis or epithelium. These benign lesions are discussed on pp 236–237. *Kaposi sarcoma* is a malignant neoplasm resulting from a herpesvirus infection that is dis-cussed on pp 250–251.

Adenovirus Keratoconjunctivitis

PATHOGENESIS. Adenoviruses can cause a variety of external ocular infections. Two syndromes of external ocular adenovirus infection, *epidemic keratoconjunctivitis (EKC)* and *pharyngoconjunctival fever (PCF),* have been described. Although patients often present with clinical features typical of one of these syndromes, they occa-sionally manifest clinical features that overlap both. External ocular adenovirus infections are acute and generally self-limited; however, chronic infections have been rarely reported.

The associated keratitis may have both an epithelial component in the early stages and a subepithelial component, usually presenting in later stages. Epithelial keratitis is caused by active viral replication within epithelial cells. In contrast, subepithelial infiltrates are likely caused by an immune response to viral antigens deposited in the superficial corneal stroma. Light and electron microscopy of sub-epithelial infiltrates reveals lymphocytes, degenerated collagen fibrils, and scarring but no virus particles.

CLINICAL PRESENTATION. EKC has been reported worldwide from 11 virus serotypes; serotypes 8, 11, and 19 are the most common causative strains. Virus transmission occurs through direct or indirect contact with infected individuals. Epidemics of adenovirus conjunctivitis commonly occur through transmission of the virus in schools, workplaces, and physicians' offices. Contaminated fingers, contact instru-ments such as tonometer tips, and swimming pool water are common modes of virus transmission.

Patients with EKC experience acute onset of watery discharge, photophobia, and mild foreign body sensation. Ocular signs include preauricular adenopathy and mixed papillary/follicular conjunctivitis, occasionally with hemorrhage and mem-brane formation (Figs VIII-3, VIII-4). Conjunctival follicles may be masked by chemo-sis. The peak intensity of the conjunctivitis occurs 5–7 days after the onset of symp-toms; the fellow eye is involved in at least 50% of cases.

Adenovirus keratitis progresses through six stages characterized by an orderly sequence of superficial epithelial keratitis, deep epithelial keratitis, and subepithe-

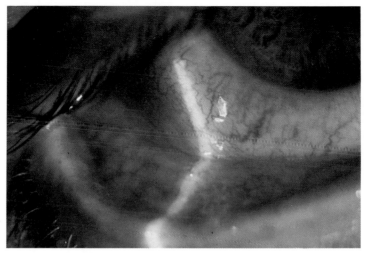

FIG VIII-3—Prominent follicular reaction on inferior tarsal conjunctiva in adenovirus conjunctivitis.

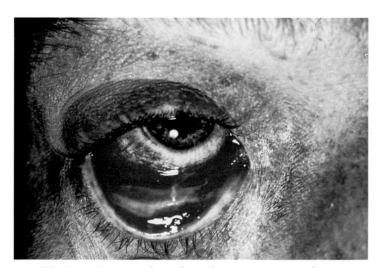

FIG VIII-4—Conjunctival pseudomembrane in a patient with EKC.

lial infiltrates (Table VIII-1; Figs VIII-5 through VIII-7). Chronic complications, including symblepharon formation and tear drainage obstruction from punctal or canalicular occlusion, may occasionally occur following severe membranous adenoviral conjunctivitis.

TABLE VIII-1

STAGES OF ADENOVIRUS KERATITIS

STAGE	INVOLVEMENT	INTERVAL FROM ONSET (DAYS)
0	Diffuse PEE	1–3
I	Diffuse PEK	4–7
II	Deep PEK	6–10
III	Deep PEK, anterior stromal	8–14
IV	Anterior stromal	12–18
V	Anterior stromal, epithelial changes	weeks to months

PEE = punctate epithelial erosions (slightly depressed gray-white spots that stain readily with fluorescein and poorly with rose bengal)

PEK = punctate epithelial keratitis (elevated, granular, opalescent epithelial cells that stain brilliantly with rose bengal and poorly with fluorescein)

PCF is often indistinguishable from EKC. Usually caused by adenovirus serotypes 3, 4, and 7, the disease manifests as an acute follicular conjunctivitis with an associated upper respiratory tract infection and fever. The conjunctivitis follows a clinical course similar to EKC, although punctate epithelial keratitis and subepithelial infiltrates are less common.

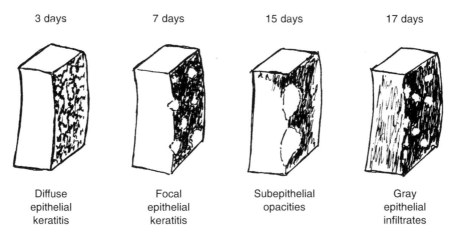

3 days	7 days	15 days	17 days
Diffuse epithelial keratitis	Focal epithelial keratitis	Subepithelial opacities	Gray epithelial infiltrates

FIG VIII-5—Schematic drawing illustrating the different types of keratitis seen with adenovirus keratoconjunctivitis.

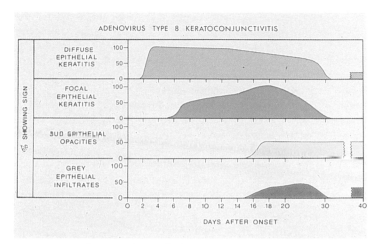

ADENOVIRUS TYPE 8 KERATOCONJUNCTIVITIS

DAYS AFTER ONSET

FIG VIII-6—Durations of various forms of adenovirus keratitis. (Reproduced with permission from Dawson CR, Hanna L, Wood TR, et al. Adenovirus type 8 keratoconjunctivitis in the United States. *Am J Ophthalmol.* 1970;69:473–480.)

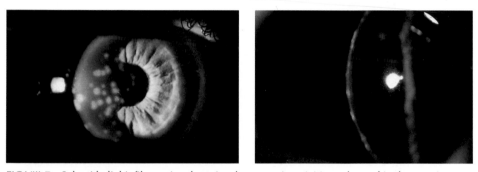

FIG VIII-7—Subepithelial infiltrates in adenovirus keratoconjunctivitis are located in the anterior stroma (never in the deep stroma). They are small and uniform in size and shape. Neovascularization of the cornea does not occur.

LABORATORY EVALUATION. Diagnosis is usually based on clinical features, and only selected cases are confirmed. Rapid immunodetection of adenovirus antigen may aid in diagnosis in confusing cases or in epidemic outbreaks. Viral cultures can be performed, but the cost and time required present obstacles to routine use. The sensitivity of both types of tests is highest within the first week of acute disease, when viral shedding is maximal.

MANAGEMENT. Therapy of adenovirus keratoconjunctivitis is mainly supportive. Cold compresses and topical vasoconstrictors may provide symptomatic relief. Little clinical evidence supports use of topical antibiotics, since secondary bacterial infection is uncommon. Despite in vitro activity of several antiviral agents against adenovirus species, clinical trials of these agents have been unsuccessful in reducing the severity of the conjunctivitis or preventing keratitis. Topical interferon has not proven useful in treating the disease but may limit spread to the fellow eye.

The use of topical corticosteroids to treat external ocular adenoviral infections is controversial. Topical steroid therapy has been reported to play a causative role in chronic adenovirus keratoconjunctivitis. Furthermore, acute follicular conjunctivitis can be caused by herpes simplex virus (see discussion below). To avoid complications that may result from steroid treatment of herpes simplex virus keratoconjunctivitis, topical steroids should probably be avoided until a specific diagnosis of adenovirus keratoconjunctivitis is made based on clinical features or laboratory tests. Indications for topical corticosteroid therapy for adenovirus keratoconjunctivitis include the following:

☐ Conjunctival membrane or pseudomembrane

☐ Marked foreign body sensation and chemosis

☐ Reduced vision due to epithelial or subepithelial keratitis

To minimize steroid-related complications, the dosage of topical corticosteroids should be tapered to once a day or to every other day as rapidly as possible. Subepithelial infiltrates may worsen or recur as topical steroids are weaned or discontinued too rapidly. The role of topical nonsteroidal anti-inflammatory agents is unclear.

Patients with external ocular adenovirus infections should be informed of the natural course of the disease to allay anxiety they may experience if severe conjunctival chemosis or eyelid edema develops. Most patients with ocular adenovirus infections are contagious for at least 7 days; therefore, patients should be advised to avoid direct personal contact for at least 1 week following onset of symptoms to prevent spread of infection.

Enterovirus and Coxsackievirus Conjunctivitis

Acute hemorrhagic keratoconjunctivitis is caused by a picornavirus, usually enterovirus 70 but occasionally coxsackievirus A24. Acute hemorrhagic conjunctivitis is characterized by acute onset of severe unilateral or bilateral follicular conjunctivitis with the following:

☐ Bulbar and tarsal conjunctival hemorrhages

☐ Chemosis

☐ Eyelid edema

☐ Profuse mucopurulent discharge

☐ Preauricular adenopathy

☐ Fine punctate epithelial keratitis similar to stage I EKC

The disease is highly contagious and occurs in large and rapidly spreading epidemics. Several epidemics of acute hemorrhagic conjunctivitis have been reported in the United States. The disease is self-limited and usually lasts 10 days or less.

Herpes Simplex Virus Blepharitis, Conjunctivitis, Epithelial Keratitis, and Stromal Keratitis

PATHOGENESIS. Herpes simplex virus (HSV) is a DNA virus that commonly infects humans. Two distinct but antigenically related strains of HSV exist: type 1 (HSV-1) and type 2 (HSV-2). Epidemiologic studies have found that 50%–90% of adult humans in the United States have serum antibodies to HSV-1. HSV infection is spread by direct contact of the epidermis or mucous membranes with infectious secretions. HSV-1 generally causes infection above the waist (orofacial and ocular), and HSV-2 is generally sexually transmitted and causes genital infections. HSV-1 occasionally causes genital infection as a result of orogenital sexual activity. Similarly, HSV-2 may infect the eye by means of direct contact with infected genital secretions, or it may be transmitted to neonates as they pass through the birth canal of a mother with genital HSV-2 infection. Neonatal HSV-2 infection may be confined to the skin or mucous membranes including the eye, or it may cause a more severe systemic infection, which can be fatal if encephalitis develops. BCSC Section 6, *Pediatric Ophthalmology and Strabismus,* discusses herpes infection in neonates in greater detail.

Approximately 0.15% of the United States population has a history of external ocular HSV infection. Recurrent HSV keratitis may result in permanent corneal scarring and irregularity, and HSV keratitis has been reported to be one of the most frequent causes of infective corneal blindness in the United States.

Primary HSV-1 infection in humans occurs most commonly on the mucocutaneous areas of the head, those body surfaces innervated by cranial nerve V. It characteristically manifests as a nonspecific upper respiratory tract infection. At the time of primary infection, HSV may spread from the epithelial site of infection to sensory nerve endings in the infected tissue, where the virus is then transported down the nerve axon to the cell body located in a sensory ganglion. The virus genome then enters the nucleus of a neuron, where it persists in a latent nonpathogenic state. Primary infection of any of the three branches of cranial nerve V can result in latent infection of sensory neurons within the trigeminal ganglion that supplies all three branches. This interneuronal ("backdoor") spread of HSV in the trigeminal ganglion occurs either at the time of initial infection or during reactivation. Therefore, patients may develop recurrent ocular HSV disease without ever having had primary ocular HSV infection.

Primary ocular infections CLINICAL PRESENTATION. Primary ocular HSV infection typically manifests as a unilateral blepharokeratoconjunctivitis. The conjunctival inflammatory response is usually follicular and accompanied by a palpable preauricular lymph node. Occasionally, conjunctival membranes develop. Cutaneous vesicles on the eyelid skin or margin develop in the majority of cases (Fig VIII-8). Approximately two thirds of patients with primary ocular HSV infection develop epithelial keratitis, which consists of scattered punctate epithelial lesions or one or more epithelial dendrites. Stromal keratitis and uveitis develop in fewer than 10% of patients with primary ocular HSV infection. In one study HSV was cultured from the conjunctiva of 25% of patients with acute follicular conjunctivitis not associated with an epidemic.

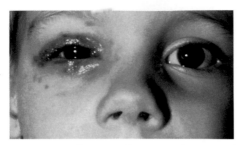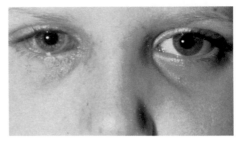

FIG VIII-8—*Left,* Primary herpes simplex virus infection involving the eye, with vesicles on the eyelid margin and acute conjunctivitis. *Right,* Acute follicular conjunctivitis without associated skin lesions, caused by primary herpes simplex virus infection.

It may sometimes be difficult to distinguish acute follicular conjunctivitis caused by HSV from that caused by adenovirus. Signs that can be used to distinguish HSV keratitis from adenovirus keratitis include the following:

☐ The distinctive dendritic morphology of HSV keratitis

☐ The presence in primary HSV of cutaneous vesicles

☐ The lack of an associated epidemic

☐ Unilaterality (only 10% of HSV keratitis cases are bilateral, whereas the majority of adenovirus keratoconjunctivitis cases have bilateral involvement)

LABORATORY EVALUATION. In cases in which a clinical diagnosis cannot be made, laboratory tests (culture or antigen detection) may be helpful. Serologic testing is generally of limited value in establishing a diagnosis because over 90% of the adult population shows serologic evidence of HSV-1 infection. Therefore, a single positive IgG titer is nondiagnostic, whereas a negative result may be helpful in excluding HSV-related disease (on a retrospective basis). A minimum fourfold rise in antibody titer and/or the presence of IgM class antibodies may be helpful in making a retrospective diagnosis of primary infection.

MANAGEMENT. Although primary ocular HSV infection is a self-limited condition, topical antiviral therapy with trifluridine or vidarabine or oral antiviral therapy with acyclovir, valacyclovir, or famciclovir for 1 week is used to limit corneal epithelial involvement and, although unproven, possibly reduce the risk of recurrences (Table VIII-2).

Recurrent ocular infection PATHOGENESIS. Recurrent HSV infection may occur as a result of reactivation of latently infected cells. Traditionally, recurrent lytic HSV infection was thought to be caused by reactivation of the virus in the sensory ganglion that travels down the nerve axon to the sensory nerve endings, where the virus would be transferred to epithelial cells on the ocular surface or cornea. If favorable conditions existed in the epithelium, viral replication and cell lysis could occur, producing clinical manifestations.

Recently, HSV-specific nucleic acid sequences have been detected, and HSV has been cultured from corneal buttons excised from patients with chronic herpetic

TABLE VIII-2

ANTIVIRAL AGENTS IN ANTERIOR SEGMENT HERPES SIMPLEX VIRUS DISEASE

AGENT	MECHANISM OF ACTION	ADMINISTRATION	ACUTE DOSAGE[1]
Vidarabine	Purine analogue Inhibits DNA polymerase	Ophthalmic: 3% ointment	5×/day for 14 days
Trifluridine	Pyrimidine analogue Inhibits DNA polymerase and thymidylate synthase	Ophthalmic. 1% solution	8×/day for 14 days
Acyclovir	Pyrimidine analogue	Ophthalmic: 3% ointment[2]	5×/day for 14 days
	Activated by a viral thymidine kinase to inhibit viral DNA polymerase	Dermatologic: 5% ointment	6×/day for 7 days
		Oral: 200, 400, and 800 mg	400 mg 5×/day
Famciclovir	Similar to acyclovir	Oral: 500 mg	500 mg 3×/day for 7 days
Valacyclovir	Similar to acyclovir	Oral: 500 mg	1 g 3×/day for 7 days in immuno-competent patients

[1] Dosage for chronic suppression is lower.
[2] Not commercially available in the United States.
(Modified from Parrish CM. Herpes simplex virus eye disease. In: *Focal Points: Clinical Modules for Ophthalmologists.* San Francisco: American Academy of Ophthalmology; 1997;15:2.)

keratitis, without evidence of lytic epithelial infection at the time therapeutic penetrating keratoplasty was performed. These data suggest that the human cornea may be a site of latency and a potential source of recurring clinical ocular disease.

CLINICAL PRESENTATION. The several different types of recurrent ocular HSV infection include the following:

□ Blepharoconjunctivitis

□ Dendritic and geographic epithelial keratitis

□ Nonnecrotizing and necrotizing stromal keratitis

□ Iridocyclitis

The strain of infecting virus and the genetic constitution of the host contribute to the disease pattern and severity of ocular HSV infection.

Blepharoconjunctivitis. Eyelid and/or conjunctival involvement may occur in patients with recurrent ocular HSV infection. Blepharoconjunctivitis may or may not accompany epithelial keratitis, and it can be treated for 7–10 days with topical or oral antivirals.

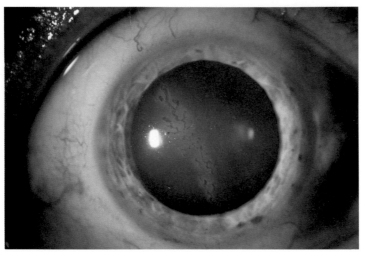

FIG VIII-9—Corneal epithelial dendrite caused by herpes simplex virus.

Dendritic and geographic epithelial keratitis. CLINICAL PRESENTATION. Patients with dendritic epithelial keratitis may be asymptomatic or experience mild foreign body sensation, photophobia, redness, and blurred vision. Recurrent HSV epithelial keratitis often has a dendritic, or dichotomously branching, shape. The lesions may begin as discrete punctate epithelial keratitis, then coalesce into dendritic-shaped lesions consisting of swollen, opaque epithelial cells within several days. The tips of the dendrite's branches have a characteristic bulblike morphology referred to as *terminal bulbs* (Fig VIII-9).

A very narrow ulcer typically develops in the center of the dendrite within several days of onset, as a result of lysis or desquamation of virus-infected cells. The opaque cells at the edge of the central ulcer stain brilliantly with rose bengal and moderately with fluorescein. Fluorescein will pool in the central ulceration of epithelial dendrites.

Geographic-shaped epithelial ulcers occasionally develop by centrifugal spread of HSV from a central dendrite toward the peripheral cornea. Risk factors for developing geographic ulcers include the strain of infecting virus, topical or systemic immunosuppressive therapy, and HIV infection (Fig VIII-10).

Patients with HSV epithelial keratitis may develop a ciliary flush and mild conjunctival infection. Mild stromal edema and subepithelial infiltrates may develop beneath epithelial keratitis. The subepithelial infiltrates often mirror the shape of the overlying epithelial lesion and have been termed *ghost dendrites.* They may serve as a marker for recent epithelial keratitis in patients who are examined after the epithelial lesion has resolved.

Sectoral or diffuse reduction in corneal sensation often develops following HSV epithelial keratitis. The distribution of corneal hypoesthesia is related to the extent, duration, severity, and number of recurrences of herpetic keratitis. Sectoral corneal anesthesia may be difficult to detect clinically and is not a reliable sign of herpetic disease.

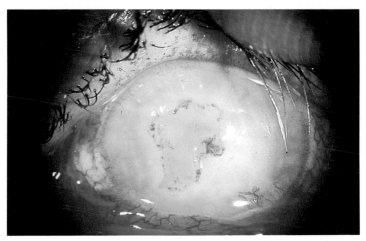

FIG VIII-10—Geographic, ameboid-shaped corneal ulcer stained with rose bengal and fluorescein demonstrates cells containing replicating virus at ulcer margin. (Reproduced with permission from Parrish CM. Herpes simplex virus eye disease. In: *Focal Points: Clinical Modules for Ophthalmologists*. San Francisco: American Academy of Ophthalmology; 1997;15:2.)

Other conditions that may produce dendritic epithelial lesions include the following:

- Varicella virus (varicella and herpes zoster ophthalmicus, see below)
- Healing epithelial defects
- Soft contact lens wear
- Epstein-Barr virus (rare)
- Tyrosinemia type II (very rare)

LABORATORY EVALUATION. A specific clinical diagnosis of HSV as the cause of dendritic keratitis can usually be made on the presence of characteristic features of HSV epithelial dendrites (central location, rose bengal staining pattern, and terminal bulbs). In cases lacking specific clinical signs, tissue culture and/or antigen detection techniques may be helpful in establishing the diagnosis. These techniques have been reported to have equal sensitivity and specificity for diagnosis of HSV epithelial keratitis.

MANAGEMENT. Most cases of HSV epithelial keratitis resolve spontaneously within 3 weeks. The rationale for treating is to decrease corneal damage secondary to lytic viral infection and the virus-inspired immunologic response. Some studies have reported that minimal wiping debridement of HSV epithelial keratitis with a dry cotton-tipped applicator or cellulose sponge can speed resolution and decrease the load of infectious virus and viral antigens that may be presented to the immune system, inducing stromal keratitis. Impression cytology of dendritic epithelial keratitis has been reported to remove virus-infected cells with less trauma to the epithelial basement membrane. This method can also be used for antigen detection studies.

Antiviral therapy is an effective treatment for epithelial disease and can be used in combination with epithelial debridement. Topical trifluridine 1% solution eight times daily or vidarabine 3% ointment five times daily have equal efficacy in treatment of HSV dendritic epithelial keratitis; however, trifluridine is more effective than vidarabine for treatment of geographic epithelial keratitis. Treatment of HSV epithelial keratitis with topical antivirals should be discontinued in 8–10 days to avoid toxicity to the ocular surface, which frequently accompanies the use of these medications. Acyclovir 3% ointment has been reported to be equally effective and less toxic than trifluridine and vidarabine for treatment of epithelial keratitis, but the ointment is currently available commercially only as a 5% topical dermatologic treatment. The topical ophthalmic 3% form is not available in the United States. Oral acyclovir is available, and a dose of 2 g per day for 10 days has been reported to be as effective as topical antivirals for treatment of epithelial keratitis. This treatment regimen is more expensive than topical antivirals, but it may be considered in patients with frequent recurrences of epithelial disease or tear drainage obstruction who are particularly susceptible to toxicity from the topical medications. Oral acyclovir does not, however, reduce the risk of stromal keratitis following resolution of HSV epithelial keratitis.

Stromal keratitis and uveitis. PATHOGENESIS. HSV stromal keratitis is the form of recurrent herpetic ocular disease associated with the greatest visual morbidity. Stromal keratitis accounts for about one fourth of all forms of HSV ocular infections. Stromal keratitis may occur with epithelial keratitis or may occur subsequently to epithelial keratitis, and it can be the first clinical manifestation of HSV eye disease. There is a strong positive correlation between the occurrence of prior stromal keratitis and the risk of again developing stromal keratitis.

Herpetic stromal keratitis is thought to be caused by a cell-mediated immunologic response to herpesvirus infection of keratocytes. It is not known whether the immune response is stimulated by concurrent or previous epithelial infection, by residual viral antigens in the corneal stroma following epithelial disease, or by a smoldering low-grade lytic HSV infection in keratocytes or inflammatory cells in the corneal stroma. Reports of the recovery of infectious virus and detection of HSV antigens and DNA in the corneas of patients with chronic herpetic stromal keratitis suggest that persistent stromal infection may be an important factor for induction and progression of herpetic stromal keratitis. Granulomatous or nongranulomatous iridocyclitis frequently accompanies necrotizing stromal keratitis, but it may occur independently of epithelial or stromal disease. Elevated IOP caused by trabeculitis and patchy atrophy of the iris pigment epithelium and stroma may be seen in patients with HSV iridocyclitis. Infectious virus has been cultured from the anterior chamber of patients with herpetic iridocyclitis, and its presence is positively correlated with ocular hypertension.

CLINICAL PRESENTATION. Two different clinical forms of herpetic stromal keratitis occur: nonnecrotizing and necrotizing. *Nonnecrotizing stromal keratitis* appears as a homogenous translucent cellular infiltration that may be accompanied by stromal edema and surrounding ring infiltrates (Fig VIII-11). Generally, this type of stromal keratitis is not associated with stromal vascularization. One type of nonnecrotizing stromal keratitis termed *disciform keratitis* presents as a disc-shaped zone of corneal edema, often without stromal inflammatory cell infiltrate (Fig VIII-12). Keratic precipitates are frequently found adherent to the endothelium in the area of stromal edema, and iridocyclitis may occur. Severe cases of disciform keratitis may be accompanied by marked stromal edema as well as epithelial microcystic edema and

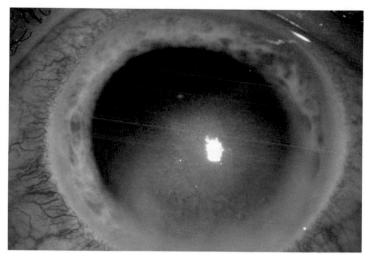

FIG VIII-11—Nonnecrotizing herpes simplex virus stromal keratitis.

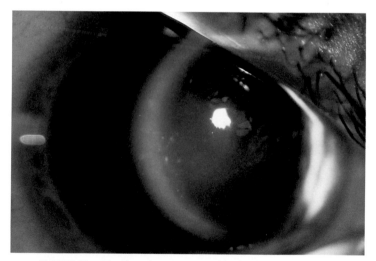

FIG VIII-12—Disciform keratitis caused by herpes simplex virus.

bullae. Persistent bullous keratopathy is a rare complication of chronic or recurrent herpetic disciform keratitis.

Necrotizing stromal keratitis appears as single or multiple cheesy white necrotic infiltrates (Fig VIII-13). It frequently incites stromal vascularization, which appears as one or more leashes of mid- to deep stromal blood vessels extending from the peripheral cornea into the area of stromal infiltration.

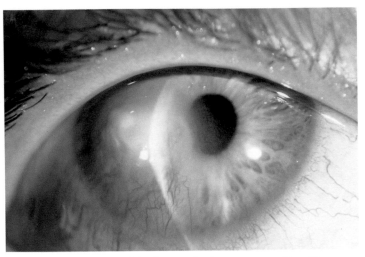

FIG VIII-13—Necrotizing herpes simplex virus stromal keratitis.

MANAGEMENT. For years controversy has surrounded the optimal management of HSV stromal keratitis. Conflicting results have been reported in uncontrolled retrospective studies regarding the efficacy of topical corticosteroids. Some studies have reported a decrease in stromal infiltration and improved visual acuity with combined corticosteroid and antiviral therapy. Other studies have suggested that topical corticosteroids may increase the severity of herpetic stromal keratitis, prolong its course, and predispose the patient to secondary complications. Recently, a multicenter clinical trial, the Herpetic Eye Disease Study (HEDS), compared the effects of topical trifluridine plus either a topical corticosteroid or a placebo in patients with herpes simplex stromal keratitis. Corticosteroid therapy was shown to reduce the risk of persistent or progressive stromal keratouveitis.

The strategy for topical corticosteroid therapy of stromal keratitis should be frequent initial administration (every 1–4 hours) followed by tapering of the dose based on the clinical response. Frequently, there will be a threshold dosage below which stromal inflammation will flare. Therefore, patients should be tapered to the lowest possible steroid dosage that controls their inflammation. Concentrations of corticosteroid less than those commercially available may suppress inflammation in some cases, and these can be prepared by serially diluting 1/8% commercial preparations.

Topical or oral antivirals are recommended for prophylaxis of epithelial disease in patients receiving topical steroids for stromal keratitis to prevent or limit lytic epithelial keratitis if a recurrence should develop while the patient is using frequent topical steroid applications. The optimal dose of topical antiviral for prophylaxis has not been determined; however, prophylactic antivirals are probably not required when the steroid dose is decreased to the equivalent of one drop of 1/8% prednisolone per day. Cycloplegics are frequently helpful in decreasing pain or photophobia associated with herpetic stromal keratitis and uveitis.

Uncontrolled clinical series have suggested that oral acyclovir may have added therapeutic benefits when used with topical corticosteroids for treatment of stromal keratitis and uveitis. The HEDS clinical trial evaluated the efficacy of oral acyclovir in treating patients with stromal keratitis receiving topical corticosteroids and trifluridine, and no statistically or clinically significant beneficial effect from oral acyclovir was found in the treatment of HSV non-necrotizing stromal keratitis. Oral acyclovir can be substituted for topical antiviral prophylaxis when topical corticosteroids are used for stromal keratitis, for prophylaxis in patients who develop clinical toxicity from topical agents, and as an adjunct to topical treatment for some patients with herpetic iridocyclitis. Chronic suppression for 1 year with oral acyclovir 400 mg twice daily prevents recurrent HSV eye disease, including epithelial keratitis and stromal keratitis in patients who have had a recent episode in the prior year.

Barron BA, Gee L, Hauck WW, et al. Herpetic Eye Disease Study. A controlled trial of oral acyclovir for herpes simplex stromal keratitis. *Ophthalmology*. 1994;101: 1871–1882.

The Herpetic Eye Disease Study Group. Acyclovir for the prevention of recurrent herpes simplex virus eye disease. *N Engl J Med*. 1998;300:300–306.

Liesegang TJ. Biology and molecular aspects of herpes simplex and varicella-zoster virus infections. *Ophthalmology*. 1992;99:781–799.

Parrish CM. Herpes simplex virus eye disease. In: *Focal Points: Clinical Modules for Ophthalmologists*. San Francisco: American Academy of Ophthalmology; 1997;15:2.

Wilhelmus KR, Gee L, Hauck WW, et al. Herpetic Eye Disease Study. A controlled trial of topical corticosteroids for herpes simplex stromal keratitis. *Ophthalmology*. 1994; 101:1883–1895.

Complications of herpetic eye disease   A number of complications of recurrent herpetic keratitis can result in visual morbidity. Herpes simplex virus dermatoblepharitis may complicate *mycosis fungoides,* a cutaneous T-cell lymphoma.

Epithelial complications. Diffuse *punctate* or *vortex epitheliopathy* may occur from topical antiviral toxicity. This problem can persist for weeks to months following cessation of topical antiviral agents. *Recurrent epithelial erosions* may develop in areas of previous herpetic epithelial keratitis. Trauma to the basement membrane from vigorous debridement of infected epithelial cells may serve as a predisposing factor for recurrent epithelial erosions. This problem can be treated with nonpreserved lubricants, patching, or bandage contact lenses. *Nonhealing trophic epithelial defects* may develop in patients with corneal anesthesia. *Trophic ulcers* are usually round or oval and are located in the central or inferior cornea. The edges of *neurotrophic ulcers* are gray and elevated, have a rolled appearance, and do not stain with rose bengal. Neurotrophic ulcers should be treated with copious nonpreserved lubricant drops of ointments, eyelid patching, and bandage contact lenses. Ulcers that do not heal with these therapies will frequently heal with a tarsorrhaphy. Corneal stromal thinning and perforation may occasionally occur in association with nonhealing trophic epithelial defects.

Stromal complications. Visually significant *corneal stromal scarring* and *irregular astigmatism* may develop in patients with chronic or recurrent stromal keratitis. *Surface irregularity* and *stromal opacification* may diminish gradually in some patients. Patients whose visual acuity is limited by irregular astigmatism may benefit from a carefully fitted gas-permeable hard contact lens, although the possibility that contact lenses might induce recurrences of herpetic keratitis must be considered.

Lipid keratopathy may develop in patients with chronic stromal keratitis with corneal stromal vascularization. Topical corticosteroids have been found to inhibit progression of stromal lipid deposition. Laser photocoagulation has not been successful in occluding stromal blood vessels in patients with herpetic keratitis and lipid keratopathy.

SURGICAL TREATMENT. Penetrating keratoplasty may be indicated in patients with visually significant stromal scarring or corneal perforation resulting from neurotrophic ulcers or necrotizing stromal keratitis. If possible, small descemetoceles or perforations in inflamed eyes should be treated conservatively with therapeutic tissue adhesive and bandage contact lenses, and penetrating keratoplasty should be deferred until the eye is less inflamed. Stromal inflammation, ulceration, or graft failure may develop in inflamed eyes with herpetic keratitis undergoing tectonic penetrating keratoplasty.

The prognosis for successful optical penetrating keratoplasty approaches 80% in eyes without signs of active inflammation for at least 6 months prior to surgery. Intensive topical corticosteroid therapy may reduce vascularization prior to penetrating keratoplasty and reduce the risk of graft rejection, and it should be continued postoperatively. The dosage is based on the amount of ocular inflammation. Cases with severe postoperative inflammation may require periocular and/or oral corticosteroids to reduce inflammation.

Controversy persists regarding the use of prophylactic antiviral therapy following penetrating keratoplasty. In reported clinical series of penetrating keratoplasty for herpetic keratitis the frequency of recurrent epithelial keratitis has ranged from 6% to 75% of cases, and the majority of these recurrences occurred within the first year following surgery. Antiviral therapy appeared to decrease the percentage of epithelial recurrences. Because allograft rejection accompanied epithelial recurrences in 25% of cases, antiviral therapy also appears to be associated with improved graft survival. Oral acyclovir may be preferable to chronic topical antivirals in patients with recent penetrating keratoplasty to prevent epithelial toxicity.

Varicella-Zoster Virus Dermatoblepharitis, Conjunctivitis, Epithelial Keratitis, and Stromal Keratitis

Varicella PATHOGENESIS. Varicella-zoster is morphologically identical to HSV. The differentiating features of the two conditions are listed in Table VIII-3. Like HSV, varicella-zoster virus (VZV) is capable of establishing latency after primary infection, and disease may be caused by reactivation of latent virus. *Chickenpox*, the primary human infection, occurs by direct contact of airborne droplets from cutaneous lesions or respiratory secretions and is highly contagious to susceptible individuals. Varicella typically develops during childhood and is usually a mild, self-limited disease. The infection manifests with fever, malaise, and a cutaneous exanthem that typically lasts 7–10 days.

CLINICAL PRESENTATION. The rash of chickenpox begins as macules and progresses to papules, vesicles, and finally pustules that dry and crust. Mild ocular involvement may develop. A papillary conjunctivitis, occasionally with membrane formation, is the most common ocular manifestation. Small vesicles may develop on the eyelid margins or bulbar conjunctiva. Punctate or dendritic epithelial keratitis may occur concurrently with skin lesions. Subepithelial infiltrates, stromal keratitis, disciform

TABLE VIII-3

DIFFERENTIATING FEATURES OF HERPES SIMPLEX VIRUS AND
VARICELLA-ZOSTER VIRUS EYE DISEASES

	HERPES SIMPLEX VIRUS	VARICELLA-ZOSTER VIRUS
Dermatomal distribution	Incomplete	Complete
Pain	Less pain	More pain
Dendrite morphology	Large dendrites with central ulceration and terminal bulbs	Small, medusa-like dendrites without central ulceration or terminal bulbs; dendritic mucous plaques may occur late and are associated with decreased corneal sensation
Skin scarring	Rare	Frequent
Postherpetic neuralgia	Rare	Common
Iris atrophy	Patchy, generally not sectoral	Sectoral
Bilateral involvement	Rare	Never
Recurrent lytic epithelial keratitis	Common	Never
Corneal hypoesthesia	Sectoral or diffuse, correlated with number of recurrences	Frequent

keratitis, uveitis, and elevated intraocular pressure may develop following epithelial keratitis. Varicella keratitis is self-limited and does not recur. Corneal scarring is a rare complication.

MANAGEMENT. Primary prevention consists of varicella vaccine administration in susceptible hosts (nonimmune adults and immunodeficient, immunosuppressed, or atopic children). The symptoms and duration of viral shedding may be mitigated by administration of oral acyclovir. Severe disciform stromal keratitis that causes substantial reduction in vision may be treated with topical corticosteroids. Prompt treatment is especially important in an amblyopia-susceptible age group.

Herpes zoster ophthalmicus PATHOGENESIS. Varicella-zoster virus establishes latency in sensory neural ganglia after primary infection. In most cases zoster (shingles) represents endogenous reactivation of latent varicella-zoster virus. Cutaneous zoster lesions may rarely develop in patients who harbor latent virus after exposure to exogenous varicella-zoster virus through contact with patients who have active varicella infection. Twenty percent of adults experience zoster. Age is the most common predisposing factor; most patients are in their sixth to ninth decades. The majority of individuals developing zoster are healthy with no specific predisposing factors; however, zoster may be triggered by malignancy, HIV infection, surgery, trauma, irradiation, immunosuppressive therapy, or debilitating systemic disease.

Zoster manifests as a painful vesicular dermatitis localized to a dermatome supplied by a spinal or cranial sensory ganglion. Patients may experience a prodrome of fever and malaise, which can be accompanied by warmth, erythema, and hyper-

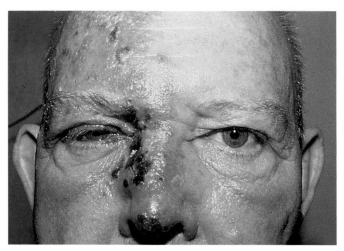

FIG VIII-14—Herpes zoster ophthalmicus with involvement of the nasociliary branch of the ophthalmic division (V$_1$) of cranial nerve V (Hutchinson's sign).

esthesia in the affected dermatome. Zoster may occur in any dermatome, but the most commonly affected dermatomes are T3 through L3 and those supplied by cranial nerve V. The ophthalmic division (V$_1$) of CN V is affected more often than the maxillary and mandibular branches, and infection in the ophthalmic branches is referred to as *herpes zoster ophthalmicus (HZO)* whether or not the eye is involved (Fig VIII-14). The zoster exanthem begins as a maculopapular eruption, followed by development of vesicles. The vesicles become yellow pustules in 3–4 days, then dry and crust in 10–12 days. Zoster dermatitis involves deeper layers of the skin than does chickenpox, and it may result in eschars that can resolve with extensive scarring and pigmentation. Ischemia caused by vasculitis contributes to tissue damage in involved areas. Hematogenous dissemination occasionally occurs in patients with HZO.

CLINICAL PRESENTATION. Zoster dermatitis is accompanied by pain and dysesthesia. The pain usually decreases as lesions resolve; however, neuralgia in the affected dermatome can continue from months to years. This pain is usually mild to moderate, but it can be incapacitating and has led to suicide.

Ocular involvement is common with HZO, occurring in more than 70% of patients. It is most likely to appear with infection of the nasociliary branch of cranial nerve V$_1$. However, ocular involvement may develop with infection limited to the frontal or lacrimal branches of CN V, and it has also been reported to occur with zoster of the maxillary (V$_2$) or mandibular (V$_3$) branches.

Infection and inflammation secondary to zoster can affect virtually all adnexal, ocular, and orbital tissues. Eyelid vesicular eruption can lead to secondary bacterial infection, eyelid scarring, marginal notching, loss of cilia, trichiasis, and cicatricial entropion. Scarring and occlusion of the lacrimal puncta or canaliculi may occur.

Episcleritis or scleritis associated with zoster may be either nodular or diffuse and can persist for months.

Corneal involvement in HZO assumes many forms. Dendritic epithelial keratitis caused by infectious virus is the most common early manifestation. Variant forms, consisting of multifocal or persistent dendrites that are positive for VZV, may be seen in patients with AIDS. Elevated noninfectious mucous plaques, often resembling dendrites, may occur weeks to months after resolution of skin lesions. Diminished corneal sensation, a predisposing factor for development of neurotrophic keratitis, develops in up to 50% of cases. Noninfectious corneal inflammation may result in sectoral pannus, nummular subepithelial infiltrates, stromal keratitis, and disciform edema. Chronic stromal inflammation can lead to vascularization, corneal opacification, lipid keratopathy (Fig VIII-15), corneal thinning, and irregular astigmatism. Sterile corneal stromal ulceration and perforation are not uncommon in cases which have corneal anesthesia, nonhealing epithelial defects, and persistent stromal inflammation.

Anterior uveitis, which is frequently associated with elevated IOP and sectoral iris atrophy, develops more frequently in patients with dendritic and stromal keratitis. Cataracts may develop in cases with chronic uveitis. Focal choroiditis, occlusive retinal vasculitis, and retinal detachment have been reported. However, patients with HZO rarely develop ipsilateral acute retinal necrosis (ARN); this condition is more commonly associated with zoster in dermatomes remote to the distribution of CN V.

Orbital or central nervous system involvement as a result of an occlusive arteritis may be associated with HZO. Vasculitis may lead to eyelid ptosis, orbital edema, and proptosis. Papillitis or retrobulbar optic neuritis may also develop. Cranial nerve palsies have been reported to occur in up to one third of cases of HZO, with cranial nerve III (oculomotor) most commonly affected. Cranial nerve involvement may occur within the orbit or the cavernous sinus.

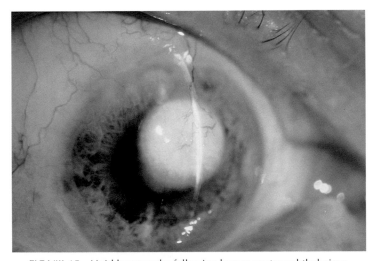

FIG VIII-15—Lipid keratopathy following herpes zoster ophthalmicus.

MANAGEMENT. Oral acyclovir therapy for HZO was found in randomized clinical trials to

□ Reduce virus shedding from vesicular skin lesions

□ Decrease systemic dissemination of virus

□ Ameliorate the incidence and severity of the most common ocular complications: dendritic keratitis, stromal keratitis, and uveitis

Unfortunately, oral acyclovir has little effect on the incidence, severity, or duration of postherpetic neuralgia.

The currently recommended dosage of oral acyclovir for HZO is 800 mg five times per day for 10 days, starting within 72 hours of the onset of skin lesions. Topical antiviral medications have not been found to be effective for treatment of HZO. Cutaneous lesions should be treated with moist compresses and topical antibiotics to loosen crusts and avoid secondary bacterial infection. Topical corticosteroids and cycloplegics may be used for stromal keratitis, disciform keratitis, or uveitis resulting in pain or decreased vision. Oral corticosteroids on a tapering dosage over 3 weeks have been recommended by dermatologists for treatment of patients with HZO, particularly those over age 60, to reduce the incidence of postherpetic neuralgia.

Postherpetic neuralgia may respond to capsaicin 0.25% ointment applied to the involved skin twice daily. Tricyclic antidepressants may also be helpful in treating postherpetic neuralgia. These medications are started initially at low doses, which are then increased if patients experience a response. Copious amounts of non-preserved topical lubricants may be useful for persistent punctate epitheliopathy. Nonpreserved lubricant ointments, bandage contact lenses, or tarsorrhaphy may be required for nonhealing neurotrophic corneal epithelial defects.

Epstein-Barr Virus Dacryoadenitis, Conjunctivitis, and Keratitis

PATHOGENESIS. Epstein-Barr virus (EBV) is a ubiquitous herpesvirus that infects the majority of humans by early adulthood. The virus is capable of establishing a persistent nonpathogenic infection in the human lacrimal gland.

CLINICAL PRESENTATION. EBV is the most common cause of acute *dacryoadenitis,* characterized by inflammatory enlargement of one or both lacrimal glands. Acute follicular conjunctivitis, Parinaud oculoglandular syndrome, and bulbar conjunctival nodules have been reported in patients with acute infectious mononucleosis caused by EBV. Multiple corneal epithelial dendrites involving the central and peripheral cornea have been reported in a patient with infectious mononucleosis, and EBV has been implicated as a causative agent of both epithelial and stromal keratitis. Several types of corneal stromal keratitis have been observed in patients with infectious mononucleosis:

□ Multiple focal anterior subepithelial infiltrates similar to those occurring in adenovirus infection

□ Multiple granular ring-shaped or nummular opacities scattered throughout the anterior midstroma (Fig VIII-16)

□ Mid- to deep peripheral stromal infiltrates with vascularization

MANAGEMENT. EBV stromal keratitis is generally self-limited; however, patients with significant irritation or reduced vision may respond to topical corticosteroids.

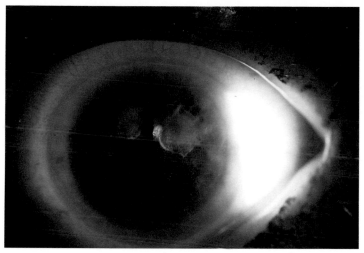

FIG VIII-16—Epstein-Barr virus stromal keratitis.

Other Viral Infections of the Ocular Surface

Mumps virus used to be a common cause of dacryoadenitis and conjunctivitis, but it has become rare because of widespread Immunization. Similarly, measles conjunctivitis and epithelial keratitis is uncommon in regions where childhood Immunization is extensive. Vaccinia blepharoconjunctivitis and epithelial keratitis, a complication of vaccination for smallpox, has also become rare with the waning of this practice.

Viruses that infect the upper respiratory tract, such as influenza virus, occasionally cause conjunctivitis, but the eye disease is mild and generally an unimportant aspect of the systemic illness. Exposure to animals can lead to unusual occurrences, such as Newcastle disease conjunctivitis among handlers of infected birds.

Microbial and Parasitic Infections of the Eyelid Margin and Conjunctiva

Staphylococcal Blepharitis

PATHOGENESIS. Inflammation of the eyelid margins, termed *blepharitis,* is one of the most common causes of external ocular irritation. Blepharitis can have an infectious or inflammatory etiology; the most common causes of blepharitis are staphylococcal infection (usually caused by *S aureus* but occasionally other species) and irritation from oily meibomian gland secretions or seborrheic blepharitis. The symptoms, signs, and treatment of infectious staphylococcal blepharoconjunctivitis and meibomian gland dysfunction overlap considerably. In general, the term *staphylococcal blepharitis* refers to cases in which bacterial infection of the eyelids (and frequently the conjunctiva) is predominant. *Meibomian gland dysfunction* and *seborrheic blepharitis* designate the presence of chronic abnormal oily secretions producing irritative effects in the eyelid margin and conjunctiva. Clinical features that may aid in the differential diagnosis of these entities are summarized in Table VIII-4.

TABLE VIII-4

	STAPHYLOCOCCAL	MEIBOMIAN GLAND DYSFUNCTION	SEBORRHEIC
Location	Anterior eyelid	Posterior eyelid	Anterior eyelid
Loss and whitening of lashes	Frequent	(–)	Rare
Eyelid crusting	Hard, fibrinous scales; hard, matted crusts (often accompany ulcerative form)	+/–	Oily or greasy
Eyelid ulceration	Occasional	(–)	(–)
Conjunctivitis	Papillary (occasionally with mucopurulent discharge)	Mild to moderate injection, papillary tarsal reaction	Mild injection, follicular or papillary tarsal reaction
Keratitis	Inferior PEE,* marginal infiltrates, vascularization, phlyctenulosis	Inferior PEE, marginal infiltrates, vascular pannus	Inferior PEE
Aqueous tear deficiency	Occasional	Occasional	Occasional
Rosacea	(–)	+ +	+

+ : 0%–33%, + + : 34%–66%.
*PEE: punctate epithelial erosions.

CLINICAL PRESENTATION. Staphylococcal blepharitis is seen more commonly in younger individuals. Symptoms include burning, itching, foreign body sensation, and crusting, particularly upon awakening. Symptoms of irritation and burning tend to peak in the morning and improve as the day progresses, presumably as the crusted material that accumulates on the eyelid margin overnight dissipates.

Typical clinical manifestations include hard, brittle fibrinous scales and hard, matted crusts surrounding individual cilia on the anterior eyelid margin (Fig VIII-17). Small ulcers of the anterior eyelid margin may be seen when the hard crusts are removed. Injection and telangiectasis of the anterior and posterior eyelid margins, white lashes (poliosis), lash loss (madarosis), and trichiasis may be seen in varying degrees, depending on the severity and duration of the blepharitis.

Aqueous tear deficiency is found in some patients with staphylococcal blepharitis. Excessive secretion of bacterially modified lipid products into the tear film can increase instability and accentuate evaporative losses, thus further compounding any associated dry eye state. See also discussion in chapter VI, pp 79–88.

Chronic conjunctivitis A unilateral or bilateral conjunctivitis that persists for more than 3 weeks is considered chronic. When conjunctivitis accompanies blepharitis, as it frequently does, the condition is known as *staphylococcal blepharoconjunctivitis*. This association is marked by a chronic papillary reaction of the tarsal conjunctiva, particularly the inferior tarsal conjunctiva near the eyelid margin, as well

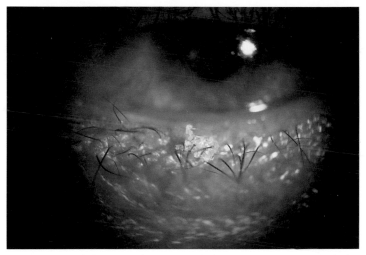

FIG VIII-17—Staphylococcal blepharitis with collarettes surrounding eyelashes.

as injection of the bulbar and tarsal conjunctiva. Chronic conjunctivitis tends to be associated with mild conjunctival injection and scant mucopurulent discharge.

Specific clinical signs are commonly seen in patients with chronic conjunctivitis caused by certain bacterial species. *S aureus* is often associated with matted golden crusts and ulcers on the anterior eyelid margin, inferior punctate keratopathy, marginal corneal infiltrates, and, rarely, conjunctival or corneal phylctenules. *Moraxella lacunata* may produce a chronic angular blepharoconjunctivitis with crusting and ulceration of the skin in the lateral canthal angle and papillary or follicular reaction on the tarsal conjunctiva. *Moraxella* angular blepharoconjunctivitis is frequently associated with concomitant *S aureus* blepharoconjunctivitis.

Conjunctival swabs for culture and sensitivity should be performed in cases that do not respond to initial empirical antibiotic therapy. In cases of persistent chronic unilateral conjunctivitis refractory to therapy, masquerade syndrome (conjunctival malignancy) and factitious illness should be ruled out.

Keratitis Several forms of keratitis may develop in association with staphylococcal blepharoconjunctivitis.

Punctate epithelial keratopathy manifests as erosions that stain with fluorescein. Frequently, the distribution of the keratopathy is mostly inferior, and it sometimes coincides with the contour of the eyelids across the corneal surface. Occasionally, a diffuse pattern may be observed, and asymmetric or unilateral keratopathy is not uncommon. The degree of corneal involvement can be markedly out of proportion to the severity of the eyelid disease, a circumstance that can lead to diagnostic confusion. Marginal corneal infiltrates may be the most distinctive clinical finding (Fig VIII-18) (see also pp 213–214).

Phlyctenulosis is sometimes observed in children and young adults with staphylococcal blepharoconjunctivitis. The appearance of phlyctenules represents a cell-

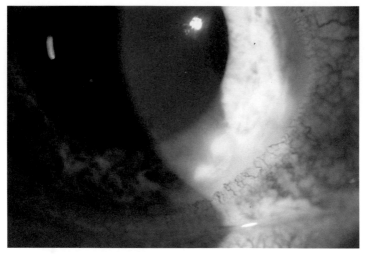

FIG VIII-18—Staphylococcal marginal corneal infiltrate.

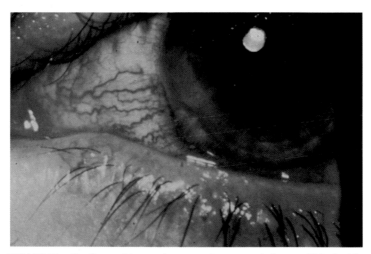

FIG VIII-19—Confluent phlyctenules secondary to staphylococcal blepharitis.

mediated, or delayed, hypersensitivity reaction to staphylococcal cell wall components. Bulbar conjunctival phlyctenules manifest as round, elevated focal inflammatory nodules fed by a leash of vessels, usually occurring at or near the limbus (Fig VIII-19). They typically become necrotic and ulcerate centrally, then spontaneously involute over a period of 2–3 weeks. Following resolution, limbus based triangular fibrovascular scars, more often on the inferior than the superior cornea, may indicate previous phlyctenulosis. Corneal involvement occurs with recurrences and centripetal migration of successive inflammatory lesions, accompanied by a wedge-shaped pannus. Occasionally, such inflammation leads to corneal thinning and, rarely, perforation.

LABORATORY EVALUATION. Eyelid and conjunctival cultures can be performed in suspected cases of staphylococcal blepharoconjunctivitis with a doubtful clinical diagnosis or a poor response to empiric treatment. Swabs should be directly plated onto prewarmed solid blood agar media (with L-shaped streaks to designate the lids and C-shaped streaks to designate the conjunctiva). If solid media is not available, specimens should be placed into transport media and immediately sent to a qualified microbiology laboratory for processing. The characteristic laboratory finding in staphylococcal blepharoconjunctivitis is a heavy, confluent growth of *Staphylococcus aureus.* Nevertheless, the finding of a light to moderate growth of bacteria and/or the isolation of staphylococcal species other than *S aureus* does not exclude the diagnosis, particularly if a predominant manifestation of the disease is punctate epithelial keratopathy, marginal infiltrates, or phlyctenulosis. Susceptibility testing may be useful in guiding treatment in cases that have been refractory to empiric antibiotic therapy.

MANAGEMENT. Treatment consists of antibacterial and anti-inflammatory measures. Eyelid hygiene, consisting of warm water or baby shampoo scrubs, may aid in reducing bacterial colonization and accumulation of sebaceous secretions. Eyelid scales or crusts can be removed with a moistened cotton-tipped applicator or a face cloth sudsed with a dilute concentration of baby shampoo. Following scrubs, a thin film of antibiotic ointments may be applied to the eyelid margins with a cotton-tipped applicator. Since aqueous tear deficiency and/or lipid-induced tear film instability is frequently present, the use of artificial tears may be beneficial.

Cases with a prominent conjunctivitis component should be treated with an antibiotic solution. Treatment for staphylococcal blepharitis is frequently prolonged and repeated, a consideration in selecting a topical antibiotic. In order to minimize toxicity and resistance, a well-tolerated, relatively narrow spectrum antimicrobial agent effective against the majority of staphylococci should be selected. Antibiotics meeting these criteria include bacitracin, erythromycin, and sulfacetamide. These agents are preferred over aminoglycosides, which can have variable activity against *Staphylococcus* and can produce corneal and conjunctival toxicity, and over fluoroquinolones, which tend to induce high-level resistance with prolonged use.

Anti-inflammatory therapy consists of limited and judicious use of mild doses of topical corticosteroids in selected cases. Corticosteroids should be reserved for patients who have a strong inflammatory component with little active infection. Patients with routine staphylococcal blepharitis or blepharoconjunctivitis may obtain more rapid symptomatic relief with the use of adjunctive topical corticosteroids, but the potential risks include prolonging or worsening the infection or inducing steroid-related side effects. Therefore, corticosteroid use in routine cases is discouraged.

Corticosteroids have little therapeutic benefit for toxic-related punctate epithelial keratopathy. In contrast, marginal infiltrates and phlyctenulosis are entities that have a strong immunologic component and can thus respond to topical corticosteroid therapy. In these cases the response to eyelid hygiene and antibiotic therapy alone should first be assessed. If after a few days (in the case of marginal infiltrates) or weeks (in the case of phlyctenulosis) the therapeutic effect is inadequate, a time-limited course of a mild dose of corticosteroid can be prescribed. Chronic or indefinite use of corticosteroids should be avoided.

Hordeoleum PATHOGENESIS. Hordeola are inflammatory or infectious nodules that develop in the eyelid. Most frequently, they result from inspissation and secondary infection of sebaceous glands. As discussed on p 73, those occurring on the anterior eyelid in the glands of Zeis or lash follicles are called *external hordeola,* or *styes.* Hordeola occurring at the posterior eyelid from meibomian gland inspissation are termed *internal hordeola.* Either type is associated with a localized purulent abscess, usually caused by *S aureus.*

CLINICAL PRESENTATION. Hordeola present as painful, tender, red nodular masses near the eyelid margin. They may rupture, producing a purulent drainage. Hordeola are generally self-limited, improving spontaneously over the course of 1–2 weeks. Internal hordeola occasionally evolve into *chalazia,* which are chronic granulomatous nodules centered around sebaceous glands, usually the meibomian glands. Chalazia are discussed on pp 71–73.

LABORATORY EVALUATION AND MANAGEMENT. Cultures are not indicated for isolated, uncomplicated cases of hordeolum. Warm compresses may relieve symptoms and facilitate drainage. Topically applied antibiotics are generally not effective and therefore not indicated unless an accompanying infectious blepharoconjunctivitis is present. Systemic antibiotics are indicated only in rare cases of secondary eyelid cellulitis. Incision and drainage may be required for large or persistent lesions.

Fungal and Parasitic Infections of the Eyelid Margin

Demodex is a genus of mites that are normal commensal parasites of humans. They can commonly be seen by slit-lamp biomicroscopy as waxy sleeves around eyelashes or as cylinders extending from sebaceous glands of the eyelid margin. The role of these parasites in the pathogenesis of blepharitis is unclear. Other organisms that survive on lipids of eyelid glands, such as *Malassezia furfur,* have also been incriminated in certain types of blepharitis.

A focal granuloma or dermatitis affecting the eyelid or conjunctiva can be caused by very rare infection, including the following:

□ Blastomycosis

□ Sporotrichosis

□ Rhinosporidiosis

□ Cryptococcosis

□ Leishmaniasis

□ Ophthalmomyiasis

Lice infestation of the eyelids and eyelashes, also known as *pediculosis* and *phthiriasis,* is an uncommon condition affecting adolescents and young adults caused by the pubic louse and its ova. Delousing of the cilia can be performed with forceps, but pubic hairs are usually treated with a pedulocide. An ointment can smother the lice. Bed linen and clothing should be cleaned and dried at the highest temperature setting.

Bacterial Conjunctivitis in Children and Adults

PATHOGENESIS. A bacterial etiology is a relatively uncommon cause of conjunctivitis. Bacterial conjunctivitis is the result of bacterial overgrowth and infiltration of the conjunctival epithelial layer and sometimes the substantia propria as well. The source of infection is either direct contact with an infected individual's secretions (usually through eye-hand contact) or the spread of infection from the organisms colonizing the patient's own nasal and sinus mucosa.

Although usually self-limited, bacterial conjunctivitis can occasionally be severe and sight-threatening when caused by virulent bacterial species such as *Neisseria gonorrhoeae* or *Streptococcus pyogenes*. In rare cases it may presage life-threatening systemic disease, as with conjunctivitis caused by *N meningitidis*. Direct infection and inflammation of the conjunctival surface, bystander effects on adjacent tissues such as the cornea, and the host's acute inflammatory response and long-term reparative response all contribute to the pathology.

CLINICAL PRESENTATION AND MANAGEMENT. Bacterial conjunctivitis should be suspected in patients with conjunctival inflammation and a purulent discharge. The rapidity of onset and severity of conjunctival inflammation and discharge are suggestive of the possible causative organism. Table VIII-5 shows the clinical classification of bacterial conjunctivitis based on these parameters.

Acute purulent conjunctivitis This form of bacterial conjunctivitis is characterized by an acute (less than 3 weeks in duration), self-limited infection of the conjunctival surface that evokes an acute inflammatory response with purulent discharge. Cases may occur spontaneously or in epidemics. The most common etiologic pathogens are *Streptococcus pneumoniae, S aureus, and H influenzae*. The relative frequency with which each of these organisms is isolated depends in part on the patient's age and geographic location.

TABLE VIII-5

CLINICAL CLASSIFICATION OF BACTERIAL CONJUNCTIVITIS

COURSE OF ONSET	SEVERITY	COMMON ORGANISMS
Slow (days to weeks)	Mild–moderate	*Staphylococcus aureus* *Moraxella lacunata* *Proteus* species Enterobacteriaceae *Pseudomonas*
Acute or subacute (hours to days)	Moderate–severe	*Haemophilus influenzae* biotype III* *Haemophilus influenzae* *Streptococcus pneumoniae* *Staphylococcus aureus*
Hyperacute (<24 hours)	Severe	*Neisseria gonorrhoeae* *Neisseria meningitidis*

*Previously referred to as *Haemophilus aegyptius*.

Streptococcus pneumoniae is usually the most common cause of acute purulent bacterial conjunctivitis. Moderate purulent discharge, eyelid edema, chemosis, conjunctival hemorrhages, and occasionally inflammatory membranes on the tarsal conjunctivae are often associated with acute conjunctivitis caused by *Streptococcus pneumoniae*. Corneal ulceration rarely occurs.

H influenzae conjunctivitis occurs in young children, sometimes in association with otitis media, and in adults, particularly those chronically colonized with *H influenzae* (e.g., smokers or patients with chronic bronchopulmonary disease). Acute purulent conjunctivitis caused by *H influenzae* biotype III (previously referred to as *H aegyptius*) resembles that caused by *Streptococcus pneumoniae*; however, conjunctival membranes do not develop, and peripheral corneal epithelial ulcers and stromal infiltrates occur more commonly.

S aureus may produce an acute blepharoconjunctivitis. The discharge tends to be somewhat less purulent than that seen in pneumococcal conjunctivitis, and the associated signs are generally less severe.

Gram-stained smears and culture of the conjunctiva need not be performed in uncomplicated cases of suspected bacterial conjunctivitis but should be performed in the following:

□ Certain compromised hosts such as neonates or debilitated or immunocompromised individuals

□ Severe cases of purulent conjunctivitis to differentiate it from hyperpurulent conjunctivitis, which generally requires systemic therapy

□ Cases unresponsive to initial therapy

Most cases of acute purulent conjunctivitis can be managed with empiric antibiotic therapy. However, most cases of infectious conjunctivitis are viral in etiology. Therefore, uncomplicated cases that are equivocal or cases likely to represent a viral conjunctivitis should *not* be routinely treated with empiric antibiotics. If empiric antibiotic therapy is prescribed, it should be based on the Gram-stained morphology of the conjunctival smear, if available. Cultures of the nose or throat may be performed if an associated sinusitis or pharyngitis is present. Even if no overt sinusitis, rhinitis, or pharyngitis is present, nasal or throat swabs should be considered in cases of relapsing conjunctivitis, because the persistence of organisms colonizing the respiratory mucosa may be the source of infection.

Acute purulent conjunctivitis caused by gram-positive organisms should be treated with topical erythromycin or polymyxin B/bacitracin ointment or polymyxin B/trimethoprim solution. Cases with gram-negative coccobacilli on Gram-stained smears are probably caused by *Haemophilus* species and should be treated with polymyxin B/trimethoprim. Topical aminoglycosides or ciprofloxacin should be reserved for cases refractory to initial therapy. Supplemental oral antibiotics are recommended for patients with acute purulent conjunctivitis associated with pharyngitis, for conjunctivitis-otitis syndrome, and for *Haemophilus* conjunctivitis in children.

Gonococcal conjunctivitis   This condition presents with the explosive onset of severe purulent conjunctivitis: massive exudation; severe chemosis; and in untreated cases corneal infiltrates, melting, and perforation. The organism most commonly responsible for hyperpurulent conjunctivitis is *Neisseria gonorrhoeae* (Fig VIII-20). Gonococcal conjunctivitis is a sexually transmitted disease resulting from direct genital-eye transmission, genital-hand-ocular contact, or maternal-neonate transmission during vaginal delivery.

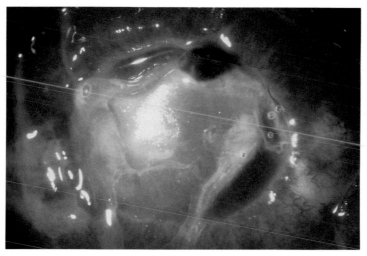

FIG VIII-20—Peripheral corneal ulceration and perforation occurring several days after onset of hyperacute conjunctivitis caused by *N gonorrhoeae.*

The disease is characterized by rapid progression, copious purulent conjunctival discharge, marked conjunctival hyperemia and chemosis, and eyelid edema. Gonococcal conjunctivitis may be associated with preauricular lymphadenopathy and the formation of conjunctival membranes. Keratitis, the principal cause of sight-threatening complications, has been reported to occur in 15%–40% of cases. Corneal involvement may consist of diffuse epithelial haze, epithelial defects, marginal infiltrates, and peripheral ulcerative infectious keratitis that can rapidly progress to perforation.

Gonococcal conjunctivitis should be treated with systemic antibiotics. Topical ocular antibiotics can supplement but not replace systemic therapy. Current treatment regimens for gonococcal conjunctivitis reflect the increasing prevalence of penicillin-resistant *N gonorrhoeae* (PRNG) in the United States. Ceftriaxone, a third-generation cephalosporin, is highly effective against PRNG. Gonococcal conjunctivitis without corneal ulceration may be treated on an outpatient basis with one intramuscular ceftriaxone (1 g) injection. Patients with corneal ulceration should be admitted to the hospital and treated with intravenous ceftriaxone (1 g IV every 12 hours) for 3 consecutive days. Patients with penicillin allergy can be given spectinomycin (2 g IM) or oral fluoroquinolones (ciprofloxacin 500 mg or ofloxacin 400 mg orally bid for 5 days).

Erythromycin ointment, bacitracin ointment, gentamicin ointment, and ciprofloxacin solution have been recommended for topical therapy. Just as important as systemic therapy for the treatment of severe cases is the copious, frequent (every 30–60 minutes) irrigation of the conjunctival sac with normal saline. Such lavages help to remove inflammatory cells, proteases, and debris that may be toxic to the ocular surface and contribute to corneal melting.

Up to one third of patients with gonococcal conjunctivitis have been reported to have concurrent chlamydial venereal disease. Because of this frequent association, it is advisable to place patients on supplemental oral antibiotics for treatment of chlamydial infection. These medications include tetracycline 500 mg orally qid for 1 week, doxycycline 100 mg orally bid for 1 week, minocycline 100 mg orally bid for 1 week, erythromycin 250 mg qid for 1 week, or azithromycin 1 g orally once.

Preferred Practice Patterns Committee, Cornea Panel. *Conjunctivitis.* San Francisco: American Academy of Ophthalmology; 1998.

Bacterial Conjunctivitis in Neonates

Neisseria gonorrhoeae causes the most severe neonatal conjunctivitis. Fortunately, *N gonorrhoeae* is currently responsible for fewer than 1% of all cases of neonatal conjunctivitis in the industrialized countries. In order of decreasing prevalence, the causes of neonatal conjunctivitis are as follows:

- *Chlamydia trachomatis*
- *Streptococcus viridans*
- *Staphylococcus aureus*
- *Haemophilus influenzae*
- Group D *Streptococcus*
- *Moraxella catarrhalis*
- *Escherichia coli* and other gram-negative rods
- *Neisseria gonorrhoeae*

Neonatal gonococcal conjunctivitis The infrequency of neonatal gonococcal conjunctivitis has been attributed to effective prenatal screening for maternal gonococcal genital infection and prophylactic antimicrobial therapy for conjunctivitis in newborns. Infants with gonococcal conjunctivitis typically develop bilateral conjunctival discharge 3–5 days after parturition. The discharge may be serosanguineous during the first several days, and a copious purulent exudate may develop later. Corneal ulceration, corneal perforation, and endophthalmitis have been reported as complications of untreated neonatal gonococcal conjunctivitis. Infected infants may also have other localized gonococcal infections including rhinitis and proctitis. Disseminated gonococcal infection with arthritis, meningitis, pneumonia, and sepsis resulting in death of the infant is a rare complication.

The currently recommended treatment for neonatal gonococcal conjunctivitis is a single intramuscular ceftriaxone (125 mg) injection or cefotaxime (25 mg/kg) IV or IM every 8–12 hours for 7 days. Either of these regimens should be combined with saline irrigation of the conjunctiva and application of topical erythromycin ointment.

Neonatal chlamydial conjunctivitis Chlamydial conjunctivitis in neonates differs clinically from adult chlamydial conjunctivitis in the following ways:

- No follicular response appears in newborns
- The amount of mucopurulent discharge is greater in newborns
- Membranes on the tarsal conjunctiva can develop in newborns
- Intracytoplasmic inclusions are seen in a greater percentage of Giemsa-stained conjunctival specimens in newborns
- The infection in newborns is more likely to respond to topical medications

Both Gram and Giemsa stains of conjunctival scrapings are recommended in neonates with conjunctivitis to identify *C trachomatis* and *N gonorrhoeae*, as well as other bacteria as causative agents. Other *Chlamydia*-associated infections such as pneumonitis and otitis media can accompany inclusion conjunctivitis in the newborn. Therefore, systemic erythromycin (12.5 mg/kg oral or IV qid for 14 days) is recommended, even though inclusion conjunctivitis in the newborn usually responds to topical erythromycin or sulfacetamide.

Chlamydial Conjunctivitis

PATHOGENESIS. *Chlamydia trachomatis* is an obligate intracellular bacterium that causes several different conjunctivitis syndromes, each is associated with different serotypes of *C trachomatis:*

□ Trachoma: serotypes A–C

□ Adult and neonatal inclusion conjunctivitis: serotypes D–K

□ Lymphogranuloma venereum: serotypes L1, L2, and L3

Rare cases of keratoconjunctivitis in humans have been reported caused by *Chlamydia* species that typically infect animals, such as *Chlamydia psittaci,* an agent generally associated with disease in parrots, and the feline pneumonitis agent.

CLINICAL PRESENTATION AND MANAGEMENT. Trachoma and adult inclusion conjunctivitis are discussed individually below.

Trachoma   Trachoma is an infectious disease occurring in communities with poor hygiene and inadequate sanitation. It affects approximately 400 million individuals worldwide and is the leading cause of preventable blindness. Trachoma is currently endemic to the Middle East and In impoverished regions of many countries. In the United States it occurs sporadically among American Indians and in mountainous areas of the South. Evidence suggests that the common housefly and other household fomites are important vectors for transmitting *Chlamydia,* and patients with trachoma are repeatedly infected. Other bacteria that cause secondary bacterial infections in patients with trachoma are spread by these fomites as well.

The initial symptoms of trachoma include foreign body sensation, redness, tearing, and mucopurulent discharge. A severe follicular reaction develops, most prominently in the superior tarsus conjunctiva but sometimes appearing in the superior and inferior fornices, inferior tarsal conjunctiva, semilunar fold, and limbus. In acute trachoma, follicles on the superior tarsus may be obscured by diffuse papillary hypertrophy and inflammatory cell infiltration. Large tarsal follicles in trachoma may become necrotic and eventually heal with significant scarring. Linear or stellate scarring of the superior tarsus (*Arlt's line*) typically occurs (Fig VIII-21). Involution and necrosis of follicles may result in limbal depressions known as *Herbert's pits* (Fig VIII-22). Corneal findings in trachoma include epithelial keratitis, focal and multifocal peripheral and central stromal infiltrates, and superficial fibrovascular pannus, which is most prominent in the superior third of the cornea but may extend centrally into the visual axis (Fig VIII-23).

Clinical diagnosis of trachoma requires at least two of the following clinical features:

□ Conjunctival follicles on the upper tarsal conjunctiva

□ Limbal follicles and their sequelae (Herbert's pits)

□ Typical tarsal conjunctival scarring

□ Vascular pannus most marked on the superior limbus

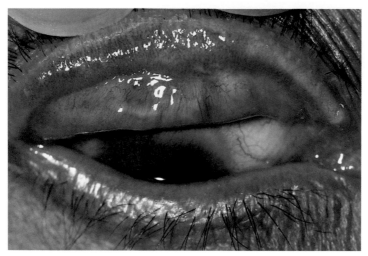

FIG VIII-21—Linear scarring of the superior tarsal conjunctiva (Arlt's line) in a patient with old trachoma.

Severe conjunctival and lacrimal gland duct scarring from chronic trachoma can result in aqueous tear deficiency, tear drainage obstruction, trichiasis, and entropion.

The World Health Organization (WHO) has introduced a simple severity grading system for trachoma based on the presence or absence of five key signs:

- Follicular conjunctival inflammation
- Diffuse conjunctival inflammation
- Tarsal conjunctival scarring
- Trichiasis
- Corneal opacification

The WHO grading system was developed for use by trained personnel other than ophthalmologists to assess the prevalence and severity of trachoma in population-based surveys in endemic areas.

Thylefors B, Dawson CR, Jones BR, et al. A simple system for the assessment of trachoma and its complications. *Bull World Health Organ.* 1987;65:477–483.

Active trachoma is treated with topical and oral tetracycline or erythromycin. Topical tetracycline 1% or erythromycin ointment should be administered twice daily for 2 months. Oral tetracycline in a dosage of 1.5–2.0 g daily in divided doses should be administered for 3 weeks. Erythromycin is recommended for treatment of the rare cases of trachoma that are clinically resistant to tetracycline. Azithromycin, a long-acting macrolide, may have utility for mass treatment programs because of the prolonged duration of action of single-dose administration. The management of the complications of trachoma may include tear substitutes for dry eye and eyelid procedures for entropian or trichiasis.

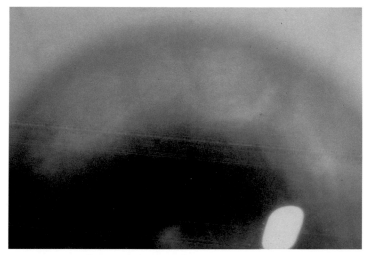

FIG VIII-22—Trachoma exhibiting Herbert's pits of the superior limbus (round to oval, relatively lucent areas within pannus).

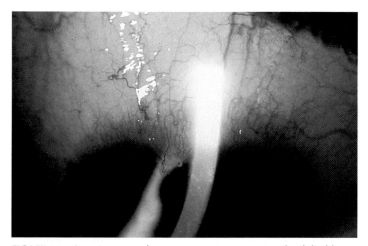

FIG VIII-23—Superior corneal micropannus in a patient with adult chlamydial conjunctivitis.

Adult chlamydial conjunctivitis This sexually transmitted disease is often found in conjunction with chlamydial urethritis or cervicitis. It is most prevalent in sexually active adolescents and young adults. The eye is usually infected by direct or indirect contact with infected genital secretions, although other modes of transmission may include shared eye cosmetics and inadequately chlorinated swimming pools. Onset of conjunctivitis is typically 1–2 weeks after ocular inoculation and is not as acute as adenovirus keratoconjunctivitis. Often patients may complain of mild symptoms for weeks to months.

External signs of adult inclusion conjunctivitis include a follicular conjunctival response that is most prominent in the lower palpebral conjunctiva and fornix, scant mucopurulent discharge, and palpable preauricular adenopathy. Follicles in the bulbar conjunctiva and semilunar fold are frequently present, and these are a helpful and specific sign in patients who have not been using topical medications associated with development of bulbar follicles. Inflammatory conjunctival membranes do not develop in chlamydial keratoconjunctivitis.

Corneal involvement may consist of fine or coarse epithelial infiltrates, occasionally associated with subepithelial infiltrates. The keratitis is more likely to be found in the superior cornea but may also occur centrally and resemble adenovirus keratitis. A micropannus, usually extending less than 3 mm from the superior cornea, may develop.

Left untreated, adult chlamydial conjunctivitis often resolves spontaneously in 6–18 months. Currently, one of the following antibiotic regimens is recommended:

□ Oral tetracycline 250 mg qid for 3 weeks

□ Doxycycline 100 mg bid for 3 weeks

□ Oral erythromycin 500 mg qid for 3 weeks

A single oral dose of azithromycin 1 g may be effective. Patients with laboratory-confirmed chlamydial conjunctivitis and their sexual contacts should be evaluated for coinfection with other sexually transmitted diseases such as syphilis or gonorrhea before antibiotic treatment is started. Sexual partners should be concomitantly treated to avoid reinfection.

Cat-Scratch Disease

Granulomatous conjunctivitis with regional lymphadenopathy is a very uncommon condition called *Parinaud oculoglandular syndrome.* Cat-scratch disease accounts for most cases, but other rare causes include the following:

□ Tularemia

□ Lymphogranuloma venereum

□ Tuberculosis

□ Sporotrichosis

□ Syphilis

□ Mediterranean spotted fever

PATHOGENESIS. *Bartonella henselae* lives on cats and their fleas and can apparently be transferred to human skin or mucous membrane by a scratch or bite. Local infection causes a granulomatous reaction. Systemic spread from a skin lesion can result in encephalitis and optic neuritis.

CLINICAL PRESENTATION. Unilateral follicular conjunctivitis with one or more gelatinous lesions develops on the conjunctiva about 1 week after inoculation; 1–2 weeks later preauricular, submandibular, and cervical nodes enlarge and can become suppurative.

LABORATORY EVALUATION. Most cases are diagnosed by histopathologic examination of a conjunctival biopsy. A reference laboratory can help to identify the organism by culture or PCR. Specific antibody can also be detected.

MANAGEMENT. Oral antibacterial treatment generally includes erythromycin, doxycycline, or a fluoroquinolone.

Microsporidal Keratoconjunctivitis

Microsporida are intracellular protozoa that can infect the conjunctival and corneal epithelium in immunosuppressed individuals with AIDS. Patients may also have disseminated microsporidiosis involving the sinuses, respiratory tract, or gastrointestinal tract.

Encephalitozoon hellem and *E cuniculi* cannot be seen within the conjunctiva, although chronic conjunctivitis is typical. Punctate epithelial keratopathy is manifested by a coarse granularity of the corneal epithelium that extends to the limbus. The corneal stroma remains clear, with no or minimal iritis. Scrapings of the ocular surface can be stained to reveal acid-fast spores. Electron microscopy is used to classify the spores and meronts. Medical treatment includes topical fumagillin and oral albendazole.

Loiasis

Conjunctivitis can be caused by *Loa loa* and other subconjunctival nematodes that burrow subcutaneously after the bite of an infected vector. A migrating worm moves under the skin at about 1 cm/min but is most conspicuous when it is seen or felt wriggling under the bulbar conjunctiva. Extraction of the filarial worm cures the conjunctivitis; it is followed by antiparasitic treatment for widespread infestation.

Microbial and Parasitic Infections of the Cornea and Sclera

Bacterial Keratitis

Bacterial infection is a common sight-threatening condition. Some cases have explosive onset and rapidly progressive stromal inflammation. Untreated, it often leads to progressive tissue destruction with corneal perforation or extension of infection to adjacent tissue. Bacterial keratitis is frequently associated with risk factors that disturb the corneal epithelial integrity. Common predisposing factors include the following:

□ Contact lens wear

□ Trauma

□ Contaminated ocular medications

□ Impaired defense mechanisms

□ Altered structure of the corneal surface

The most frequent risk factor for bacterial keratitis in the United States is contact lens wear, which has been identified as such in 19%–42% of patients who develop culture-proven microbial keratitis. Epidemiologic studies have estimated the annual incidence of cosmetic contact lens–related ulcerative keratitis at 0.21% for individuals using extended-wear soft lenses and 0.04% for patients using daily-wear soft lenses. The risk of developing microbial keratitis increases significantly (approximately tenfold) in patients who wear their contact lenses overnight and is positively correlated with the number of consecutive days lenses are worn without removal.

PATHOGENESIS. Bacteria have multiple mechanisms of adherence. For example, *S aureus* uses adhesins to bind to collagen and other components of the exposed Bowman's layer and stroma, while *P aeruginosa* can bind to molecular receptors exposed on injured epithelial cells. A clone of bacteria initially proliferates, then—within hours—invades the cornea between stromal lamellae. Corneal inflammation begins with the local production of cytokines and chemokines that enable diapedesis and migration of neutrophils into the peripheral cornea from the limbal vessels. Some microorganisms produce proteases that disrupt the extracellular matrix. Enzymes released by neutrophils and activation of corneal matrix metalloproteinases exacerbate inflammatory necrosis. With antimicrobial control of bacterial replication, wound healing processes begin that may be accompanied by neovascularization and scarring. Progressive inflammation, on the other hand, may lead to corneal perforation.

CLINICAL PRESENTATION. Rapid onset of pain is accompanied by conjunctival injection, photophobia, and decreased vision in patients with bacterial corneal ulcers. The rate of progression of these symptoms depends on the virulence of the infecting organism. Bacterial corneal ulcers typically show a sharp epithelial demarcation with underlying dense, suppurative stromal inflammation that has indistinct edges and is surrounded by stromal edema. *P aeruginosa* typically produces stromal necrosis with a shaggy surface and adherent mucopurulent exudate (Fig VIII-24). An endothelial inflammatory plaque, marked anterior chamber reaction, and hypopyon frequently occur.

Infections caused by slow-growing, fastidious organisms such as mycobacteria or anaerobes may have a nonsuppurative infiltrate and intact epithelium. Infectious crystalline keratitis, an example of this type of infection, presents as densely packed, white branching aggregates of organisms in the virtual absence of a host inflammatory response. It is believed to develop when a sequestered colony of slow-growing organisms develops after midstromal implantation in a cornea with compromised inflammatory responses. Corticosteroid use, contact lens use, and infections in a

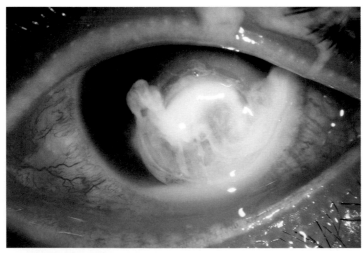

FIG VIII-24—Suppurative ulcerative keratitis caused by *P aeruginosa*.

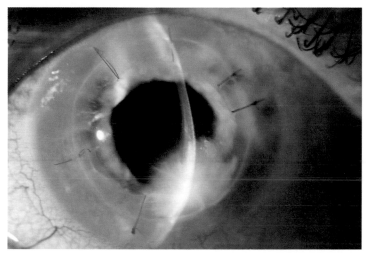

FIG VIII-25—Infectious crystalline keratopathy in a corneal graft caused by α-hemolytic *Streptococcus* species.

corneal graft can all create a predisposition to this infection. Infectious crystalline keratopathy has been reported with a number of bacterial species, most commonly α-hemolytic *Streptococcus* species (Fig VIII-25).

LABORATORY EVALUATION. A wide variety of bacterial species may cause microbial keratitis. The prevalence of a particular causative organism depends on the geographic location and risk factors for the infection. Common and uncommon organisms causing bacterial keratitis are listed in Table VIII-6.

Because keratitis can be caused by a wide variety of organisms, many of which have unique antimicrobial sensitivity profiles, it can be difficult to determine clinically whether a corneal ulcer has an infectious etiology. Prior to initiating anti-

TABLE VIII-6

CAUSES OF BACTERIAL KERATITIS

COMMON ORGANISMS	UNCOMMON ORGANISMS
Staphylococcus aureus	*Neisseria* species
Staphylococcus epidermidis	*Moraxella* species
Streptococcus pneumoniae and other *Streptococcus* species	*Mycobacterium* species
	Nocardia species
Pseudomonas aeruginosa (most common organism in soft contact lens wearers)	Non-spore-forming anaerobes
	Corynebacterium species
Enterobacteriaceae *(Proteus, Enterobacter, Serratia)*	

microbial therapy for cases of suspected bacterial keratitis, the clinician should conduct microbiological diagnostic tests.

Traditionally, a Kimura spatula has been used to scrape the area of corneal involvement to obtain specimens for stained smears and cultures. However, swabs have been reported to be as effective as a spatula for culturing corneal ulcers. Because growth patterns on culture media vary among different bacterial species, the material obtained from the corneal ulcer should be used to inoculate microscope slides for stained smears and several different culture media (Table VIII-7). This wide-ranging approach may aid in recovery and identification of the causative organism. A Gram stain is usually sufficient to identify most bacterial species. Additional diagnostic stains may be indicated for rare bacterial species (mycobacteria), *Acanthamoeba,* and fungi. Mycobacteria are frequently identified in acid-fast stains, whereas acridine orange and calcofluor white are excellent for amoebae and fungi.

If the patient has already been treated with topical antibiotics, the medication should be stopped for 12–24 hours prior to culturing in order to enhance recovery of viable organisms. However, antimicrobial therapy should not be discontinued in severe or rapidly progressive corneal ulcers. An antibiotic removal device, which contains resins to bind antibiotics that might inhibit bacterial growth, may be considered in these cases.

In addition to culturing cornea, it is often helpful to culture the eyelids, conjunctiva, topical ocular medications, contact lenses, and contact lens cases and solutions as well, because any of these might provide a clue to the causative organ-

TABLE VIII-7

RECOMMENDED STAINS AND CULTURE MEDIA FOR MICROBIAL KERATITIS

SUSPECTED ORGANISM	STAIN	MEDIA
Aerobic bacteria	Gram Acridine orange	Blood agar Chocolate agar Thioglycollate broth
Anaerobic bacteria	Gram Acridine orange	Anaerobic blood agar Phenylethyl alcohol agar in anaerobic chamber Thioglycollate broth
Mycobacteria	Gram Acid-fast Lectin	Blood agar Lowenstein-Jensen agar
Fungi	Gram Acridine orange Calcofluor white	Blood agar (25°C) Sabouraud agar (25°C) Brain-heart infusion (25°C)
Acanthamoeba	Acridine orange Calcofluor white	Nonnutrient agar with *E coli* overlay Blood agar Buffered charcoal-yeast extract agar

ism in the event that corneal cultures are negative. This approach can also help identify the source of the infection.

MANAGEMENT. Currently, no single antibiotic agent is effective against all bacterial species causing microbial keratitis. If one type of bacteria is identified on a stained diagnostic smear, then appropriate single-agent antimicrobial therapy can be considered (Table VIII-8). If no organisms, rare bacteria, or multiple types of bacteria are visualized on stained smears, then initial broad-spectrum antibiotic therapy is indicated.

The route of antibiotic administration should be based on the severity of the keratitis. Frequent (every 15–30 minutes) fortified topical antibiotics are now used for bacterial keratitis. Fortified antibiotic solutions produce therapeutic antibiotic concentrations in the corneal stroma, while commercially available antibiotic solutions may result in subtherapeutic stromal antibiotic concentrations. In severe cases therapeutic stromal concentrations of antibiotic may be achieved more rapidly by initially administering the antibiotic drop every 5 minutes for 30 minutes as a loading dose. Subconjunctival and IV antibiotics in addition to frequent topical antibiotics are indicated in cases with suspected scleral and/or intraocular extension of infection. A collagen corneal shield can be used to enhance tear film retention and corneal drug penetration.

Modification of initial antimicrobial therapy should be based on clinical response, not the results of antimicrobial sensitivity testing. Determination of antibiotic sensitivity or resistance in traditional antimicrobial sensitivity tests is based on antibiotic concentrations achievable in the serum by oral or parenteral administration. Often, antibiotic concentrations greatly exceeding the mean inhibitory concentrations of bacteria are achieved in the corneal stroma following frequent fortified antibiotic administration. An alternate antibiotic regimen should be considered in patients who do not show clinical response or who develop toxicity from the agent(s) used initially. Modification of antibiotic therapy in these cases should be based on antimicrobial sensitivity testing. Several clinical parameters are useful to monitor clinical response to antibiotic therapy:

□ Blunting of the perimeter of the stromal infiltrate

□ Decreased density of the stromal infiltrate

□ Reduction of stromal edema and endothelial inflammatory plaque

□ Reduction in anterior chamber inflammation

□ Reepithelialization

The frequency of topical antibiotic administration should slowly be tapered as the stromal inflammation resolves.

Combination therapy with cefazolin or vancomycin and an aminoglycoside (tobramycin or gentamicin) provides excellent broad-spectrum antimicrobial coverage, and this approach remains the mainstay of therapy. The antibiotics should initially be given every hour, then tapered in frequency according to the clinical response. Fortified antibiotics can generally be discontinued after 10–14 days, and a broad-spectrum, nonfortified antibiotic given four times daily can be substituted during the final, additional week of therapy. Disadvantages of fortified antibiotics include ocular irritation, cost, and the inconvenience of extemporaneously preparing a non–commercially available solution.

TABLE VIII-8

INITIAL THERAPY OF BACTERIAL KERATITIS

ORGANISM	ANTIBIOTIC	TOPICAL DOSE	SUBCONJUNCTIVAL DOSE
Gram-positive cocci	Cefazolin	50 mg/ml	100 mg in 0.5 ml
	Vancomycin*	50 mg/ml	25 mg in 0.5 ml
Gram-negative rods	Tobramycin	9–14 mg/ml	20 mg in 0.5 ml
	Ceftazidime	50 mg/ml	100 mg in 0.5 ml
	Fluoroquinolones	3 mg/ml	Not available
No organism or multiple types of organisms	Cefazolin with	50 mg/ml	100 mg in 0.5 ml
	Tobramycin or	9–14 mg/ml	20 mg in 0.5 ml
	Fluoroquinolones	3 mg/ml	Not available
Gram-negative cocci	Ceftriaxone	50 mg/ml	100 mg in 0.5 ml
	Ceftazidime	50 mg/ml	
Mycobacteria	Amikacin	20 mg/ml	20 mg in 0.5 ml

*For resistant *Staphylococcus* species.

Notes for Table VIII-8: Preparation of Topical Antibiotics

Cefazolin 50 mg/ml
1. Add 9.2 ml of Tears Naturale artificial tears to a vial of cefazolin in 1 g (powder for injection).
2. Dissolve. Take 5 ml of this solution and add it to 5 ml of artificial tears.
3. Refrigerate and shake well before instillation.

Vancomycin 50 mg/ml
1. Add 10 ml of 0.9% sodium chloride for injection USP (no preservatives) or artificial tears to a 500-mg vial of vancomycin to produce a solution of 50 mg/ml.
2. Refrigerate and shake well before instillation.

Ceftazidime 50 mg/ml
1. Add 9.2 ml of artificial tears to a vial of ceftazidime 1 g (powder for injection).
2. Dissolve. Take 5 ml of this solution and add it to 5 ml of artificial tears.
3. Refrigerate and shake well before instillation.

Tobramycin 14 mg/ml
1. Withdraw 2 ml of tobramycin injectable vial (40 mg/ml).
2. Add 2 ml to a tobramycin ophthalmic solution (5 ml) to give a 14 mg/ml solution.
3. Refrigerate and shake well before instillation.

An alternative to combination therapy is the use of fluoroquinolone monotherapy, which is most appropriate in compliant patients with less severe ulcers (e.g., less than 3 mm in diameter, midperipheral or peripheral, and not associated with thinning to greater than 50% of stromal thickness). Fluoroquinolones (e.g., ciprofloxacin 0.3%, ofloxacin 0.3%) must be administered every hour to maximize therapeutic effect. Because first-generation fluoroquinolones such as ciprofloxacin and ofloxacin typically have variable activity against streptococci, documented streptococcal infections should be treated with a cell wall–active agent (e.g., cefazolin, vancomycin, or penicillin G) rather than a fluoroquinolone, regardless of in vitro susceptibility data that may suggest fluoroquinolone susceptibility.

Corticosteroids The role of corticosteroid therapy for bacterial keratitis is controversial. It is well recognized that tissue destruction in microbial keratitis is a result of a combination of the direct effects of lytic enzymes and toxins produced by the infecting organism as well as the damage caused by the inflammatory reaction directed at the microorganisms. An intense suppurative inflammatory reaction consisting predominantly of polymorphonuclear leukocytes is induced by many of the bacteria that cause microbial keratitis. Neutrophils are capable of causing significant tissue destruction by generation of free radicals as well as liberation of proteolytic enzymes, including collagenases and gelatinases that will dissolve the corneal stroma. The rationale for use of corticosteroids for bacterial keratitis is to decrease the tissue destruction caused by these neutrophils.

Several studies using animal models of bacterial keratitis have demonstrated that concurrent use of topical corticosteroids does not impair the killing effect of bactericidal antibiotics against susceptible microorganisms. Clinical series evaluating the effectiveness of corticosteroids for treatment of human bacterial keratitis have reported either no treatment effect or more rapid resolution of stromal inflammation than resulted from antibiotic therapy alone.

However, the use of topical corticosteroids following presumed resolution of Gram-negative bacterial keratitis (especially that caused by *P aeruginosa*) has been documented to promote a relapse of the infection. Presumably, virulent organisms that require a low inoculum to establish infection may remain viable in small numbers for some time following clinical resolution of the infection. If the immune system is impaired by administration of topical corticosteroids before clearance of these organisms can be effected, recurrent infection may result. Topical corticosteroids should therefore be used for treatment of bacterial keratitis with extreme caution and only in exceptional circumstances. Recommendations have been made that the following requisites be met prior to instituting corticosteroid therapy for bacterial keratitis:

□ Corticosteroids should not be used in the initial phase of the treatment, at least until an etiologic organism has been identified, the organism shows in vitro sensitivity to the antibiotics used for treatment, and the patient has shown a favorable clinical response to antibiotic therapy

□ The patient must be able to return for frequent follow-up examinations

□ The infection is not caused by *P aeruginosa* or other virulent or difficult-to-eradicate organism

Corticosteroid drops may be started in moderate dosages (prednisolone acetate or phosphate 1% every 4–6 hours), and the patient should be monitored at 24 and 48 hours after initiation of therapy. If the patient shows no adverse effects, the frequency of administration may possibly be increased for a short period of time, then the medication can be tapered based on the clinical response.

Surgery Penetrating keratoplasty for treatment of bacterial keratitis is indicated if the disease progresses despite therapy, descemetocele formation or perforation occurs, or the keratitis is unresponsive to antimicrobial therapy. The involved area should be identified preoperatively, and an attempt should be made to circumscribe all areas of infection. Peripheral iridectomies are indicated, since patients may develop seclusion of the pupil from inflammatory pupillary membranes. Interrupted sutures are recommended. The patient should be treated with appropriate antibiotics, cycloplegics, and intense topical corticosteroids postoperatively. See chapters XXIII–XXIV for a discussion of penetrating keratoplasty in greater detail.

Matoba AY. Infectious keratitis. In: *Focal Points: Clinical Modules for Ophthalmologists.* San Francisco: American Academy of Ophthalmology; 1992;10:8.

Poggio EC, Glynn RJ, Schein OD, et al. The incidence of ulcerative keratitis among users of daily-wear and extended-wear soft contact lenses. *N Engl J Med.* 1989; 321:779–783.

Preferred Practice Patterns Committee, Cornea Panel. *Bacterial Keratititis.* San Francisco: American Academy of Ophthalmology; 1995.

Schein OD, Glynn RJ, Poggio EC, et al. The relative risk of ulcerative keratitis among users of daily-wear and extended-wear soft contact lenses. A case-control study. Microbial Keratitis Study Group. *N Engl J Med.* 1989;321:773–778.

Stern GA, Buttross M. Use of corticosteroids in combination with antimicrobial drugs in the treatment of infectious corneal disease. *Ophthalmology.* 1991;98:847–853.

Fungal Keratitis

PATHOGENESIS. Fungal keratitis is less common than bacterial keratitis, generally representing less than 5%–10% of corneal infections in reported clinical series from the United States. Filamentous fungal keratitis occurs more frequently in warmer, more humid parts of the United States than in other regions of the country. Trauma to the cornea with plant or vegetable material is the leading risk factor for fungal keratitis. Another risk factor is corticosteroid therapy; corticosteroids appear to reduce the resistance of the cornea to fungal infection and potentiate existing fungal infections of the cornea. The frequent use of topical corticosteroids during the past three decades has been implicated as a cause of the increased incidence of fungal keratitis during that period.

CLINICAL PRESENTATION. Patients with fungal keratitis tend to have fewer inflammatory signs and symptoms during the initial period than those with bacterial keratitis. Filamentous fungal keratitis frequently manifests as a gray-white, dry-appearing infiltrate that has a delicate filamentous or feathery edge (Fig VIII-26). Superficial lesions may appear as gray-white strands elevating the surface of the cornea. Occasionally, multifocal or satellite infiltrates may be present, although these are less common than previously reported. Large or deep fungal infiltrates are often accompanied by an endothelial plaque and hypopyon.

As the keratitis progresses, intense suppuration may develop and the lesions may resemble bacterial keratitis. At this point rapidly progressive hypopyon and anterior chamber inflammatory membranes may develop. Extension of fungal infection into the anterior chamber is often seen in cases with rapidly progressive anterior chamber inflammation. Occasionally, fungus may invade the iris or posterior chamber, and angle-closure glaucoma may develop from inflammatory pupillary block. See also BCSC Section 10, *Glaucoma.*

Yeast keratitis is most frequently caused by *Candida* species. This form of fungal keratitis manifests as a focal, dense suppuration that resembles keratitis induced by gram-positive bacteria.

MANAGEMENT. Natamycin 5% suspension is recommended for treatment of most cases of filamentous fungal keratitis, particularly those caused by *Fusarium* spp, which are the most common causative agents for exogenous fungal keratitis occurring in the southern United States. Topical miconazole 10% is the agent of choice to combat *Paecilomyces lilacinus.* Topical amphotericin B 0.15% solution is recom-

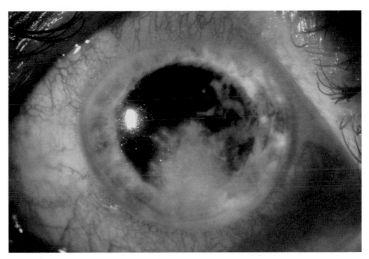

FIG VIII-26—Fungal keratitis caused by *Fusarium solani* with characteristic dry white stromal infiltrate with feathery edges.

mended for filamentous keratitis caused by *Aspergillus* spp as well as yeast keratitis. Oral ketoconazole (200–600 mg/day) should be considered as adjunctive therapy for severe filamentous fungal keratitis, and oral fluconazole (200–400 mg/day) for severe yeast keratitis.

Mechanical debridement may be beneficial for cases of superficial fungal keratitis. Fungal infiltration of the deep corneal stroma is frequently unresponsive to topical antifungal therapy, since the penetration of these agents is poor. Cases with progressive disease despite maximal topical and/or oral antifungal therapy may require therapeutic penetrating keratoplasty to prevent scleral or intraocular extension of the fungal infection. Both of these conditions carry a very poor prognosis for salvaging the eye.

Acanthamoeba *Keratitis*

PATHOGENESIS. Acanthamoebae are free-living ubiquitous protozoa found in freshwater and soil. They are resistant to killing by freezing, desiccation, and levels of chlorine routinely used in municipal water supplies, swimming pools, and hot tubs. They may exist as mobile trophozoites or dormant cysts. The majority (70%) of reported cases of amoebic keratitis have been associated with contact lens use. Homemade saline solution prepared by dissolving saline tablets in distilled water appeared to be the source of infecting *Acanthamoeba* in many cases of contact lens–related amoebic keratitis until saline tablets were taken off the U.S. market in the 1980s.

CLINICAL PRESENTATION. Patients with amoebic keratitis commonly have severe ocular pain, photophobia, and a protracted, progressive course. Frequently, they have shown no therapeutic response to a variety of topical antimicrobial agents. *Acanth-*

amoeba infection is often localized to the corneal epithelium in early cases and may manifest as a diffuse punctate epitheliopathy or dendritic epithelial lesion. Cases with epithelial dendrites are often misdiagnosed as herpetic keratitis and treated with antiviral agents and/or corticosteroids. Stromal infection typically occurs in the central cornea, and early cases have a gray-white superficial nonsuppurative infiltrate. As the disease progresses, a partial or complete ring infiltrate in the paracentral cornea is frequently observed (Fig VIII-27). Enlarged corneal nerves termed *radial perineuritis* may be noted as well as focal nodular or diffuse scleritis.

LABORATORY EVALUATION. Diagnosis of *Acanthamoeba* keratitis is made by visualizing amoebae in stained smears or by culturing organisms obtained from corneal scrapings. The highest diagnostic yield occurs relatively early in the course of the disease, when the organisms are localized to the epithelium. Later in the course of the disease, the organisms penetrate into deeper layers and may be difficult to isolate from superficial scraping. Lamellar corneal biopsy may be required to establish the diagnosis in these cases. In contact lens–associated cases the contact lenses and contact lens case should be examined.

Amoebae are visualized in smears stained with Giemsa, periodic acid–Schiff (PAS), calcofluor white, or acridine orange stains. Nonnutrient agar with *E coli* or *E aerogenes* overlay is the preferred media for culturing amoebae, although organisms frequently grow well on blood agar plates and on buffered charcoal-yeast extract agar. Characteristic trails form as the motile trophozoites travel across the surface of the culture plate. Confocal in vivo microscopy can also be used to demonstrate organisms, particularly the cyst forms.

MANAGEMENT. Early diagnosis of *Acanthamoeba* keratitis is the most important prognostic indicator of a successful treatment outcome. Unfortunately, many cases are treated initially for herpetic keratitis. Not only is the delay in diagnosis detrimental, but the use of corticosteroids is highly correlated with a poor outcome. Clinical

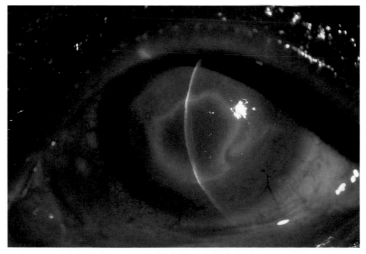

FIG VIII-27—Ring infiltrate in *Acanthamoeba* keratitis.

features that suggest *Acanthamoeba* keratitis rather than herpes simplex keratitis include the following:

- Noncontiguous or multifocal pattern of granular epitheliopathy and subepithelial opacities (unlike contiguous, dendritic pattern in HSV keratitis)

- Disproportionately severe pain, probably secondary to perineural inflammation (unlike hypoesthesia and disproportionately mild pain secondary to trigeminal nerve involvement in HSV)

- Presence of epidemiologic risk factors such as contact lens use or exposure to possibly contaminated freshwater

- Failure to respond to initial antiviral therapy

Cases diagnosed during the early, epithelial stage of the disease respond well to epithelial debridement, followed by a relatively short (3–4 months) course of anti-amoebic therapy. The prognosis for visual recovery with only mild residual stromal involvement is very good. Once stromal infiltrates appear, however, eradication of organisms is more difficult, and treatment may be needed for 6–12 months.

A number of antimicrobial agents have been recommended for therapy of *Acanthamoeba* keratitis based on their in vitro amoebicidal effects as well as their clinical effectiveness. Agents used for topical administration include

- Diamidines: propamidine, hexamidine

- Biguanides: polyhexamethylene biguanide (polyhexanide), chlorhexidine

- Aminoglycosides: neomycin, paromomycin

- Imidazoles/triazoles: miconazole, clotrimazole, ketoconazole, itraconazole

Most of these agents are effective against the free-living trophozoite form of the organism but have reduced efficacy in killing cysts. No consensus as to which of these agents are optimal exists, but successful resolution has been achieved with a biguanide with or without a diamidine. Treatment with topical corticosteroids is of uncertain long-term benefit and may contribute to prolonged persistence of viable cysts.

Penetrating keratoplasty is reserved for cases progressing despite maximal medical therapy and showing evidence of severe stromal melting with threatened perforation. The risk for recurrence in this setting is very high. Even in apparently quiet, treated eyes, optical penetrating keratoplasty procedures are associated with a high risk of recurrence if performed within the first year after the onset of infection. The presumed pathogenesis of such recurrences is the persistence of an occasional, residual viable cyst in an eye with compromised immunity as the result of the presence of an allograft and the use of topical corticosteroids postoperatively. Therefore, it is advisable to perform any elective penetrating keratoplasty procedure only after a full course of amoebicidal therapy has been completed and a minimum of 6 months of disease-free follow-up thereafter has been documented.

Microsporidal Stromal Keratitis

Nosema corneum is an intracellular protozoon that can very rarely infect the corneal stroma after traumatic inoculation. Granulomatous inflammation can lead to necrotic thinning and perforation. Penetrating keratoplasty is the only available treatment.

Corneal Stromal Inflammation Associated With Systemic Infections

Nonsuppurative stromal keratitis can be caused by the following:

☐ Reiter syndrome

☐ Congenital or acquired syphilis

☐ Lyme disease

☐ Tuberculosis

☐ Hansen disease (leprosy)

☐ Onchocerciasis

Refer to the index for further discussion of these conditions.

Microbial Scleritis

PATHOGENESIS. Bacterial and fungal infections of the sclera are very rare. Most cases result from extension of microbial keratitis involving the peripheral cornea. Trauma and contaminated foreign bodies (including a scleral buckle) are possible risk factors. Bacterial scleritis has also occurred in sclera damaged by previous pterygium surgery, especially when beta irradiation or mitomycin-C has been used (Fig VIII-28). Bacteria and fungi can also invade tissue of the eye wall surrounding a scleral surgical wound, but endophthalmitis is more likely in this setting. Scleral inflammation can also be a feature of syphilis, tuberculosis, and leprosy. Diffuse or nodular scleritis is an occasional complication of varicella-zoster virus eye disease.

LABORATORY EVALUATION. Suppurative scleritis is evaluated in a way similar to microbial keratitis. Smears and cultures are obtained before antimicrobial therapy is begun. The work-up of nonsuppurative scleritis is guided by the history and physical examination, as described in chapter X.

MANAGEMENT. Topical antimicrobial therapy is begun, just as for microbial keratitis. Subconjunctival injection and intravenous antibiotics are often used because of the difficulty in controlling microbial scleritis. The role of debridement and cryotherapy is unclear.

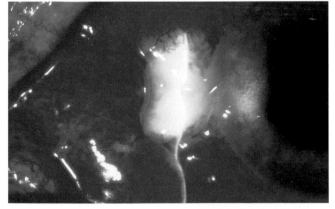

FIG VIII-28—Bacterial scleritis occurring 2 weeks after pterygium surgery.

PART 4

IMMUNE-MEDIATED DISORDERS OF THE EYELIDS, CONJUNCTIVA, CORNEA, AND SCLERA

CHAPTER IX

Ocular Immunology

Immunologic Features of the Outer Eye

The immune system of the ocular surface, cornea, and sclera encompasses systemic and mucosal immunity. The normal conjunctiva contains immunoglobulins, polymorphonuclear leukocytes, lymphocytes, plasma cells, and mast cells within the subepithelial tissue. The epithelium contains Langerhans' cells, which are dendritic cells capable of functioning like tissue macrophages. The normal cornea contains Langerhans' cells and lymphocytes in the peripheral epithelium and anterior stroma and immunoglobulins in the stroma. Table IX-1 shows the distribution of immunologic and inflammatory cells in the epithelium and substantia propria. Some of the cells listed in the table are explained below. The normal cornea is an immunologically privileged site because it lacks blood vessels and lymphatics. It interacts with the immune system primarily through the limbal vessels and the anterior chamber. Antigens that are released into the aqueous humor bypass the regional lymph nodes and can result in tolerance.

McClellan KA. Mucosal defense of the outer eye. *Surv Ophthalmol.* 1997;42:233–246.

Streilein JW. Regional immunology of the eye. In: Pepose JS, Holland GN, Wilhelmus KR, eds. *Ocular Infection and Immunity.* St Louis: Mosby; 1996:19–32.

TABLE IX-1

IMMUNOLOGIC COMPONENTS OF THE EXTERNAL EYE

CELL	EPITHELIUM	SUBSTANTIA PROPRIA
Langerhans' cells	+	+
Helper T cells	+	+
Suppressor T cells	+	+
B cells and plasma cells	−	+
Neutrophils	+	+
Eosinophils	−	−
Mast cells	−	+

Many immunoglobulins are also normally present in the tear film; dimeric IgA predominates. Antibody levels drop during lacrimal gland atrophy and increase in patients with allergic disorders of the external eye. Also present in the tears are components of the complement cascade. Complement can be activated through the classic pathway beginning with C4 serum alteration and through the alternate pathway involving C3. BCSC Section 9, *Intraocular Inflammation and Uveitis,* discusses all the elements of the immune system mentioned above in greater detail with illustrations.

Lymphocytes of the immune system include *natural killer (NK) cells, B cells,* and *T cells.* NK cells are responsible for innate immunity against tumor cells and virus-infected cells, while B cells and T cells are the key components of clonally specific adaptive immune responses. NK cells are large lymphocytes lacking immunoglobulin (Ig) and the T-cell antigen receptor (TCR) but possessing CD6, the receptor for the Fc portion of IgG, and CD56. B cells are defined by their surface Ig. T cells are classified into subsets based on their activity and by their transmembrane TCR, which targets antigen displayed by antigen-presenting cells or binds bacterial superantigens directly. T-cell phenotypes include cytotoxic (CD8+) T cells, helper (CD4+) T cells, and suppressor (CD8+) T cells. Because the correlation between function and CD expression is not absolute, T cells are also classified by their cytokine profile. For example, T cells that produce interleukin-2 (IL-2), interferon-γ, and tumor necrosis factor–β are called *Th1 cells*; and T cells that produce IL-4, IL-5, IL-9, IL-10, and IL-13 are *Th2 cells.*

Cellular immunity involves proteins encoded by the major histocompatibility complex on chromosome 6. *Human leukocyte antigens (HLA)* are glycoproteins with a molecular weight groove that can hold a linear peptide antigen for display to the TCR. They include class I antigens coded by the HLA-A, -B, and -C loci and class II antigens coded by HLA-DP, -DQ, and -DR loci. With a different allele for each gene pair and considering multiple chains of class II HLA molecules, an individual would express 6 different class I HLA molecules (2 HLA-A, 2 HLA-B, and 2 HLA-C) and 10 class II HLA molecules (2 HLA-DP, 4 HLA-DQ, and 4 HLA-DR). HLA antigens are epidemiologically associated with some immune-mediated ocular diseases (Table IX-2).

TABLE IX-2

HLA ASSOCIATIONS WITH SOME OCULAR DISORDERS

DISORDER	HUMAN LEUKOCYTE ANTIGEN (HLA)
Atopic dermatitis and keratoconjunctivitis	A1, A3, A9, B5, B8, B12
Ocular cicatricial pemphigoid	B12, DR4, DQ7
Stevens-Johnson syndrome	A33, B12, B44, DR53
Sjögren syndrome	B8, DR3
Rheumatoid arthritis	D4
Wegener granulomatosis	DR1, DR2, DQ1

TABLE IX-3

SOLUBLE MEDIATORS OF OCULAR INFLAMMATION

GROUP	EXAMPLE	ACTION
Kinin-forming system	Bradykinin	Increases vascular permeability
Clotting and fibrinolytic systems	Fibrin	Enhances leukocyte activity
Complement	C5a	Promotes leukocyte recruitment
Vasoactive amines	Histamine	Dilates blood vessels
Eicosanoids	Leukotriene B_4	Promotes leukocyte recruitment
Neuropeptides	Substance P	Promotes leukocyte recruitment
Cytokines	Interleukin-1	Promotes leukocyte recruitment
Cell adhesion molecules	P-Selectin	Promotes leukocyte recruitment
Leukocyte enzymes	Cathepsin	Degrades proteins
Leukocyte oxidants	Hydrogen peroxide	Oxidizes free radicals
Corneal proteases	Collagenase	Degrades proteins

Cytotoxicity is mediated by class II–restricted cytotoxic T (Tc) cells that are activated by the antigenic epitope in conjunction with class I antigens. The helper response involves antigen presentation in conjunction with class II antigens. Activated T cells elaborate lymphokines. They include molecules that regulate

□ Lymphocytes (e.g., interleukin-2)

□ Phagocytes (e.g., leukocyte migration inhibition factor)

□ Target cells (e.g., tumor necrosis factor–β)

Various soluble mediators are listed in Table IX-3.

Hendricks RL, Tang Q. Cellular immunity and the eye. In: Pepose JS, Holland GN, Wilhelmus KR, eds. *Ocular Infection and Immunity.* St Louis: Mosby; 1996:71–95.

Waldrop JC, Mondino BJ. Humoral immunity and the eye. In: Pepose JS, Holland GN, Wilhelmus KR, eds. *Ocular Infection and Immunity.* St Louis: Mosby; 1996:33–49.

Hypersensitivity Reactions of the Conjunctiva, Cornea, and Sclera

Hypersensitivity involves normal protective mechanisms that become excessive or destructive because of increased antigenic exposure or heightened immune status. Hypersensitivity reactions are typically classified into several basic mechanisms grouped as Types I–V (Type V is not discussed; see BCSC Section 9, *Intraocular Inflammation and Uveitis*). These mechanisms, as shown in Figure IX-1, are useful in explaining the pathogenesis of several immune-mediated disorders (Table IX-4). Multiple reactions can occur during ocular inflammation associated with many immunologic disorders, such as sarcoidosis.

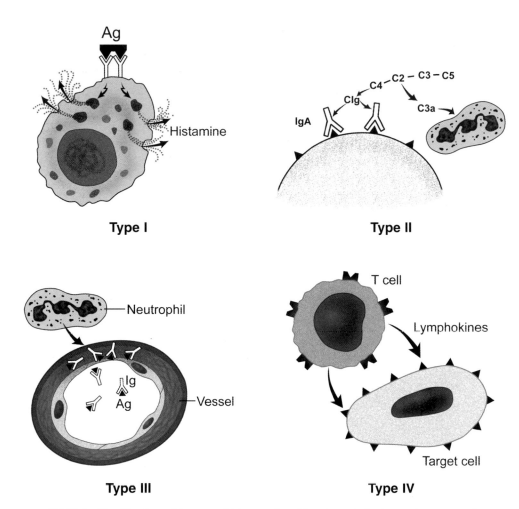

FIG IX-1—Classifications of hypersensitivity reactions. Type I anaphylactic reactions are mediated by IgE antibodies bound to mast cells. Type II cytolytic or cytotoxic reactions are mediated by immunoglobulins that activate complement. Type III immune-complex reactions occur when antigen-antibody complexes accumulate in a tissue and activate the complement cascade to attract leukocytes. Type IV cell-mediated immune reactions are mediated by T cells that release lymphokines to attract macrophages. (Illustration by Christine Gralapp.)

Anaphylactic or Atopic Reactions (Type I)

A Type I reaction involves antigen-antibody interactions. An antigen binds with two adjacent IgE molecules on a mast cell, resulting in the release of histamine and other preformed mediators and the synthesis of prostaglandins and leukotrienes. The pathogenesis of an allergic reaction begins with antigen-presenting B cells interacting with Th2 cells that release interleukin-4 (IL-4) and other cytokines. Atopy is

TABLE IX-4

HYPERSENSITIVITY REACTIONS AND OCULAR DISEASE

TYPE	OCULAR DISEASE
I	Allergic conjunctivitis Atopic keratoconjunctivitis and dermatitis
II	Ocular cicatricial pemphigoid Mooren ulcer
III	Scleritis
IV	Contact dermatitis Phlyctenulosis

associated with an inherited mutation in the receptor for IL-4 that enhances IgE production by B cells and increases the number of helper T cells. Other atopy-susceptibility genes are also under study. Along with the increased B-cell production of IgE, other features of atopy are a decreased level of suppressor T cells and the production of autoantibodies to β-adrenergic receptors. Treatment usually includes mast-cell inhibitors, antihistamines, vasoconstrictors, and cyclo-oxygenase inhibitors (Table IX-5).

TABLE IX-5

SOLUBLE MEDIATORS RELEASED BY MAST CELLS AND EOSINOPHILS

SUBSTANCE	ACTION
Released by mast cells	
Histamine	Vasodilation and increased capillary permeability
Heparin	Anticoagulation
Tryptase	Complement activation
Eosinophil chemotactic factor	Eosinophil chemotaxis
Neutrophil chemotactic factor	Neutrophil chemotaxis
Platelet-activating factor	Vasodilation and increased capillary permeability
Prostaglandins (PGD$_2$)	Vasodilation
Leukotrienes (LTB$_4$)	Leukocyte chemotaxis
Released by eosinophils	
Major basic protein	Mast cell degranulation
Cationic protein	Epithelial cytotoxicity
Peroxidase	Epithelial cytotoxicity
Eotaxin	Eosinophil chemotaxis
Platelet-activating factor	Vasodilation and increased capillary permeability
Leukotrienes (LTC$_4$)	Increased capillary permeability
Slow-reacting substance of anaphylaxis	Increased capillary permeability

Cytotoxic Hypersensitivity (Type II)

A Type II reaction involves interaction of immunoglobulins with antigens that are closely associated with cells. Cell lysis occurs by complement activation, neutrophil recruitment, and lymphocyte recruitment. Killer (K) cells are involved in antibody-dependent cell cytotoxicity. The presence and location of the autoantigen determines the form of the autoimmune disease. For example, in ocular cicatricial pemphigoid several antigens along the conjunctiva basement membrane zone can react with IgG or IgA autoantibodies. Treatment may involve immunosuppression with cytotoxic and other agents.

Immune-Complex Reactions (Type III)

A Type III reaction follows the deposition of antigen-antibody complexes in ocular tissue with complement activation and neutrophil recruitment. The Arthus reaction involves vasculitis from immune-complex deposition in small blood vessels. Immune complexes can fix complement that attracts polymorphonuclear leukocytes. The pathophysiology of scleritis and other ocular manifestations of vasculitis involve immune complexes, but the antigens are usually unknown. Treatment may include local and systemic corticosteroids.

Delayed Hypersensitivity (Type IV)

Type IV cell-mediated immunity involves sensitized T lymphocytes. Antigens interact with receptors on the surface of T lymphocytes and result in the release of lymphokines. Contact dermatitis is a delayed hypersensitivity reaction caused by a lipid-soluble, low-molecular-weight hapten that penetrates the skin to Langerhans' cells in the basal layer where the antigen is presented on an HLA-DR molecule to Th1 cells. Treatment of ocular inflammatory diseases involving delayed hypersensitivity usually includes a corticosteroid.

Patterns of Immune-Mediated Ocular Disease

Conjunctiva

The conjunctiva is a mucosa-associated lymphoid tissue. Humoral immunity involves IgA, and cellular immunity is dominated by CD4+ T cells. Serosal mast cells that contain neutral proteases are normally present in the conjunctiva; mucosal mast cells with granules containing only tryptase are increased in the conjunctiva of atopic patients. Mast-cell degranulation produces conjunctival redness, chemosis, mucous discharge, and itching.

Cornea

The normal cornea can exhibit neither an acute allergic reaction, as it contains no mast cells, nor a typical Arthus reaction, as there are no blood vessels. The cornea does participate in immune reactions, however, by way of humoral and cellular immune elements that enter the periphery from the limbal blood vessels.

The cornea can act as an immunologic blotter, soaking up antigens from the ocular surface. This phenomenon was first described by Wessely in 1911 when foreign antigen was injected into the cornea of a previously sensitized animal. A ring-shaped infiltrate formed in the corneal stroma concentric to the limbus, much like an antigen-antibody complex in an immunodiffusion test. Still occasionally referred to as a *Wessely immune ring,* an arc of immune precipitates contains complements and neutrophils. Circulating antibodies are not required if sufficient local antibody production is stimulated by antigens deposited in the cornea. The antigen may be a drug, as in the peripheral corneal infiltrates associated with a neomycin reaction, or an unknown substance, as in the corneal infiltrates that occasionally occur in contact lens wearers.

Sclera

Nearly one half of patients with scleritis have an associated systemic immunologic or connective tissue disease. Immune-complex deposition, granulomatous inflammation, and occlusive vasculitis are involved in the pathogenesis of scleral inflammation.

> Chandler JW. Ocular surface immunology. In: Pepose JS, Holland GN, Wilhelmus KR, eds. *Ocular Infection and Immunity.* St Louis: Mosby; 1996:104–111.

Diagnostic Approach to Immune-Mediated Ocular Disorders

Many immune mediated ocular disorders are a component of a systemic disease. Investigation must begin with a complete history, including a review of systems, and a general physical examination. Diagnostic tests can be selected to further narrow the differential diagnosis (Table IX-6).

Chapter V, Diagnostic Approach to Ocular Surface Disease, discusses and illustrates the specific morphological characteristics that can be found on conjunctival or

TABLE IX-6

LABORATORY TESTS FOR SUSPECTED SYSTEMIC
IMMUNE-MEDIATED DISEASE

TEST	ANTIBODY MEASURED
Rheumatoid factor (RF)	Autoantibody (IgG, IgA, or IgM) against epitopes on the Fc portion of IgG
Antinuclear antibody (ANA)	Antibodies against cell nuclear antigens (DNA-histone, double-stranded DNA, single-stranded DNA, histone, RNA, nuclear ribonucleoprotein, etc.)
Antineutrophil cytoplasmic antibodies (ANCA)	Autoantibody (IgG) against cytoplasmic antigen (either cytoplasmic proteinase-3 or perinuclear antigens) of neutrophils

corneal specimens through microscopic examination following standard staining procedures. Table IX-7 shows the clinical interpretation of the findings produced by the procedures described in chapter V for immune-mediated keratoconjunctivitis.

TABLE IX-7

CLINICAL INTERPRETATION OF OCULAR SURFACE CYTOLOGY
FOR IMMUNE-MEDIATED KERATOCONJUNCTIVITIS

FINDING	EXAMPLES
Predominance of neutrophils	Severe allergic or atopic conjunctivitis
Predominance of lymphocytes and monocytes	Chronic toxic or allergic conjunctivitis
Eosinophils	Acute allergic conjunctivitis
Basophils or mast cells	Vernal conjunctivitis
Keratinized epithelial cells	Ocular cicatricial pemphigoid Stevens-Johnson syndrome

CHAPTER X

Clinical Approach to Immune-Related Disorders of the External Eye

Immune-Mediated Diseases of the Eyelid

Contact Dermatoblepharitis

PATHOGENESIS. Topical application of ophthalmic medications and contact with cosmetics and environmental substances can occasionally trigger allergic reactions. These may occur acutely as anaphylactic reactions or have a delayed onset. Anaphylactic reactions are Type I IgE-mediated hypersensitivity reactions. Contact blepharoconjunctivitis is a Type IV cell-mediated, or delayed hypersensitivity, reaction that may begin 24–72 hours following instillation of a topical medication.

CLINICAL PRESENTATION. Type I (immediate) hypersensitivity reactions typically occur within minutes after application of an allergen. They are associated with itching, eyelid erythema and swelling, and conjunctival redness and chemosis (Fig X-1). Occasionally, patients may develop signs of systemic anaphylaxis. Ocular anaphylactic reactions are rare, but they have followed instillation of topical anesthetics and antibiotics such as bacitracin, cephalosporins, penicillin, sulfacetamide, and tetracycline.

Delayed Type IV hypersensitivity reactions to medications may begin 24–72 hours following instillation of a topical drug. Patients are often sensitized by previous exposure to the offending drug or preservative. An acute eczema with erythema, a leatherlike thickening, and scaling of the eyelid develop (Fig X-2). Chronic sequelae of contact blepharoconjunctivitis include hyperpigmentation, dermal scarring, and lower eyelid ectropion. A papillary conjunctivitis and a mucoid or mucopurulent discharge may develop. Punctate epithelial erosions may be noted on the inferior cornea. Medications that are commonly associated with contact blepharoconjunctivitis are

□ Cycloplegics such as atropine and homatropine

□ Aminoglycosides such as neomycin, gentamicin, and tobramycin

□ Antiviral agents such as idoxuridine and trifluridine

□ Preservatives such as thimerosal and ethylenediaminetetraacetic acid (EDTA)

MANAGEMENT. Treatment of hypersensitivity reactions requires identification and discontinuation of the offending agent. Rechallenge may be helpful in confirming a suspected medication. Type I hypersensitivity reactions should be treated with allergen

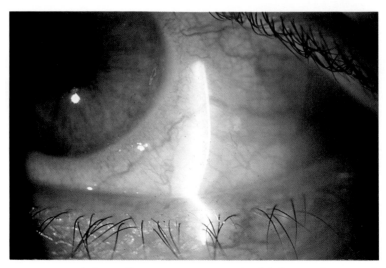

FIG X-1—Anaphylactic allergic reaction to topical ophthalmic medication with acute conjunctival hyperemia and chemosis.

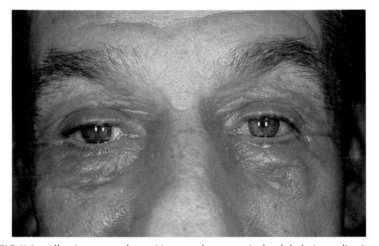

FIG X-2—Allergic contact dermatitis secondary to topical ophthalmic medication.

avoidance or discontinuation. Adjunctive therapy may involve the use of cold compresses, topical antihistamines, mast-cell stabilizers, and topical nonsteroidal anti-inflammatory agents. Topical vasoconstrictors, either alone or in combination with antihistamines, may provide acute symptomatic relief but have been incriminated as causes of chronic blepharoconjunctivitis.

Delayed hypersensitivity reactions are also treated with allergen withdrawal. In severe cases of Type IV hypersensitivity reactions, a brief course of topical corticosteroids applied to the eyelids and periocular skin may speed resolution of eyelid and conjunctival inflammation.

Atopic Dermatitis

PATHOGENESIS. Atopic dermatitis is a chronic condition that usually begins in infancy or childhood. Environmental irritants, climatic changes, and psychologic factors may play a role in genetically susceptible individuals. Immune changes involved in the pathogenesis of atopic dermatitis include increased IgE hypersensitivity, increased histamine release from mast cells and basophils, and impaired cell-mediated immunity. The reason for sustained dysregulation of immune responses is unknown.

CLINICAL PRESENTATION. Diagnostic criteria for atopic dermatitis include the presence of pruritus, the appearance of lesions on the eyelid and other sites (e.g., joint flexures in adolescents and adults; face and extensor surfaces in infants and young children), and a personal or family history of other atopic disorders such as asthma or allergic rhinitis. Other ocular findings may include periorbital darkening, exaggerated eyelid folds, ectropion, and chronic conjunctivitis. The appearance of the skin lesions varies depending on the age of the patient. Infants typically have an erythematous rash; children tend to have eczematoid dermatitis with secondary lichenification from scratching; and adults have scaly patches with dry skin.

MANAGEMENT. Allergens in the environment and in foods should be minimized when possible. Moisturizing lotions and petrolatum gels can be useful in skin hydration. Acute lesions can be controlled with a topical corticosteroid cream or ointment, but its use should be limited to avoid skin thinning. Oral antipruritic agents such as antihistamines and mast-cell stabilizers can alleviate itching.

Immune-Mediated Disorders of the Conjunctiva

Hay Fever Conjunctivitis and Perennial Allergic Conjunctivitis

PATHOGENESIS. Hay fever (seasonal) and perennial allergic conjunctivitis are Type I IgE-mediated immediate hypersensitivity reactions. The allergen is typically airborne. It enters the tear film and comes into contact with conjunctival mast cells that bear allergen-specific IgE antibodies. Degranulation of mast cells releases histamine and a variety of other inflammatory mediators that promote vasodilation, edema, and recruitment of other inflammatory cells such as eosinophils. The activation and degranulation of mast cells in a presensitized individual can be triggered within minutes of allergen exposure.

CLINICAL PRESENTATION. Patients with hay fever conjunctivitis often suffer from other atopic conditions such as allergic rhinitis and asthma. Symptoms develop rapidly after exposure to the allergen and consist of itching, eyelid swelling, conjunctival hyperemia and chemosis, and mucoid discharge. Intense itching is a hallmark symptom. Attacks are usually short-lived and episodic.

LABORATORY EVALUATION. The diagnosis of hay fever conjunctivitis is generally made clinically, although scraping of the conjunctiva can be performed in order to observe the characteristic eosinophils or their granules. Challenge testing with a panel of allergens can be performed using either the conjunctiva or the skin as the responding tissue.

MANAGEMENT. Treatment efforts should first be directed at avoidance or abatement of allergen exposure. Thorough cleaning of carpets, linens, and bedding can be effective in removing accumulated allergens such as animal dander and house dust mites. Treatment should be based on the severity of patient symptoms and consists of one or more of the following:

- Cold compresses
- Topical vasoconstrictors
- Topical antihistamines
- Topical nonsteroidal anti-inflammatory medications
- Judicious, selective use of topical corticosteroids

Artificial tears may be of benefit in diluting and flushing allergens and other inflammatory mediators present on the ocular surface.

Topical vasoconstrictors, alone or in combination with antihistamines, may provide acute symptomatic relief. However, their use for more than 5–7 consecutive days may predispose to rebound phenomenon characterized by tachyphylaxis, compensatory chronic vascular dilatation, and rebound conjunctival hyperemia.

Topical mast-cell stabilizing agents such as cromolyn sodium and lodoxamide tromethamine may be useful for treatment of seasonal allergic conjunctivitis, but their primary role is in prophylaxis. Mast-cell stabilizers that are currently available are ineffective in the acute phase of hay fever conjunctivitis because of their slow onset of effect. Oral antihistamines may provide symptomatic relief in some patients. Hyposensitization injections can be beneficial if the offending allergen has been identified.

Vernal Keratoconjunctivitis

PATHOGENESIS. Usually a seasonally recurring, bilateral inflammation of the conjunctiva, vernal keratoconjunctivitis occurs predominantly in male children who frequently but not invariably have a personal or family history of atopy. The disease may persist year-round in tropical climates. The immunopathogenesis appears to involve both Type I and Type IV hypersensitivity reactions. The conjunctival inflammatory infiltrate in vernal conjunctivitis consists of eosinophils, lymphocytes, plasma cells, and monocytes.

CLINICAL PRESENTATION. Symptoms consist of itching, blepharospasm, photophobia, blurred vision, and copious mucoid discharge. Clinically, two forms of vernal conjunctivitis may be seen, *palpebral* and *limbal*. The inflammation in palpebral vernal is located predominantly on the palpebral conjunctiva, where a diffuse papillary hypertrophy develops, usually more prominently on the upper than the lower region. Bulbar conjunctival hyperemia and chemosis may occur. In more severe cases giant papillae resembling "cobblestones" may develop on the upper tarsus (Fig X-3).

Limbal vernal may develop alone or in association with palpebral vernal. It occurs predominantly in patients of African or Asian descent. In limbal vernal the limbus has a thickened, gelatinous appearance with scattered opalescent mounds and vascular injection (Fig X-4). Horner-Trantas dots, whitish dots that represent

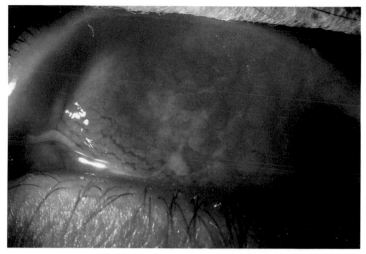

FIG X-3—Giant papillae of palpebral vernal conjunctivitis.

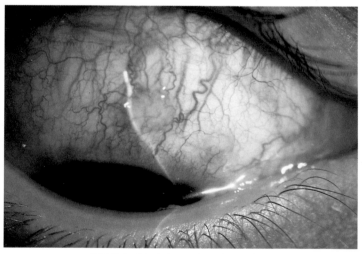

FIG X-4—Limbal vernal conjunctivitis.

macroaggregates of degenerated eosinophils and epithelial cells, may be observed in the hypertrophied limbus of patients with limbal vernal.

Several different types of corneal changes may also develop in vernal conjunctivitis. Punctate epithelial erosions in the superior and central cornea are frequently observed. Pannus occurs most commonly in the superior cornea, but occasionally 360° corneal vascularization may develop. Noninfectious epithelial ulcers with an

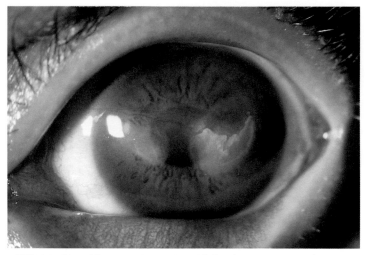

FIG X-5—Vernal keratoconjunctivitis with focal nonsuppurative keratitis.

oval or shield shape and underlying stromal opacification may develop in the superior or central cornea (Fig X-5). An association between vernal conjunctivitis and keratoconus has been reported, possibly in part as a result of frequent rubbing of itchy eyes.

MANAGEMENT. Therapy should be based on the severity of the patient's symptoms and of the ocular surface disease. Mild cases may be successfully managed with topical antihistamines. Climatotherapy such as the use of home air-conditioning or relocation to a cooler environment can promote improvement of the condition. Patients with moderate to severe disease may respond to topical mast-cell stabilizers such as cromolyn sodium or lodoxamine tromethamine. In patients with seasonal exacerbations these drops should be given four times a day starting at least 1 month prior to the usual time of symptomatic onset. Patients with year-round disease can be maintained chronically on mast-cell stabilizer drops. Topical nonsteroidal anti-inflammatory preparations such as ketorolac 0.5% may offer adjunctive benefit.

Severe cases may require the use of topical corticosteroids or topical immunomodulatory agents such as cyclosporine. Both have been shown to be effective in reducing inflammation and patient symptoms. Because of the likelihood that patients will develop steroid-related complications from chronic administration, however, corticosteroids should be reserved for exacerbations with moderate to severe discomfort and/or decreased visual acuity. During these exacerbations, intermittent (pulse) therapy is very effective: topical steroids are used at relatively high frequency (e.g., every 2 hours) for 5–7 days, then rapidly tapered. Because of the propensity of particles of suspended steroid (such as prenisolone acetate) to lodge between papillae, the use of less potent but soluble steroids such as dexamethasone phosphate is preferred. Corticosteroids should be discontinued between attacks. To minimize indiscriminate use for relief of mild symptoms the patient and family must be thoroughly informed of the potential dangers of chronic topical steroid therapy.

Cooperative patients can be offered an alternative to topical delivery that avoids the problem of continuing self-medication: supratarsal injection of corticosteroid. The supratarsal subconjunctival space is located superior to the upper border of the superior tarsus and is most easily reached by everting the upper eyelid. This space is free of the subepithelial adhesions that bind the superior palpebral conjunctiva to the tarsal plate. After the upper eyelid is everted and the supratarsal conjunctiva has been preanesthetized, supratarsal injection of 0.5–1.0 ml of either a relatively short-acting steroid such as dexamethasone phosphate (4 mg/ml) or a depot steroid such as triamcinolone acetonide (40 mg/ml) can be performed.

Topical cyclosporine 2% given twice daily can also be used for the treatment of refractory cases of vernal keratoconjunctivitis. Cyclosporine exerts an immuno-modulatory effect on both the afferent and efferent limbs of the cellular immune response. Reported side effects include punctate epithelial keratopathy and ocular surface irritation. Although systemic absorption after topical instillation is minimal, experience with this agent is limited, and the use of topical cyclosporine in vernal keratoconjunctivitis should therefore probably be reserved for the most severe cases.

Atopic Keratoconjunctivitis

PATHOGENESIS. Keratoconjunctivitis may occur in patients who have or have had atopic dermatitis. Approximately one third of patients with atopic dermatitis develop one or more manifestations of atopic keratoconjunctivitis. Atopic individuals demonstrate signs of Type I immediate hypersensitivity responses but also have depressed systemic cell-mediated immunity. As a consequence of this altered immunity, they are susceptible to herpes simplex virus keratitis and to colonization of the eyelids with Staphylococcus aureus. Complications related to this predisposition to infection may contribute to or may compound the primary immunopathogenic manifestations.

CLINICAL PRESENTATION. The ocular findings are similar to those of vernal kerato-conjunctivitis with the following differences:

□ Seasonal exacerbation is minimal

□ The papillae are more apt to be small or medium sized, rather than giant

□ The papillae occur in the upper and lower palpebral conjunctiva (Fig X-6)

□ Milky conjunctival edema is often present

□ Extensive corneal vascularization and opacification can occur (Fig X-7)

□ Eosinophils seen in conjunctival cytology are less numerous and are less often degranulated

□ Conjunctival scarring often occurs and is sometimes so extensive as to produce symblepharon formation

□ Characteristic posterior subcapsular and/or multifaceted or shield-shaped anterior subcapsular lens opacities may occasionally develop

MANAGEMENT. Treatment of atopic keratoconjunctivitis involves allergen avoidance and the use of pharmacotherapeutic agents similar to those used in the treatment of vernal keratoconjunctivitis. Additionally, patients should be carefully monitored for infectious disease complications that may warrant specific therapy, such as secondary staphylococcal infections.

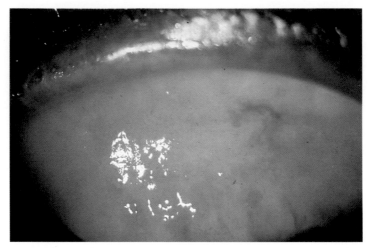

FIG X-6—Atopic keratoconjunctivitis with small and medium-sized papillae and edema of the tarsal conjunctiva.

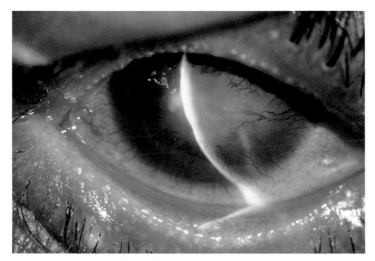

FIG X-7—Severe corneal vascularization and scarring in a patient with atopic keratoconjunctivitis.

Liesegang TJ. Atopic keratoconjunctivitis. In: Pepose JS, Holland GN, Wilhelmus KR, eds. *Ocular Infection and Immunity.* St Louis: Mosby; 1996:376–390.

Ligneous Conjunctivitis

PATHOGENESIS. Ligneous conjunctivitis is a rare, idiopathic, chronic disorder characterized by the formation of firm ("woody"), yellowish fibrinous membranes on the conjunctival surface. These membranes composed of an admixture of fibrin, epithelial cells, and mixed inflammatory cells adhere to the conjunctival surface. Bacteria can be sporadically isolated from cultures of the membranes but probably represent incidental, colonizing microorganisms rather than the etiologic agents, as is the case with infectious membranous conjunctivitis.

CLINICAL PRESENTATION. Ligneous conjunctivitis affects all ages. Patients present with symptoms of ocular irritation and foreign body sensation. The cardinal finding consists of yellowish platelike masses that overlie one or more of the palpebral surfaces and are readily visible with eversion of the eyelid. Ligneous conjunctivitis is generally bilateral.

MANAGEMENT. Cultures can be taken upon initial diagnosis to exclude a bacterial pseudomembranous or membranous conjunctivitis. Surgical excision with or without adjunctive cryotherapy has been advocated. However, recurrences are frequent. Anecdotal successes have been reported with the use of a variety of pharmacologic agents, including topical corticosteroids and cyclosporine, but no single treatment has been shown to be consistently effective or superior. Many cases of ligneous conjunctivitis eventually resolve spontaneously after months to a few years.

Contact Lens–Induced Conjunctivitis

PATHOGENESIS. The pathogenesis of contact lens–induced conjunctivitis is not fully understood. Patients with ocular prostheses and exposed monofilament sutures have shown reactions similar to those seen in patients with contact lens–induced conjunctivitis, suggesting that an immune-related response may result from

□ Repeated mechanical trauma of the superior tarsus by the sharp or rough surface of a contact lens, prosthesis, or suture

□ Hypersensitivity reaction to the contact lens or other foreign material

□ Hypersensitivity reaction to antigenic material adherent to the contact lens or prosthesis

□ A combination of these factors

The histologic findings in contact lens–induced conjunctivitis are similar to those observed in vernal keratoconjunctivitis. An abnormal accumulation of mast cells, basophils, and eosinophils is noted in the epithelium and/or the substantia propria of the superior tarsus. Abnormally elevated concentrations of immunoglobulins, specifically IgE, IgG, and IgM, and complement components have been found in the tears of affected patients. These findings suggest a combined mechanical and immunologically mediated pathophysiology for contact lens–induced conjunctivitis. It is recognized that surface deposits on worn contact lenses are a risk factor for development and persistence of this condition.

CLINICAL PRESENTATION. Some patients who wear contact lenses, in particular extended-wear soft contact lenses, may develop inflammatory symptoms, including redness, itching, and mucoid discharge. One or more of the following signs may be seen during biomicroscopic examination of contact lens wearers with these symptoms:

□ Mild papillary reaction (<0.3-mm-diameter papillae) on the superior tarsal conjunctiva

□ Punctate epithelial erosions

□ Peripheral corneal infiltrates and vascularization

At the more severe end of the spectrum of contact lens–related inflammation is the entity known as *giant papillary conjunctivitis (GPC)*. GPC tends to develop earlier and more frequently in soft contact lens wearers than in hard contact lens wearers. Symptoms include contact lens intolerance, itching, excessive mucous discharge, blurred vision from mucous coating of the contact lens, contact lens decentration, and conjunctival redness. In rare instances bloody tears and ptosis secondary to inflammation of the superior tarsal conjunctival may be observed.

The signs of GPC consist of hyperemia, thickening, and abnormally large papillae (diameter >0.3 mm) on the superior tarsal conjunctiva (Fig X-8). The morphological appearance of the superior tarsal papillae may be variable in GPC. In some cases the giant papillae cover the entire central tarsus from the posterior eyelid margin to the upper border of the tarsal plate, while involvement in other cases may be less extensive. Occasionally, only a few giant papillae appear surrounded by smaller papillae. Long-standing or involuted giant papillae on the superior tarsus can resemble follicles.

The symptoms of GPC generally resolve with the discontinuation of contact lens wear. The tarsal conjunctival hyperemia and thickening may resolve in several weeks, but papillae or dome-shaped scars on the superior tarsus can persist for months to years.

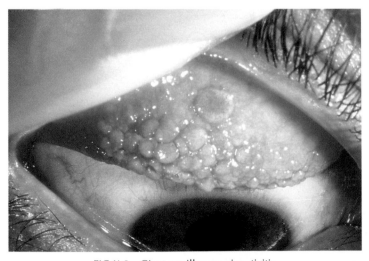

FIG X-8—Giant papillary conjunctivitis.

MANAGEMENT. The goal of GPC treatment is to enable patients to continue wearing contact lenses. Therapeutic strategies include discarding the offending contact lenses and refitting the patient with new ones, improving lens hygiene, and treating conjunctival inflammation with drugs. Simply fitting the patient with new contact lenses frequently resolves GPC. Daily-wear rather than extended-wear soft contact lenses should be encouraged. Periodic planned replacement of soft contact lenses is often beneficial and can easily be accomplished by switching the patient to disposable contact lenses that are worn on a daily-wear basis and discarded every day or every 2 weeks. Reducing daily wear time or instituting a 1-month contact lens holiday are additional measures that can be helpful in many cases.

Patients should be encouraged to clean their soft contact lenses daily using agents free of preservatives, particularly thimerosal, and to rinse and store lenses in nonpreserved sterile saline solution. Disinfection of contact lenses with a hydrogen peroxide system appears to be the method best tolerated by the inflamed conjunctiva. Regular enzymatic treatment of contact lenses with papain or subtilisin A may remove inciting contact lens deposits, and it is also well tolerated. If GPC persists in soft contact lens wearers despite following these treatment strategies, then consideration can be given to fitting the patient with rigid gas-permeable contact lenses, which are associated with lower incidence of GPC.

Pharmacologic therapy can be helpful in the management of patients with GPC. Mast-cell stabilizers such as cromolyn sodium have been reported to improve early mild GPC but have not been successful in advanced severe cases. However, once advanced cases of GPC have been brought under control, maintenance therapy with topical mast-cell inhibitors may prevent further exacerbations. Topical corticosteroids, while effective in GPC, have a limited role because of potential side effects associated with long-term use and because use of topical corticosteroids simultaneously with contact lens wear is hazardous.

Stevens-Johnson Syndrome (Erythema Multiforme Major) and Toxic Epidermal Necrolysis

PATHOGENESIS. Immune-complex deposition in the dermis and conjunctival stroma is probably the cause of erythema multiforme. Inciting agents most commonly include drugs such as sulfonamides, anticonvulsants, salicylates, penicillin, ampicillin, and isoniazid; or infectious organisms, such as herpes simplex virus, streptococci, adenovirus, and occasionally mycoplasma.

Distinctive pathologic changes of *Stevens-Johnson syndrome* are subepithelial bullae and subsequent scarring. The most severe form of this condition is referred to as *toxic epidermal necrolysis (TEN)*. TEN, which occurs more commonly in children and people with AIDS, has more superficial inflammation and produces less scarring. It is characterized by interepithelial bullae and extensive sloughing of epidermis, often with conjunctival scarring.

CLINICAL PRESENTATION. The term *erythema multiforme* refers to an acute inflammatory vesiculobullous reaction of the skin and mucous membranes. When these hypersensitivity disorders involve just the skin, the term *erythema multiforme minor* is used; when the skin and mucous membranes are involved, the condition is known as *Stevens-Johnson syndrome,* or *erythema multiforme major,* which accounts for 20% of all patients with erythema multiforme. The incidence of Stevens-Johnson syndrome has been shown in population-based studies to be about five cases per million per year. Recent reports have suggested that patients with AIDS are at a higher risk of developing erythema multiforme, particularly patients treated for *Pneumocystis carinii* pneumonia.

Stevens-Johnson syndrome occurs most commonly in children and young adults and in females more often than males. Fever, arthralgia, malaise, and upper or lower respiratory symptoms are usually sudden in onset. Skin eruption follows within a few days with a classic "target" lesion consisting of a red center surrounded by a pale ring and then a red ring, although maculopapular or bullous lesions are also common. The mucous membranes of the eyes, mouth, and genitalia may be affected by bullous lesions with membrane or pseudomembrane formation. New lesions may appear over 4–6 weeks with approximate 2-week cycles for each crop of lesions. The primary ocular finding is a mucopurulent conjunctivitis and episcleritis (Table X-1). Bullae and extensive areas of necrosis can develop (Fig X-9). Late ocular complications are caused by cicatrization resulting in conjunctival shrinkage, trichiasis, and tear deficiency. Cicatricial pemphigoid has been reported as a sequela of Stevens-Johnson syndrome (see below).

MANAGEMENT. Management of Stevens-Johnson syndrome is mainly supportive. The mainstay of therapy is ocular lubrication with artificial tears and ointments and vigilance for the early manifestations of ocular infections. Improved supportive therapy and, in some cases, administration of systemic corticosteroids have reduced the high mortality rate previously associated with this condition. However, the role of corticosteroids remains controversial. Most authorities recommend treating severe cases with oral prednisone, starting with 1 mg/kg/day. Even when used for short periods of time, however, high doses of systemic corticosteroids (primarily when administered intravenously) can be associated with serious complications: sepsis, gastrointestinal hemorrhage, electrolyte imbalance, and even sudden death. The efficacy of topical corticosteroids for the ocular manifestations of this condition has not been established. Lubrication with drops and ointment can prevent nosocomial complications in debilitated patients.

TABLE X-1

OCULOCUTANEOUS IMMUNE-MEDIATED REACTIONS

CONDITION	CAUSES	EYE	SKIN	OTHER
Stevens-Johnson syndrome	Drugs Infection	Conjunctival erosion Conjunctivitis Episcleritis	Blisters	Fever Respiratory lesions
Toxic epidermal necrolysis	Drugs Infections	Blepharodermatitis Conjunctivitis Corneal exposure	Blisters Necrosis	Fever Respiratory lesions Gastrointestinal lesions
Angioedema	Drugs Foods Insect sting	Eyelid edema	Facial edema Urticaria	Cardiorespiratory distress

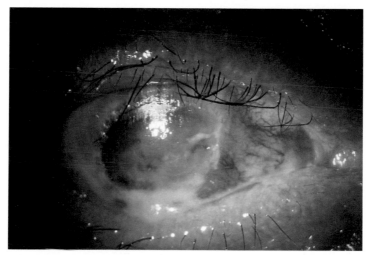

FIG X-9—Stevens-Johnson syndrome with associated ocular disease.

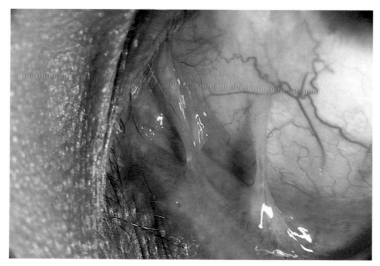

FIG X-10—Symblepharon formation (adhesion between the globe and palpebral conjunctiva) secondary to the conjunctival scarring of Stevens-Johnson syndrome (erythema multiforme major); virtually identical adhesions occur in ocular cicatricial pemphigoid.

Symblephara may form during the acute phase, because the raw, necrotic palpebral and bulbar conjunctival surfaces can adhere to one another (Fig X-10). Some authors recommend daily lysis of the symblephara and the use of symblepharon rings, but the long-term results of this therapy may be disappointing.

Late eyelid sequelae, such as entropion, trichiasis, and loss of the fornices, can be surgically corrected after the disease is quiescent. All efforts are aimed at avoiding secondary corneal complications. Because of the altered ocular surface and the corneal neovascularization that frequently develops in these patients, penetrating keratoplasty has an extremely poor prognosis and is generally reserved for progressive thinning or perforation. Favorable results in desperate cases have been achieved with the use of a keratoprosthesis, although its long-term stability may be problematic. Unfortunately, many patients suffering from this condition are young and are left with lifelong ocular morbidity.

Holland EJ, Hardten DR. Stevens-Johnson syndrome. In: Pepose JS, Holland GN, Wilhelmus KR, eds. *Ocular Infection and Immunity.* St Louis: Mosby; 1996:416–425.

Wilkins J, Morrison L, White CR Jr. Oculocutaneous manifestations of the erythema multiforme/Stevens-Johnson syndrome/toxic epidermal necrolysis spectrum. *Dermatol Clin.* 1992;10:571–582.

Ocular Cicatricial Pemphigoid

PATHOGENESIS. The cause of cicatricial pemphigoid (CP) is unknown. Antibody activates complement with subsequent breakdown of the conjunctival membrane. Pemphigoid may represent a cytotoxic (Type II) hypersensitivity, in which cell injury results from autoantibodies directed against a cell surface antigen in the BMZ. Cellular immunity may also play a role. HI A-DR4 has been associated with this condition. A similar clinical picture *(pseudopemphigoid)* has been associated with the chronic use of certain topical ophthalmic medications. Case reports have implicated pilocarpine, epinephrine, timolol, idoxuridine, echothiophate iodide, and demecarium bromide. The principal difference between pseudopemphigoid and true pemphigoid is that in the former further progression of the disease generally ceases once the offending agent is recognized and removed. The differential diagnosis of cicatrizing conjunctivitis includes four major categories:

□ Postinfectious conditions that follow severe episodes of trachoma, adenovirus conjunctivitis, or streptococcal conjunctivitis

□ Autoimmune or presumably autoimmune reactions, such as sarcoidosis, scleroderma, lichen planus, Stevens-Johnson syndrome, dermatitis herpetiformis, epidermolysis bullosa, atopic blepharoconjunctivitis, and practolol-induced cicatrizing conjunctivitis

□ Prior conjunctival trauma

□ Severe blepharoconjunctivitis caused by rosacea and other disorders

The diagnosis of unilateral CP should be made with caution, since other diseases, including many of those listed above, may masquerade as CP. Finally, linear IgA dermatosis, a rare dermatologic condition, can result in an ocular syndrome that is clinically identical to cicatricial pemphigoid and requires similar treatment.

CLINICAL PRESENTATION. Cicatricial pemphigoid is a chronic cicatrizing conjunctivitis of autoimmune etiology. Although it is a chronic vesiculobullous disease primarily involving the conjunctiva, it frequently affects other mucous membranes, including the mouth and oropharynx, genitalia, and anus. The skin is involved as well in appoximately 15% of the cases. Pemphigoid should not be confused with pemphigus vulgaris, a skin disease that rarely affects the eyes and with rare exceptions does not cause conjunctival scarring.

Cicatricial pemphigoid affects women more than men by a 2:1 ratio. Patients are usually older than 60 and rarely younger than 30. They frequently present with recurrent attacks of mild and nonspecific conjunctival inflammation with an occasional mucopurulent discharge. In its early phases CP may present with conjunctival hyperemia, edema, ulceration, and tear dysfunction. However, in many cases this insidious disease in its early stages produces bland, nonspecific symptoms with minimal overt physical findings. Oral mucosal lesions may be a clue that can lead to early diagnosis.

Transient bullae of the conjunctivae rupture, leading to subepithelial fibrosis, particularly of the medial eye. Loss of goblet cells, shortening of the fornices, symblepharon formation, and, on occasion, restricted ocular motility can follow. An inferior forniceal depth of less than 8 mm is abnormal and should prompt further evaluation. Subtle inferior symblephara can be detected when the lower eyelid is pulled down while the patient looks up (Fig X-11). Fine gray-white linear opacities, best seen with an intense but thin slit beam, appear in the deep conjunctiva.

Recurrent attacks of conjunctival inflammation can lead to destruction of goblet cells and eventually obstruction of the lacrimal gland ductules. The resultant aqueous and mucous tear deficiency leads to keratinization of the already-thickened conjunctiva. Conjunctival bullae may rupture, exposing underlying stroma and leading to symblepharon formation. Entropion and trichiasis develop as scarring progresses, leading to abrasions, corneal vascularization, further scarring, ulceration, and epidermalization of the ocular surface (Fig X-12). Although the clinical course is variable, progressive deterioration in untreated cases usually occurs. Remissions and exacerbations are common. Surgical intervention can incite to further scarring but may be essential for the management of entropion and trichiasis.

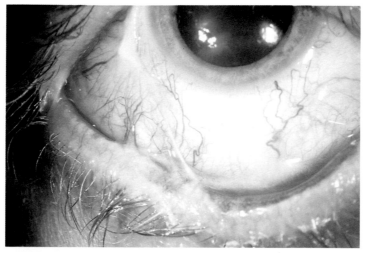

FIG X-11—Inferior symblepharon as a result of ocular cicatricial pemphigoid.

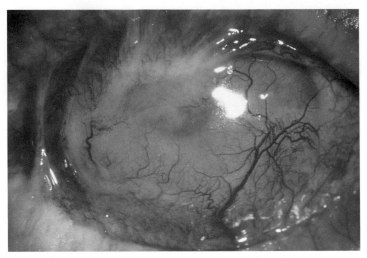
FIG X-12—Advanced cicatricial pemphigoid.

LABORATORY EVALUATION. Although ocular pemphigoid is a bilateral disease, one eye may be more severely involved than the other. Pathologic support for a diagnosis of pemphigoid can be obtained from a conjunctival biopsy sent for immunofluorescent or immunohistochemical analysis. Biopsy specimens should be obtained from an actively affected area of the conjunctiva or, if diffuse involvement is present, from near the inferior conjunctival fornix. Conjunctival biopsies may or may not be positive for immunoreactants in pseudopemphigoid. Immunofluorescent and immunohistochemical staining techniques can demonstrate C3, IgG, IgM, and/or IgA localized in the basement membrane zone (BMZ) of the conjunctiva in pemphigoid (Fig X-13). Circulating anti–basement membrane antibody has been identified in the sera of some patients with pemphigoid.

MANAGEMENT. Therapy with systemic corticosteroids has limited success. Oral corticosteroids can be used in combination with any of the agents discussed below, although usually for only brief periods of time, measured in months, in severe cases. Since progression is often slow, careful clinical staging of the disease and photodocumentation in differing positions of gaze is essential for evaluation of the disease course and response to therapy. Severity and staging of pemphigoid can be judged by recording the extent of shortening of the inferior fornix depth and the extent of symblepharon along the inferior fornix in quartiles (0%–25%, 25%–50%, 50%–75%, and 75%–100%).

Diaminodiphenylsulfone (dapsone), a drug previously used to treat Hansen disease and dermatitis herpetiformis, has been advocated as the initial drug of choice in milder cases. It must be used cautiously in patients with glucose-6-phosphate dehydrogenase (G6PD) deficiency or sulfa allergy.

Cyclophosphamide (Cytoxan) has been used for CP in a manner patterned after its use in treatment of Wegener granulomatosis. Cyclophosphamide remains a main-

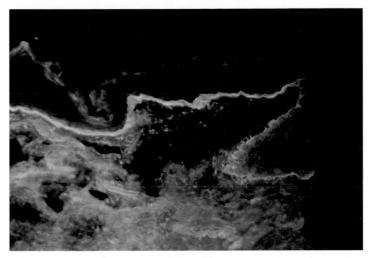

FIG X-13—Immunofluorescent staining of basement membrane in a patient with cicatricial pemphigoid.

stay of therapy in moderate to severe disease. The usual therapeutic dose is 1.5–2.0 mg/kg/day in divided doses. The therapeutic target is a reduction in white blood count to the range of 2000–3000 cells per μl. Cytotoxic therapy can bring about disease remission. Consultation with an internist or oncologist is recommended for the administration of immunosuppressive agents such as cyclophosphamide. Azathioprine (Imuran) has been used as an alternate agent when cyclophosphamide cannot be tolerated, although the success rate with azathioprine is lower.

Topical corticosteroids may suppress the immediate inflammatory response and acute exacerbations. Topical vitamin A has been shown to reverse, to some extent, the keratinization resulting from the squamous metaplasia associated with this condition.

Other measures, such as surgical correction of eyelid deformities and intraocular surgery, are most successful when disease activity has been under control for an extended period of time. Hard palate and buccal mucosal grafting can be useful techniques in fornix reconstruction. Cryotherapy of the eyelids and other measures aimed at control of trichiasis are essential. Punctal occlusion, which may already have resulted from cicatrization, can be useful in the management of any associated dry eye condition. Keratoprosthesis has been used with limited success.

Foster CS. Cicatricial pemphigoid. *Trans Am Ophthalmol Soc.* 1986;84:527–663.

Mondino BJ. Ocular cicatricial pemphigoid. In: Pepose JS, Holland GN, Wilhelmus KR, eds. *Ocular Infection and Immunity.* St Louis: Mosby; 1996:408–415.

Tauber J, Sainz de la Maza M, Foster CS. Systemic chemotherapy for ocular cicatricial pemphigoid. *Cornea.* 1991;10:185–195.

Other Immune-Mediated Diseases of the Skin and Mucous Membranes

Ocular ciatricial pemphigoid accounts for most cases of chronic cicatrizing conjunctivitis. Other immune-mediated disorders that can rarely affect the conjunctiva include linear IgA bullous dermatosis, dermatitis herpetiformis, epidermolysis bullosa, lichen planus, paraneoplastic pemphigus, pemphigus vulgaris, and pemphigus foliaceus.

Graft-versus-host disease is a complication of bone marrow transplantation. The ocular complications include conjunctival and corneal epithelial erosions, aqueous tear deficiency, and cicatricial lagophthalmos.

Immune-Mediated Diseases of the Cornea

Thygeson Superficial Punctate Keratitis (SPK)

PATHOGENESIS. The etiology of Thygeson superficial punctate keratitis is unknown. Although many of the clinical features resemble a viral infection of the epithelium, attempts to confirm viral particles by electron microscopy or culture have been unsuccessful. Patients with Thygeson SPK have been found to have an increased frequency of HLA antigen DR3. The response of the lesions of Thygeson SPK to corticosteroid therapy suggests that some immunopathologic component is likely in the pathogenesis.

CLINICAL PRESENTATION. This condition, first reported by Thygeson in 1950, is characterized by recurrent episodes of tearing, foreign body sensation, photophobia, and reduced vision. It affects children to older adults and is typically bilateral, although it may develop initially in one eye. The hallmark finding is multiple (up to 40) corneal epithelial lesions, which are noted during exacerbations. The epithelial lesions are round or oval conglomerates of gray, granular opacities associated with minimal conjunctival reaction, in contrast to adenovirus keratoconjunctivitis. High magnification reveals each opacity to be a cluster of multiple smaller pinpoint opacities (Fig X-14). A characteristic feature is the waxing and waning appearance of individual epithelial opacities, which change in location and number over time. The

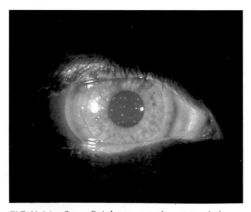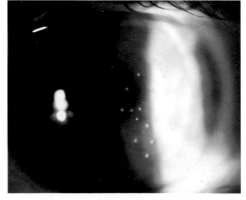

FIG X-14—Superficial punctate keratitis of Thygeson; with higher magnification each lesion is seen to consist of several minute dots.

greatest density of these lesions typically appears in the central cornea. The punctate epithelial lesions stain with fluorescein and rose bengal.

No conjunctival inflammatory reaction is noted during exacerbations, but occasionally patients will have mild bulbar conjunctival injection. Rarely, a mild subepithelial opacity may develop underlying the epithelial lesion, more commonly in patients who have received topical antiviral therapy.

MANAGEMENT. Supportive therapy with artificial tears and bandage soft contact lenses is often adequate in milder cases. Treatment alternatives for persistently symptomatic cases include topical corticosteroids. Idoxuridine has been associated with increased risk of subepithelial scarring in Thygeson SPK and is therefore contraindicated. The value of trifluridine therapy remains unclear; some authors report benefit while others find none.

If a topical steroid is prescribed, only a very mild preparation need be used (e.g., fluorometholone 0.1% or medrysone 1%). Treatment with corticosteroids may hasten resolution, but the lesions frequently recur in the same or different locations on the cornea after the topical steroids are stopped. Anecdotal reports suggest that use of topical corticosteroids may prolong the duration of disease to more than 15 years, a duration that is uncommon in cases never treated with steroids. Topical cyclosporine given twice daily is also effective in causing regression of the lesions, usually within 2–3 weeks.

> Schwab IR, Thygeson P. Thygeson superficial punctate keratopathy. In: Pepose JS, Holland GN, Wilhelmus KR, eds. *Ocular Infection and Immunity.* St Louis: Mosby; 1996:403–407.

Interstitial Keratitis Associated with Infectious Diseases

PATHOGENESIS. Interstitial keratitis (IK) is a nonsuppurative inflammation of the corneal stroma that features cellular infiltration and usually vascularization without primary involvement of the epithelium or endothelium. Most cases result from an immunologic response to infectious microorganisms or their antigens in the corneal stroma. The topographic distribution (diffuse versus focal or multifocal) and depth of the stromal infiltration, in addition to associated systemic signs, are helpful in determining the cause of IK.

Congenital syphilis was the first infection to be linked with interstitial keratitis. Herpes simplex virus, which accounts for most cases of stromal keratitis, is discussed on pp 141–150. Varicella-zoster virus keratitis is discussed on pp 150–154. Other microorganisms that rarely produce stromal inflammation include

- *Mycobacterium tuberculosis*
- *M leprae*
- *Borrelia burgdorferi* (Lyme disease)
- Rubeola (measles)
- Epstein-Barr virus (infectious mononucleosis)
- *Chlamydia trachomatis* (lymphogranuloma venereum)
- *Leishmania* species
- *Onchocerca volvulus* (onchocerciasis)

Syphilitic interstitial keratitis CLINICAL PRESENTATION. Syphilitic interstitial keratitis may be caused by congenital or acquired syphilis. Most cases are associated with congenital syphilis. Manifestations of congenital syphilis that occur early (within the first 2 years of life) are infectious, resembling secondary syphilis in adults. Interstitial keratitis is an example of a late, immune-mediated manifestation of congenital syphilis. Affected children typically show no evidence of corneal disease until the first or second decade of life, when a subacute or acute stromal keratitis lasting weeks first develops. However, these patients may have other nonocular signs of congenital syphilis:

- Dental deformities: notched (Hutchinson) incisors and mulberry molars
- Bone and cartilage abnormalities: saddle nose, palatal perforation, saber shins, and frontal bossing
- Cranial nerve VIII (vestibulocochlear) deafness
- Rhagades (circumoral radiating scars)
- Mental retardation

Congenital syphilitic keratitis is usually bilateral (80%), although both eyes may not be affected simultaneously. Initial symptoms are pain, tearing photophobia, and perilimbal injection. The inflammation may last for weeks if left untreated. Sectoral superior stromal inflammation and keratic precipitates are typically seen early. As the disease progresses, the peripheral stroma thickens and deep stromal neovascularization develops. Eventually, the inflammation spreads centrally, and corneal opacification and edema may develop. In some cases, the deep corneal vascularization becomes so intense that the cornea appears pink, hence the term *salmon patch*. Sequelae of stromal keratitis include corneal scarring, thinning, and ghost vessels in the deepest layers of the stroma (Fig X-15). Visual acuity may be reduced because of irregular astigmatism and stromal opacification.

Stromal keratitis rarely develops in acquired syphilis, and it is typically unilateral (60%) when it does occur. The ocular findings are similar to those seen in congenital syphilitic keratitis. Uveitis is the most common ocular manifestation of acquired syphilis. See also BCSC Section 9, *Intraocular Inflammation and Uveitis.*

LABORATORY EVALUATION AND MANAGEMENT. The diagnosis can be confirmed serologically with the rapid plasmin reagin test and a treponeme-specific antibody test (FTA-ABS or MHA-TP). Ocular inflammation during the acute phase should be treated with cycloplegic agents and topical corticosteroids in order to limit stromal inflammation and late scarring. The systemic syphilis infection should be treated with penicillin or an appropriate alternative antibiotic according to a protocol appropriate for either congenital or acquired syphilis. The necessity of lumbar puncture in syphilitic interstitial keratitis is uncertain.

Reiter syndrome   Reiter syndrome is a systemic disorder characterized by a triad of ocular (conjunctivitis, iridocyclitis, or keratitis), urethral, and joint inflammation. These manifestations can appear simultaneously or separately in any sequence. Less common manifestations include keratoderma blennorrhagicum, a scaling skin eruption; balanitis; aphthous stomatitis; fever; lymphadenopathy; pneumonitis; pericarditis; and myocarditis. Attacks are self-limited, lasting from 2 to several months, but they may recur periodically over the course of several years. Reiter syndrome may occur after gram-negative bacterial dysentery (most frequently associated with *Salmonella, Shigella,* and *Yersinia*) or after nongonococcal urethritis caused by *Chlamydia trachomatis.* More than 75% of patients with Reiter syndrome are HLA-B27 positive. See BCSC Section 9, *Intraocular Inflammation and Uveitis,* for discus-

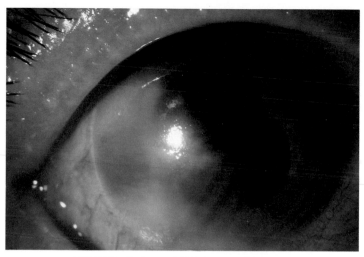

FIG X-15—Active syphilitic interstitial keratitis.

sion of HLA-B27–related diseases and illustrations of nonocular manifestations of Reiter syndrome.

A bilateral papillary conjunctivitis with mucopurulent discharge is the most common ocular finding in Reiter syndrome; it has been reported in 30%–60% of patients. The conjunctivitis is self-limited, lasting for days to weeks. Mild nongranulomatous iritis has been reported to occur in 3%–12% of patients. Various forms of keratitis may rarely occur, including diffuse punctate epithelial erosions, superficial or deep focal infiltrates, and superficial or deep vascularization. Reiter syndrome should be considered in any case of chronic, nonfollicular, mucopurulent conjunctivitis with negative cultures.

Treatment is mainly palliative. Corneal infiltrates and vascularization often respond to topical steroids. Systemic antibiotic treatment of chlamydial urethritis or bacterial dysentery may be beneficial.

Cogan Syndrome

PATHOGENESIS. Cogan syndrome is an autoimmune disorder that produces stromal keratitis, vertigo, and hearing loss. The etiology of Cogan syndrome is obscure but shares some clinicopatholgic features with polyarteritis nodosa.

CLINICAL PRESENTATION. Cogan syndrome typically occurs in young adults, the majority of whom have had an upper respiratory infection 1–2 weeks prior to the onset of ocular or vestibuloauditory symptoms (vertigo, tinnitus, and hearing loss). The earliest corneal findings are pseudoguttata and bilateral faint white subepithelial infiltrates similar to those occurring in viral keratoconjunctivitis but located in the peripheral cornea. Multifocal nodular infiltrates may develop in the posterior cornea later in the course of this condition. Some patients develop a systemic vasculitis (polyarteritis nodosa).

LABORATORY EVALUATION. When the cause of stromal keratitis is not apparent, VDRL or RPR and FTA-ABS or MHA-TP are obtained (VDRL and RPR may become nonreactive in congenital syphilis). Other infectious syndromes should also be considered.

MANAGEMENT. The acute keratitis of Cogan syndrome is treated with frequent topical steroids. Oral steroids are recommended for the treatment of vestibuloauditory symptoms, because they improve the long-term prognosis for recovery of normal hearing. Cytotoxic agents may also have a therapeutic role.

Toxic Medication Reaction

PATHOGENESIS. Toxic conjunctivitis or keratoconjunctivitis may occur as a complication of exposure to various substances. Topically applied ophthalmic medications can result in a dose-dependent cytotoxic effect on the ocular surface. The epithelium of the conjunctiva and cornea may show punctate staining or erosive changes indicative of direct toxicity. A conjunctival reaction may be observed in the form of either a papillary reaction (vascular dilation) or follicular response (lymphocytic and plasma cell hyperplasia). An immunologic response can produce subepithelial corneal infiltrates.

CLINICAL PRESENTATION. Toxicity should be suspected in cases of ocular surface inflammation when patients have been using topical medications. Although these reactions generally occur after long-term use (weeks to months) of a drug, they may occur sooner in individuals with delayed tear clearance from aqueous tear deficiency or tear drainage obstruction.

Toxic reactions of the ocular surface can take different forms. A generalized injection of the tarsal and bulbar conjunctiva may be associated with a mild to severe papillary reaction of the tarsal conjunctiva, mucopurulent discharge, and punctate keratitis. Occasionally, the discharge may be severe and mimic bacterial conjunctivitis. The reaction can occur in only one eye even though the medication has been applied to both, most commonly in patients with impaired lacrimal outflow in the involved eye.

In its mildest form toxic keratitis consists of punctate epithelial erosions of the inferior cornea. A diffuse punctate epitheliopathy, occasionally in a whorl pattern, may be observed in more severe cases. This vortex or hurricane pattern reflects the centripetal migration of epithelial cells, which is revealed in toxicity because of the epithelial irregularity and punctate whitening keratopathy produced by the offending agent. The most severe cases may involve a corneal epithelial defect of the inferior or central cornea, stromal opacification, and neovascularization. This severe type of corneal disease is seen with extensive damage to the limbal stem cells. A sign of limbal stem-cell deficiency is effacement of the palisades of Vogt. Prolonged use of medication or administration of antifibrotic agents (e.g., use of topical mitomycin drops) may be the cause. Use of topical mitomycin-C has a very low therapeutic ratio, and even if prescribed in correct dosages for brief periods, the drug can result in prolonged, irreversible stem-cell damage and the resultant chronic keratopathy. Localized administration of mitomycin-C using a cellulose microsponge to the surgical field (as in trabeculectomy or pterygium excision) incurs a substantially lower risk and is the preferred method of antifibrotic administration.

A different type of toxic keratitis manifests as peripheral corneal infiltrates located in the epithelium and anterior stroma, leaving a clear zone between them and the limbus. Conjunctival and/or corneal toxic reactions are typically seen following use of aminoglycoside antibiotics, antiviral agents, or medications preserved with benzalkonium chloride or thimerosal.

Another manifestation of external ocular toxicity is chronic follicular conjunctivitis. Generally, the follicular reaction involves both the upper and lower palpebral conjunctiva, but the follicles are usually most prominent on the inferior tarsus and fornix. Bulbar follicles are uncommon but highly suggestive of a toxic etiology when present. The medications most commonly associated with toxic follicular conjunctivitis include atropine, antiviral agents, miotics (particularly phospholine iodide), sulfonamides, epinephrine (including dipivefrin), apraclonidine (Iopidine), and vasoconstrictors. Inferior punctate epithelial erosions may occasionally accompany toxic follicular conjunctivitis.

With chronic use of topical medications, the conjunctiva shows an increased number of chronic inflammatory cells and fibroblasts. Any medication may potentially cause this low-grade inflammatory response, although the chronic use of miotics for the treatment of glaucoma is the most common setting. Fine wisps of subepithelial fibrosis are not unusual in patients who have undergone chronic miotic therapy. The best way to observe them is to scan the conjunctiva with a very thin slit beam. The use of red-free ("green") illumination can sometimes help in the delineation of the fine, whitish wisps of fibrous strands. Although asymptomatic subconjunctival fibrosis is not uncommon with chronic topical drug use, a small minority of affected patients will develop an insidiously progressive and more severe type of subconjunctival scarring that can lead to forniceal contraction, symblepharon formation, and, eventually, corneal pannus. Such an entity is termed *drug-induced cicatricial pemphigoid,* or *pseudopemphigoid.*

MANAGEMENT. Treatment of toxicity requires discontinuation of the offending topical medications. Severe cases may take months to resolve completely. The failure of symptoms and signs to resolve within a period of days to a few weeks should therefore not be considered inconsistent with a toxic etiology. Patients with toxic medication reaction who are experiencing significant ocular irritation may find relief with nonpreserved topical lubricant drops or ointment.

Drug-induced pemphigoid should be confirmed with a conjunctival biopsy, which will often (but not always) demonstrate the characteristic diffuse immunofluorescent staining indicative of antibody deposition at the conjunctival basement membrane. Withdrawal of the medication is generally followed by a lag of weeks to months before stabilization of progressive scarring can be achieved. If clinical observation and photographic documentation demonstrate clinical progression despite discontinuation of the medication, chemotherapy with diaminodiphenysulfone or cytotoxic agents may be necessary.

Marginal Corneal Infiltrates Associated with Blepharoconjunctivitis

PATHOGENESIS. The limbus plays an important role in immune-mediated corneal disorders. Frequently, immune-related corneal changes occur in a peripheral location adjacent to the limbus, which is the interface between the conjunctival and episcleral vasculature and the avascular cornea. Thus circulating immune cells, immune complexes, and complement tend to deposit adjacent to the terminal capillary loops of the limbal vascular arcades, producing a variety of immune phenomena that manifest in the corneal periphery. Predisposing causes include

□ Blepharoconjunctivitis

□ Contact lens wear

□ Trauma

□ Endophthalmitis

CLINICAL PRESENTATION AND MANAGEMENT. Marginal infiltrates (also referred to as *catarrhal infiltrates*) usually occur where the eyelid margins intersect with the corneal surface: the 10, 2, 4, and 8 o'clock positions. Marginal infiltrates in staphylococcal blepharitis are typically gray-white, well circumscribed, and located approximately 1 mm inside the limbus, with a characteristic clear zone of cornea between the infiltrate and the limbus (see Figure VIII-18). In chronic disease superficial blood vessels may cross the clear interval into the area of infiltration. The epithelium overlying marginal infiltrates may be intact, show punctate epithelial erosions, or be ulcerated. Stromal opacification, peripheral corneal thinning, and/or pannus may develop following resolution of the acute marginal infiltrates. Treatment is discussed on p 159.

Peripheral Ulcerative Keratitis Associated with Systemic Immune-Mediated Diseases

PATHOGENESIS. Autoimmune-related peripheral keratitis occasionally develops in patients who have systemic autoimmune disease. Peripheral ulcerative keratitis occurs most often in association with rheumatoid arthritis but may be seen with related diseases such as Wegener granulomatosis, systemic lupus erythematosus, polyarteritis nodosa, ulcerative colitis, relapsing polychondritis, and others. Biopsy of conjunctival tissue adjacent to marginal keratolysis typically shows evidence of immune-mediated vasoocclusive disease.

CLINICAL PRESENTATION. A history of connective tissue disease is generally present, although the ocular finding of peripheral corneal melting may be the first sign of the underlying systemic illness. Autoimmune peripheral ulcerative keratitis generally correlates with exacerbations of systemic disease activity. Follow-up of these patients reveals that a high proportion suffer severe disease-related morbidity and mortality.

Autoimmune peripheral ulcerative keratitis may be bilateral and extensive, but it is usually unilateral and limited to one sector of the peripheral cornea (Fig X-16). The initial lesions appear in a zone within 2 mm of the limbus and are accompanied by varying degrees of vasoocclusion of the adjacent limbal vascular networks. The epithelium is absent in the affected area, and the underlying stroma is thin. Ulceration may or may not be associated with cellular infiltrate in the corneal stroma, and the adjacent conjunctiva can be minimally or severely inflamed.

MANAGEMENT. The goals of therapy are to provide local supportive therapy to decrease melting, improve wetting, and promote reepithelialization; and to suppress the underlying systemic disorder. The keratolysis will stop if the epithelium can be made to heal by means of lubricants, patching, or a bandage soft contact lens. Topical collagenase inhibitors such as sodium citrate 10% and systemic collagenase inhibitors such as tetracycline are of possible value. Topical corticosteroids have variable effects and in some cases may delay reepithelialization, predispose to superinfection, and exacerbate melting. Lesions with a prominent inflammatory

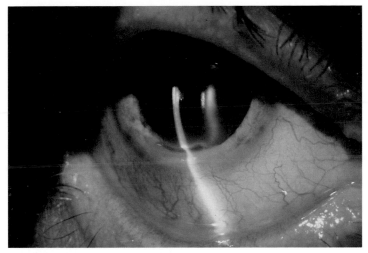

FIG X-16—Peripheral ulcerative keratitis as a result of rheumatoid disease.

infiltrate may respond initially to topical corticosteroids, but corneal thinning without a prominent inflammatory infiltrate will often not benefit. Excision or recession of adjacent limbal conjunctiva is often followed by healing of the ulcer, probably because the procedure eliminates a source of inflammatory cells and collagenolytic enzymes.

Definitive treatment often requires institution or escalation of systemic therapy, including immunosuppressive therapy using cytotoxic agents such as cyclophosphamide or immunomodulatory agents such as cyclosporine. Severe, rapidly melting cases may require intravenous therapy with high-dose cyclophosphamide, with or without corticosteroid therapy. Threatened perforation should be treated with temporizing measures such as cyanoacrylate glue and bandage contact lens placement until systemic therapy has been initiated, since lamellar or penetrating grafts are also susceptible to melting. Once control of the underlying disease process has been gained, reconstructive keratoplasty can be performed (see chapters XXIII–XXIV). Conjunctival flaps should be avoided, since the melting could potentially be accelerated by bringing the conjunctival vasculature in even closer proximity to the corneal lesion.

Mooren Ulcer

PATHOGENESIS. Although the etiology of this peripheral ulcerative keratitis is unknown, evidence is mounting that autoimmunity plays a key role. The following have been found in patients with Mooren ulcer:

□ Deficiency of suppressor T cells

□ Increased level of IgA

□ Increased concentration of plasma cells and lymphocytes in the conjunctiva adjacent to the ulcerated areas

□ Tissue-fixed immunoglobulins and complement in the conjunctival epithelium and peripheral cornea

215

At least 25%–100% of the resident cells in Mooren ulcer specimens express major histocompatibility class II antigens. It has been suggested that autoreactivity to a cornea-specific antigen may play a role in the pathogenesis of this disorder, and humoral and cell-mediated immune mechanisms may be involved in the initiation and perpetuation of corneal destruction. The proximity of the ulcerative lesion to the limbus probably has pathophysiologic importance, since resection or recession of the limbal conjunctiva can often have a beneficial therapeutic effect.

Though the cause is unknown, precipitating factors include accidental trauma or surgery and exposure to parasitic infection. The inflammation associated with antecedent injury or infection may have altered corneal epithelial and conjunctival antigen, to which autoantibodies are then produced.

CLINICAL PRESENTATION. Mooren ulcer is a chronic, progressive, painful, idiopathic ulceration of the peripheral corneal stroma and epithelium. Typically, the ulcer starts in the periphery of the cornea and spreads circumferentially and then centripetally, with a leading undermined edge of de-epithelialized tissue (Fig X-17). A slower movement of ulceration proceeds toward the sclera. The eye is inflamed and pain can be intense, with photophobia and tearing. Perforation may occur with minor trauma or during secondary infection. Extensive vascularization and fibrosis of the cornea is likely.

Two clinical types of Mooren ulcer have been described. Unilateral Mooren ulcer occurs in an older patient population. Sex distribution is equal in this form, which has a slow course of progression.

A second type of Mooren ulcer is more common in Africa. This form is usually bilateral, rapidly progressive, and poorly responsive to medical or surgical intervention (Fig X-18). Central corneal ulceration and perforation is frequent. Many of the

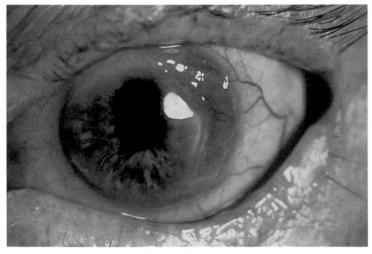

FIG X-17—Mooren ulcer.

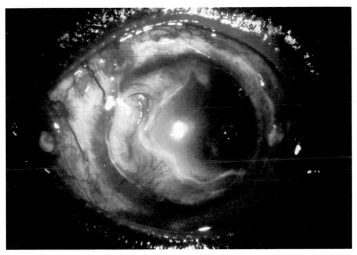

FIG X-18—Mooren ulcer with severe superior limbal ulceration and thinning.

patients with this atypical form of Mooren ulcer also have coexistent parasitemia. It is possible that Mooren ulcer in this subgroup of West African males may be triggered by antigen-antibody reaction to helminthic toxins deposited in the limbal cornea during the bloodborne phase of parasitic infection.

MANAGEMENT. The multiplicity of therapeutic strategies employed against Mooren ulcer underscores the relative lack of effective treatment. Topical steroids, contact lenses, collagenase inhibitors such as acetylcysteine (Mucomyst 10%) and L-cysteine (0.2 molar), topical cyclosporine, limbal conjunctival excision, and lamellar keratoplasty have all been tried with variable success. Systemic immunosuppressives such as oral corticosteroids, cyclophosphamide, methotrexate, and cyclosporine have shown some promise in selected cases. Hepatitis C–associated cases of Mooren ulcer have responded to interferon therapy.

Immune-Mediated Diseases of the Sclera

Episcleritis

PATHOGENESIS. Episcleritis is a self-limited, generally benign inflammation of the episcleral tissues. The pathophysiology of this disorder remains obscure. An underlying systemic cause is found in a minority of patients.

CLINICAL PRESENTATION. Episcleritis is a transient, self-limited disease of adults, usually 20–50 years of age. The chief complaint is usually ocular redness without irritation, which typically persists for days to a few weeks, then resolves spontaneously. Slight tenderness may be present. The disease occurs most commonly in the exposure zone of the eye, often in the area of a pingueculum, and it may recur in the same or different locations. About one third of patients have bilateral disease at one time or another.

Episcleritis is diagnosed clinically by localizing the site of inflammation to the episclera. Unlike the deeper inflamed blood vessels involved in scleritis, inflamed episcleral vessels

- Radiate posteriorly from the limbus
- Have a salmon pink color in natural sunlight
- Can be moved over the deeper sclera with a cotton-tipped applicator
- Will blanch with topical phenylephrine

Episcleral edema without underlying scleral edema may be seen with a thin slit-lamp beam. Episcleritis is classified as simple (diffuse injection) or nodular. In simple episcleritis the inflammation is localized to one sector of the globe in 70% of cases, and the entire episclera is inflamed in 30% of cases. A localized mobile nodule develops in nodular episcleritis (Fig X-19). Small peripheral corneal opacities can be observed adjacent to the area of episcleral inflammation in 10% of patients. Episcleritis generally resolves without producing any lasting destructive effects on tissues of the eye.

MANAGEMENT. A diagnostic work-up for underlying causes (e.g., autoimmune connective tissue disease, gout, herpes zoster, syphilis, tuberculosis, rosacea) is rarely indicated except after multiple recurrences. Episcleritis generally clears without treatment, but topical or oral nonsteroidal anti-inflammatory agents may be prescribed for patients bothered by pain. Topical vasoconstricting agents may reduce the redness but should be used sparingly to avoid rebound phenomenon. The use of topical corticosteroids should be avoided in this benign, self-limited condition.

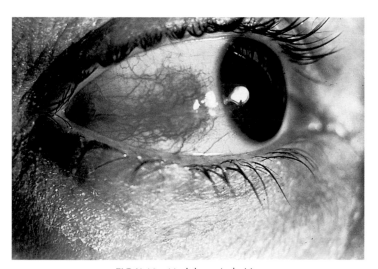

FIG X-19—Nodular episcleritis.

Scleritis

PATHOGENESIS. Scleritis is a much more severe ocular inflammatory condition than episcleritis. It is caused by an immune-mediated (typically immune-complex) vasculitis that inflames and destroys the sclera. Scleritis is frequently associated with an underlying systemic immunologic disease; about one third of patients with diffuse or nodular scleritis and two thirds with necrotizing scleritis have a detectable connective tissue or autoimmune disease. Scleritis causes significant pain and may lead to structural alterations of the globe and visual morbidity. It is exceedingly rare in children, occurring most often in the fourth to sixth decades of life, and is more common in women. More than half of scleritis cases are, or become, bilateral.

CLINICAL PRESENTATION. The onset of scleritis is usually gradual, extending over several days. Most patients with scleritis develop severe boring, or piercing, ocular pain, which may worsen at night and occasionally awaken them from sleep. The pain may be referred to other regions of the head on the involved side, and the globe is often tender to touch. The inflamed sclera has a violaceous hue best seen in natural sunlight. Inflamed scleral vessels have a crisscross pattern, adhere to the sclera, and cannot be moved with a cotton-tipped applicator. Scleral edema, often with overlying episcleral edema, is noted by slit-lamp examination. Scleritis can be classified clinically based on the anatomical location (anterior or posterior sclera) and appearance of scleral inflammation (Table X-2).

Diffuse or nodular anterior scleritis   *Diffuse anterior scleritis* is characterized by a zone of scleral edema and redness. A portion of the anterior sclera (<50%) is involved in 60% of cases, and the entire anterior segment is involved in 40% of cases (Fig X-20). In *nodular anterior scleritis* the scleral nodule is a deep red to purple color, immobile, and separated from the overlying episcleral tissue, which is elevated by the nodule (Fig X-21).

TABLE X-2

SUBTYPES AND PREVALENCE OF SCLERITIS

LOCATION	SUBTYPE	PREVALENCE
Anterior sclera	Diffuse scleritis	40%
	Nodular scleritis	44%

	Necrotizing scleritis
	  with inflammation
	  without inflammation (scleromalacia perforans)
		14%
		(10%)
		(4%)

Posterior sclera		2%

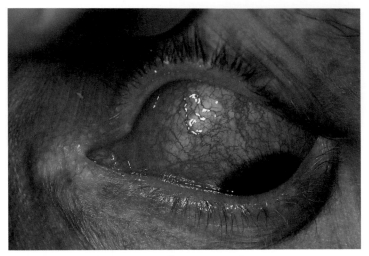

FIG X-20—Diffuse anterior scleritis.

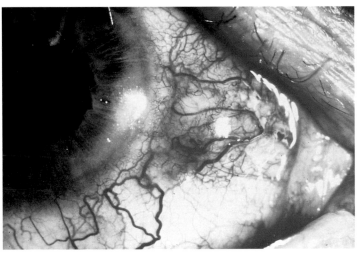

FIG X-21—Nodular scleritis.

Necrotizing scleritis   Necrotizing scleritis is the most destructive form of scleritis. Of the patients affected 60% develop ocular and systemic complications; 40% suffer loss of vision; and up to 30% die within 5 years of onset, usually as a result of complications of vasculitis.

Patients typically present with severe pain out of proportion to the inflammatory signs. Most commonly, a localized patch of inflammation is noted initially, with

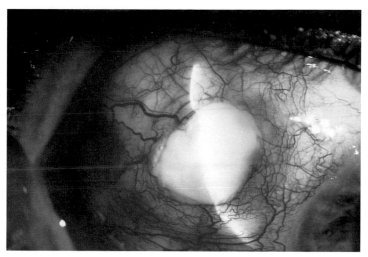

FIG X-22—Necrotizing scleritis.

the edges of the lesion more inflamed than the center. A less common presentation (25% of cases) is an avascular edematous patch of sclera and overlying episclera (Fig X-22). Untreated, necrotizing scleritis may spread posteriorly to the equator and circumferentially until the entire anterior globe is involved. Severe loss of tissue may result if treatment is not intensive and prompt. The sclera may have a blue-gray appearance and show an altered deep episcleral blood vessel pattern (large anastomotic blood vessels that may circumscribe the involved area) after the inflammation subsides.

Necrotizing scleritis without signs of inflammation (scleromalacia perforans) This form of scleritis occurs predominantly in patients with long-standing rheumatoid arthritis (55% of cases). Signs of inflammation are minimal, and generally no pain accompanies this type of scleritis. As the disease progresses, the sclera thins and the underlying dark uveal tissue becomes visible (Fig X-23). In many cases the uvea is covered with only thin connective tissue and conjunctiva. Large abnormal blood vessels surround and cross the areas of scleral loss. A bulging staphyloma develops if the IOP is elevated; spontaneous perforation is rare, although these eyes may rupture with minimal trauma.

Posterior scleritis Posterior scleritis can occur in isolation or concomitant with anterior scleritis. Patients present with pain, tenderness, proptosis, visual loss, and occasionally with restricted motility. Choroidal folds, exudative retinal detachment, papilledema, and angle-closure glaucoma secondary to choroidal thickening may develop. Retraction of the lower eyelid may occur in upgaze, presumably caused by infiltration of muscles in the region of the posterior scleritis. The pain may be referred to other parts of the head, and the diagnosis can be missed in the absence of associated anterior scleritis. Demonstration of thickened posterior sclera by echography,

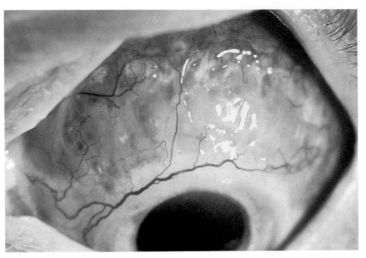

FIG X-23—Scleromalacia perforans in a patient with long-standing rheumatoid arthritis.

computed tomography (CT), or magnetic resonance imaging (MRI) may be helpful in establishing the diagnosis. Most often no related systemic disease can be found in patients with posterior scleritis.

Complications of scleritis   Complications are frequent and include peripheral keratitis (37%), uveitis (30%), cataract (7%), glaucoma (18%), and scleral thinning (33%). Anterior uveitis may occur as a spillover phenomenon in eyes with anterior scleritis. Posterior uveitis occurs in all patients with posterior scleritis and may occur in anterior scleritis when the overlying sclera is inflamed. Although one third of patients with scleritis have evidence of scleral translucency and/or thinning, frank scleral defects are seen only in the most severe forms of necrotizing disease and in the late stages of scleromalacia perforans.

The following forms of corneal involvement may develop in conjunction with scleritis:

□ *Acute stromal keratitis.* Superficial and midstromal infiltrates appear in the peripheral cornea and sometimes centrally. Vascularization and opacification of the involved stroma may ensue in the absence of treatment. In nodular or sectoral scleritis the corneal changes are usually localized to the area of inflammation.

□ *Sclerokeratitis.* The peripheral cornea becomes opacified by fibrosis and lipid deposition. Fibers in the involved area may reflect light and resemble the sugar

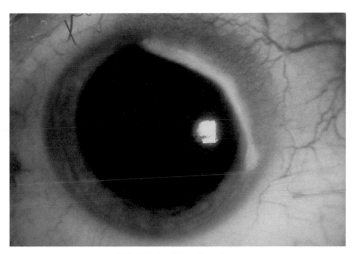

FIG X-24—Sclerokeratitis.

crystals of cotton candy (Fig X-24). The area of involvement may gradually move centrally, resulting in opacification of a large segment of cornea. Vascularization is often seen in the involved area. In nodular scleritis these changes are localized to the area of scleral involvement. This type of keratitis commonly accompanies herpes zoster sclerokeratitis.

□ *Marginal keratolysis ("melting")*. A peripheral crescentic corneal ulcer, or gutter, may develop in patients with scleritis adjacent to the limbus. The peripheral corneal stroma may be infiltrated or appear clear. Commonly, corneal ulceration occurs adjacent to an area of scleritis; however, in some cases adjacent scleral inflammation may be minimal. Marginal keratolysis is most commonly seen in patients who have autoimmune connective tissue disease, especially rheumatoid arthritis, or a systemic vasculitis such as Wegener granulomatosis.

LABORATORY EVALUATION. Scleritis can occur in association with various systemic infectious diseases, including syphilis, tuberculosis, herpes zoster, and Hansen disease. It is most frequently seen in association with autoimmune connective tissue diseases such as rheumatoid arthritis, systemic lupus erythematosus, and ankylosing spondylitis and with vasculitides such as Wegener granulomatosis and polyarteritis nodosa. Metabolic diseases such as gout may also be associated with scleritis. More than one half of patients with scleritis have an associated identifiable systemic disease.

Since patients with certain forms of scleritis, especially necrotizing scleritis with inflammation, have an increased mortality rate, its presence should be recognized as a manifestation of a potentially fatal systemic disease. The work-up of scleritis should therefore include a complete physical examination, with attention to the joints, skin, and cardiovascular and respiratory systems. The following laboratory tests are recommended:

- Complete blood count (CBC) with differential
- Erythrocyte sedimentation rate (ESR)
- Circulating immune complexes
- Serum autoantibody screen (antinuclear antibodies, anti–DNA antibodies, rheumatoid factor)
- Urinalysis
- Serum uric acid
- Syphilis serology
- Chest x-ray

Additional laboratory tests may be indicated based on the clinical findings.

MANAGEMENT. Topical corticosteroids may occasionally reduce ocular inflammation in mild cases of diffuse anterior and nodular scleritis. When these are not effective, oral nonsteroidal anti-inflammatory medications such as indomethacin (Indocin), naproxen (Naprosyn), or diclofenac (Voltaren) frequently are effective. If scleritis does not respond to these treatments, then oral corticosteroids may be required. Although subconjunctival steroids may be effective in reducing scleral inflammation, they have been reported to cause scleral necrosis when used for scleritis.

Necrotizing scleritis and sclerokeratitis are considered ocular manifestations of systemic vasculitis, and sytemic immunosuppressive therapy has been recommended for these conditions. Oral and/or high-dose (pulse) IV steroids may be effective for some cases of necrotizing scleritis or sclerokeratitis. If no therapeutic response is observed with corticosteroids, however, systemic cytotoxic immunosuppressive therapy (cyclophosphamide, azathioprine, methotrexate) or cyclosporine is recommended. Cyclophosphamide is the drug of choice for ocular involvement in patients with Wegener granulomatosis. Patients receiving systemic immunosuppressive therapy for scleritis should be monitored closely for systemic complications associated with these drugs. Provision of antituberculosis coverage may be necessary for PPD-positive patients.

Dubord PJ, Chalmers A. Scleritis and episcleritis: diagnosis and management. In: *Focal Points: Clinical Modules for Ophthalmologists*. San Francisco: American Academy of Ophthalmology; 1995;13:9.

Foster CS, Sainz de la Maza M. *The Sclera*. New York: Springer-Verlag; 1994.

PART 5

NEOPLASTIC DISORDERS OF THE EYELIDS, CONJUNCTIVA, AND CORNEA

CHAPTER XI

Tumor Cell Biology and Diagnostic Approaches to Neoplastic Disorders

The Eyelid Skin and Ocular Surface

Microanatomy

The anatomy of the eyelids and the ocular surface and the pathologic processes that affect these tissues should be reviewed. BCSC Section 2, *Fundamentals and Principles of Ophthalmology,* and Section 4, *Ophthalmic Pathology and Intraocular Tumors,* provide the necessary background regarding these areas.

The skin of the upper eyelid is the thinnest of the body, and it continues to thin with aging. The epidermis of the eyelid skin is composed of keratinocytes arranged in layers: basal, prickle, squamous, granular, and keratin. Basal keratinocytes contain a variable amount of melanin pigment. *Dendritic melanocytes* and *Langerhans' cells* are scattered throughout the epidermis. *Nevus cells* are modified melanocytes found in clumps in the epidermis and dermis that have varying degrees of pigmentation depending on their expression of tyrosinase and melanogenic activity. Basal epidermal cells produce a basement membrane to which they attach by hemidesmosomes. Downward projections of the epidermis into the dermis are called *rete ridges,* and the corresponding upward projections of the dermis are called *dermal ridges,* or *dermal papillae* (Fig XI-1). The dermis of the eyelid skin lacks well-defined papillae and consists of a thin layer of fibrovascular tissue containing hair follicles, sebaceous glands, and sweat glands but no fat. The dermis is loosely attached to the underlying orbicularis oculi muscle, except at the eyelid creases, canthi, and margins.

The epithelium of the conjunctiva and cornea includes basal cells, wing cells, and superficial cells but lacks granular and keratin layers. Goblet cells, melanocytes, and Langerhans' cells are present in the conjunctival epithelium. Pigmented and nonpigmented nevus cells are found in nests of the conjunctival epithelium and substantia propria. Langerhans' cells and occasional melanocytes are present in the peripheral cornea. Basal epithelial cells produce a basement membrane to which they attach by hemidesmosomes. The substantia propria of the conjunctiva and the stroma of the cornea consist of fibrous tissue.

Stem Cells and Cell Turnover

Stem cells for skin and mucous membranes are present in the basal layer, located in certain niches sheltered from environmental insults. Epidermal stem cells reside in rete ridges; conjunctival epithelial stem cells are present in the fornix; and corneal

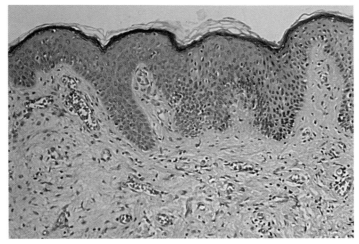

FIG XI-1—Normal eyelid skin, with typical downward projections of epidermis and upward projections of dermis. (Hematoxylin-eosin, ×100.)

epithelial stem cells are clustered at the limbus. The eyelid epidermis is replaced every 2 weeks, and conjunctival and corneal epithelial cells are replaced every week. How the homeostatic sequence—the shedding of superficial cells, division of basal cells, and migration of stem cells—occurs is currently under study.

Histopathologic Processes and Conditions

A *tumor* is a tissue mass that may be caused by inflammation, fibrovascular proliferation, cystic enlargement, or neoplasia. The most common growths of the external eye, such as pterygia and chalazia, are reactive rather than neoplastic. True neoplasms of the eyelids and ocular surface are disturbances of squamous epidermis or epithelium, melanocytes, or altered mesenchymal cells. Neoplastic tumors are associated with various cellular and tissue reactions, which are defined in Table XI-1.

Neoplasia is the unregulated proliferation of cells in a tissue. The pattern of growth can be described clinically or histologically. For example, a papilloma is any epidermal or epithelial growth that extends outward in a multilobulated pattern and that contains a central vascular core in each lobule. A neoplasm may be benign or malignant. Histopathologic criteria that differentiate benign from malignant neoplasms are based on cellular and nuclear morphology and on tissue organization (Table XI-2).

Dysplasia is a term that indicates a trend toward malignancy; it is characterized by acanthosis, cellular atypia, and abnormal polarity. *Anaplasia* is severe dysplasia that indicates malignancy. Lesions classified as precancerous are those in which malignant transformation has taken place at a cellular level but no invasion has occurred. For example, intraepithelial neoplasia is a malignancy that has not invaded beneath the epidermal or epithelial basement membrane or shown metastasis.

TABLE XI-1

CELLULAR AND TISSUE REACTIONS

HISTOPATHOLOGIC TERM	DEFINITION
Hypertrophy	Increase in size of cells or tissue without increase in number of cells
Hyperplasia	Increase in number of cells in excess of normal but not progressive
Metaplasia	Transformation of one type of tissue into another
Atrophy	Decrease in size of cells or tissue
Necrosis	Secondary death of cells or tissue
Apoptosis	Normal or abnormal programmed death of cells
Dysplasia	Abnormal growth of cells
Neoplasia	Unregulated increase in number of cells

TABLE XI-2

HISTOPATHOLOGIC FEATURES OF NEOPLASIA

HISTOPATHOLOGIC TERM	DEFINITION	IMPLICATION
Acanthosis	Thickening of the squamous layer, as a result of increased mitosis of basal cell layer	Active cell proliferation, whether benign, preinvasive, or malignant
Hyperkeratosis	Increased thickness of the keratin layer of the epidermis (also called *epidermalization* when occurring on mucosal epithelium)	Active cell proliferation, whether benign, preinvasive, or malignant (called *leukoplakia* when a visible white plaque is seen on the conjunctiva)
Parakeratosis	Hyperkeratosis in which nuclei persist in the superficial cells	Active cell proliferation, whether benign, preinvasive, or malignant
Dyskeratosis	Keratinization of individual cells that lie within the epidermis or epithelium, rather than at the surface	Active cell proliferation, whether benign, preinvasive, or malignant
Cellular atypia	Increased nucleus-to-cytoplasm ratio (hyperchromasia); nucleus may be increased in size or number, be abnormally shaped, or have abnormal mitotic figures	Isolated atypical cells may indicate premalignant lesions; abundant atypical cells occur in malignancy
Abnormal polarity	Loss of normal transition from basal cells to superficial cells, and all epidermal or epithelial cells look alike	Mild loss of normal cell maturation may indicate premalignant lesions; disorganized architecture occurs in malignancy

Carcinoma indicates invasion of dysplastic cells beneath the basement membrane and/or metastatic spread. Malignant neoplasms invade and destroy surrounding tissue and may metastasize to form secondary centers of neoplastic growth.

Overview of Oncogenesis

Replicating cells are a necessary component of neoplasia. Most cancers of the eyelids and ocular surface are *carcinomas,* tumors of epithelial cells that continually replicate. *Sarcomas* are less common, partially because the rate of turnover of connective tissue cells is lower.

Oncogenesis is a multistep process. Table XI-3 gives examples of risk factors that can lead to neoplasms. Tumors are initiated by the following:

□ Mutagens or carcinogens that alter cellular DNA

□ Oncogene activation

□ Loss of genetically controlled tumor suppression (e.g., by alterations of the p53 gene on chromosome 17)

Heredity can also play a role; in basal cell carcinoma, for example, alterations in the gene encoding either a membrane-bound protein or the surface protein that it controls may allow the latter molecule to activate cancerous cell division. Promoters that induce inflammation can alter cellular metabolism and increase replication of initiated cells to form benign tumors. BCSC Section 2, *Fundamentals and Principles of Ophthalmology,* discusses these concepts in Part 3, Genetics, and defines many of the terms in the accompanying glossary.

TABLE XI-3

EXAMPLES OF INITIATING CAUSES OF NEOPLASMS
OF THE EYELID AND OCULAR SURFACE

RISK FACTOR	BENIGN	PREINVASIVE/INVASIVE
Physical/chemical exposure (e.g., sunlight)	Squamous cell papilloma Nevus	Actinic keratosis Basal cell carcinoma Lentigo maligna Melanoma
Virus	Molluscum contagiosum Verruca Conjunctival papilloma	Kaposi sarcoma Conjunctival/corneal intraepithelial neoplasia (CIN) Squamous cell carcinoma

Heredity	Neurofibromatosis
	Muir-Torre syndrome
	Gardner syndrome
	Multiple endocrine
	   neoplasia (MEN) syndromes
	Lipoid proteinosis
	Benign hereditary intraepithelial
	   dyskeratosis
		Basal cell nevus syndrome
		Xeroderma pigmentosum

Aberrant regulation of the normal cell cycle with impaired DNA repair mechanisms results in a heterogeneous population of transformed phenotypes. In carcinogenesis the irreversible DNA changes in a subpopulation of cells are partially attenuated by apoptosis of genetically damaged cells. Even though apoptotic cells are more common in rapidly growing tumors, however, an imbalance favoring proliferation over apoptosis produces neoplastic growth.

Growth factors can result in uncontrolled proliferation with malignant transformation and angiogenesis. Local invasion and metastasis involve additional genetic changes with imbalanced regulation of extracellular matrix (e.g., basement membrane) degradation, adhesion, and motility.

The immune system has some control on neoplastic growth. The rare occurrence of spontaneous regression of a tumor in a healthy individual may be related to immune surveillance, and, conversely, immunosuppressed patients have an increased risk of lymphomas and other cancers. Cell-mediated tumor immunity involves the following:

□ Lymphocytes that attack tumor cells

□ Activated macrophages that secrete tumor necrosis factors, proteolytic enzymes, and free radicals

□ Neutrophils

Cancer cells can, however, avoid immune-mediated destruction; for example, by expressing surface ligands that induce apoptosis of T cells.

Antigens expressed by tumor cells include those of the normal cell of origin as well as other tumor-associated antigens. Dedifferentiated cells that fail to suppress genes connected with embryogenesis may express antigens associated with an earlier developmental stage of the parent cell line. Examples are carcinoembryonic antigen and α-fetoprotein. Tumor-specific antigens may be particular to a given neoplastic cell type or may cross-react with other neoplasms of the same histogenesis. Histopathologic diagnosis of certain ocular neoplasms (e.g., melanoma and lymphoma) can be facilitated using monoclonal antibodies to specific epitopes of neoplastic cells.

Ksander BR, Murray TG. Immunology of ocular tumors. In: Pepose JS, Holland GN, Wilhelmus KR, eds. *Ocular Infection and Immunity.* St Louis: Mosby; 1996:157–182.

Diagnostic Approaches

Noninvasive Investigation

Many neoplastic lesions of the eyelid or ocular surface have typical clinical features, and an accurate diagnosis can often be made before histopathologic confirmation. Determining whether the lesion is congenital or acquired can be helpful, and the clinician should investigate the time of onset and growth pattern. History-taking can also help the examiner learn whether an acquired tumor may have arisen from sun exposure, a previous injury, a preexisting lesion, or systemic disease.

External inspection, palpation, and slit-lamp biomicroscopy should be used to distinguish epithelial and subepithelial lesions, cystic and solid tumors, and the presence of inflammation. Malignancy should be suspected in cases of rapid growth, changing color, chronic inflammation, ulceration, or bleeding. Regional lymph nodes should be checked. Periodic observation and sequential photographs are used to follow presumed benign lesions such as nevi.

Biopsy Decisions and Techniques

Biopsy is considered for any suspicious lesion. A biopsy may be *incisional,* removing a representative portion of the lesion, or *excisional,* removing the entire lesion with adjacent normal margins. A *shave biopsy* is a type of excisional biopsy for removing a superficial lesion of the epidermis or outer dermis. Microscopic control using frozen sections or Mohs' resection technique can ensure completeness of an excisional biopsy (see BCSC Section 4, *Ophthalmic Pathology and Intraocular Tumors*).

Primary excisional biopsy is undertaken for small lesions that are symptomatic or suspected to be malignant. If a biopsy is planned, an excisional biopsy is often preferred to completely remove the lesion. An incisional biopsy is reserved for large lesions where extensive, reconstructive surgery would be required. The choice of whether to primarily close or to use a skin or mucous-membrane graft depends on the extent of surgery.

The excision should be deep enough to contain the lesion and a small amount of adjacent nonaffected tissue. Lesions of the eyelid skin are usually excised, when possible, by a small ellipse aligned along orbicularis fibers (Fig XI-2). A lesion of the eyelid margin is often removed with a wedge resection (Fig XI-3). Frozen sections are then obtained to determine completeness of excision. A limbal lesion can be removed with a lamellar conjunctivosclerectomy (Fig XI-4). Gentle handling to avoid crushing is essential. Marking the tissue and making a diagram when cutting appropriate cross sections help to orient the pathologist.

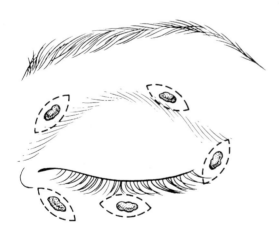

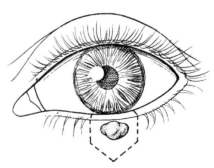

FIG XI-2—Placement of incisions for excisional biopsy of eyelid lesions. (Illustration by Christine Gralapp.)

FIG XI-3—Placement of incisions for excisional biopsy of eyelid margin lesion. (Illustration by Christine Gralapp.)

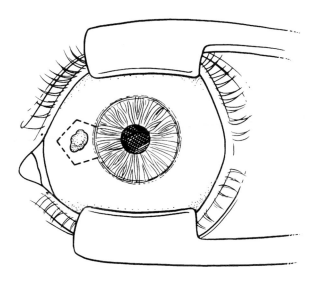

FIG XI-4—Excisional biopsy of conjunctival lesion. (Illustration by Christine Gralapp.)

Approximately 80% of cutaneous eyelid lesions are benign. The diagnosis by an experienced ophthalmologist of malignancy or premalignancy is approximately 90% predictive of subsequent histopathologic evaluation. If the initial histopathologic findings do not agree with the clinical impression, repeat biopsy should be considered.

Management

Therapeutic approaches include surgery, cryotherapy, radiotherapy, and chemotherapy. Drugs that inhibit viral replication, kill proliferating cells, block angiogenesis, or clot blood vessels feeding a tumor are under development. Consultation with a tumor board, a multidisciplinary group of physicians that meets to review cancer cases, can aid in the decision-making process of cancer care. See also BCSC Section 7, *Orbit, Eyelids, and Lacrimal System*.

Shields JA, Shields CL, De Potter P. Surgical management of conjunctival tumors. *Arch Ophthalmol.* 1997;115:808–815.

Clinical Approach to Neoplastic Disorders of the Conjunctiva and Cornea

Approximately 1 person in 2500 seeks ophthalmic care for a tumor of the eyelid or ocular surface each year, totaling about 100,000 per year in the United States. Benign neoplasms are at least three times more frequent than malignant lesions. Most of these tumors arise from the eyelid skin and are discussed in BCSC Section 4, *Ophthalmic Pathology and Intraocular Tumors,* and Section 7, *Orbit, Eyelids, and Lacrimal System.*

Neoplastic tumors of the conjunctiva and cornea are considered together because the lesions often affect both tissues in a similar fashion. These lesions are classified by the type of cell, such as epithelium, melanocytes and nevus cells, vascular endothelium and mesenchymal cells, and lymphocytes. Many are analogous to lesions affecting the eyelid (Table XII-1). Several infectious and inflammatory lesions of the conjunctiva, limbus, and cornea are associated with exophytic growth. Lesions discussed elsewhere in this volume are hordeolum; various granulomatous reactions such as chalazion, sarcoidosis, cat-scratch disease, and lymphogranuloma venereum; and corneal keloid (consult the index). See also BCSC Section 4, *Ophthalmic Pathology and Intraocular Tumors.*

> Kaufman HE, Barron BE, McDonald MB. *The Cornea.* 2nd ed. Boston: Butterworth-Heinemann; 1998:597–632.

> Smolin G, Thoft RA, eds. *The Cornea: Scientific Foundations and Clinical Practice.* 3rd ed. Boston: Little, Brown; 1994:579–595.

Cysts of the Epithelium

Epithelial Inclusion Cyst

These cysts may occur from an obstructed duct or infolding of normal conjunctival crypts. One or more small conjunctival cysts are very commonly seen in the lower fornix of healthy people (Fig XII-1).

PATHOGENESIS. Like epidermal cysts of the eyelids, cysts of conjunctival epithelium can be congenital or can develop during life. Many small cysts are likely formed by apposition of conjunctival folds. Large, single cysts are usually a result of epithelium implanted into the substantia propria by trauma, surgery, or inflammation.

CLINICAL FINDINGS. Conjunctival inclusion cysts are clear and are lined by normal conjunctival epithelium. A corneal epithelial inclusion cyst can occur if trauma or

Table XII-1

Comparison Between Some Cutaneous and Mucosal Manifestations
of Neoplastic and Pigmentary Conditions

EYELID	CONJUNCTIVA
Surface lesions	
Epidermal inclusion cyst	Epithelial inclusion cyst
Squamous cell papilloma	Squamous cell papilloma
Actinic keratosis	Mild conjunctival intraepithelial neoplasia
Intraepidermal squamous cell carcinoma	Severe conjunctival intraepithelial neoplasia
Squamous cell carcinoma	Squamous cell carcinoma
Pigmentary lesions	
Freckle	Freckle
Dermal melanocytosis	Ocular melanocytosis
Nevus	Nevus
Junctional	Junctional
Compound	Compound
Intradermal	Subepithelial
Lentigo maligna	Primary acquired melanosis
Melanoma	Melanoma

surgery displaces ocular surface epithelium into the stroma. Lymphangiectasia may look like an inclusion cyst of the bulbar conjunctiva.

MANAGEMENT. Because the cyst will recur after simple puncture if its epithelial wall remains, complete excision or marsupialization is necessary.

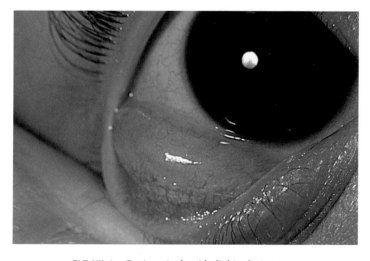

FIG XII-1—Conjunctival epithelial inclusion cyst.

TABLE XII-2

NEOPLASTIC TUMORS OF OCULAR SURFACE EPITHELIUM

BENIGN	PREINVASIVE	MALIGNANT
Papilloma	Conjunctival and corneal intraepithelial neoplasia	Squamous cell carcinoma
Pseudoepitheliomatous hyperplasia		Mucoepidermoid carcinoma
Benign hereditary intraepithelial dyskeratosis		

Tumors of Epithelial Origin

Table XII-2 lists the epithelial tumors of the conjunctiva and cornea.

> Margo CE. Nonpigmented lesions of the ocular surface. In: *Focal Points: Clinical Modules for Ophthalmologists.* San Francisco: American Academy of Ophthalmology; 1996;14:9.

> Warner MA, Jakobiec FA. Squamous neoplasms of the conjunctiva. In: Krachmer JF, Mannis MJ, Holland EJ, eds. *Cornea.* St Louis: Mosby; 1997;2:701–714.

Benign Epithelial Tumors

Conjunctival papilloma The two forms of conjunctival papilloma—sessile or pedunculated—have etiologic, histologic, and clinical differences. Papillomatous growth of conjunctival intraepithelial neoplasia is discussed below.

PATHOGENESIS. Human papillomavirus (HPV), usually subtype 6 or 11, initiates a neoplastic growth of epithelial cells with vascular proliferation that gives rise to a verruca vulgaris (wart) of the eyelid skin or a pedunculated papilloma of the conjunctiva (Fig XII-2). In contrast, a sessile lesion, which has a higher tendency to develop into a dysplastic or carcinomatous lesion, is caused by HPV subtype 16 or 18. HPV 16 produces a protein that interferes with the normal cell cycle and inhibits cellular apoptosis. This oncogenic virus strain is also associated with human cervical carcinoma.

CLINICAL FINDINGS. A pedunculated conjunctival papilloma is a fleshy, exophytic growth with a fibrovascular core. It often arises in the inferior fornix but can also present on the tarsal or bulbar conjunctiva or along the semilunar fold. The lesion emanates from a stalk and has a multilobulated appearance with smooth, clear epithelium and numerous underlying tiny, superficial corkscrew blood vessels. Multiple lesions sometimes occur, and the lesion may be extensive in patients with HIV infection.

A sessile papilloma is more typically found at the limbus and has a flat base. The surface glistens, and numerous red dots resembling a strawberry appear. Spread

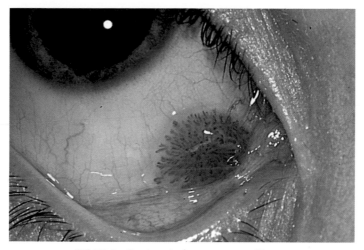

FIG XII-2—Conjunctival squamous papilloma.

onto the adjacent cornea can occur. Signs of dysplasia are keratinization (leuko-plakia), inflammation, and invasion. A very rare variant is an inverted papilloma.

MANAGEMENT. Many conjunctival papillomas regress spontaneously. A peduncu-lated papilloma that is small, cosmetically acceptable, and nonirritating may be observed, although spontaneous resolution can take months to years. An incomplete excision can stimulate growth. Cryotherapy, excision with cryotherapy to the base, or excision with mitomycin-C application is sometimes curative, but recurrences are frequent. Surgical manipulation should be minimal to reduce the risk of disseminat-ing virions to other conjunctival sites. Interferon injections have been tried with vari-able success. The use of antisense oligonucleotides is under investigation.

A sessile limbal papilloma may also be observed. If the lesion enlarges or shows clinical features suggesting dysplastic or carcinomatous growth, then excisional biopsy with adjunctive cryotherapy is recommended.

Pseudoepitheliomatous hyperplasia   Somewhat common on the eyelid, pseudo-epitheliomatous hyperplasia and keratoacanthoma are rarely diagnosed clinically on the conjunctiva. Pseudoepitheliomatous hyperplasia can be found histologically in the conjunctival epithelium overlying a pterygium or pinguecula.

Benign hereditary intraepithelial dyskeratosis   This very rare inherited condition of the bulbar conjunctiva begins in infancy. It is an autosomal dominant disorder of mucosal squamous cell maturation that occurs in descendants of a triracial family from North Carolina. Bilateral horseshoe-shaped plaques affect the nasal and/or tem-poral bulbar conjunctiva and sometimes extend onto the peripheral cornea. Similar leukoplakic lesions may involve the buccal mucosa. The tumors are benign and have no malignant potential, although they may recur following excision.

Preinvasive Epithelial Lesions

Conjunctival intraepithelial neoplasia Conjunctival intraepithelial neoplasia (CIN) is analogous to actinic keratosis of the eyelid. The neoplastic process, which does not invade the underlying basement membrane, is sometimes called mild CIN, or *squamous dysplasia,* if atypical cells involve only part of the epithelium; and it is called severe CIN, or *carcinoma in situ,* when cellular atypia extends throughout the epithelial layer (Figs XII-3, XII-4). (Squamous cell carcinoma, illustrated in Figure XII-4, is discussed below.)

PATHOGENESIS. The relative contribution of human papillomavirus infection, sunlight exposure, and host factors has not been determined. The lesion most commonly develops on exposed areas of the bulbar conjunctiva, at or near the limbus, of fair-skinned, older people who have been exposed to petroleum products or tobacco smoke or to the sun over long periods of time. Rapid growth has occurred when the lesion is present in a person with AIDS.

CLINICAL FINDINGS. Conjunctival intraepithelial neoplasia is characterized by the following:

□ Gelatinous thickening of the epithelium as a result of acanthosis and dysplasia

□ Varying degrees of leukoplakia that is caused by hyperkeratosis, parakeratosis, and dyskeratosis

□ Abnormal vascularization

□ Mild inflammation

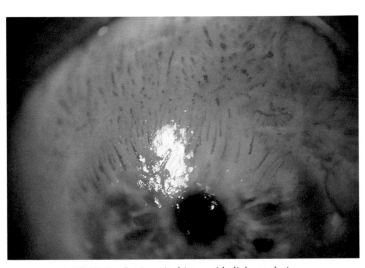

FIG XII-3—Conjunctival intraepithelial neoplasia.

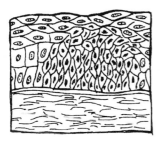
Mild conjunctival
intraepithelial neoplasia
(squamous dysplasia)

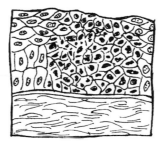
Severe conjunctival
intraepithelial neoplasia
(carcinoma in situ)

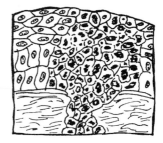
Squamous cell carcinoma

FIG XII-4—Conjunctival epithelial neoplasia.

This slow-growing tumor nearly always begins at the limbus but can spread to affect other areas of the ocular surface or extend onto the cornea. Rose bengal eyedrops may help to define the extent of the lesion, since dysplastic cells stain with a punctate stippling.

LABORATORY EVALUATION. HPV can be detected by immunohistochemistry, in situ hybridization, and polymerase chain reaction. HPV subtypes 6, 8, and 11 are associated with benign growth, while HPV subtypes 16 and 18 are associated with dysplasia and malignant neoplasia.

MANAGEMENT. Excisional biopsy is usually recommended, although lesions may recur in up to one third of eyes, sometimes many years later. Lesions with dysplastic cells at the excision margin recur sooner and more often than completely excised lesions. Adjunctive cryotherapy, irradiation, or use of mitomycin-C might reduce the likelihood of recurrence. Use of topical interferon and other antiviral agents is under investigation.

Corneal intraepithelial neoplasia The cornea adjacent to intraepithelial neoplasia of the conjunctiva, whether papillomatous or leukoplakic, can also be affected. Sometimes, the conjunctival or limbal component is not clinically apparent, and only ground-glass corneal epithelial changes are seen.

PATHOGENESIS. Human papillomavirus infection is suspected to be the initiating cause of corneal epithelial dysmaturation and of epithelial dysplasia.

CLINICAL FINDINGS. An abnormal, translucent, gray epithelial sheet usually has a broad base at the limbus and extends onto the cornea with fimbriated margins and pseudopodialike extensions (Fig XII-5). Free islands of frosted epithelium are sometimes present on the cornea. Neovascularization does not occur.

MANAGEMENT. Corneal involvement is treated by gently scraping away the opalescent epithelium from the underlying Bowman's layer. Bowman's layer should not be

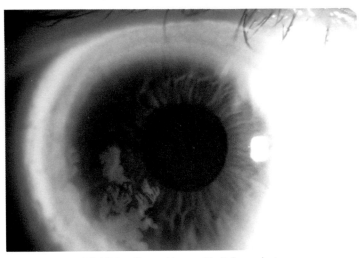

FIG XII-5—Corneal intraepithelial neoplasia.

excised. Excision of the grossly normal but often histologically abnormal adjacent limbal tissues is important, even if the lesion appears to be primarily corneal. Cryotherapy or irradiation of the remaining adjacent conjunctiva (and underlying sclera) can destroy abnormal cells that might remain, probably reducing the likelihood of recurrence.

Malignant Epithelial Lesions

Squamous cell carcinoma   This plaquelike or papillary growth occurs in horizontal bulbar conjunctiva in the interpalpebral fissure zone of older individuals.

PATHOGENESIS. Ultraviolet radiation is the main influence on the development of squamous cell carcinoma, but viral and genetic factors may also play a role. Invasion occurs under the conjunctival portion of the tumor, more aggressively in HIV-infected individuals.

CLINICAL FINDINGS. A broad base is usually present along the limbus, and the lesion tends to grow outward with sharp borders and often has surface leukoplakia (Fig XII-6). While histologic invasion beneath the epithelial basement membrane is present, growth usually remains superficial, infrequently penetrating the sclera or Bowman's layer. Pigmentation can occur in dark-skinned patients. Engorged conjunctival vessels feed the tumor. Adenoid squamous cell carcinoma is a variant that arises in sun-exposed conjunctiva and may be more common in tropical regions. It presents with inflammation, is locally invasive, and can metastasize.

MANAGEMENT. When possible, complete local excision of the tumor accompanied by cryotherapy is the treatment of choice. This procedure may require lamellar dissection into the sclera and aggressive cryotherapy. If neglected, squamous cell carcinoma can eventually invade the interior of the eye, where the tumors can exhibit vigorous growth. Invasion of the iris or trabecular meshwork provides the tumor with

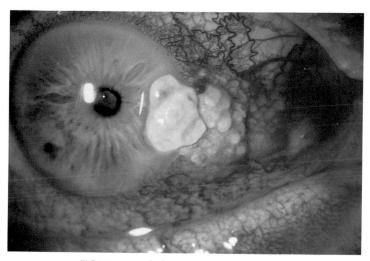

FIG XII-6—Limbal squamous cell carcinoma.

access to the systemic circulation and may be the route by which metastases occur. Extensive invasion can necessitate orbital exenteration, and radiation therapy might sometimes be indicated as an adjunct.

> Lee GA, Hirst LW. Ocular surface squamous neoplasia. *Surv Ophthalmol.* 1995; 39:429–450

Mucoepidermoid carcinoma This tumor is a very rare carcinoma of the limbal conjunctiva, fornix, and caruncle that clinically resembles an aggressive variant of squamous cell carcinoma. In addition to neoplastic epithelial cells, malignant goblet cells can be demonstrated with mucin stains. Compared to squamous cell carcinoma, mucoepidermoid carcinoma is more likely to invade the globe or orbit. Treatment is wide surgical excision; adjuvant therapy can include cryotherapy and radiotherapy.

> Carrau RL, Stillman E, Canaan RE. Mucoepidermoid carcinoma of the conjunctiva. *Ophthalmic Plast Reconstruct Surg.* 1994;10:163–168.

Other carcinomas Spindle cell carcinoma is a very rare tumor of the bulbar or limbal conjunctiva in which the anaplastic cells appear spindle-shaped like fibroblasts. Basal cell carcinoma arising from the conjunctiva is also very rare.

Glandular Tumors of the Conjunctiva

Oncocytoma

A slow-growing cystadenoma may arise from metaplasia of ductal and acinar cells of accessory lacrimal glands. These benign tumors most often arise from the caruncle in elderly individuals, although the most common tumors of the caruncle are papillomas and nevi.

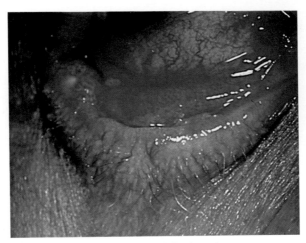

FIG XII-7—Sebaceous gland carcinoma.

Dacryoadenoma

This very rare benign proliferation of lacrimal cells originates from the conjunctival epithelium.

Sebaceous Gland Carcinoma

Sebaceous adenocarcinoma   Sebaceous gland carcinoma accounts for approximately 1% of all eyelid tumors and for 5% of eyelid malignancies. It affects older individuals, women more than men, and Asians more than others. It masquerades as a benign eyelid lesion such as a chalazion and as chronic unilateral blepharitis or conjunctivitis (Fig XII-7).

PATHOGENESIS. Most sebaceous gland carcinomas of the eyelid arise from a meibomian gland, but some develop from the glands of Zeis, sebaceous glands of the caruncle, and pilosebaceous glands of the eyelids and eyebrows. Stepwise genetic damage may explain the multifocal nature of sebaceous carcinoma and its gradual progression from dysplasia to cancer in long-standing disease. Mutational inactivation of p53 may be involved. Human papillomavirus infection, previous radiation therapy, and exposure to carcinogens are possible risk factors. Lesions are more common on the upper eyelid than the lower and tend to involve the eyelid margin.

CLINICAL FINDINGS. The clinical appearance is variable, as the tumor tends to spread beneath the surface. It may be associated with inflammation and is occasionally multicentric. A typical presentation is a painless, slowly enlarging, very firm nonmobile yellowish nodule. When it arises from a meibomian gland or a gland of Zeis at the eyelid margin, intraepithelial pagetoid spread into the conjunctiva with inflammation may mask the site of origin and seriously delay the diagnosis.

MANAGEMENT. A full-thickness biopsy is performed for histopathologic confirmation. Mapping biopsies may be needed because of skip areas. Wide excision may be necessary, sometimes requiring exenteration or extensive reconstructive surgery. Adjunctive radiotherapy can be given. Complications of the disease include orbital invasion, recurrence, and metastases. A poor prognosis, with a 10-year mortality of approximately 25%, is associated with a duration longer than 6 months, extensive tumor dedifferentiation and invasion, and incomplete excision.

Tumors of Neuroectodermal Origin

Table XII-3 lists the ocular surface tumors arising from melanocytes, nevus cells, and other neuroectodermal cells. Some pigmented lesions of the globe are normal. For example, a *pigment spot of the sclera* is a collection of melanocytes associated with an intrascleral nerve loop or perforating anterior ciliary vessel. The term *melanosis* refers to excessive pigmentation without an elevated mass that may be congenital (whether epithelial or subepithelial) or acquired (whether primary or secondary).

Helm CJ. Melanoma and other pigmented lesions of the ocular surface. In: *Focal Points: Clinical Modules for Ophthalmologists.* San Francisco: American Academy of Ophthalmology; 1996;14:11.

McLean IW. Melanocytic neoplasms of the conjunctiva. In: Krachmer JH, Mannis MJ, Holland EJ, eds. *Cornea.* St Louis: Mosby; 1997;2:715–722.

TABLE XII-3

NEOPLASTIC TUMORS AND RELATED CONDITIONS OF
NEUROECTODERMAL CELLS OF THE OCULAR SURFACE

CELL OF ORIGIN	BENIGN	PREINVASIVE/MALIGNANT
Epithelial melanocytes	Freckle Benign acquired melanosis	Primary acquired melanosis Melanoma
Subepithelial melanocytes	Ocular melanocytosis Blue nevus Melanocytoma	Melanoma
Nevus cells	Intraepithelial nevus Compound nevus Subepithelial nevus	Melanoma
Neural and other cells	Neurofibroma	Leiomyosarcoma

Benign Pigmented Lesions

Freckle A conjunctival ephelis is a flat brown patch, usually of the bulbar conjunctiva near the limbus. It is more common in darkly pigmented individuals and is present from an early age. Larger lesions are called *lentigo* or *benign acquired melanosis.*

Benign acquired melanosis Increasing pigmentation of the conjunctiva of both eyes is a common occurrence in middle-aged individuals with dark skin. This pigmentation, which affects predominantly blacks, is often most apparent in the bulbar conjunctiva within the interpalpebral fissure zone and at the limbus. The stimulus to melanocytic hyperplasia is unknown but may be related to sunlight exposure, like solar lentigo of the skin; secondary melanosis also frequently occurs over any elevated mass of the conjunctiva. Secondary acquired melanosis is characterized by light brown pigmentation of the perilimbal and interpalpebral bulbar conjunctiva. Streaks and whorls called *striate melanokeratosis* sometimes extend into the peripheral corneal epithelium. Some cases resemble a junctional nevus. Conjunctival pigmentation can also occur from epinephrine, silver, and mascara.

Ocular melanocytosis Congenital melanosis of the deep conjunctiva or superficial sclera occurs in about 1 in every 2500 individuals and is more common in the black, Hispanic, and Asian populations.

PATHOGENESIS. Ocular melanocytosis consists of focal proliferation of subepithelial melanocytes (blue nevus).

CLINICAL FINDINGS. Patches of episcleral pigmentation appear slate gray through the normal conjunctiva (Fig XII-8). A diffuse nevus of the uvea is seen as increased pigmentation of the iris and choroid. About one half of patients with ocular melanocytosis have ipsilateral dermal melanocytosis (nevus of Ota), a proliferation of dermal melanocytes in the periocular skin of the first and second dermatomes of cranial nerve V. The combined ocular and cutaneous pigmentations are referred to as *oculodermal melanocytosis.* Approximately 5% of cases are bilateral.

MANAGEMENT. Secondary glaucoma occurs in the affected eye in 10% of patients. Malignant transformation is possible but rare and seems to occur only in white patients. Malignant melanoma can develop in the skin, conjunctiva, uvea, or orbit. The lifetime risk of uveal melanoma in a patient with ocular melanocytosis is about 1 in 400, much greater than the risk of 1 in 13,000 of the general population.

Nevus Nevocellular nevi of the conjunctiva are hamartia that arise during childhood and adolescence. A nevus can be junctional, compound, or subepithelial.

PATHOGENESIS. Pure intraepithelial nevi are rare except in children, and these junctional nevi may be difficult to distinguish histopathologically from primary acquired melanosis. The subepithelial nevus of the conjunctiva is the equivalent of the intradermal nevus of the skin.

CLINICAL FINDINGS. A nevus near the limbus is usually almost flat. Those appearing elsewhere on the bulbar conjunctiva, semilunar fold, caruncle, or eyelid margin tend to be elevated. Pigmentation of conjunctival nevi is variable; they are often light tan

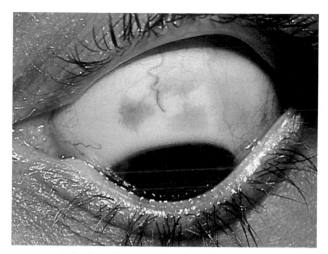

FIG XII-8—Congenital ocular melanocytosis.

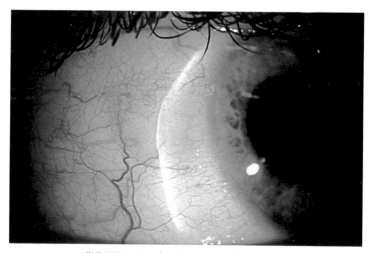

FIG XII-9—Amelanotic conjunctival nevus.

or amelanotic (Fig XII-9). About one fourth lack pigment. A subepithelial nevus often has a cobblestone appearance. Small epithelial inclusion cysts occur within about half of all conjunctival nevi, particularly within compound or subepithelial ones, and this finding is often used to exclude malignancy.

Secretion of mucin by goblet cells in the inclusion cysts can cause a nevus to enlarge, producing a false impression of malignant change. Nevi in adolescents may change around the age of puberty; cellular proliferation causes the nevus to enlarge, which produces secondary lymphocytic inflammation and can cause clinical and histologic confusion with other entities. When inflamed, an amelanotic, vascularized nevus may resemble an angioma.

MANAGEMENT. Conjunctival nevi have a high prevalence of junctional activity. Even so, they rarely become malignant. Nevertheless, excision is so easy that surgery of suspicious lesions is often preferred to prolonged observation or sequential photography, unless the patient is too young to undergo the procedure without being given general anesthesia. Because nevi are rare on the palpebral conjunctiva, pigmented neoplasms on the tarsus or in the fornix are generally excised.

Preinvasive Pigmented Lesions

Primary acquired melanosis This acquired pigmentation of the conjunctival epithelium is analogous to lentigo maligna of the skin (Hutchinson's freckle), a preinvasive intraepidermal lesion of sun-exposed skin. The term *primary acquired melanosis (PAM)* refers to flat, brown lesions of the conjunctival epithelium that are commonly encountered in clinical practice (Fig XII-10). By definition, the condition differs from congenital pigmented lesions and from secondary acquired melanosis, such as that caused by Addison disease, radiation, or pregnancy. Table XII-4 compares the various pigmentary lesions of the conjunctiva. Most idiopathic types of acquired melanosis remain benign, but rare cases show cellular atypia and can be a precursor of conjunctival melanoma.

PATHOGENESIS. Intraepithelial conjunctival melanocytes proliferate in middle-aged white individuals for an unknown reason. Pigmentation in an individual with dark skin is called benign acquired melanosis rather than PAM, but the two conditions may be related.

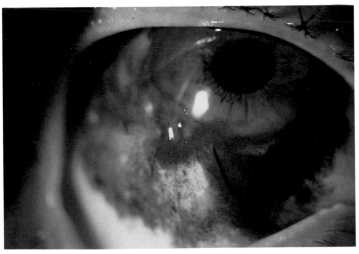

FIG XII-10—Primary acquired melanosis.

TABLE XII-4

CLINICAL COMPARISON OF CONJUNCTIVAL PIGMENTARY LESIONS

LESION	ONSET	AREA	LOCATION	MALIGNANT POTENTIAL
Freckle	Youth	Small	Conjunctiva	No
Benign acquired melanosis	Adulthood	Patchy or diffuse	Conjunctiva	No
Conjunctival nevus	Youth	Small	Conjunctiva	Low (conjunctival melanoma)
Ocular and oculodermal melanocytosis	Congenital	Patchy or diffuse	Under conjunctiva	Yes (uveal melanoma)
Primary acquired melanosis	Middle age	Diffuse	Conjunctiva	Yes (conjunctival melanoma)

CLINICAL FINDINGS. Multiple flat, brown, intermittently waxing and waning patches of unilateral pigmentation appear within the superficial conjunctiva. Changing size may be associated with inflammation or may be the result of hormonal influences. Malignant transformation is probably rare but should be suspected when a lesion shows nodularity, enlargement, or increased vascularity.

MANAGEMENT. The best treatment for this condition remains undetermined. An excisional biopsy should be considered for large or progressive or dark lesions or lesions of the palpebral conjunctiva. When lesions show substantial atypia on histopathologic examination, the clinician should check the margins carefully and perform additional resection until the lesion is completely removed. For lesions that show atypia or malignancy, cryotherapy can be a useful adjunct, and topical mitomycin-C solution is reported to be possibly effective. Regional lymph nodes should be palpated regularly.

McLean IW. Melanocytic neoplasms of the conjunctiva. In: Krachmer JA, Mannis MJ, Holland EJ, eds. Cornea. St Louis: Mosby; 1997;2:715–722.

Malignant Pigmented Lesions

Melanoma   With a prevalence of approximately 1 per 2 million in the population of European ancestry, conjunctival melanomas make up less than 1% of ocular malignancies. Conjunctival melanomas are very rare in blacks and Asians. Although malignant melanoma of the conjunctiva can metastasize, it has a better prognosis than cutaneous melanoma.

PATHOGENESIS. Conjunctival melanomas may arise from nevi, from primary acquired melanosis, or de novo (although some of these may be PAM without clinically detectable pigmentation). Intralymphatic spread increases the risk of metastasis.

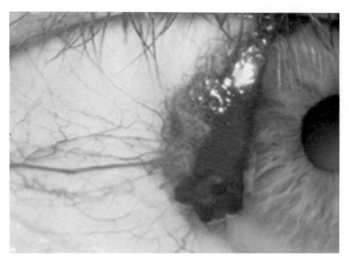

FIG XII-11—Malignant melanoma of the limbal conjunctiva. (Reproduced with permission from Helm CJ. Melanoma and other pigmented lesions of the ocular surface. In: *Focal Points: Clinical Modules for Ophthalmologists*. San Francisco: American Academy of Ophthalmology; 1996;14:11. Photograph courtesy of Thomas Pettit, MD.)

Rarely, an underlying ciliary body melanoma can extend through the sclera. Cutaneous melanoma can very rarely metastasize to the conjunctiva.

CLINICAL FINDINGS. Although conjunctival melanomas can arise in palpebral conjunctiva, they are most common in bulbar conjunctiva or at the limbus (Fig XII-11). The degree of pigmentation is variable. Since heavy vascularization is common, these tumors are likely to bleed easily. They grow in a nodular fashion but can also invade the globe and extend posteriorly into the orbit. The behavior of conjunctival melanoma remains relatively unpredictable in individual cases. Outcome is partly determined by the site involved: bulbar conjunctival melanomas have a better prognosis than melanomas of the palpebral conjunctiva, fornix, or caruncle. Cytologic risk factors for metastasis are large tumors, multicentricity, epithelioid cell type, and lymphatic invasion.

MANAGEMENT. An excisional biopsy should be considered for any suspicious pigmented epibulbar lesions; biopsy does seem not to increase the risk of metastasis. Treatment usually consists of complete local excision, supplemented with cryotherapy to the conjunctival margins and scleral base. Topical mitomycin-C has been used after excision and cryotherapy to treat residual disease. Orbital exenteration is reserved as palliative treatment for advanced, aggressive tumors. Fatal metastases are more likely with thick tumors, multifocal tumors, and melanoma arising in the caruncle or palpebral conjunctiva. The role of radiotherapy or excision of regional lymph nodes has not been determined.

Seregard S. Conjunctival melanoma. *Surv Ophthalmol.* 1998;42:321–350.

Singh AD, Campos OE, Rhatigan RM, et al. Conjunctival melanoma in the black population. *Surv Ophthalmol.* 1998;43:127–133.

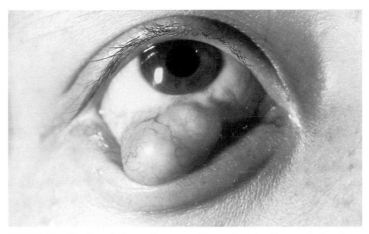

FIG XII-12—Conjunctival neurilemoma. (Reproduced with permission from Charles NC, et al. Conjunctival neurilemoma. Report of 3 cases. *Arch Ophthalmol.* 1997;115:547–549. Photograph courtesy of Norman Charles, MD.)

Neurogenic and Smooth Muscle Tumors

Peripheral nerve-sheath tumors such as *neurofibroma, Schwannoma,* and *neuroma* have been reported under the conjunctiva, especially in multiple endocrine neoplasia (MEN). A neurofibroma of the conjunctiva or eyelid is almost always a manifestation of neurofibromatosis, an autosomal dominant phakomatosis (see BCSC Section 6, *Pediatric Ophthalmology and Strabisimus*). A *neurilemoma* is a very rare tumor of the conjunctiva that originates from Schwann cells of a peripheral nerve sheath (Fig XII-12). *Leiomyosarcoma* is a very rare limbal lesion with the potential for orbital invasion.

Vascular and Mesenchymal Tumors

Vascular lesions of the eyelid margin or conjunctiva are generally a benign hamartoma or a secondary reaction to infection or other stimulus (Table XII-5).

Benign Tumors

Hemangioma   Isolated capillary and cavernous hemangiomas of the bulbar conjunctiva are very rare and are more likely to represent extension from adjacent structures. The palpebral conjunctiva is frequently involved with an eyelid capillary hemangioma. Diffuse hemangiomatosis of the palpebral or forniceal conjunctiva indicates an orbital capillary hemangioma. A cavernous hemangioma of the orbit may present initially under the conjunctiva.

   Nevus flammeus, a congenital lesion described as a port-wine stain, may occur alone or as part of Sturge-Weber syndrome, in which case it is associated with ocu-

TABLE XII-5

NEOPLASTIC TUMORS OF BLOOD VESSELS OF THE EYELID AND CONJUNCTIVA*

HAMARTOMA	REACTIVE	MALIGNANT
Nevus flammeus	Pyogenic granuloma	Kaposi sarcoma
Capillary hemangioma	Glomus tumor	Angiosarcoma
Cavernous hemangioma	Intravascular papillary endothelial hyperplasia	

* Tumors are not listed in a particular order, and lesions in one column do not necessarily correspond to those in parallel columns.

lar vascular hamartomas, secondary glaucoma, and/or leptomeningeal angiomatosis. Some cases are a result of a genetic mutation coding for the vascular endothelial protein receptor for angiopoietin-1 that controls the assembly of perivascular smooth muscle. *Ataxia-telangiectasia* is a syndrome of epibulbar telangiectasis, cerebellar abnormalities, and immune alterations.

Inflammatory vascular tumors   Inflammatory conjunctival lesions often have vascular proliferation. *Pyogenic granuloma,* a common type of reactive hemangioma, is misnamed since it is not suppurative and does not contain giant cells. Pyogenic granuloma follows minor trauma or surgery, which can stimulate exuberant healing tissue with many fibroblasts (granulation tissue) and proliferating capillaries that grow in a radiating pattern. This rapidly growing lesion is intensely red, pedunculated, and smooth (Fig XII-13). It bleeds easily. Topical or intralesional corticosteroids can be of some benefit. Excision with cauterization to the base is usually curative. Primary closure of the wound may minimize recurrence. Treatment of a recurrent pyogenic granuloma includes reexcision, conjunctival autograft, cryotherapy, irradiation, or administration of topical corticosteroids or topical antimetabolites.

   Subconjunctival granulomas may form around parasitic and mycotic infectious foci. They have also occurred with connective tissue diseases such as rheumatoid arthritis. Sarcoid nodules appear as tan-yellow knots that can resemble follicles. *Juvenile xanthogranuloma* is a histiocytic disorder that can present as a conjunctival mass. A *fibrous histiocytoma*, composed of fibroblasts and histiocytes with lipid vacuoles, very rarely arises on the conjunctiva or limbus. *Nodular fasciitis* is a very rare benign tumor in the eyelid or under the conjunctiva that features a nodule of fibrovascular tissue.

Malignant Tumors

Kaposi sarcoma   This malignant neoplasm of vascular endothelium involves the skin and mucous membranes. Internal organs are occasionally involved as well.

PATHOGENESIS. Kaposi sarcoma is caused by human herpesvirus type 8 and is most often associated with AIDS. Three histologic types are described depending on the appearance of vascular endothelium and the number of spindle cells.

CLINICAL FINDINGS. On the eyelid skin Kaposi sarcoma presents as a violet-brown papule. Orbital involvement produces eyelid and conjunctival edema. In the con-

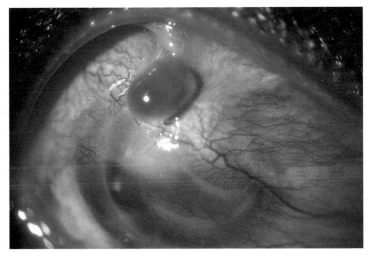

FIG XII-13—Pyogenic granuloma.

junctiva it presents as a reddish blue, vascularized, subconjunctival lesion. Lesions are most often found in the inferior fornix and may be nodular or diffuse (Fig XII-14).

MANAGEMENT. Treatment may not be curative. Options for controlling symptoms include surgical debulking, cryotherapy, and radiotherapy. Local or systemic chemotherapy may be required, and topical interferon has been used.

Other malignant tumors Malignant mesenchymal lesions that rarely involve the conjunctiva are liposarcoma, leiomyosarcoma, and rhabdomyosarcoma.

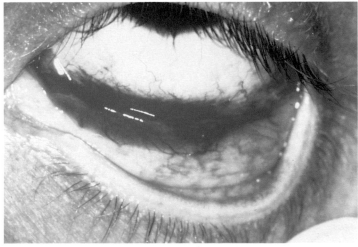

FIG XII-14—Kaposi sarcoma of the conjunctiva. (Reproduced with permission from *Ophthalmology.* 1983;90:859–873. Photograph courtesy of Gary N. Holland, MD.)

251

Lymphatic and Lymphocytic Tumors

Lymphoid tumors of the conjunctiva vary from benign to malignant neoplasia. Many of these lesions have overlapping clinical and pathologic features. About 20% of patients with a conjunctival lymphoid tumor have detectable extraocular lymphoma.

Lymphangiectasia appears on the eye as a group of irregularly dilated lymphatic channels of the bulbar conjunctiva. It may be a developmental anomaly or can follow trauma or inflammation. Anomalous communication with a venule can lead to spontaneous blood-filled lymphatic vessels with subconjunctival hemorrhage. Lymphangiomas are proliferations of lymphatic channel elements.

Lymphangioma

Like a capillary hemangioma, this hamartoma is usually present at birth and may slowly enlarge. The lesion appears as a patch of vesicles with edema. Intralesional hemorrhage, producing a "chocolate cyst," makes differentiation from a hemangioma difficult.

Lymphoid Hyperplasia

PATHOGENESIS. Formerly called *reactive hyperplasia,* this benign-appearing yet autonomous accumulation of lymphocytes and other leukocytes may be a low-grade B-cell lymphoma, but etiology is unknown.

CLINICAL FINDINGS. This mass presents clinically as a minimally elevated salmon-colored subepithelial tumor with a pebbly appearance corresponding to follicle formation (Fig XII-15). It is often moderately or highly vascularized. Primary localized amyloidosis can look like lymphoid hyperplasia.

MANAGEMENT. Lymphoid hyperplasia may resolve spontaneously, but it can be treated with local excision, topical corticosteroids, or radiation. Biopsy specimens require special handling to complete many of the unusual histochemical and immunologic studies. Because a patient with an apparently benign polyclonal lymphoid lesion has the potential to develop a systemic lymphoma, general medical consultation is advisable.

Lymphoma

A neoplastic lymphoid lesion of the conjunctiva is generally a monoclonal proliferation of B cells.

PATHOGENESIS. A lymphoma can arise in or home in on the conjunctival mucosa–associated lymphoid tissue. Some lymphomas are limited to the conjunctiva; others occur in conjunction with systemic malignant lymphoma. Some are polyclonal, but most conjunctival lymphomas are monoclonal B-cell lymphomas. Conjunctival plasmacytoma, Hodgkin lymphoma, and T-cell lymphomas are very rare.

CLINICAL FINDINGS. Aside from a lack of lymphoid follicles and an absence of much vascularity, non-Hodgkin lymphoma has the same clinical appearance as benign lymphoid hyperplasia. It often appears as a salmon pink mass of the conjunctiva that is freely movable on the globe (Fig XII-16). An epibulbar mass fixed to the under-

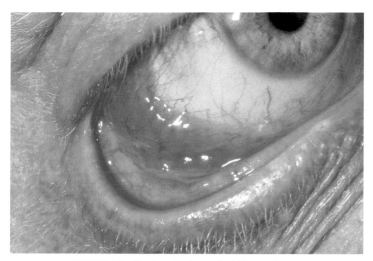

FIG XII-15—Conjunctival lymphoid hyperplasia.

lying sclera is a sign of extrascleral extension of uveal lymphoid neoplasia. Most patients with conjunctival lymphoma are either over 50 years of age or immuno-suppressed. Patients with AIDS have an increased risk of non-Hodgkin lymphomas and Burkitt lymphoma.

LABORATORY EVALUATION AND MANAGEMENT. Patients should be referred for a systemic evaluation to include lymph node palpation, chest radiography, whole body

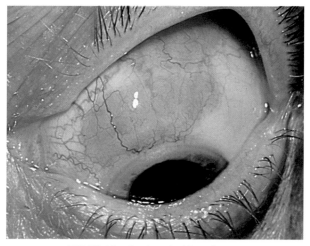

FIG XII-16—Conjunctival lymphoma.

CT scan, CBC, bone marrow biopsy, bone scan, and liver-spleen scan. Cytogenetic indicators, such as B-cell lymphoma gene rearrangement, may aid in determining prognosis. Incisional biopsy is performed for histopathologic diagnosis. Local radiation therapy or cryotherapy is often used, and systemic chemotherapy may be indicated in some cases.

Metastatic Tumors

Metastatic tumors to the conjunctiva are extremely rare but have arisen from cancer of the breast, lung, and elsewhere, including cutaneous melanoma. Metastatic lesions to the uveal tract, orbit, or paranasal sinuses can extend into the conjunctiva. Metastases or leukemic infiltrates to the limbus or cornea are also extremely rare. Immunoglobulin associated with multiple myeloma has been found in the corneal stroma.

Warner MA, Jakobiec FA. Subepithelial neoplasms of the conjunctiva. In: Krachmer JA, Mannis MJ, Holland EJ, eds. *Cornea.* St Louis: Mosby; 1997;2:723–743.

Epibulbar Choristomas

A *hamartoma* is a congenital tumor resulting from abnormal tissue residing at its normal site. Nevi and hemangiomas are hamartomas that are discussed above. A *choristoma* is a heterotopic congenital lesion that results from normal tissue residing in an abnormal location. The most common episcleral choristoma is a *dermoid.* Although present at birth, a choristoma in the eyelid or orbit may not be apparent until later in life.

Epidermoid and Dermoid Cyst

A *congenital epidermoid cyst* is a somewhat rare choristomatous anomaly caused by displacement of normal embryonic tissue. An epidermoid cyst containing accessory skin structures in its wall is called a *dermoid cyst* (Fig XII-17). Epidermoid and dermoid cysts most commonly occur near the frontozygomatic suture and, less often, the nasofrontal suture. A *scleral cyst* occurs at the inferotemporal limbus. Excision is recommended when an epidermoid or dermoid cyst causes or threatens amblyopia or produces a cosmetic deformity.

Dermoid Choristoma

This congenital lesion typically occurs on the inferotemporal globe or temporal limbus as a smooth, elevated, solid mass embedded in the superficial sclera or cornea (Fig XII-18). About 1 in 10,000 individuals is affected.

PATHOGENESIS. A dermoid choristoma occurs from faulty development of the eyelid folds and consists of displaced embryonic tissue that was destined to become skin. Dermoids are composed of fibrous tissue (and occasionally hair with sebaceous glands) that is covered by conjunctival epithelium. *Epibulbar dermoids* are solid,

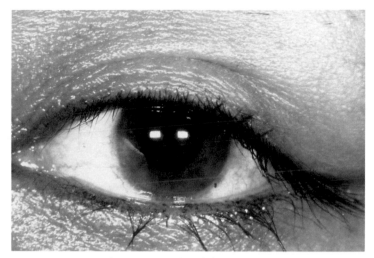

FIG XII-17—Dermoid cyst. (Reproduced from Marines HM, Patrinely JR. Benign eyelid tumors. *Ophthalmol Clin North Am.* 1992;5:243–260.)

rather than cystic, and have not been fully entrapped beneath the surface, unlike dermoid cysts.

CLINICAL FINDINGS. Dermoids are well-circumscribed, porcelain-white, round to oval lesions that occur most often at the inferotemporal limbus, but they can also be found anywhere else on the globe, the central cornea, the subconjunctival space, or

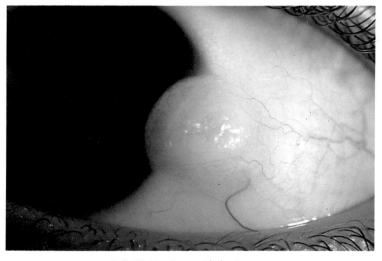

FIG XII-18—Dermoid choristoma.

in the orbit. A limbal dermoid often has an arcuslike deposition of lipid along its corneal border. Severe corneal astigmatism caused by dermoids can lead to aniso-metropic amblyopia.

Dermoids can be a hallmark of a congenital malformation such as Goldenhar syndrome (oculoauriculovertebral dysplasia), a sporadic or autosomal dominant syndrome of the first branchial arch comprising a triad of epibulbar dermoids, facial anomalies such as a coloboma of the upper eyelid and anomalies of the ear (preauricular skin tags and aural fistulae), and vertebral anomalies. One family with corneal dermoids has X-linked inheritance, mapped to Xp22.1–p22.2. BCSC Section 6, *Pediatric Ophthalmology and Strabismus,* discusses and illustrates Goldenhar syndrome in greater detail.

MANAGEMENT. Dermoids grow along with the child and the eye and have virtually no malignant potential. The elevated portion of a dermoid may be excised, but the lesion often extends deep into underlying tissues. Lamellar keratoplasty can improve the cosmetic appearance (Fig XII-19).

Dermolipoma

A dermolipoma is a pale yellow dermoid that contains adipose tissue. It extends more posteriorly than a dermoid and typically occurs superotemporally. This choristoma should be distinguished from herniation of orbital fat.

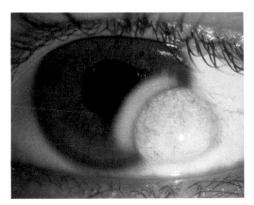
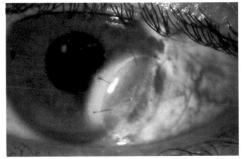

FIG XII-19—A limbal dermoid (left) can be partially excised and replaced by corresponding lamellar donor tissue (right). (Reproduced from Mader TH, Stulting D. Technique for the removal of limbal dermoids. *Cornea.* 1998;17:66–67. Photographs courtesy of Thomas H. Mader, MD, FACS.)

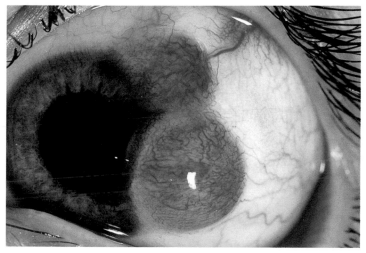

FIG XII-20—Complex choristomas showing rose coloring caused by presence of richly vascularized ectopic lacrimal gland tissue. (Reproduced with permission from Margo CE. Nonpigmented lesions of the ocular surface. In: *Focal Points: Clinical Modules for Ophthalmologists.* San Francisco: American Academy of Ophthalmology; 1996;14:9.)

Ectopic Lacrimal Gland

Lacrimal gland tissue occurring outside of the lacrimal fossa may be associated with a complex choristoma or occur alone as pink, vascularized tissue. An epibulbar lacrimal choristoma is richly vascularized and can become inflamed (Fig XII-20).

Other Choristomas

A *complex choristoma*, usually on the superotemporal globe, has multiple tissues, including cartilage, bone, lacrimal gland lobules, hair follicles, hair, sebaceous glands, and adipose tissue. An *osseous choristoma* is a solitary nodule of bone surrounded by fibrous tissue that is also located superotemporally. A *neuroglial choristoma* is more diffuse. A *phakomatous choristoma* is subcutaneous nodule in the inferomedial eyelid composed of disorganized lens cells.

PART 6

CONGENITAL ANOMALIES
OF THE CORNEA AND SCLERA

CHAPTER XIII

Basic Concepts of Congenital Anomalies of the Cornea and Sclera

Normal Prenatal Development of the Eyelids, Conjunctiva, and Cornea

Just as with the eye as a whole, three parts of the primitive embryo contribute to the development of the external eye: *neuroectoderm, neural crest cells,* and *surface ectoderm.* Mesoderm provides only the endothelium of the vasculature, the orbicularis muscles of the eyelids, and the temporal portion of the sclera. The optic primordium appears at day 24 of gestation in the neural folds (Table XIII-1). The optic vesicle evaginates at day 25, and neural crest cells migrate to surround it. The vesicle induces development of the lens placode from the surface ectoderm at day 28.

In the second month of gestation the optic and lens vesicles invaginate, and two layers of corneal epithelium originating from the surface ectoderm form over the lens vesicle. The first wave of neural crest cells migrates centrally, separating the lens vesicle from the surface ectoderm and forming the primitive corneal endothelium and acellular corneal stroma (Figs XIII-1, XIII-2). In the sixth week the eyelid folds appear. At the seventh week a second wave of neural crest mesenchyme invades the corneal stroma posteriorly, then anteriorly. This wave condenses as sclera, which then begins posterior migration. In the eighth week the third wave of neural crest mesenchyme advances to form the primitive anterior chamber, iris stroma, and pupillary membrane. In the twelfth week the eyelid folds meet and fuse, allowing the conjunctiva and corneal epithelium to develop away from amniotic fluid.

In the third month of gestation iris and ciliary body, cilia, goblet cells, and meibomian glands become evident. Endothelium thins to one layer. Descemet's membrane has become a continuous structure by 12 weeks. In the fourth month characteristic banding of Descemet's membrane begins, and the keratocytes realign and assume a spindle shape. Collagen lamellae are laid down in a spiral, orthogonal pattern proceeding from posterior to anterior. The corneal epithelium develops wing cells and appears more orderly than the conjunctiva. Aqueous humor forms and moves anteriorly. Iris sphincter muscle develops from the neuroectoderm, and the Zeiss and Moll glands form in the eyelids.

In the fifth month scleral fibrils have formed around the axonal bundles of the optic nerve. Keratinization of the eyelid margin from within the pilosebaceous complex causes the eyelids to begin to separate anteriorly. Full separation is present in the sixth month, when dilator muscle of the iris also becomes apparent. In the seventh month the fibrous lamina cribosa is fully formed and the pupillary membrane begins to atrophy. At birth the pupillary membrane has regressed, and the cornea has

TABLE XIII-1

HUMAN ANTERIOR SEGMENT DEVELOPMENT

MO	WEEK	DAY	LENGTH OF EMBRYO (MM)	EVENT
1	3	22	2–3.5	Optic sulci present in forebrain
	4	24	2.4–4.5	Optic vesicles form
				Lens placode thickens
		26	3.0–5.0	Neural crest mesenchyme surrounds optic vesicle
2	5	28		Optic cup and lens pit form invaginations
				Surface ectoderm formed
				Lens and corneal epithelial basement membranes are fused
	6	40	11–14	*First wave of neural crest cells forms corneal endothelium*
		41		Eyelid folds develop
	7	44	13–17	Anterior chamber forming
		49	24	*Second wave forms stromal keratocytes and sclera*
	8	54	25	Lacrimal gland buds from conjunctiva
				Acellular corneal stroma present
				Episclera (Tenon's layer) becoming evident
			35–40	*Third wave forms iris and pupillary membrane*
3	10		43–48	Conjunctiva forming from eyelid and cornea
				Anterior banded Descemet's membrane forms
				Sclera condenses from anterior to posterior
	12		48–52	Cilia form
			50–55	Krause, Wolfring glands form from conjunctival recess
			52	Goblet cells formed
			80	Meibomian glands form
4			87	Sclera forms lamina cribosa
				Collagen fibrils appear as lamellae and take on adult form
				Aqueous is formed
			80–100	Glands of Moll and Zeiss form
			170	Eyelids keratinized
5			320	Anterior eyelid border opens
6			385	Posterior eyelid opens

grown from 2 mm in diameter at 3 months to 9.5–10.5 mm and assumed its typical lenticular shape, although it will not reach adult size for 1–2 years. The lacrimal gland is present but reflex tearing is absent until about 3 weeks after birth, and the gland continues to grow for 3–4 years. Lacrimal drainage does not begin until near or shortly after birth and can be delayed for several months.

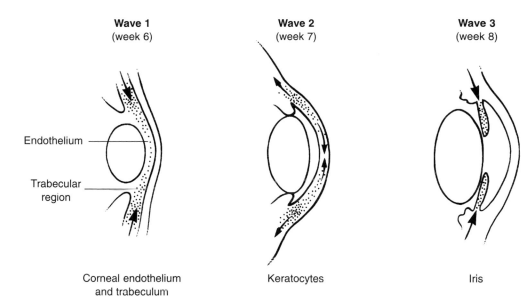

Wave 1 (week 6)	Wave 2 (week 7)	Wave 3 (week 8)
Corneal endothelium and trabeculum	Keratocytes	Iris

FIG XIII-1—The three waves of neural crest cell migration during embryogenesis. Wave 1, trabecular meshwork and corneal endothelium; wave 2, corneal stroma and keratocytes; wave 3, iris. (Illustration by Christine Gralapp, modified from Bahn CF, Falls HF, Varley GA, et al. Classification of corneal endothelial disorders based on neural crest origin. *Ophthalmology.* 1984;91:559.)

Causes of Congenital Corneal Anomalies

Congenital anomalies manifest as alterations in gross morphology evident at the time of birth. They may be sporadic or familial and unilateral or bilateral and may or may not be heritable. They are the result of abnormal development during embryonic or fetal life caused from various genetic influences and local or environmental effects.

Ocular anomalies can occur with a constellation of cranial, facial, or somatic abnormalities, making it difficult to incriminate a specific chromosomal abnormality, intrauterine infection, or maternal toxin as the cause. Ocular structures are most at risk in the period of organogenesis from 18 to 60 days. Anomalies occur when either intrinsic or extrinsic factors disrupt the intricate sequencing of embryonic events. *Intrinsic factors* include

□ Altered, defective, or imperfect genes

□ Impaired cellular induction and proliferation

□ Defective cell migration

□ Cell death

□ Abnormal extracellular substrates

□ Inadequate differentiation

□ Physical constraint

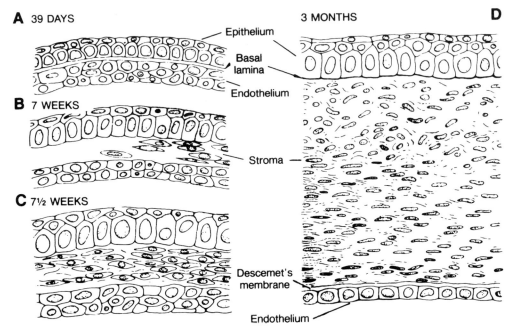

A 39 DAYS

Epithelium

Basal lamina

Endothelium

B 7 WEEKS

Stroma

C 7½ WEEKS

3 MONTHS

D

Descemet's membrane

Endothelium

FIG XIII-2—Development of cornea in central region. *A,* At day 39, two-layered epithelium rests on basal lamina and is separated from endothelium (two to three layers) by narrow acellular space. *B,* At week 7, mesenchymal cells from periphery migrate into space between epithelium and endothelium. *C,* Mesenchymal cells (future keratocytes) are arranged in four to five incomplete layers by 7½ weeks, and a few collagen fibrils are present among cells. *D,* By 3 months, epithelium has two to three layers of cells, and stroma has about 25–30 layers of keratocytes that are arranged more regularly in the posterior half. Thin, uneven Descemet's membrane lies between the most posterior keratocytes and the now single layer of endothelium. (Reproduced with permission from Cook CS, Ozanics V, Jakobiec FA. Prenatal development of the eye and its adnexa. In: Tasman W, Jaeger EA, ed. *Duane's Foundations of Clinical Ophthalmology.* Philadelphia: Lippincott; 1991.)

Extrinsic factors include health of the mother and the nature of the teratogen as well as its timing and degree.

Teratogens are infectious, pharmacologic, chemical, or physical agents that lead to defects in the developing embryo or fetus. The term means, literally, "induce a monster." Confirmed ocular teratogens with effects on the anterior segment other than cataract include the following:

☐ Radiation

☐ Fetal alcohol syndrome

☐ Rubella

☐ Cytomegalovirus

☐ Syphilis

☐ Herpes simplex virus

☐ Maternal diabetes

☐ Maternal ingestion of thalidomide, antiseizure medications, coumarin anticoagulants, and retinoic acid

Many other chemicals and environmental factors are suspected but not confirmed teratogens. No topical administration of ophthalmic medication is suspected or confirmed to produce a teratogenic effect. *Mutagens* are chemical or physical agents that induce a heritable change in offspring as opposed to acting directly on the developing embryo. BCSC Section 2, *Fundamentals and Principles of Ophthalmology*, discusses the issues covered in this chapter and the next chapter in depth in Part 2, Embryology. A helpful glossary and numerous illustrations are included. Part 3, Genetics, in the same volume discusses mutations in detail.

Diagnostic Approach

Diagnosis of congenital anomalies requires careful ophthalmic and general examination. The infant should be sedated if required. The examination should include the following:

- Documentation of eyelid and orbit orientation, formation, and anatomy
- Measurement of corneal diameter horizontally and vertically
- Biomicroscopy of the cornea with attention to the limbus, Bowman's membrane, stromal clarity, and Descemet's membrane
- Gonioscopy if cornea clarity allows
- Assessment of iris and pupil shape
- Investigation of lens anomalies and posterior segment
- Documentation of intraocular pressure
- Echography of the posterior segment if no view of anterior chamber or fundus is possible

See also BCSC Section 6, *Pediatric Ophthalmology and Strabismus*, "Rapport with Children: Tips for a Pediatric Examination."

Once an anomaly is identified, thorough family and prenatal histories should be explored with the parents to separate familial from sporadic causes. The presence of antimongoloid or pronounced mongoloid slant of the palpebral fissures, colobomas, epicanthal folds, hypertelorism, multiple systemic malformations, ptosis, strabismus, or mental retardation should prompt consultation with a geneticist and molecular ophthalmologist to identify familial syndromes or chromosomal abnormalities and to provide genetic counseling and prognostic information to patients or parents. The preliminary findings dictate which tests should subsequently be used: biochemical and chromosomal analysis, CT and MRI, tissue biopsies, and echography are the common choices. Prenatal diagnosis is very rarely attempted for ocular anomalies present in the parents or siblings.

Kim T, Palay DA. Developmental abnormalities of the cornea. In: Krachmer JH, Mannis MJ, Holland EJ, eds. *Cornea*. St Louis: Mosby; 1997;2:871–884.

McKusick VA. *Mendelian Inheritance in Man: A Catalog of Human Genes and Genetic Disorders*. 11th ed. Baltimore: The Johns Hopkins University Press; 1994. See also the *Online Mendelian Inheritance in Man* website (under OMIM Allied Resources): http://www3.ncbi.nlm.nih.gov/omim/ Bethesda: National Center for Biotechnology Information, National Library of Medicine; 1996.

Wilson FM. Congenital anomalies of the cornea and conjunctiva. In: Smolin G, Thoft RA, eds. *The Cornea: Scientific Foundations and Clinical Practice*. 3rd ed. Boston: Little, Brown; 1994:535–553.

CHAPTER XIV

Clinical Aspects of Congenital Anomalies of the Cornea and Sclera

Congenital anomalies are also discussed in depth in BCSC Section 6, *Pediatric Ophthalmology and Strabismus*. Chapter XIX of that volume covers diseases of the cornea and anterior segment. See also BCSC Section 2, *Fundamentals and Principles of Ophthalmology*, which discusses these anomalies in Part 2, Embryology.

Abnormalities of the Globe and Sclera

Cryptophthalmos

"Hidden eye" is a very rare condition with fewer than 150 reported cases. It is usually bilateral. The eyelids and associated structures of the brows and lashes fail to form *(ablepharon)*. The cornea is merged with the epidermis, and the anterior chamber, iris, and lens are variably formed or absent (Fig XIV-1). *Pseudocryptophthalmos* occurs when the eyelids and associated structures form but fail to separate *(ankyloblepharon)*.

PATHOGENESIS. The pathogenesis of this syndrome is unknown. The inward migration of all three waves of neural crest cells fails to occur. Similarities with maternal hypovitaminosis A in animal models suggest that pathogenesis may be related to retinoic acid metabolism.

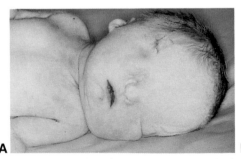
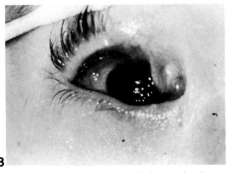

A   B

FIG XIV-1—*A,* Complete cryptophthalmos, both eyes. *B,* Incomplete cryptophthalmos of right eye with eyelid fused to cornea superonasally.

CLINICAL FINDINGS. Cryptophthalmos demonstrates equal sex distribution and equal occurrence in male and female siblings, consanguinity in families with more than one affected child, and lack of vertical transmission—strongly suggesting autosomal recessive inheritance. Ocular findings include the following:

- Dermoid transformation of the cornea and conjunctiva into skin
- Absence of the eyelid structures, lacrimal glands, and canaliculi
- Absence or transformation into connective tissue of the iris, Schlemm's canal, trabecular meshwork, anterior chamber, and lens

Cryptophthalmos syndrome includes any nonocular malformation associated with cryptophthalmos. Fraser syndrome (cryptophthalmos-syndactyly) may occur with anophthalmos and normal eyelids and, frequently, renal agenesis.

MANAGEMENT. Cryptophthalmos requires surgical intervention only for cosmesis or relief of pain from absolute glaucoma. Pseudocryptophthalmos may benefit from eyelid separation, but ongoing management of the reconstructed eyelids to prevent secondary complications will be necessary.

Microphthalmos

Microphthalmos is a small disorganized globe (Fig XIV-2). The condition is common and sometimes confused with the very rare syndrome of *anophthalmos,* or total absence of ocular tissues.

PATHOGENESIS. Normal embryonic development proceeds through at least the formation of the optic vesicle. Multiple associations have been made with microphthalmos including trisomies of almost every chromosome (typically trisomy 13) and maternal infections and exposure to toxins and radiation. Inheritance is confirmed as autosomal dominant, autosomal recessive, and X-linked. Terminal deletion with a breakpoint at Xp22.2 is lethal for males. One family is confirmed to have a translocation of the short arm of chromosome 16 [t(2;16)(p22.3;p13.3)].

CLINICAL FINDINGS. Associated ocular abnormalities may include leukomas, anterior segment disorders, retinal dysplasia, colobomas, cysts, marked internal dys-

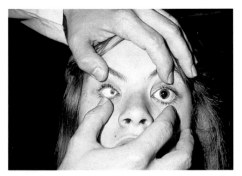

FIG XIV-2—Severe microcornea and microphthalmos OD. Both irides are colobomatous.

genesis, persistent fetal vasculature (PFV), small orbit, ptosis, and blepharophimosis. Systemic associations are numerous, including mental retardation and dwarfism among many others.

MANAGEMENT. Associated conditions should be sought and managed appropriately, and genetic counseling should be considered. A cosmetic shell or contact lens may be indicated in selected patients.

> Goldberg MF. Persistent fetal vasculature (PFV): an integrated interpretation of signs and symptoms associated with persistent hyperplastic primary vitreous (PHPV). *Am J Ophthalmol.* 1997;124:587–626.

Nanophthalmos

This uncommon finding involves a small, functional eye with relatively normal internal organization and proportions. Axial length is 15.0–20.5 mm with proportional transverse and sagittal measurements. A normal-sized lens leads to crowding of the anterior segment.

PATHOGENESIS. Cause is unknown and both autosomal dominant and recessive traits have been reported.

CLINICAL FINDINGS. Patients have high hyperopia, narrow palpebral fissures, thickened sclera, and crowded anterior segments with occasional glaucoma that may be caused by narrow angles or goniodysgenesis.

MANAGEMENT. Hyperopia and glaucoma are managed medically in the standard way. Cataract surgery may be complicated by uveal effusion syndrome unless scleral windows are created.

Blue Sclera

The striking clinical picture of blue sclera is related to generalized thinning with increased visibility of underlying uvea. This anomaly must be distinguished from the slate gray appearance of ocular melanosis bulbi and from acquired causes of scleral thinning such as rheumatoid arthritis or staining from minocycline treatment.

PATHOGENESIS. Genetic mutations and altered proteins have been identified for two syndromes associated with blue sclera:

□ *Osteogenesis imperfecta type I* is a somewhat common, dominantly inherited, generalized connective tissue disorder characterized mainly by bone fragility and blue sclerae. "Functional null" alleles of COL1A1 on chromosome 17 or COL1A2 on chromosome 7 lead to reduced amounts of normal type I collagen in most cases.

□ *Ehlers-Danlos syndrome type VI (EDS VI)* is a somewhat rare syndrome with autosomal recessive inheritance characterized by joint hyperextensibility, moderate to severe kyphoscoliosis, cardiac anomalies, and skin abnormalities of easy bruisability, abnormal scarring, and soft distensibility. EDS VI is associated with molecular defects in the gene for lysyl hydroxylase (PLOD) on 1p36.3–p36.2 in some patients.

□ A third syndrome of brittle cornea, blue sclera, keratoglobus, and joint hyperextensibility may be the same as EDS VI with a normal level of lysyl hydroxylase.

CLINICAL FINDINGS. All three syndromes may share similar manifestations of fractures from minor trauma in childhood, kyphoscoliosis, joint extensibility, and elastic skin. Decreased hearing and tinnitus may also occur.

MANAGEMENT. Regular hearing evaluations after adolescence are recommended. Postmenopausal women should engage in a long-term physical therapy program to strengthen the paraspinal muscles. Estrogen and progesterone replacement, adequate calcium intake, and perhaps calcitonin or fluoride may be specifically indicated for these patients. Fractures are treated with standard methods. See also Table XVI-7.

Abnormalities of Size and Shape of the Cornea

Microcornea

This somewhat common condition refers to a clear cornea of normal thickness whose diameter is less than 10 mm (or 9 mm in a newborn). If the whole anterior segment is small, the term *anterior microphthalmos* applies. If the entire eye is small and malformed, the term microphthalmos is used in contrast to nanophthalmos, in which the eye is small but otherwise normal.

PATHOGENESIS. Cause is unknown and may be related to fetal arrest of growth of the cornea in the fifth month. Alternatively, it may be related to overgrowth of the anterior tips of the optic cup, which leaves less space for the cornea to develop.

CLINICAL FINDINGS. Microcornea may be transmitted as an autosomal dominant or recessive trait with equal sex predilection. Dominant transmission is more common. Because their corneas are relatively flat, patients with microcornea are usually hyperopic and have a higher incidence of angle-closure glaucoma. Of patients who avoid angle-closure glaucoma, 20% develop open-angle glaucoma later in life. Important ocular anomalies often associated with microcornea include persistent fetal vasculature, congenital cataracts, anterior segment dysgenesis, and optic nerve hypoplasia. Significant systemic associations include myotonic dystrophy, fetal alcohol syndrome, achondroplasia, and Ehlers-Danlos syndrome.

MANAGEMENT. If an isolated finding, microcornea has an excellent visual prognosis with spectacles to treat the hyperopia resulting from the flat cornea. Concurrent ocular pathology such as cataract, PFV, and glaucoma may require treatment following the usual procedures for those conditions.

Megalocornea

This rare condition is a nonprogressive corneal enlargement that is not the result of congenital glaucoma. Affected subjects have histologically normal corneas measuring 13.0–16.5 mm in diameter (Fig XIV-3).

PATHOGENESIS. The cornea has normal thickness, endothelial cell count, and clarity but may be steeper keratometrically. The etiology may be related to failure of the optic cup to grow and of its anterior tips to close, leaving a larger space for the cornea to fill. Alternatively, megalocornea may represent arrested buphthalmos and exaggerated growth of the cornea in relation to the rest of the eye. An abnormality in collagen production is suggested by the association of megalocornea with systemic disorders of collagen synthesis.

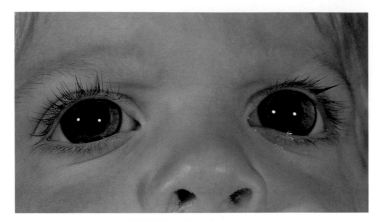

FIG XIV-3—Megalocornea.

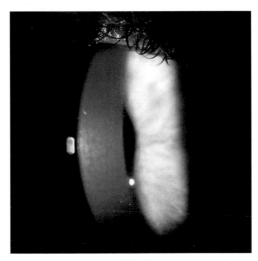

FIG XIV-4—Posterior crocodile shagreen in megalocornea.

CLINICAL FINDINGS. Megalocornea may be associated with iris translucency (di-aphany), miosis, microcoria, goniodysgenesis, cataract, ectopia lentis, arcus lip-oides, mosaic corneal dystrophy (central cloudy dystrophy of François) (Fig XIV-4), and glaucoma (but not congenital glaucoma). It is usually bilateral and X-linked recessive and is probably located in the Xq21.3–q22 region; 90% of patients are male. Sporadic, autosomal recessive, and dominant cases have also been reported.

Systemic associations include craniosynostosis, frontal bossing, hypertelor-ism, facial anomalies, dwarfism, facial hemiatrophy, mental retardation, hypotonia, Down syndrome, Marfan syndrome, Alport syndrome, osteogenesis imperfecta, mucolipidosis type II, or occasionally other genetic syndromes. Anterior megalophthalmos is the most common familial form of megalocornea, which includes bilateral megalocornea, ciliary ring enlargement, and secondary effects of iridodonesis, miosis, atrophy of iris stroma, and frequently cataractous lens.

> Vail DT. Adult hereditary anterior megalophthalmos in glaucoma: a definite disease entity. *Arch Ophthalmol.* 1937;6:39.

MANAGEMENT. Congenital glaucoma must be ruled out by intraocular pressure testing and careful biomicroscopy. Ultrasonography may be of value in determining the short vitreous length, deep lens and iris position, and normal axial length that distinguish megalocornea from buphthalmos caused by congenital glaucoma. Myopia and with-the-rule astigmatism are managed as in unaffected patients.

Cornea Plana

This rare condition refers to a flat cornea where the radius of curvature is less than 43 diopters (D), and readings of 20–30 D are common. Corneal curvature that is the same as the adjacent sclera is pathognomonic. Sclerocornea also features flat corneas, but it is distinguished by the loss of transparency as well (see Figure XIV-10).

PATHOGENESIS. Similar to sclerocornea, the second wave of neural crest cells between weeks 7 and 10 fails to form the limbal anlage and differentiates into tissue resembling sclera instead of corneal stroma. The absence of the limbus is associated with failure of the corneal curve to develop.

CLINICAL FINDINGS. Cornea plana is often seen in association with sclerocornea or microcornea. Other associated ocular or systemic abnormalities include cataracts, anterior and posterior colobomas, or Ehlers-Danlos syndrome. Cornea plana usually produces hyperopia, but any refractive error may exist because of variations in globe size. Angle-closure glaucoma occurs because of a morphologically shallow anterior chamber, and open-angle glaucoma occurs because of angle abnormalities. Both dominant and the more severe recessive forms exist. Three fourths of isolated cases appear in Finnish patients with both the autosomal recessive and dominant forms linked to chromosome 12q21 (CNA2 loci).

MANAGEMENT. Refractive errors are neutralized and glaucoma must be considered. Loss of central clarity may indicate penetrating keratoplasty, but cornea plana increases risk of graft rejection and postkeratoplasty glaucoma.

Generalized Posterior Keratoconus

The entire posterior corneal curvature is increased in this very rare anomaly, while the anterior corneal surface remains normal.

PATHOGENESIS. Generalized posterior keratoconus is probably related to mesenchymal dysgenesis and developmental arrest.

CLINICAL FINDINGS. The condition is unilateral and nonprogressive, and the cornea is thin but typically clear. All reported cases are in females, but they are thought to be sporadic.

MANAGEMENT. Observation may be the only required management as vision is usually unaffected.

Keratectasia and Congenital Anterior Staphyloma

These very rare unilateral conditions are both characterized by protrusion of the opaque cornea between the eyelids at birth. They differ only in the presence of a uveal lining of the cornea in congenital anterior staphyloma.

PATHOGENESIS. Intrauterine perforation from an infection or from thinning following secondary failure of neural crest cell migration results in dermoid transformation of the cornea to stratified squamous epithelium, sparing the eyelids and conjunctiva. Keratectasia is probably not the result of abnormal development but rather intrauterine keratitis or vitamin deficiency and subsequent corneal perforation. Histopathologically, Descemet's membrane and endothelium are absent, and a uveal lining is present (except in keratectasia). The cornea is variably thinned and scarred and the anterior segment disorganized with the lens occasionally adherent to the posterior cornea resembling unilateral Peters anomaly.

CLINICAL FINDINGS. An opaque, bulging cornea is accompanied by a deep anterior segment. These cases are typically unilateral, and all are sporadic with no familial or systemic association.

MANAGEMENT. Except in very mild cases, visual prognosis is poor because of associated severe damage to the anterior segment. Penetrating keratoplasty is rarely warranted, and enucleation may be required for the blind, glaucomatous, painful eye.

Dysgenesis of the Anterior Segment

Abnormalities of Corneal Structure and/or Clarity

Posterior embryotoxon   This condition involves a thickened and centrally displaced anterior border ring of Schwalbe. Schwalbe's ring represents the junction of the trabecular meshwork with the termination of Descemet's membrane, and it is visible in 8%–30% of normal eyes as a whitish, relucent, irregular ridge 0.5–2.0 mm central to the limbus. The term *posterior embryotoxon* is used when Schwalbe's ring is visible by external examination (Fig XIV-5). Posterior embryotoxon is usually inherited as a dominant trait. The eye is usually normal but can manifest a number of other anterior segment anomalies that are part of ocular or systemic syndromes, such as Alagille syndrome (arteriohepatic dysplasia), X-linked ichthyosis, and familial aniridia.

Axenfeld-Rieger syndrome   The conditions previously referred to as *Axenfeld anomaly* and *syndrome* and *Rieger anomaly* and *syndrome* have overlapping findings and have now been grouped into a single entity known as *Axenfeld-Rieger syndrome*. This syndrome represents a spectrum of disorders, characterized by an anteriorly displaced Schwalbe's line (posterior embryotoxon) with attached iris strands, iris hypoplasia, and glaucoma in 50% of the cases occurring in late childhood or in adulthood (Fig XIV-6). Skeletal, cranial, facial, and dental abnormalities may be associated.

Transmission is usually dominant (75%) for the Axenfeld-Rieger group, but it can be sporadic. Evidence suggests that more than one genetic form of Rieger syndrome exists, and that one form (Rieger syndrome type 1) is caused by mutations in a homeobox transcription factor gene (see BCSC Section 2, *Fundamentals and Principles of Ophthalmology*, Part 3, Genetics). Linkage studies indicated that a second type of Rieger syndrome (Rieger syndrome type 2) maps to chromosome 13q14.

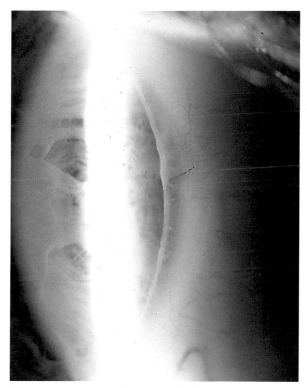

FIG XIV-5—Posterior embryotoxon displaying a prominent and anteriorly displaced Schwalbe's ring.

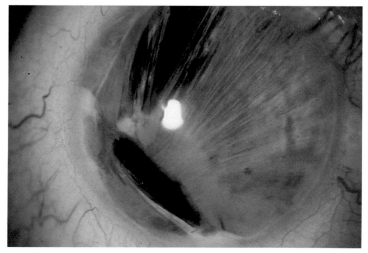

FIG XIV-6—Axenfeld-Rieger syndrome exhibiting iris atrophy, corectopia, and pseudopolycoria.

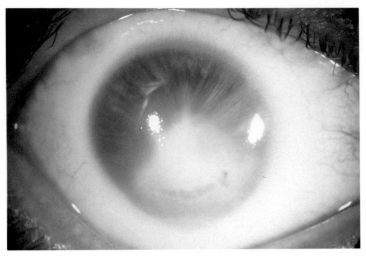

FIG XIV-7—Peters anomaly.

Peters anomaly   This spectrum of disorders includes a central corneal leukoma with defects in the posterior stroma, Descemet's membrane, and the corneal endothelium. In some cases the lens remains clear, but strands of iris tissue from the iris collarette may attach to the posterior border of the leukoma (Fig XIV-7). An anterior cataract may also be present, or lens attachment to the posterior cornea may be seen.

Peters anomaly is most often sporadic but may be recessive or occasionally dominant. Mutations at the PAX6 gene are found in heterogeneous anterior segment malformations, including Peters anomaly. Eighty percent of cases are bilateral, and more than half have glaucoma. When systemic abnormalities such as congenital cardiac defects, cleft lip and palate, craniofacial dysplasia, and skeletal changes also occur, the condition is called *Peters-plus syndrome.*

Kivlin JD, Apple DJ, Olson RJ, et al. Dominantly inherited keratitis. *Arch Ophthalmol.* 1986;104:1621–1623.

Circumscribed posterior keratoconus   The presence of a localized central or paracentral indentation of the posterior cornea without any protrusion of the anterior surface characterizes circumscribed posterior keratoconus. Often a variable amount of overlying stromal haze also appears. Loss of stromal substance can lead to corneal thinning approaching one third of normal (Figs XIV-8, XIV-9). Descemet's membrane and endothelium are usually present in the area of defect. Most cases appear in females and are unilateral, nonprogressive, and sporadic. Astigmatism and/or amblyopia may occur.

Arcus juvenilis   This deposition of lipid in the peripheral corneal stroma occasionally occurs as a congenital anomaly. It usually involves only a sector of the peripheral cornea and is not associated with abnormalities of serum lipid.

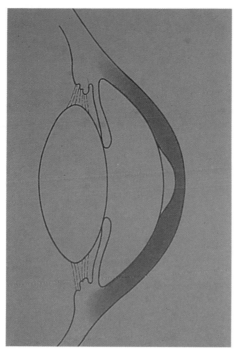

FIG XIV-8—Circumscribed posterior keratoconus. Schematic diagram shows loss of central stromal thickness, normal anterior corneal curvature, and a central posterior corneal crater.

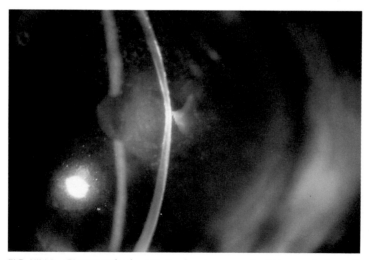

FIG XIV-9—Circumscribed posterior keratoconus. A slit-lamp photograph shows loss of stromal thickness, stromal haze, and posterior corneal crater.

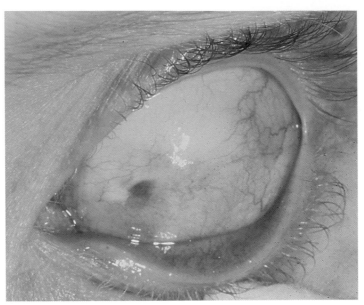

FIG XIV-10—Sclerocornea.

Sclerocornea This nonprogressive, noninflammatory scleralization of the cornea may be limited to the corneal periphery, or the entire cornea may be involved. The limbus is usually ill-defined, and superficial vessels that are extensions of normal scleral, episcleral, and conjunctival vessels cross the cornea (Fig XIV-10). No sex predilection is evident, and 90% of cases are bilateral. Half of cases are sporadic with the remainder being either dominant or recessive, which is more severe. The most common associated ocular finding is cornea plana in 80% of the cases.

Congenital hereditary stromal dystrophy (CHSD) This rare dominant stationary dystrophy presents at birth with central superficial corneal clouding. The anterior corneal stroma exhibits an ill-defined flaky or feathery appearance. The cornea is clear peripherally. No edema, photophobia, or tearing occurs, but the opacities can be sufficiently dense to cause a reduction in vision.

Posterior amorphous corneal dysgenesis This very rare autosomal dominant stromal dystrophy is bilaterally symmetrical. It appears early in life and may be congenital. Examination reveals diffuse gray-white stromal opacities concentrated in the posterior stroma. Although the central cornea is most heavily involved, the lesions extend to the limbus. The epithelium appears normal, but Descemet's membrane shows involvement, with focal areas of endothelial disruption. Other findings include central corneal thinning, hypermetropia, flattened corneal topography, anterior iris abnormalities, and fine iris processes extending to Schwalbe's line for 360°. A peripheral variant features a clear central cornea, but these patients do not show the iris processes. The dystrophy is either nonprogressive or slowly progressive. The corneal thinning produces little irregular astigmatism, and visual acuity remains good.

Dunn SP, Krachmer JH, Ching SST. New findings in posterior amorphous corneal dystrophy. *Arch Ophthalmol.* 1984;102:236–239.

Congenital hereditary endothelial dystrophy (CHED) CHED may be the cause of bilateral congenital corneal edema, but other causes such as birth trauma and congenital glaucoma must be ruled out. Two forms of CHED are recognized. The more common autosomal recessive type (CHED 2) presents at birth, remains stationary, and is accompanied by nystagmus. The bluish white cornea may be two to three times normal thickness and have a ground-glass appearance, but this finding is not associated with tearing or photophobia. There may be diffuse nonbullous epithelial edema. A uniform thickening of Descemet's membrane may exist, but no guttate changes are present.

The dominant form (CHED 1) presents in the first or second year of life, although expressivity is variable. It is slowly progressive and accompanied by pain, photophobia, and tearing, but nystagmus is not present. The cornea exhibits a diffuse, blue-gray, ground-glass appearance (Fig XIV-11). The primary abnormality is thought to be a degeneration of endothelial cells during or after the fifth month of gestation.

Either form of CHED is thought to be another example of anterior segment dysgenesis, probably caused by abnormal differentiation of neural crest ectoderm that forms corneal endothelium. CHED has no consistent associations with other systemic abnormalities, although axial myopia is common in these patients. Its gene locus is mapped to the pericentric region of chromosome 20 (20p11.2–q11.2).

Toma NM, Ebenezer, ND, Inglehearn CF et. al. Linkage of congenital hereditary endothelial dystrophy to chromosome 20. *Hum Mol Genet.* 1995;4:2395–2398.

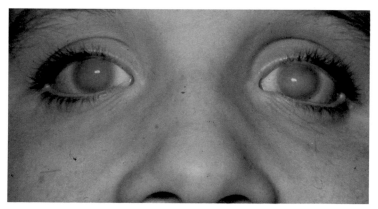

FIG XIV-11—Congenital hereditary endothelial dystrophy.

Congenital Corneal Opacities in Hereditary Syndromes and Chromosomal Aberrations

Mucopolysaccharidoses (MPS) and *mucolipidoses* are disorders caused by abnormal carbohydrate metabolism. Corneal clouding and haziness may be present in early life in varying degrees in many of these entities, including Scheie syndrome (MPS IS) and Hurler syndrome (MPS IH). A more detailed discussion of these conditions appears in chapter XVI.

Secondary Abnormalities Affecting the Fetal Cornea

Intrauterine Keratitis: Bacterial and Syphilitic

Maternally transmitted congenital infections can cause ocular damage in several different ways:

□ Through direct action of the infecting agent, which damages tissue

□ Through a teratogenic effect resulting in malformation

□ Through a delayed reactivation of the agent after birth, with inflammation that damages developed tissue

A posterior corneal defect called *von Hippel internal corneal ulcer* may follow intrauterine inflammation. Often, signs of inflammation may still be present after birth, including corneal infiltrates and vascularization, keratic precipitates, and uveitis. The iris adhesions are extensive and may arise from areas apart from the collarette, and the lens is usually involved. Corneal ulcers and endophthalmitis were common complications of gonococcal ophthalmia neonatorum before the widespread use of silver nitrate prophylaxis and antibiotics. Neonatal conjunctivitis is discussed on pp 164–165.

Congenitally acquired syphilis infections caused by the *Treponema pallidum* spirochete can lead to fetal death or premature delivery. A variety of systemic manifestations have been described. *Interstitial keratitis* can develop in the first decade of life in children with untreated congenital syphilis. It presents as a rapidly progressive corneal edema followed by abnormal vascularization in the deep stroma adjacent to Descemet's membrane. The cornea may assume a salmon pink color because of intense vascularization, giving rise to the term *salmon patch*. Over several weeks to months, blood flow through these vessels gradually ceases, leaving empty "ghost" vessels in the corneal stroma.

Congenital Corneal Keloid

Corneal keloids are relatively rare lesions most commonly described following corneal perforation or trauma. Congenital corneal keloids, often bilateral, have been described in Lowe disease (oculocerebrorenal syndrome). They can be seen in association with cataracts, aniridia, and glaucoma and may represent a developmental anomaly with failure of normal differentiation of corneal tissue. Histopathologic examination reveals thick collagenase bundles haphazardly arranged with focal areas of myofibroblastic proliferation.

Congenital Glaucoma

Primary congenital glaucoma is evident either at birth or within the first few years of life. It is believed to be caused by dysplasia of the anterior chamber angle without other ocular or systemic abnormalities. Characteristic findings in the newborn include the triad of epiphora, photophobia, and blepharospasm. External eye examination may reveal buphthalmos with corneal enlargement greater than 12 mm in diameter during the first year of life. (The normal horizontal corneal diameter is 9.5–10.5 in full-term infants.) Corneal edema is present in 25% of affected infants at birth and in more than 60% by the sixth month. It may range from mild haze to dense opacification in the corneal stroma because of elevated IOP. Tears in Descemet's membrane called *Haab's striae* may occur acutely as a result of corneal stretching. They are typically oriented horizontally or concentric to the limbus. BCSC Section 6, *Pediatric Ophthalmology and Strabismus,* also discusses pediatric glaucoma.

Birth Trauma

Progressive corneal edema developing during the first few postnatal days, accompanied by vertical or oblique posterior striae, may be caused by birth trauma (Fig XIV-12). Ruptures occur in Descemet's membrane and the endothelium. Healing usually takes place, leaving a hypertrophic ridge of Descemet's membrane. The edema may or may not clear; if it does clear, the cornea can again become edematous at any time later in life. High astigmatism and amblyopia may be associated. Congenital glaucoma can present with similar findings and should be considered in the differential diagnosis.

Iridocorneal Endothelial Syndrome (ICF)

This spectrum of disorders is characterized by varying degrees of corneal edema, glaucoma, and iris abnormalities (Fig XIV-13).

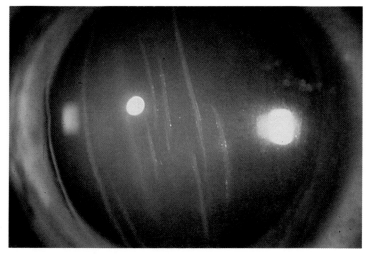

FIG XIV-12—Birth trauma demonstrating vertical ruptures of Descemet's membrane secondary to traumatic delivery.

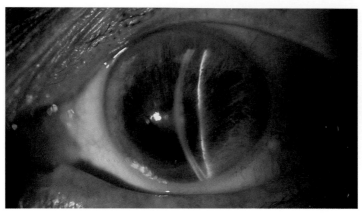

FIG XIV-13—Iridocorneal endothelial syndrome with corectopia.

PATHOGENESIS. The pathogenesis of ICE syndrome is unknown but appears to involve an abnormal clone of endothelial cells that takes on ultrastructural characteristics of epithelial cells. The condition appears to represent an acquired maldifferentiation of a group of endothelial cells, although the abnormal clone could originate at birth or before. Varying degrees of endothelialization take place in the anterior chamber angle and on the iris surface. The possibility that a herpes simplex virus infection may be responsible has been raised.

CLINICAL FINDINGS. When the pathology is confined to the inner corneal surface, corneal edema may result from subnormal endothelial pump function, producing the Chandler variant of ICE syndrome. Frequently, the border between the abnormal and normal endothelium can be seen at the slit lamp using specular reflection. When the abnormal endothelium migrates over the anterior chamber angle, the resultant peripheral anterior synechiae and outflow obstruction produce glaucoma. When the abnormal endothelium spreads onto the surface of the iris, the resulting contractile membrane may produce iris atrophy, corectopia, and polycoria, hallmarks of the essential iris atrophy variant of ICE syndrome. The Cogan-Reese (or iris nevus) variant shows multiple pigmented iris nodules, also produced by the contracting endothelial membrane.

This congenital syndrome becomes apparent most commonly in middle-aged females and is almost always unilateral. Asymmetric posterior polymorphous dystrophy, as well as other causes of unilateral corneal edema, must be included in the differential diagnosis of ICE syndrome.

MANAGEMENT. Penetrating keratoplasty is an effective treatment for the corneal component of this syndrome. Glaucoma is an important feature of the ICE syndrome. Long-term graft clarity is dependent on the successful control of IOP, which can be difficult (see BCSC Section 10, *Glaucoma*).

Patel A, Kenyon KR, Hirst LW, et al. Clinicopathologic features of Chandler's syndrome. *Surv Ophthalmol.* 1983;27:327–344.

PART 7

CORNEAL DYSTROPHIES AND METABOLIC DISORDERS INVOLVING THE CONJUNCTIVA, CORNEA, AND SCLERA

CHAPTER XV

Molecular Genetics of Corneal Dystrophies and Metabolic Disorders

This chapter includes an introduction to the genetic basis of disease and its role in diagnosis. See BCSC Section 2, *Fundamentals and Principles of Ophthalmology,* Part 3, for a more extensive review of genetics.

Principles of Genetics

Linkage refers to the process by which a known marker is used to implicate an unknown marker by their proximity on the chromosome. The mapping of different phenotypes to a specific genetic locus has enhanced our fundamental understanding of the pathogenesis of many corneal dystrophies and diseases with complex, multigenic origins. Many diseases have been mapped to specific areas of the genome, and linkages can be used to establish the potential carrier state of parents or siblings and, thereby, allow specific genetic counseling.

Diagnostic tests are emerging that can analyze the genetic material of ocular pathogens. For example, the polymerase chain reaction (PCR) is currently used to detect viral nucleic acids in patients infected with herpes simplex virus. In the future such tests will likely be used to identify and determine the correct antimicrobial agent for specific pathogens that are difficult to culture with conventional techniques.

Structure of Chromosomes and Genes

The nuclear material of human cells condenses into chromosomes during cell division. *Chromosomes* are composed primarily of protein and *deoxyribonucleic acid (DNA).* DNA is a giant, highly ordered molecule in a double-helical configuration consisting of deoxyribose (5-carbon sugar) molecules linked by phosphates and carrying one nitrogenous base each. The nitrogenous base is either a *purine* (adenine or guanosine) or a *pyrimidine* (thymine or cytosine). An individual sugar-phosphate unit with its nitrogen base is called a *nucleotide (nt).*

In double-stranded helical DNA each nitrogen base can form a hydrogen bond only with a specific counterpart: thymine (T) always pairs with adenine (A) and guanine (G) with cytosine (C), so TA, AT, GC, and CG are the possible combinations. These combinations are known as *base pairs (bp).* Three billion base pairs make up human DNA. The nucleotides are arranged on each strand in a complementary manner with a polarity from the 5′ to 3′ ends. A full, double-stranded 7-bp fragment of DNA is written

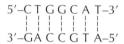

The genetic code determines the composition of cellular proteins in an elegant manner. The 20 amino acids are the building blocks of proteins, and each amino acid is specified by a grouping of 3 nucleotides (a *codon*) on the chromosome. There are 64 possible combinations of nucleotides, so some amino acids have more than one codon (i.e., the code is degenerate).

Ribonucleic acid (RNA) is a second type of nucleic acid found primarily in the cytoplasm. It contains the sugar ribose instead of deoxyribose and substitutes uracil (U) for the thymine nitrogenous base. Single-stranded RNA is formed by the process of *transcription* from double-stranded DNA in the nucleus. The DNA strand has some regions that do not code for protein and some that regulate the coding.

A region of the DNA that is ultimately translated into protein consists of *exons* and *introns,* which are spliced out of the RNA before it leaves the nucleus. Removal of the introns creates *messenger RNA (mRNA),* the functional blueprint of the genetic code, which leaves the nucleus and goes to the ribosomes. *Transfer RNA (tRNA)* binds to the mRNA in a complementary fashion, aligning the specific amino acids in the correct sequence for protein synthesis.

Genes are the smallest segments of DNA containing individual units of information that code for a single trait or a single polypeptide chain. Some functional proteins require more than one gene product (e.g., hemoglobin). The relative linear sequence of the genes is known as the *genetic map*. The specific site on the chromosome occupied by the gene is termed its genetic map *locus*. Each gene is from 500 to more than 2 million base pairs long with an average of 1000 base pairs. The distance between genes is expressed in *centimorgans (cM)*. A centimorgan is equal to approximately 1 million base pairs. The average cell contains enough genetic material for more than 6 million genes, but only about 100,000 genes contained in 22 pairs of somatic chromosomes and two sex chromosomes have been found.

Clinical Genetics

More than 4300 human diseases are known to be inherited, and 10%–15% of these are confined to the eye. Another 15% have ocular manifestations. As of this writing, 9088 genes have been determined and 6040 have been assigned to a specific locus by the Human Genome Project. Not all of the functions of these genes are known, but knowing the location has significant value both for diagnosis and for possible future linkage to a specific protein or biochemical cause of disease.

Hereditary diseases can be classified by their inheritance pattern:

□ Autosomal dominant

□ Autosomal recessive

□ X-linked

□ Y-linked

□ Mitochondrial

This classification is based on the chromosomal location and phenotypic behavior of the gene. The *genotype* of an individual refers to the biologic state of that person's genes. The *phenotype* refers to the observable physical, biochemical, molecular, or physiologic characteristics of the individual. These characteristics are determined by the genotype but may be modified by environment, maternal exposures, and other factors. Individuals can have the same phenotype but have very different genotypes (genetic heterogeneity). For example, tyrosinase-positive and tyrosinase-negative albinism have a similar phenotype, but they are not the result of mutations of the same gene. A *trait* is typically a physical characteristic that distinguishes one individual from another. A *phenocopy* is a clinical picture similar to a given phenotype but is actually the result of environmental causes without the same genotype. For example, congenital rubella retinopathy is a phenocopy of retinitis pigmentosa.

Alleles are alternate forms of a gene at the same locus on each of an identical pair of chromosomes. If the alleles are the same, the individual is *homozygous* for the gene at that locus. If the alleles are distinct from each other, the individual is *heterozygous*. If there is only one allele at a locus, the gene is termed *hemizygous*. *Polymorphisms* are genetic variations that occur at a specific locus with an appreciable frequency in the general population. These sequence variants may not have any appreciable effect on gene function, but they can be useful for mapping the gene through linkage. During meiosis, genes may "cross over" from one chromosome to the other. The likelihood that two genes, two markers of a gene, and a gene and a marker will be separated from one another during such a recombinant event is proportional to the distance between them in the genome. Thus linkage is exploited to create maps of genes and markers by observing the inheritance patterns of markers and disease phenotypes in large numbers of individuals.

A trait is *dominant* if the responsible gene is expressed even if only a single copy exists in the chromosomal pair. A trait is *recessive* if the responsible gene can be masked by a normal allele and only expressed when homozygous. A gene is either *penetrant* or *nonpenetrant* depending on whether any phenotypic effect appears in an individual. The fraction of a population with a gene that shows effect is the gene's penetrance. *Pleiotropism* is the multiple phenotypic expression of a single gene (e.g., single gene mutations on 17q11.2 cause café-au-lait spots, Lisch nodules, and neurofibromas in von Recklinghausen neurofibromatosis type 1).

Genome Database. Baltimore: Johns Hopkins University; updated on a daily basis: http://gdbwww.gdb.org/

Musarella MA. Gene mapping of ocular diseases. *Surv Ophthalmol.* 1992;36:285–312.

Diagnostic Approach

Diagnosis of corneal dystrophies and metabolic abnormalities requires suspicion based on symmetry, progression of the disease, and careful family history. Confirmation may come from the typical appearance and clinical course of the disorder or from molecular techniques.

Pedigree Analysis

The family history for ocular and nonocular conditions can be summarized in a *pedigree* chart that carefully illustrates the *proband* (first person with the recognized disease) and all of the relatives available through history and by examination (Fig XV-1). Answers regarding stillbirths, abortions, deceased members, parentage, and consanguinity must be pursued in the family history even if these may involve delicate questioning. In the United States in 1990 28% of babies were born outside legal

PEDIGREE SYMBOLS

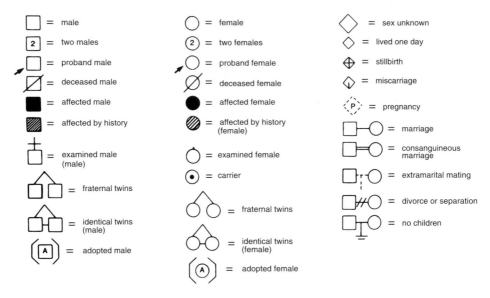

FIG XV-1—Symbols commonly used for pedigree analysis.

marriage, and the nonpaternity rate is currently 5%–15%, so difficulties in interviewing are not uncommon. The information obtained is used to determine type of inheritance and to aid in linkage analysis, and it is essential in genetic counseling.

The purpose of molecular genetics is to establish the hereditary nature of disease, to provide a link to the genome, and then to establish the specific locus and its attendant protein. These steps can help the clinician understand the pathophysiology involved and provide a specific diagnosis. For genetic linkage to be established, a disease must have a presumed hereditary basis and adequate numbers of patients and their families must have the disease. Detailed pedigree analysis over multiple generations is useful, particularly in X-linked diseases.

Molecular Biologic Techniques

Human genetic disease is related to numerical, gross structural, or point mutation changes in the chromosomes. The advent of *karyotyping*, the systematic display of chromosomes from a single cell, led to the recognition of the causes of many conditions. Numerical changes in chromosomes include trisomies or monosomies, and structural changes include deletions, isochromosome formation, inversions, translocations, and mosaicisms. Point mutations occur when one nucleotide is substituted for another. Table XV-1 shows the corneal diseases with known chromosomal abnormalities.

TABLE XV-1

CHROMOSOMAL ABERRATIONS ASSOCIATED WITH CORNEAL ANOMALIES

CORNEAL CONDITION	CHROMOSOMAL ABERRATION
Aniridia with Wilms tumor	11p13– (Miller syndrome)
Anophthalmos, cyclopia, corneal dysgenesis, sclerocornea	Trisomy 13 (Patau syndrome)
Corneal opacities	Trisomy 8 18r (ring chromosome 18) Gr (ring chromosome G) or Gq–
Corneal opacities, sclerocornea, microcornea, megalocornea	4q–
Corneal opacities, microcornea, vertically oval cornea	X0 (Turner syndrome)
Corneal opacities, anterior	Trisomy 18 (Edwards syndrome)
Keratoconus	Trisomy 21 (Down syndrome)
Megalocornea, epibulbar dermoid	5p (cri du chat syndrome)
Peters anomaly	21r (ring chromosome 21)
Posterior keratoconus	18p–
Rieger anomaly	6p–
Sclerocornea	Trisomy 10q

p– denotes deletion of the short arm of that chromosome; q– denotes deletion of the long arm.

Several methods are used to determine linkage of a disease to a specific area of a chromosome:

□ *Somatic cell hybridization* is used to map known human DNA fragments and genes with a known product to a specific locus.

□ *In situ hybridization* can also be used to identify the chromosomal location of a gene for which a cloned complementary DNA (cDNA) is available (rhodopsin was mapped to 3q21 by this method).

□ *Deletion* or *duplication mapping* correlates reduced or excess gene product with deficiency or duplication of specific segments of a chromosome (esterase D was assigned to 13q14 because of its association with retinoblastoma patients with this deletion).

□ *Linkage disequilibrium* refers to the tendency of specific alleles to occur with specific alleles of another locus on the same chromosome.

Once established, this linkage can be useful in predicting candidate genes for a specific defect. When specific genes are known, the point mutation or the resulting protein can be used for diagnosis and for genetic counseling of the family. Linkage can be valuable in diagnosis even without knowledge of the specific gene or its function.

Determination of point mutations through molecular genetics has dramatically increased with the discovery and purification of bacterial enzymes termed *restriction endonucleases*. These enzymes recognize specific nucleotide sequences and cause sharp breaks in both strands of the chromosome at those locations, which are specific to each endonuclease. The resultant fragments are useful in a variety of ways.

Recombinant DNA technology utilizes these enzymes to place fragments of human chromosomes into bacterial plasmids or other vectors to make an efficient "factory" for multiple copies of that gene. *Restriction fragment length polymorphisms (RFLP)* are created using known restriction endonucleases and then separated by agrose gel electrophoresis to determine the presence of a specific allele (polymorphism) using a radiolabeled DNA probe for a known nucleotide sequence.

Application of polymerase chain reaction to linkage analysis is accomplished using markers called *short tandem repeats (STR)*. STRs are short segments of repetitive DNA scattered throughout the genome that are frequently polymorphic. These polymorphisms can be detected by PCR amplification and polyacrylamide gel electrophoresis. STRs enable researchers to look more efficiently for linkage with even the most complex phenotypes. Genotypic data is combined with pedigree data to infer the genomic linkage of a disease gene using a statistical method known as *linkage analysis*.

The likelihood of linkage compared to independent assortment is expressed as a *LOD score*. If the likelihood is 1000:1, the LOD is 3 (logarithm to base 10 of 1000). LOD scores of 3 or higher are significant indicators of linkage. The recombination frequency is equal to the number of recombinant offspring divided by the total number of offspring observed. Expressed as a percentage, this number approximates the separation of the two observed traits (the marker and the suspected gene) in centimorgans. One cM equals 1% recombination and, as mentioned earlier, represents a physical distance of approximately 1 million base pairs. Distance between the marker and suspected gene is expressed as θ (theta) where $\theta = 0.2$ (20 cM).

The first linkage of disease to human chromosome was the observation that protanopia was linked to the X chromosome. In 1937 hemophilia was observed to be linked to congenital color deficiency, and in 1963 the Coppock cataract was the first autosomal gene to be linked (to the Duffy blood group locus on chromosome 1). Presently, over 250 genes are linked annually. Table XV-2 lists corneal dystrophies and conditions with known linkages.

TABLE XV-2

CORNEAL CONDITIONS WITH KNOWN LINKAGES

CORNEAL CONDITION	GENE LINKAGE
Meesmann dystrophy	12q12–q13 (keratin-3 mutation)
Avellino dystrophy	5q31 (βig-h3 gene)
Granular dystrophy	5q31 (βig-h3 gene)
Lattice type I dystrophy	5q31 (βig-h3 gene)
Lattice type IIIA	5q31 (βig-h3 gene)
Reis-Bückler dystrophy	5q31 (βig-h3 gene)
Thiel-Behnke dystrophy	10q24
Macular dystrophy	16q22
Schnyder central crystalline dystrophy	1p36–p34.1
Congenital hereditary endothelial dystrophy (CHED)	20p11.2–q11.2
Posterior polymorphous dystrophy (PPMD)	20p11.2–q11.2
Cornea plana	12q21 (CNA2)
Rieger anomaly	4q25–q26
Megalocornea (X-linked)	Xq21.3–q22
Peters anomaly	11p (PAX6 gene)
Aniridia	11p (PAX6 gene)
Fish eye disease	16 (LCAT deficiency)
Cystinosis	17p
Pachyonychia congenita, Jackson-Lawler type	17q12–q21
Ectodermal dysplasia, anhidrotic	Xq12.2–q13.1
Ichthyosis, X-linked	Xp22.32

CHAPTER XVI

Clinical Approach to Corneal Dystrophies and Metabolic Disorders

A *dystrophy* is a bilateral, symmetric, inherited condition that appears to have little or no relationship to environmental or systemic factors. Dystrophies begin early in life but may not become apparent until later. They tend to be slowly progressive. Corneal dystrophies can be classified according to genetic pattern, severity, histopathologic features, biochemical characteristics, or anatomical location. The anatomical scheme that classifies the dystrophies according to the levels of the cornea that are involved is the one used most often.

Anterior Corneal Dystrophies

Corneal Basement Membrane Dystrophies

Corneal epithelial basement membrane dystrophy (EBMD) Also known as *map-dot-fingerprint* or *Cogan microcystic dystrophy*, EBMD is the most common anterior corneal dystrophy. It is bilateral and may have dominant inheritance (often with incomplete penetrance) but is more often sporadic. EBMD occurs in 6%–18% of the population, more commonly in women, with increasing frequency over the age of 50 years.

PATHOGENESIS. EBMD is an abnormality of epithelial turnover, maturation, and production of basement membrane. Histopathologic findings include the following:

□ A thickened basement membrane with extension into the epithelium

□ Abnormal epithelial cells with microcysts (often with absent or abnormal hemidesmosomes)

□ Fibrillar material between the basement membrane and Bowman's layer

CLINICAL FINDINGS. Gray patches, microcysts, and/or fine lines in the central epithelial layer are seen on examination. These are usually best seen with sclerotic scatter, retroillumination, or a broad tangential beam. The findings are quite variable and may change with time. Three kinds of lesions are seen with the epithelium and its immediately subjacent basement membrane:

□ Map lines

□ Dots or microcysts

□ Fingerprint lines

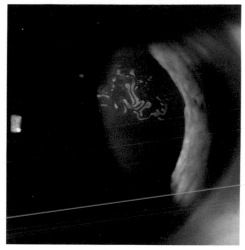
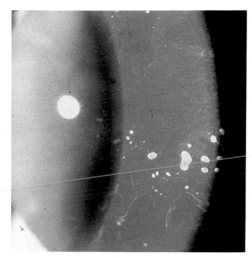

FIG XVI-1—Epithelial basement membrane dystrophy showing thick geographic map lines, or "putty marks."

FIG XVI-2—EBMD dystrophy showing microcysts and geographic map line areas.

These abnormalities occur in varying combinations and change in number and distribution from time to time. Fingerprint lines are thin, relucent, hairlike lines; several of them are often arranged in a concentric pattern so that they resemble fingerprints. Map lines are the same as fingerprint lines except thicker, more irregular, and surrounded by a faint haze; they resemble irregular coastlines or geographic borders on maps (Fig XVI-1). Maps and fingerprints consist of thickened or multilaminar strips of epithelial basement membrane. Dots are intraepithelial spaces containing the debris of epithelial cells that have collapsed and degenerated before having reached the epithelial surface (Fig XVI-2). The gray-white dots have discrete edges. When they are very prominent, the term *Cogan microcystic dystrophy* may be used.

Symptoms that are related to recurrent epithelial erosions and to transient blurred vision are more common in patients older than 30 but can be seen at any age. It is estimated that 10% of patients with EBMD will have corneal erosions and that 50% of patients with recurrent epithelial erosions have evidence of this anterior dystrophy. Both eyes must be examined, since evidence of the dystrophy may be found in the uninvolved eye. In some circumstances clinical findings may mimic corneal intraepithelial dysplasia, and removed material should be submitted for histopathology.

MANAGEMENT. Treatment may need to be extended for months. It consists of varying combinations of the following (see also discussion of recurrent corneal erosions in chapter VI):

- 5% sodium chloride or other lubricating ointment
- Lubricating drops
- Epithelial scraping
- Patching
- Fitting of a thin, loose bandage (soft contact) lens

Recalcitrant cases of recurrent corneal erosion may require anterior stromal puncture of the epithelium using a 20–25–gauge needle (0.1 mm is sufficient depth). Multiple small punctures disturb Bowman's layer, thereby promoting a tighter adhesion and stimulating the cornea to produce functional basement membrane complexes. The Nd:YAG laser and 5-mm diamond burr have also been reported to be effective in creating anterior stromal disturbance as treatment of recurrent erosion. Removal of damaged epithelium alone may be very effective. Phototherapeutic keratectomy (PTK) with excimer laser into the anterior 2–4 μm of Bowman's membrane after removal of the epithelium may be needed with central or recalcitrant erosions.

Meesmann (juvenile epithelial) dystrophy This rare bilateral autosomal dominant epithelial dystrophy appears very early in life.

PATHOGENESIS. Thickened epithelium and a multilaminar, thickened basement membrane with projections into the basal epithelium are seen. The epithelial cells contain an electron-dense accumulation of "peculiar substance," a fibrillogranular material of unknown composition.

CLINICAL FINDINGS. Tiny epithelial vesicles are seen extending out to the limbus, most easily with retroillumination. They appear as tiny, bubblelike blebs and are most numerous in the interpalpebral area (Fig XVI-3). The surrounding epithelium is clear. Whorled and wedge-shaped epithelial patterns have been reported. The cornea may be slightly thinned and corneal sensation may be reduced. Symptoms are limited to mild irritation and a slight decrease in visual acuity.

MANAGEMENT. Most patients require no treatment, but soft contact lens wear may be helpful if patients show frequent symptoms. Superficial PTK is useful for reducing symptoms but rarely required.

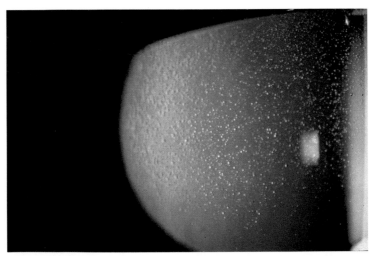

FIG XVI-3—Meesmann dystrophy, appearing as tiny, bubblelike blebs against the red reflex.

Reis-Bücklers dystrophy   This progressive autosomal dominant dystrophy appears in the first few years of life and mainly affects Bowman's layer. Reis-Bücklers dystrophy has been linked to chromosome 5q31 in the same region as granular, lattice, and Avellino (granular-lattice) dystrophies (see below).

PATHOGENESIS. A mutation occurs in the βig-h3 (human transforming growth factor β–induced) gene responsible for formation of keratoepithelin, but the exact material accumulating is unknown. Degenerative changes occur in the deep epithelium, but basement membrane is not thickened. Bowman's layer is disrupted or absent and replaced by fibrocellular tissue in an undulating, or "sawtooth," fashion that corresponds clinically to areas of subepithelial opacification. Transmission electron microscopy reveals pathognomonic "curly fibers" at the level of Bowman's membrane.

CLINICAL FINDINGS. Biomicroscopy reveals a superficial geographic, or honeycomb, gray-white reticular opacification that is greatest in the central cornea. The posterior cornea appears normal, but in advanced cases the anterior scarring can lead to surface irregularity. Symptoms often begin in the first or second decade with painful, recurrent epithelial erosions. Vision is reduced by both anterior scarring with surface irregularity and anterior stromal edema.

LABORATORY EVALUATION. Some authors divide corneal dystrophy of Bowman's membrane into two types based on the transmission electron microscopic appearance. *Type I* has rod-shaped bodies similar to granular dystrophy, and *type II* has curly fibers and is renamed *Thiel-Behnke dystrophy.* Although based on morphology, this reclassification has been substantiated by recent linkage to 10q24 gene. Thiel-Behnke may be the more prevalent form of Bowman's layer dystrophy and is typically honeycomb in appearance.

MANAGEMENT. Initial treatment is aimed at the recurrent erosions. Superficial keratectomy, lamellar keratoplasty, PTK, or rarely penetrating keratoplasty may be performed. Recurrence in the graft is common (Fig XVI-4).

Laibson PR. Anterior corneal dystrophies. In: Krachmer JH, Mannis MJ, Holland EJ, eds. *Cornea.* St Louis: Mosby; 1997;2:1033–1042.

Munier FL, Korvatska E, Djemai A, et al. Kerato-epithelin mutations in four 5q31-linked corneal dystrophies. *Nat Genet.* 1997;15:247–251.

Yee RW, Sullivan LS, Lai HT, et al. Linkage mapping of Thiel-Behnke corneal dystrophy (CDB2) to chromosome 10q23–24. *Genomics.* 1997;46:152–154.

Stromal Corneal Dystrophies

Posterior amorphous corneal dysgenesis and congenital hereditary stromal dystrophy are discussed in chapter XIV. Conditions related to those discussed below are also described later in this chapter under the heading, "Disorders of Protein Metabolism." Table XVI-1 includes information about the stromal corneal dystrophies.

Granular dystrophy and Avellino dystrophy   Granular dystrophy is one of the three most common stromal dystrophies. Transmission is autosomal dominant and the gene has been linked to chromosome 5q31 along with lattice, Avellino, and Reis-Bücklers dystrophies.

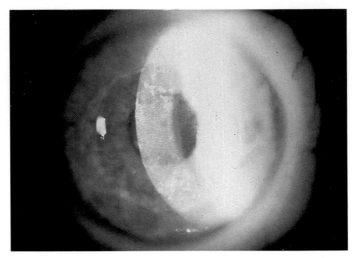

FIG XVI-4—Reis-Bücklers corneal dystrophy: recurrence in graft.

PATHOGENESIS. Microscopically, the granular material is hyaline and stains bright red with Masson trichrome stain. An electron-dense material made up of rod-shaped bodies immersed in an amorphous matrix is seen ultrastructurally. Histochemically, the deposits are noncollagenous protein that may derive from the corneal epithelium and/or keratocytes. Although the exact cause is unknown, a mutation different from that in Reis-Bücklers, lattice, and Avellino dystrophies has been identified in the βig-h3 gene responsible for formation of keratoepithelin.

TABLE XVI-1

HISTOPATHOLOGIC DIFFERENTIATION OF
GRANULAR, MACULAR, AND LATTICE DYSTROPHIES

DYSTROPHY	MASSON	ALCIAN BLUE	PAS	AMYLOID*	BIREFRINGENCE
Granular	+	−	−	−	−
Macular	−	+	−	−	−
Lattice	+	−	+	+	+

*Stains for amyloid: Congo red, crystal violet, and thioflavine T

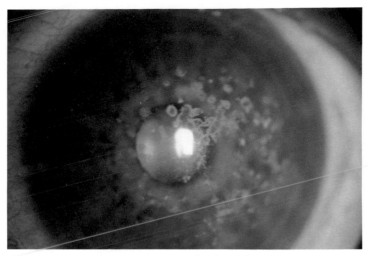

FIG XVI-5—Granular dystrophy.

CLINICAL FINDINGS. Three clinical forms are identified, but all have the same electron microscopic features. *Type I* is most frequent and corresponds to Groenouw dystrophy type I. Onset occurs early in life with crumblike opacities that broaden into a disciform appearance as the patient reaches the teens. The lesions do not extend to the limbus but can extend anteriorly through focal breaks in Bowman's layer (Fig XVI-5). The dystrophy is slowly progressive with vision rarely dropping to 20/200 after age 40. *Type II* presents in the second decade with fewer, larger ring- or disc-shaped granular deposits in the anterior stroma, sharply defined by intervening clear areas. The deposits can be found progressively deeper as the patient ages. Erosions are infrequent and vision is usually better than 20/70. *Type III* is more superficial and presents in infancy with erosions. Fine granular deposits are confined to Bowman's layer or anterior stroma. This form clinically resembles Reis-Bücklers dystrophy.

Avellino corneal dystrophy, a variant of granular dystrophy, was originally described in a small number of families who traced their roots to Avellino, Italy. The affected patients have a granular dystrophy both histologically and clinically. Lattice lesions are also present in some patients. Older patients have anterior stromal haze between deposits, which reduces visual acuity. Pathologically, both the hyaline deposits typical of granular dystrophy and the amyloid deposits typical of lattice dystrophy (see below) are seen, and Avellino dystrophy is also known as *granular-lattice dystrophy.*

The relationship among these four different phenotypes of stromal dystrophy (granular, Avellino, lattice, and Reis-Bücklers) is not fully understood, although Avellino and lattice dystrophies have the same mutations in the βig-h3 gene responsible for formation of keratoepithelin, which differ from the mutations in granular and Reis-Bücklers dystrophies.

MANAGEMENT. Early in the disease process no treatment is needed. Recurrent erosions in superficial granular dystrophy may be treated with therapeutic contact lenses, superficial keratectomy, or PTK. When visual acuity is affected, penetrating keratoplasty has a good prognosis. Recurrence in the graft (anteriorly and peripherally) may occur after many years as fine subepithelial opacities varying from original presentation.

Bron AJ. The corneal dystrophies. *Curr Opinion Ophthal.* 1990;1:333–346.

Lattice dystrophy   This autosomal dominant dystrophy is very common. Variable expression is characterized by typical glasslike branching lines in the stroma.

PATHOGENESIS. Light microscopy of lattice dystrophy demonstrates amyloid deposits concentrated most heavily in the anterior stroma. Amyloid may also accumulate in the subepithelial area, giving rise to poor epithelial–stromal adhesions. Amyloid stains rose to orange-red with Congo red dye and metachromatically with crystal violet dye, and it exhibits dichroism and birefringence. Recently, investigators have noted corneal elastotic degeneration in combination with lattice dystrophy, although it is not known if an association is present. The specific genetic defect is in the βig-h3 gene responsible for formation of keratoepithelin. This mutation is not in one of the 14 known amyloid-associated genes.

CLINICAL FINDINGS. The spectrum of corneal changes is broad, and the classic branching lattice figures may not be present in all cases. Refractile lines, central and subepithelial ovoid white dots, and diffuse anterior stromal haze appear early in life. Initially, the white dots resemble granular dystrophy. The refractile lines, so-called lattice lines, are best seen against a red reflex or with retroillumination (Fig XVI-6). The stroma can take on a ground-glass appearance, but the peripheral cornea remains clear. Recurrent epithelial erosions often occur. In addition, stromal haze and epithelial surface irregularity may decrease vision.

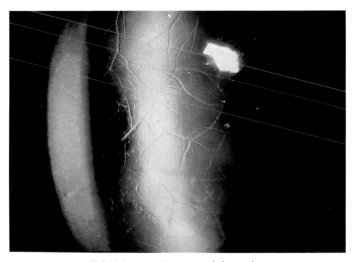

FIG XVI-6—Lattice corneal dystrophy.

This disorder is a primary localized corneal amyloidosis, in which the amyloid deposits may result from corneal epithelial cells and keratocytes. At least three types of lattice dystrophy have been identified.

Type I (Biber-Haab-Dimmer). This form is classic lattice dystrophy with onset of erosions or vision difficulty at the end of the first decade. There is no systemic amyloid deposition (see primary localized amyloidosis, p 324). Type I is linked to chromosome 5q31.

Type II (Meretoja syndrome). This form combines lattice dystrophy with coexistent systemic amyloidosis and manifests around age 20 years. In addition to lattice corneal changes, patients with Meretoja syndrome (Finnish type) have a characteristic facial mask; blepharochalasis; pendulous ears; cranial and peripheral nerve palsies; and dry, lax skin with amyloid deposition. The classic corneal lattice lines are less numerous and more peripherally located in this form. The amyloid in this condition is related to gelsolin and does not stain for type AA or AP (see p 322 for an explanation of these proteins and staining procedures). A mutation in chromosome 9q34 has been found in Meretoja syndrome.

Type III. These deposits are midstromal and larger than the deposits in age-matched individuals with type I. Type III deposits are type AP amyloid in contrast to the type AA seen in type I lattice dystrophy. The inheritance pattern appears to be autosomal recessive with symptoms delayed until the fifth to seventh decade. Recurrent erosion is uncommon in patients with type III lattice dystrophy. A variant described as type IIIa differs in some respects: recurrent erosions are common, inheritance is autosomal dominant, and this form is reported only in white patients.

MANAGEMENT. Recurrent erosions are managed with therapeutic contact lenses, superficial keratectomy, or PTK. Severe cases of lattice dystrophy with visual loss are treated with penetrating keratoplasty. Recurrence of this dystrophy in the corneal graft, usually in 2–12 years, occurs more frequently than after grafting for granular or macular dystrophy.

Macular dystrophy   This least common of the three classic stromal dystrophies differs from both lattice and granular dystrophies: it has an autosomal recessive inheritance, involves the corneal periphery, and features a decrease in vision at an earlier age. Two types are described below.

PATHOGENESIS. The deposits in macular dystrophy are glycosaminoglycan (acid mucopolysaccharide), and they stain with colloidal iron and Alcian blue. They accumulate in the endoplasmic reticulum and not in lysosomal vacuoles as seen in systemic mucopolysaccharidoses. Both types I and II have been linked to chromosome 16q22, suggesting different mutations of the same allele.

CLINICAL FINDINGS. Corneas are clear at birth and begin to cloud at ages 3–9. Patients with macular dystrophy show focal, gray-white, superficial stromal opacities that progress to involve full stromal thickness and extend to the corneal periphery. Macular spots have indefinite edges, and the stroma between the opacities is diffusely cloudy (Fig XVI-7). Involvement of Descemet's membrane and the endothelium is indicated by the presence of cornea guttatae. Epithelial erosions are possible, but symptoms usually involve decrease in vision. Central corneal thinning has been noted. The two types of macular dystrophy are based on biochemical differences.

Type I. Patients with this more prevalent form of macular dystrophy lack antigenic keratan sulfate in their cornea, serum, and cartilage. These patients have a normal synthesis of dermatan sulfate–proteoglycan. An error occurs in the synthesis of

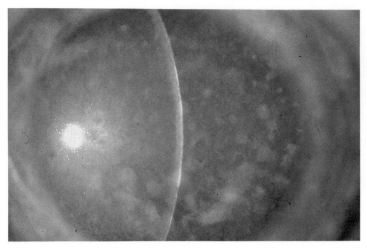

FIG XVI-7—Macular dystrophy, showing involvement to the limbus with diffuse haze.

keratan sulfate and in the activity of specific sulfotransferases involved in the sulfation of the keratan sulfate lactose aminoglycan side chain.

Type II. Patients with this form synthesize a normal ratio of keratan sulfate and dermatan sulfate–proteoglycans, but synthesis is 30% below normal. Moreover, the dermatan sulfate–proteoglycan chains are 40% shorter than normal. Clinical presentation is similar to type I.

LABORATORY EVALUATION. An enzyme-linked immunosorbent assay (ELISA) can measure sulfated keratan sulfate. This test can help in the diagnosis of macular dystrophy even in preclinical forms and carriers.

MANAGEMENT. Recurrent erosions are treated as for other stromal dystrophies, and photophobia may be relieved with tinted contact lenses. Definitive treatment is by penetrating corneal transplantation, although recurrences may be seen with both lamellar and penetrating keratoplasty.

Gelatinous droplike dystrophy (primary familial amyloidosis)   This uncommon autosomal recessive corneal dystrophy maps to chromosome 1p. It features typical amyloid occurring as subepithelial deposits (see also p 324). Electron microscopy suggests the source of the amyloid is the basal epithelial layer. Most reports are in the Japanese literature. Onset occurs in the first decade and may resemble band keratopathy, but advancing disease develops protruding, mulberry-like subepithelial deposits (Fig XVI-8). Management is similar to lattice dystrophy, and recurrence rate is very high following keratoplasty.

Schnyder central crystalline dystrophy   This rare, slowly progressive autosomal dominant stromal dystrophy appears in the first year of life but usually goes undetected at that age. It has been linked to chromosome 1p36–p34.1.

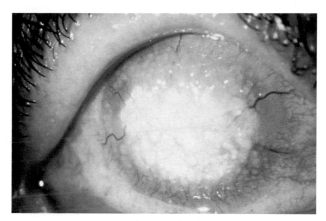

FIG XVI-8—Gelatinous droplike dystrophy.

PATHOGENESIS. Theoretically, this condition is a primary disorder of corneal lipid metabolism. Pathologically, the opacities are accumulations of unesterified cholesterol and neutral fats. Oil red O stains the neutral fats red. In the normal process of embedding tissue in paraffin, cholesterol and other fatty substances are dissolved; therefore, the pathologist must be made aware of the requirements for special stains. Electron microscopy will demonstrate abnormal accumulation of lipid and dissolved cholesterol in the epithelium, Bowman's layer, and throughout the stroma

CLINICAL FINDINGS. Involved patients may show any combination of the following:

□ Minute yellow-white crystals

□ Diffuse stromal haze

□ Dense corneal arcus

□ Type I limbal girdle of Vogt

The central opacities accumulate just beneath Bowman's layer, often in a doughnut-like or wreath configuration. The epithelium is usually uninvolved clinically and remains smooth, and the cornea does not vascularize (Fig XVI-9). Corneal arcus may develop.

LABORATORY EVALUATION. Fasting lipid profile should be done for possible hyperlipoproteinemia (type II-a, III, or IV) or hyperlipidemia. Approximately 50% of affected patients have elevated serum cholesterol.

MANAGEMENT. Crystalline dystrophy rarely reduces vision enough to require transplantation, and recurrences do occur. PTK has been used to treat decreased vision, and abnormal lipids are managed as with other affected patients.

Fleck dystrophy This uncommon nonprogressive stromal dystrophy begins very early in life and may be congenital. It can show extreme asymmetry (unilateral only) and is probably autosomal dominant.

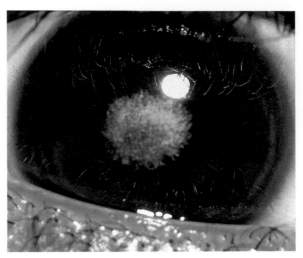

FIG XVI-9—Central crystalline dystrophy.

PATHOGENESIS. Affected keratocytes contain two abnormal substances: excess gly-cosaminoglycan, which stains with Alcian blue and colloidal iron; and lipids, demonstrated by Sudan black B and oil red O.

CLINICAL FINDINGS. Discrete, flat, gray-white, dandrufflike (sometimes ring-shaped) opacities appear throughout the stroma to its periphery. The epithelium, Bowman's layer, Descemet's membrane, and the endothelium are not involved. Symptoms are minimal, and vision is usually not reduced. However, fleck dystrophy may be associated with decreased corneal sensation, limbal dermoid, keratoconus, central cloudy dystrophy, punctate cortical lens changes, pseudoxanthoma elasticum, or atopy.

Central cloudy dystrophy This bilateral symmetrical stromal dystrophy is nonprogressive or only very slowly progressive. It is autosomal dominant. No management is required.

PATHOGENESIS. Cause is unknown. Pathologically, the collagen of the deep stroma is thrown into sawtooth folds.

CLINICAL FINDINGS. The opacity is most dense centrally and posteriorly and fades both anteriorly and peripherally (Fig XVI-10). Opacities consist of multiple nebulous, polygonal, gray areas separated by cracklike intervening clear zones. The epithelium, Bowman's layer, stromal thickness, Descemet's membrane, and endothelium are normal. Vision is usually not reduced. This condition differs from posterior crocodile shagreen (see Figure XIV-4) principally in showing a strong autosomal dominant inheritance pattern and having haze extend anteriorly into the cornea.

Mannis MJ, DeSousa LB, Gross RH. The stromal dystrophies. In: Krachmer JH, Mannis MJ, Holland EJ, eds. *Cornea.* St Louis: Mosby; 1997;2:1043–1062.

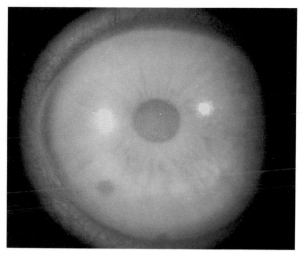

FIG XVI-10—Central cloudy dystrophy (François) showing mild stromal haze and peripheral clearing.

Smolin G. Corneal dystrophies and degenerations. In: Smolin G, Thoft RA, eds. *The Cornea: Scientific Foundations and Clinical Practice.* 3rd ed. Boston: Little, Brown; 1994:499–533.

Endothelial Dystrophies

Fuchs endothelial dystrophy This very common condition ranges from asymptomatic cornea guttata to a decompensated cornea with stromal edema, subepithelial fibrosis, and epithelial bullae. The condition shows variable autosomal dominant transmission and may be sporadic. Onset occurs after 50 years with a female preponderance.

PATHOGENESIS. Primary dysfunction of the endothelial cell manifests as increased corneal swelling and deposition of collagen and extracellular matrix in Descemet's membrane. The cause of the abnormal function is unknown, but there is a reduction in the number Na^+,K^+-ATPase pump sites or in pump function. It is not clear whether the reduction in the posterior nonbanded zone and the increase in thickness of the posterior banded zone (posterior collagenase layer) is a primary effect of endothelial dysfunction or secondary to chronic corneal edema.

CLINICAL FINDINGS. Findings vary with the severity of the disease. Cornea guttata is first evident centrally and spreads toward the periphery. Descemet's membrane becomes thickened, and folds develop secondary to stromal edema (Fig XVI-11).

Increased endothelial pigmentation is also seen. As the endothelium further decompensates, the central corneal thickness may approach 1 mm (0.52–0.56 mm is normal). Epithelial edema develops (Fig XVI-12), leading to microcystic edema, and later progresses to epithelial bullae, which may rupture.

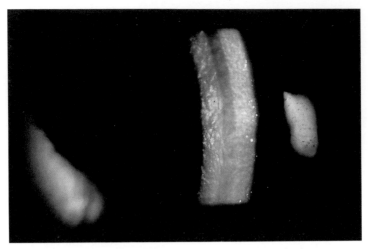

FIG XVI-11—Fuchs endothelial dystrophy showing stromal edema, Descemet's folds, and endothelial guttatae.

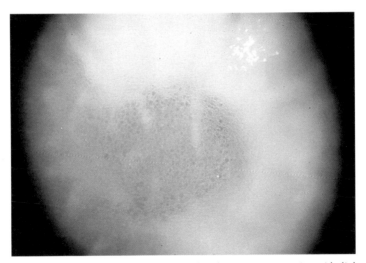

FIG XVI-12—Fuchs endothelial dystrophy showing microcystic epithelial edema.

Microscopically, the endothelial cells are noted to be larger and more polymorphic than normal and disrupted by excrescences of excess collagen, a product of the stressed endothelial cells (Fig XVI-13). Descemet's membrane is thickened. Long-standing cases lead to subepithelial fibrosis.

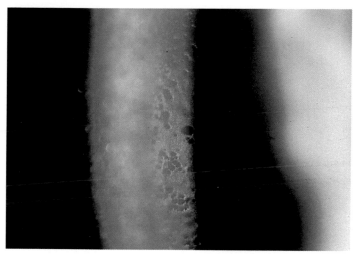

FIG XVI-13—Fuchs endothelial dystrophy. Endothelial cells are large and disrupted by numerous guttatae (specular reflection photomicrograph).

Symptoms are rare before age 50 and are related to the edema, which causes a decrease in vision and pain secondary to ruptured bullae. Symptoms are worse upon awakening, because of decreased surface evaporation during sleep. Painful episodes may subside once subepithelial fibrosis occurs.

LABORATORY EVALUATION. Specular microscopy may be helpful in diagnosing Fuchs and following the clinical course for loss of endothelial cells. Corneal pachymetry may indicate relative endothelial function and change with progression of disease. Both are useful in determining the relative safety of cataract or other intraocular surgery. Endothelial cell count <1000/mm^2 or corneal thickness >650 μm suggests caution and the possibility the cornea may decompensate with surgery.

MANAGEMENT. Treatment is first aimed at reducing corneal edema and relieving pain. Use of sodium chloride drops and ointment (5%) and measures to lower intraocular pressure (IOP) may temporarily help the edema. Lubricating drops and a soft bandage lens are useful in the treatment of ruptured bullae. In advanced cases a conjunctival flap may be considered, but restoration of vision requires corneal transplantation. Surgery should be performed before vascularization, and most authorities would recommend surgery before the entire cornea becomes edematous. Prognosis for graft survival is good.

Posterior polymorphous dystrophy (PPMD) This uncommon, slowly progressive autosomal dominant or recessive dystrophy presents early in life. It has a variable clinical spectrum and can often be asymmetric and overlooked. PPMD has been mapped to chromosome 20q11 (congenital hereditary endothelial dystrophy links to 20p11.2–q11.2).

PATHOGENESIS. The most distinctive microscopic finding is the appearance of abnormal, multilayered endothelial cells that look and behave like epithelial cells or fibroblasts. These cells

□ Show microvilli

□ Stain positively for keratin

□ Show rapid and easy growth in cell culture

□ Have intercellular desmosomes

□ Manifest proliferative tendencies

Similar changes that are not limited to the cornea are seen in iridocorneal endothelial (ICE) syndrome (see pp 279–280). A diffuse abnormality of Descemet's membrane is common including thickening, a multilaminated appearance, and polymorphous alterations.

CLINICAL FINDINGS. Careful examination of the posterior corneal surface will show any or all of the following:

□ Isolated grouped vesicles

□ Geographic-shaped discrete gray lesions

□ Broad bands with scalloped edges (Fig XVI-14)

Variable amounts of stromal edema, corectopia, or broad iridocorneal adhesions are also seen (Fig XVI-15). Fine, glasslike adhesions may be seen gonioscopically. Both angle-closure and open-angle glaucoma can occur, and 14% of patients have elc vated IOP.

LABORATORY EVALUATION. Specular microscopy may show typical vesicles and bands in contrast to the involved cells in ICE syndrome, which appear as dark areas with central highlight and light peripheral borders. Opinion is divided on the value of relying on specular microscopy alone in making the diagnosis.

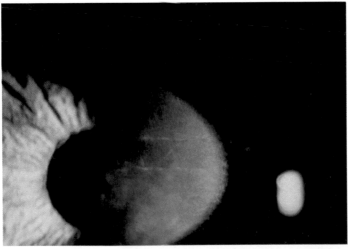

FIG XVI-14—Posterior polymorphous dystrophy showing scallop-edged endothelial band.

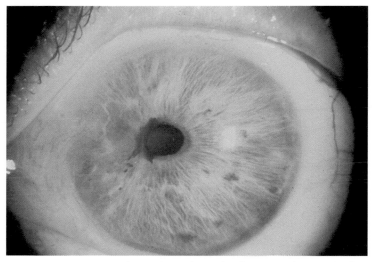

FIG XVI-15—Posterior polymorphous dystrophy showing iridocorneal adhesion and corectopia.

MANAGEMENT. Most patients are stable and asymptomatic. Mild corneal edema may be managed as with early Fuchs disease. Stromal micropuncture to induce subepithelial pannus can be used to manage localized swelling. With more severe disease glaucoma must be managed, and corneal transplants may be required. Prognosis for PK is related to the presence of visible peripheral anterior synechiae and glaucoma. PPMD may recur in the graft.

Ectatic Disorders

Keratoconus

In this common disorder (prevalence of about 50 per 100,000) the central or paracentral cornea undergoes progressive thinning and bulging, so that the cornea takes on the shape of a cone (Fig XVI-16). The hereditary pattern is not prominent or predictable, but positive family histories have been reported in 6%–8% of cases. Corneal topography of family members related to the patient with keratoconus shows subclinical keratoconus, suggesting a dominant inheritance pattern with incomplete penetrance.

PATHOGENESIS. Etiology is unknown and likely multifactorial because of the wide variety of associated syndromes and the low recurrence rate following transplantation. Histopathologically, keratoconus shows the following:

□ Fragmentation of Bowman's layer

□ Thinning of the stroma and overlying epithelium

□ Folds or breaks in Descemet's membrane

□ Variable amounts of diffuse scarring

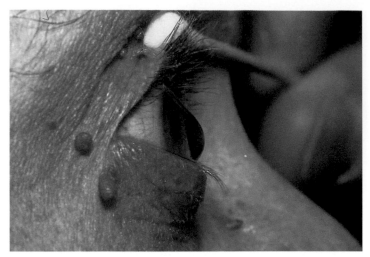

FIG XVI-16—Keratoconus.

CLINICAL FINDINGS. Nearly all cases are bilateral, but one eye may be much more severely involved. Sometimes the less affected eye shows only high astigmatism, which may be considered the minimal manifestation of keratoconus. The disease tends to progress during the adolescent years and then to stabilize when the patient has attained full growth, although progression can occur at any time. Early biomicroscopic and histopathologic findings include fibrillation of Bowman's layer, leading to breaks followed by fibrous growth and dysplasia through the break. As progression occurs, the apical thinning of the central cornea worsens, and extreme degrees of irregular astigmatism can develop. No associated inflammation occurs.

Scissoring of the red reflex on ophthalmoscopy or retinoscopy is a very early sign of keratoconus. *Rizzutti's sign,* a conical reflection on the nasal cornea when a penlight is shone from the temporal side, is another early finding (Fig XVI-17). Iron deposits are often present within the epithelium around the base of the cone and constitute a *Fleischer ring* (Fig XVI-18). This ring is brown in color and best appreciated with the cobalt blue filter. Fine, relucent, and roughly parallel striations *(Vogt lines),* or stress lines, of the stroma can be observed. Focal ruptures and flecklike scars occur in Bowman's layer.

Spontaneous perforation in keratoconus is extremely rare. But at any time a tear in Descemet's membrane can occur, resulting in the sudden development of corneal edema, or *acute hydrops.* The break in the posterior cornea usually heals spontaneously in 6–12 weeks; the corneal edema then disappears, but stromal scarring may be left in its wake. Some patients regain good vision following the resolution of hydrops, depending largely on the extent and location of the scar.

An increased prevalence of keratoconus has been reported in Down syndrome, atopy, Marfan syndrome, floppy eyelid syndrome, Leber congenital hereditary optic neuropathy, and mitral valve prolapse. Keratoconus also occurs commonly in numerous congenital anomalies of the eye.

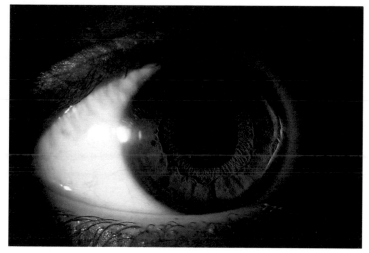

FIG XVI-17—Rizzutti's sign.

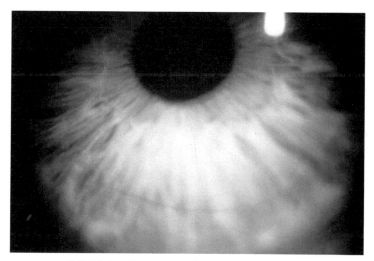

FIG XVI-18—Keratoconus showing a Fleischer ring.

LABORATORY EVALUATION. Computerized videokeratography may be helpful in detecting early keratoconus, following its progression, or assisting in fitting contact lenses. Placido-based topography shows inferior steepening in the power map, but pachymetry mapping shows the thin zone to be paracentral (Fig XVI-19).

MANAGEMENT. Some cases of keratoconus are mild enough, at least for a time, that vision can be corrected adequately with glasses. However, hard or gas-permeable

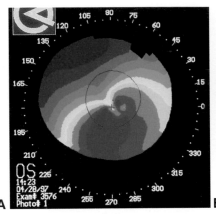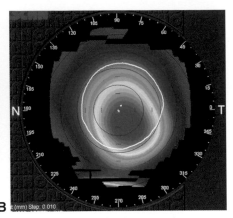

FIG XVI-19—Keratoconus. *A,* Placido disk computerized videography showing inferior steepening. *B,* Orbscan computerized videography showing a pachymetry map of the same eye as in *A.* Note the thinnest zone is near the visual axis and not where the steepest point is located.

contact lenses are far more helpful in all but the mildest cases. Their ability to neutralize the irregular corneal astigmatism often produces dramatic improvement in vision. The majority of patients with keratoconus without central corneal scarring can be fitted successfully with contact lenses using advanced techniques, and central subepithelial scar can on occasion be removed (nodulectomy), allowing continued wear of contact lenses. A multicenter study is presently examining the natural history of keratoconus and whether the type of contact lens fit (flat or vaulting the cone) determines improvement in vision or leads to earlier or more frequent surgery.

When contact lenses are no longer satisfactory, penetrating keratoplasty is the treatment of choice. The prognosis for keratoplasty in keratoconus is excellent. Thermokeratoplasty, corneal flattening by heat application, may regularize the corneal surface, but the procedure is difficult and fraught with complications. It is most often used to flatten the cornea at the time of PK to make trephination easier. Use of the argon-fluoride excimer laser is controversial, and keratoconus is considered a contraindication to elective photorefractive keratectomy (PRK), which thins an already thin cornea. However, some surgeons use PTK for central scarring, and trials of elective PRK are being closely monitored.

Hydrops is treated conservatively with topical hypertonic agents and patching or a soft contact lens. A cycloplegic agent may be needed for ciliary pain. Hydrops is not an indication for immediate surgery.

Belin MW. Optical and surgical correction of keratoconus. In: *Focal Points: Clinical Modules for Ophthalmologists.* San Francisco: American Academy of Ophthalmology; 1988;6:11.

Maguire LJ. Computerized corneal analysis. In: *Focal Points: Clinical Modules for Ophthalmologists.* San Francisco: American Academy of Ophthalmology; 1996;14:5.

Rabinowitz YS. Keratoconus. *Surv Ophthalmol.* 1998;42:297–319.

Zadnik K, Barr JT, Gordon MO, et al. Biomicroscopic signs and disease severity in keratoconus. Collaborative Longitudinal Evaluation of Keratoconus (CLEK) Study Group. *Cornea.* 1996;15:139–146.

TABLE XVI-2

NONINFLAMMATORY ECTATIC DISORDERS COMPARED AND CONTRASTED:
TYPICAL CLINICAL PRESENTATION AND APPEARANCE

	KERATOCONUS	KERATOGLOBUS	PELLUCID MARGINAL DEGENERATION
Frequency	Most common	Rare	Less common
Laterality	Usually bilateral	Bilateral	Bilateral
Age at onset	Puberty	Usually at birth	Age 20–40 years
Thinning	Inferior paracentral	Greatest in periphery	Inferior band 1–2 mm wide
Protrusion	Thinning at apex	Generalized	Superior to band of thinning
Iron line	Fleischer ring	None	Sometimes
Scarring	Common	Mild	Only after hydrops
Striae	Common	Sometimes	Sometimes

Modified from Krachmer JH, Mannis MJ, Holland EJ, eds. *Cornea.* St Louis: Mosby; 1997:1092.

Keratoglobus

This very rare, bilateral, noninflammatory condition differs from keratoconus and pellucid marginal degeneration in typically being present at birth (Table XVI-2). It is usually not hereditary. Keratoglobus is similar in appearance to keratoconus but manifests a globular rather than a conical deformation of the cornea (Fig XVI-20).

PATHOGENESIS. Keratoglobus is strongly associated with blue sclera and Ehlers-Danlos syndrome type VI (see Chapter XIV), and it may represent a defect in collagen synthesis. Histopathologically, it is characterized by absent or fragmented Bowman's layer, thinned stroma with normal lamellar organization, and thin Descemet's membrane. Unlike keratoconus, keratoglobus is not associated with atopy, hard contact lens wear, or tapetoretinal degeneration.

CLINICAL FINDINGS. Both corneas have a globular shape with very deep anterior chamber. The corneal curve may be as steep as 50–60 D, and generalized thinning appears, especially in the midperiphery, in contrast to keratoconus, which has maximal thinning at or near the apex of the protrusion. Spontaneous rupture of Descemet's membrane and corneal hydrops can occur, but iron lines, stress lines, and anterior scarring are not seen. The corneal diameter may be slightly increased. Fleischer rings are usually not present, but prominent folds and areas of thickening in Descemet's membrane are common. Keratoglobus may be associated with blue sclera, hyperextensibility of the joints, sensorineural deafness, fractures, and corneal perforation with minimal trauma (fragile cornea).

MANAGEMENT. Prognosis for successful PK is much poorer in keratoglobus, and lamellar surgery should be considered in those cases requiring intervention to main-

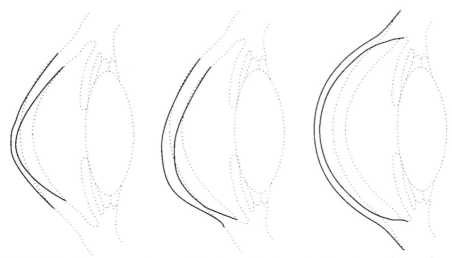

FIG XVI-20—The presence of corneal thinning and the type of contour abnormality can be helpful in recognizing the type of ectatic disorder. From left: keratoconus, pellucid marginal degeneration, keratoglobus. (Reproduced with permission from Krachmer JH, Mannis MJ, Holland EJ, eds. *Cornea*. St Louis: Mosby; 1997:1092.)

tain functional vision. Spontaneous corneal rupture has been reported, so patients must be counseled regarding the importance of protection with eye wear. High myopia is treated with spectacles to prevent amblyopia.

Pellucid Marginal Degeneration

This condition is somewhat common, nonhereditary, and bilateral. Clear, inferior, peripheral corneal thinning takes place in the absence of inflammation. Etiology is unknown.

CLINICAL FINDINGS. Protrusion of the cornea occurs above the band of thinning. At times a clear distinction between pellucid marginal degeneration and keratoconus is not possible. A cornea with keratoconus will show protrusion *at* the point of maximal thinning, but pellucid marginal degeneration will show protrusion *above* the area of maximum thinning. No vascularization or lipid deposition occurs, but posterior stromal scarring has been noted within the thinned area. Most patients are diagnosed between 20 and 40 years of age, and men and women are affected equally. Decreased vision results from high irregular astigmatism (Figs XVI-21, XVI-22). Acute hydrops has been reported.

MANAGEMENT. Treatment consists of contact lenses early in the disease, although lens fitting is more difficult in pellucid marginal degeneration than in keratoconus. Eventually, PK may be required to restore vision. Because of the location of the thin-

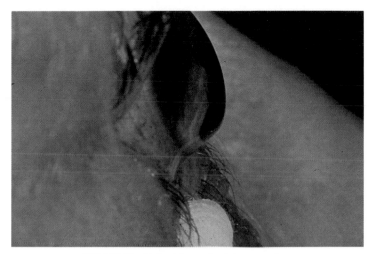
FIG XVI-21—Pellucid marginal degeneration.

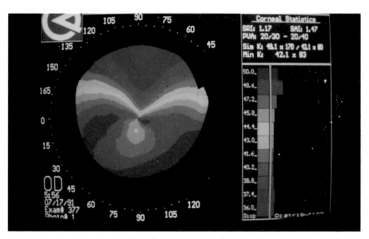
FIG XVI-22—Topogram of pellucid marginal degeneration. Note inferior steepening.

ning, the grafts tend to be large and close to the limbus, making surgery technically more difficult and the graft more prone to rejection. Recently, wedge resection or lamellar tectonic grafts have been advocated.

Feder RS. Noninflammatory ectatic disorders. In: Krachmer JH, Mannis MJ, Holland EJ, eds. *Cornea*. St Louis: Mosby; 1997;2:1091–1106.

Metabolic Disorders With Corneal Changes

Many of the corneal manifestations of systemic disease are alterations in corneal clarity caused by abnormal storage of metabolic substances within the epithelium, stroma, or endothelium. Abnormal substances typically accumulate in lysosomes or lysosome-like intracytoplasmic structures as a result of a single enzyme defect. Most of these disorders are autosomal recessive with the notable exceptions of Hunter syndrome (MPS type II) and Fabry disease, which are both X-linked recessive.

> Sugar J. Metabolic disorders of the cornea. In: Kaufman HE, Barron BA, McDonald MB. *The Cornea.* 2nd ed. Boston: Butterworth-Heinmann; 1998:391–410.

Disorders of Carbohydrate Metabolism

Mucopolysaccharidoses Systemic mucopolysaccharidoses (MPS) are rare inherited lysosomal storage diseases that result from the absence of lysosomal acid hydrolases, the enzymes that usually catabolize the glycosaminoglycans (GAGs) dermatan sulfate, heparan sulfate, and keratan sulfate.

PATHOGENESIS. While there are at least eight separate syndromes, several features are common to all. Heparan sulfate, dermatan sulfate, and keratan sulfate, the GAG normally present in highest concentration, are the accumulated metabolites. All syndromes are autosomal recessive, with the exception of the X-linked recessive Hunter syndrome, which rarely involves the cornea until old age, if at all. Hurler (MPS IH) and Scheie (MPS IS) and the intermediate syndrome (Hurler-Scheie, MPS IH/S) are all allelic for the enzyme α-L-iduronidase, with different nucleotide substitutions leading to different amino acid substitutions and markedly reduced enzyme activity (<0.1% of normal). Normally, GAGs constitute the ground substance of the cornea, but in these diseases microscopic deposits of mucopolysaccharide are found in the keratocytes and stroma and, in some cases, in the corneal epithelium and endothelium.

CLINICAL FINDINGS. Differential findings are listed in Table XVI-3. These various conditions are characterized by corneal clouding, retinopathy, and optic atrophy, although Sanfilippo syndrome only occasionally has corneal opacities, and Hunter syndrome only rarely has corneal clouding. This clouding generally involves the entire cornea and may or may not be present at birth. It is often slowly progressive from the periphery toward center and can cause serious reduction in visual acuity.

LABORATORY EVALUATION. Microscopic differentiation of the syndromes is not possible. Scheie syndrome has been studied most intensely with regard to its corneal manifestations. Histiocytes laden with abnormally accumulated storage material (gargoyle cells) are noted. Recent electron microscopic and x-ray diffraction studies demonstrate an abnormally large range of stromal fibril size (20–52 nm in contrast to normal 26 nm) and disruption of the extracellular matrix by sulfated glycosaminoglycan deposits.

Conjunctival biopsy can confirm classic histopathology, but specific diagnosis requires biochemical assay for enzymes in tears, leukocytes, cultured fibroblasts, or amniotic cells and for elevated urinary glycosaminoglycans levels.

MANAGEMENT. These conditions, as well as those discussed in the following sections, are sometimes amenable to penetrating keratoplasty, unless impairment of the patient's mental status or retinal abnormalities preclude visual improvement. The

TABLE XVI-3

DIFFERENTIAL FEATURES OF THE SYSTEMIC MUCOPOLYSACCHARIDOSES

	GENETICS	SYSTEMIC FEATURES		OCULAR FEATURES			URINARY AMP EXCESS			DEFECTIVE ENZYME
		SKELETAL DYSPLASIA	MENTAL RETARDATION	CORNEAL CLOUDING	RETINAL PIGMENTARY DEGENERATION	OPTIC ATROPHY	HEPARAN SULFATE	DERMATAN SULFATE	KERATAN SULFATE	
IH: Hurler	AR	+++	+++	+++	R	R	++	+++	−	α-L-Iduronidase
IS: Scheie (formerly MPS V)	AR	+	+	+++	R	R	++	+++	−	α-L-Iduronidase (partial)
II: Hunter										
A: Severe phenotype	XR	+++	+++	−	R	R	++	++	−	L-Iduronate sulfatase
B: Mild phenotype	XR	++	+	+*	R	R	++	++	−	L-Iduronate sulfatase
III: Sanfilippo										
A: Sulfatase-deficient	AR	+	+++	−	R	R	+++	−	−	Heparan sulfate sulfatase
B: Glucosaminidase-deficient	AR	+	+++	−	R	R	+++	−	−	N-Acetyl-α-D-glucosaminidase
C: Acetyl-CoA-α-glucosaminidase-N-acetyl-transferase deficient	AR	+	+++	−	R	R	+++	−	−	Acetyl-CoA-α-glucosaminidase N-acetyl-transferase
D: N-acetylglucosaminidase-6-sulfate sulfatase deficient	AR	+	+++	−	R	R	+++	−	−	N-acetylglucosaminidase-6-sulfate sulfatase
IV: Morquio	AR	+++	+	++	NR	R	−	−	+++	Galactosamine-6-sulfate sulfatase
V: Vacant; now MPS IS										
VI: Maroteaux-Lamy										
A: Severe phenotype	AR	+++	−	++	NR	R	−	+++	−	Arylsulfatase B
B: Mild phenotype	AR	+	−	++	NR	NR	−	+++	−	Arylsulfatase B
VII: Sly	AR	+	+	++	NR	NR	+++	+++	−	β-Glucuronidase

* Positive by slit-lamp biomicroscopy in some older patients.
AR = autosomal recessive; XR = X-linked recessive; R = reported; NR = not reported; − = absent/not elevated; + = mild; + + = moderate; + + + = marked.

prognosis for successful keratoplasty is considered guarded, as the abnormal storage material may accumulate again in the graft. Some regression of corneal clouding following successful donor stem-cell bone-marrow transplantation occurs in about one third of patients.

Diabetes mellitus   The most common disorder of carbohydrate metabolism, diabetes mellitus has nonspecific corneal manifestations of punctate epithelial erosions, basement membrane changes resembling EBMD, Descemet's folds, and decreased corneal sensation. Diabetes is discussed at length in BCSC Section 12, *Retina and Vitreous,* although the emphasis is on retinal rather than corneal aspects of the disease.

PATHOGENESIS. Diabetic patients have ultrastructural abnormalities of the basement membrane complex that contribute to problems of epithelial-stromal adhesion. These abnormalities include thickening of the multilaminar basement membrane, reduced hemidesmosome number, and decreased penetration of anchoring fibrils. Accumulation of polyols such as sorbitol by the action of aldose reductase on excess glucose may contribute to the alterations in the epithelium and endothelium and the corneal hypoesthesia seen in diabetic patients.

CLINICAL FINDINGS. Corneal epithelial surface changes and hypoesthesia occur with increasing severity (e.g., type I, insulin-dependent diabetes mellitus, as opposed to type II, non–insulin-dependent diabetes mellitus) and increasing duration of disease. Removal of diabetic epithelium at surgery results in the loss of the basal cells and basement membrane, leading to prolonged healing difficulties. Faint vertical folds in Descemet's membrane and deep stroma (Waite-Beetham lines) are not specific to diabetes mellitus but may represent early endothelial dysfunction and increased stromal hydration.

LABORATORY EVALUATION. Glycosolated hemoglobin is related to poor control of the diabetes and may correlate with poor corneal healing in addition to progressive retinopathy, but it is not routinely required for management.

MANAGEMENT. Diabetes is not a contraindication to PK or other corneal surgery. Topical aldose reductase inhibitors may prove beneficial in treating diabetic epitheliopathy. Measures that can improve diabetic epitheliopathy include the following:

□ Minimizing epithelial debridement at surgery

□ Increasing lubrication

□ Avoiding toxic medications

□ Using therapeutic contact lenses

Disorders of Lipid Metabolism and Storage

Hyperlipoproteinemias   These common conditions are associated with premature coronary artery and peripheral vascular disease. Recognition of the ocular hallmarks of these diseases as well as xanthelasma and corneal arcus can result in early intervention and reduced morbidity.

PATHOGENESIS. Extracellular deposits consist of cholesterol, cholesterol esters, phospholipids, and triglycerides.

TABLE XVI-4

GENETICALLY DETERMINED HYPERLIPOPROTEINEMIAS

PRIMARY TYPE	PREVALENCE	LIPOPROTEIN ABNORMALITY	INCREASED LIPID FRACTION	LIPEMIA RETINALIS	CORNEAL ARCUS	XANTHELASMA	INHERITANCE
I	Very rare	Chylomicrons	Triglyceride	+	–	–	8p2 AR
II	0.5%	β-lipoprotein	Cholesterol	–	+	+	AD
III	Rare	Broad-β band	Cholesterol	+	+	+	19q13.2 AR apolipo-protein E
IV	1.0%	Pre-β lipoprotein	Triglyceride	+	–	–	AD
V	Rare	Chylomicrons Pre-β	Triglyceride	+	–	–	AD

Modified from Bron AJ. Dyslipoproteinemias and their ocular manifestations. *Birth Defects.* 1976;12:257.

CLINICAL FINDINGS. Table XVI-4 gives Fredrickson's classification of five types of hyperlipoproteinemia. Types II and III are associated with early-onset xanthelasma and corneal arcus, or arcus juvenilis. Types II, III, and IV can have xanthomas involving the conjunctiva. Type III has been linked to 19q13.2 (apolipoprotein E mutation). Corneal arcus is a very common degenerative change of older patients and does not require systemic evaluation. Schnyder central crystalline dystrophy is a localized defect of lipid metabolism, but laboratory evaluation is needed to rule out concurrent systemic abnormality (see pp 298–299 earlier in this chapter).

LABORATORY EVALUATION. A fasting and alcohol-restricted lipid profile that includes cholesterol, triglycerides, and high- and low-density lipoproteins is required. Patients can then be classified phenotypically to assess their risk for atherosclerotic disease when corneal arcus is present in individuals younger than 50 years of age or is significantly asymmetric.

MANAGEMENT. Early detection gives the patient time to be referred for diet or drug treatment.

Hypolipoproteinemias Abnormal reductions in serum lipoprotein levels occur in five disorders:

☐ Lecithin–cholesterol acyltransferase (LCAT) deficiency

☐ Tangier disease

☐ Fish eye disease

☐ Familial hypobetalipoproteinemia

☐ Bassen-Kornzweig syndrome

The last two disorders do not result in corneal disease, and discussion here focuses on the first three.

PATHOGENESIS. LCAT facilitates the removal of excess cholesterol from peripheral tissues to the liver, and a deficiency would be expected to lead to accumulation of free cholesterol in the tissues. Atherosclerosis, renal insufficiency, and diffuse corneal clouding ensue. LCAT deficiency and fish eye disease are allelic variants of the same genetic locus on chromosome 16q22.1, but fish eye disease has normal levels of LCAT that do not function to aid HDL in esterifying cholesterol. Tangier disease has complete absence of serum high-density α-lipoproteins. The mRNA has been characterized, but the gene is not mapped.

CLINICAL FINDINGS. All three cornea-affecting hypolipoproteinemias are rare, autosomal recessive conditions. Familial LCAT deficiency is characterized by peripheral arcus and nebular stromal haze made up of myriad minute focal deposits of lipid that appear early in childhood but do not interfere with vision. Fish eye disease has obvious corneal clouding from minute gray-white-yellow dots that progress from the periphery to decrease vision. One source describes the eye as resembling that of a boiled fish. Tangier disease, after the Chesapeake Bay island, features very large orange tonsils; enlarged liver, spleen, and lymph nodes; hypocholesterolemia; abnormal chylomicron remnants; and markedly reduced high-density lipoproteins (HDL) in the plasma. Corneas show diffuse clouding and posterior focal stromal opacities but no arcus. Neuropathy leads to lagophthalmos and corneal sequelae. Heterozygotes show low α-lipoproteins in the serum.

LABORATORY EVALUATION AND MANAGEMENT. Serum lipid profile shows characteristic low levels of HDL. Recognition can allow the clinician to make appropriate referrals and encourage the patient to seek genetic counseling.

Sphingolipidoses These rare inherited disorders of complex lipids (gangliosides and sphingomyelin) involve the cornea in three conditions:

□ Fabry disease (angiokeratoma corporis diffusum)

□ Multiple sulfatase deficiency

□ Generalized gangliosidosis (GM$_1$ gangliosidosis type I)

PATHOGENESIS. These disorders of lipid storage are autosomal recessive with the exception of Fabry, which is X-linked recessive. They principally affect the retina and may lead to central nervous system dysfunction. Fabry disease is again an important exception. It is caused by a deficiency of α-galactosidase A, leading to the accumulation of ceramide trihexoside in the renal and cardiovascular systems. Multiple sulfatase deficiency combines features of metachromatic leukodystrophy and mucopolysaccharidosis. Affected children have subtle diffuse corneal opacities, optic atrophy, and progressive psychomotor retardation. They die in the first decade. Generalized gangliosidosis is characterized by deficiencies of β-galactosidases and the accumulation of gangliosides in the central nervous system and keratan sulfate in somatic tissues. It has been linked to chromosome 3p12–3p13. Although Tay-Sachs disease (hexosaminidase A deficiency with accumulation of GM$_2$ ganglioside) primarily involves the retina, a recent report has demonstrated pathologic changes where the corneal endothelial cells appeared distended and filled with single membrane–bound vacuoles.

CLINICAL FINDINGS. In these conditions the cornea exhibits distinctive changes, consisting of whorl-like lines (cornea verticillata) in the basal layers of the epithelium that appear to flow together to the inferior central corneal epithelium (Fig XVI-23).

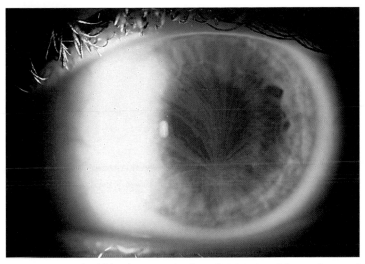

FIG XVI-23—Whorl-like deposits of sphingolipid in basal layer of corneal epithelium in patient with Fabry disease; identical deposits occur in otherwise asymptomatic female carriers of this disease.

Periorbital edema occurs in 25% of cases, posterior spokelike cataracts in 50%, and conjunctival aneurysms in 60%. Other ocular signs include papilledema, retinal or macular edema, optic atrophy, and retinal vascular dilation. The corneal changes resemble those seen in patients on long-standing oral chloroquine or amiodarone treatment. A careful drug history will help make this differentiation.

Hemizygous males with Fabry disease are more seriously affected and show the typical corneal changes. The heterozygous female is usually asymptomatic but still shows the same corneal changes. Fabry disease is also characterized by renal failure, peripheral neuropathy with painful dysesthesias in the lower extremities, and skin lesions. The skin lesions are small, round vascular eruptions that later become hyperkeratotic. They consist of an accumulation of sphingolipid within the vascular endothelium.

LABORATORY EVALUATION. In Fabry disease α-galactosidase is markedly decreased in urine and plasma. Conjunctival biopsy may be positive before cornea verticillata are apparent.

MANAGEMENT. If a female patient is diagnosed as an asymptomatic heterozygous Fabry carrier, genetic counseling should be considered. The prognosis for successful penetrating keratoplasty in these conditions is generally poor.

Mucolipidoses   These autosomal recessive conditions have features common to both mucopolysaccharidoses and lipidoses.

PATHOGENESIS. These diseases are inherited defects of carbohydrate and lipid metabolism combined. Consequently, they have something in common with the mucopolysaccharidoses as well as the sphingolipidoses. Mucopolysaccharides accumulate in the cornea and viscera, and sphingolipids are deposited in the retina and central nervous system. Currently recognized diseases in this class are the following:

- Mucolipidosis (MLS) I (dysmorphic sialidosis)
- MLS II (I-cell disease)
- MLS III (pseudo–Hurler polydystrophy)
- MLS IV
- Goldberg syndrome
- Mannosidosis
- Fucosidosis

These conditions are all autosomal recessive. Histopathologic examination of corneal scrapings has revealed the accumulation of intracytoplasmic storage material. In fucosidosis histopathologic study has revealed that, in spite of clinically normal corneas, corneal endothelial cells show the presence of cytoplasmic, membrane-bound, confluent areas of fibrillar, granular, and multilaminated deposits. A retinal cherry-red spot and retinal degeneration are also associated with many of these disorders. All are caused by a defect in lysosomal acid hydrolase enzymes.

CLINICAL FINDINGS. With the exception of mannosidosis and fucosidosis, which are oligosaccharidoses, all of these conditions are characterized by varying degrees of corneal clouding, which can often be progressive. A recent report described a patient with fucosidosis who was afflicted with recurrent episodes of severe ocular pain, tearing, and ipsilateral facial flushing. These findings were thought to be suggestive of reflex sympathetic dystrophy (pain and sympathetic hyperactivity).

LABORATORY EVALUATION. Plasma cells are vacuolated and plasma lysosomal hydrolases are elevated. In MLS IV with corneal clouding from birth, conjunctival biopsy shows fibroblast inclusion bodies that are

- Single membrane–limited cytoplasmic vacuoles containing both fibrillogranular material and membranous lamellae
- Lamellar and concentric bodies resembling those of Tay-Sachs disease

There is no evidence of mucopolysacchariduria or cellular metachromasia.

MANAGEMENT. Both PK and lamellar keratoplasty have been associated with generally poor results, probably because resurfacing is impaired by the abnormal epithelial cells. While donor limbal stem-cell transplantation has been advocated, tissue matching may be required, as graft rejection in these vascularized recipient beds is possible.

Bietti crystalline corneoretinal dystrophy

This very rare autosomal recessive condition is characterized by peripheral corneal opacities and tapetoretinal dystrophy. It is presumed to be caused by a defect in lipid metabolism.

PATHOGENESIS. Lysosomes of fibroblasts in the choroid and skin and circulating lymphocytes contain crystalline deposits, but no abnormal accumulation of cholesterol or cholesterol esters has been documented.

CLINICAL FINDINGS. Retinal crystals that are pathognomonic appear to decrease with time. Peripheral, sparkling, yellow-white spots are seen at the corneal limbus in the superficial stroma and subepithelial layers of the cornea in 75% of patients. They may fade with time.

LABORATORY EVALUATION AND MANAGEMENT. Visual fields, dark adaptation test, and ERG may be normal in early cases, but advanced cases may have decreased ERG and retinal findings of atypical retinitis pigmentosa. No specific treatment is reported.

Kenyon KR, Navon SE. Corneal manifestations of metabolic diseases. In: Krachmer JH, Mannis MJ, Holland EJ, eds. *Cornea.* St Louis: Mosby; 1997;2:897–924.

Online Mendelian Inheritance in Man website (under OMIM Allied Resources) http:www3.ncbi.nlm.nih.gov/omim/citations.html. Bethesda: National Center for Biotechnology Information, National Library of Medicine; 1996.

Disorders of Amino Acid Metabolism

Cystinosis   This rare autosomal recessive disorder is characterized by the accumulation of the amino acid cystine within lysosomes.

PATHOGENESIS. A defect in transport across the lysosomal membrane leads to accumulation of cystine.

CLINICAL FINDINGS. Cystinosis is a systemic metabolic defect that can present as an infantile, intermediate, or adult form. The infantile, or nephropathic, form features dwarfism and progressive renal dysfunction with the deposition of fine polychromatic cystine crystals in the conjunctiva, corneal stroma, and other parts of the eye. This form is uniformly fatal in the first decade of life in the absence of renal transplantation. The intermediate, or adolescent, form has less severe renal involvement, with death occurring in the second or third decade. Life expectancy is normal in the adult form. The corneal stromal crystals of cystinosis are the only positive findings. Although the crystals usually do not affect visual acuity, these patients are often afflicted with photophobia.

LABORATORY EVALUATION. Cystine crystals may be seen in conjunctival biopsy or in buffy coat of blood or bone marrow.

MANAGEMENT. Topical cysteamine drops reduce the density of the crystalline deposits and diminish corneal pain, possibly as a result of a decrease in the development of corneal erosions. Another study, however, failed to note a significant difference with the use of lower concentrations of drops. Presumably, the topically administered cysteamine reacts with the intracellular cystine, forming a cysteine-cysteamine disulfide that resembles lysine and is transported through the lysosome by the normal lysine transport system. The crystals have been observed to recur in patients who have undergone PK for clouding associated with the corneal deposits. These refractile polychromatic crystals are most dense in the peripheral cornea but are seen throughout the anterior stroma, even within the central cornea (Fig XVI-24).

The normal cornea and conjunctiva are transparent and any deposits—whether from the tear film, limbus, or aqueous humor—are easily discerned. Table XVI-5 summarizes the differential diagnosis based on the depth of corneal involvement, color and refractile character, and conjunctival involvement.

Bridges WZ, Palay DA. Corneal deposits. In: Krachmer JH, Mannis MJ, Holland EJ, eds. *Cornea.* St Louis: Mosby; 1997;1:417–428.

TABLE XVI-5

CORNEAL DEPOSITS IN DIFFERENTIAL DIAGNOSIS

TYPE	SUPERFICIAL	STROMAL	DEEP STROMAL/ENDOTHELIAL	CONJUNCTIVA
Pigmented	Cornea verticillata (Fabry disease, amiodarone)	Phenothiazines	Mercury	Tetracycline
	Striate melanokeratosis	Blood staining	Wilson disease (copper)	Adrenochrome
	Iron lines	Bilirubin	Chalcosis (copper)	
	Pigmented (noncalcific) band keratopathy	Siderosis (iron)	Chrysiasis (systemic gold)	Argyriasis
	Spheroidal degeneration	Corneal tattoo	Argyriasis (topical silver)	
	Adrenochrome		Krukenberg spindle	
	Alkaptonuria			
Nonpigmented	Subepithelial mucinous dystrophy	Granular dystrophy	Cornea farinata	Gout (urate)
	Coats white ring	Macular dystrophy	Pre-Descemet's dystrophy	
	Calcific band keratopathy	Fleck dystrophy	X-linked ichthyosis	
	Ciprofloxacin	Lipid deposition	Argyriasis (silver)	
		Mucopolysaccharidoses		
Refractile/ crystalline	Meesmann dystrophy	Lattice dystrophy	Polymorphic amyloid degeneration	Cystinosis
	Superficial amyloid	Schnyder dystrophy		
	Tyrosinemia type II	Bietti crystalline corneoretinal dystrophy		
	Intraepithelial ointment	Immunoglobulin deposition		
	Gout (urate)	Cystinosis		
		Infectious crystalline keratopathy		

Modified from Bridges WZ, Palay DA. Corneal deposits. In: Krachmer JH, Mannis MJ, Holland EJ, eds. *Cornea.* St Louis: Mosby; 1997;1:418.

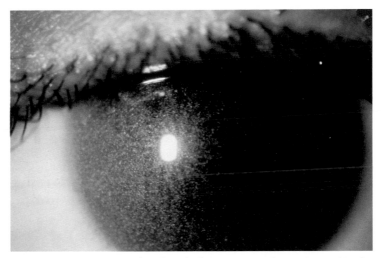

FIG XVI-24—Cystinosis. Refractile polychromatic crystals are clustered in the peripheral cornea.

Tyrosinemia   Richner-Hanhart syndrome (tyrosinemia type II) is characterized by systemic findings including hyperkeratotic lesions of palms, soles, and elbows, as well as eventual mental retardation.

PATHOGENESIS. This autosomal recessive disorder occurs secondary to an enzymatic defect of tyrosine aminotransferase that leads to excess tyrosine in the blood and urine. The elevated tyrosine probably has a direct action on lysosomal membranes, leading to release of their enzymes with characteristic changes. The gene locus is at 16q22.1–q22.3.

CLINICAL FINDINGS. Ocular changes include marked photophobia, tearing, conjunctival injection, and tarsal papillary hypertrophy. Patients develop recurrent episodes of pseudodendrites, which usually do not stain well with fluorescein or rose bengal. Continued episodes of epithelial breakdown can result in corneal vascularization and scarring. It is important to consider this disorder in the young child who may carry a diagnosis of recurrent herpes simplex virus keratitis.

LABORATORY EVALUATION. Hypertyrosinemia and tyrosinuria with normal phenylalanine level and biopsy showing soluble tyrosine aminotransferase (TAT) deficiency are diagnostic.

MANAGEMENT. Restriction of dietary intake of tyrosine and phenylalanine can reduce both the corneal and systemic changes, including mental retardation. The institution of appropriate dietary restrictions even later in life can improve the mental status.

Alkaptonuria   Alkaptonuria is a rare autosomal recessive disorder with a defect of tyrosine metabolism that maps to gene locus 3q21–q23. An unusually high frequency occurs in the Dominican Republic and Slovakia.

PATHOGENESIS. Homogentisate 1,2-dioxygenase, the enzyme necessary to degrade tyrosine and phenylalanine, is deficient. Phenylalanine and tyrosine cannot be metabolized beyond homogentisic acid, which is oxidized and polymerized into alkapton, a brown-black material similar to melanin. Alkapton then deposits in connective tissues as dark pigment known as *ochronosis*. Corneal lesions consisting of homogentisic acid are easily seen by light microscopy. Recent electron microscopic studies have shown that extracellular deposits of finely granular ochronotic pigment were seen in and around collagen fibrils. Intracellular membrane–bound ochronotic pigment granules were observed in macrophages in fibroblasts, along with two other forms of extracellular ochronotic pigment.

CLINICAL FINDINGS. Patients develop arthropathy, renal calculi, and pigmentation of cartilaginous structures including ear lobes, trachea, nose, tendons, dura mater, heart valves, and prostate. Eventually, medial and lateral rectus muscle tendons and the sclera adjacent to the tendon insertions develop smudgelike pigmentation. Darkly pigmented, dotlike opacities may appear in the corneal epithelium or in Bowman's layer near the limbus.

LABORATORY EVALUATION. Urine turns dark on standing and alkalinization. Homogentisic acid oxidase deficiency can be demonstrated.

MANAGEMENT. No specific therapy is available, although high-dose ascorbic acid is reported to reduce arthropathy in young patients. It is hoped that specific gene therapy will be available to treat this disorder in the future.

Disorders of Protein Metabolism

Amyloidosis The amyloidoses are a heterogenous group of diseases characterized by the accumulation of amyloid in various tissues and organs. Table XVI-6 summarizes ocular findings in the amyloidoses.

PATHOGENESIS. Amyloid is an eosinophilic hyaline material with five basic staining characteristics:

□ Positive staining with Congo red dye

□ Dichroism and birefringence

□ Metachromasia with crystal violet dye

□ Fluorescence in ultraviolet light with thioflavine T stain

□ Typical filamentous appearance by electron microscopy

Protein AP derives from α-globulin and is found in all amyloid fibrils. In addition, amyloid fibrils are composed of immunoglobulin light chains or fragments of light chains (especially of the variable region) and nonimmunoglobulin protein. Amyloid composed of immunoglobulin is designated AL for amyloid fibril protein and the L chain amyloid protein. Nonimmunoglobulin amyloid is designated AA for amyloid fibril protein and SAA, its serum-related protein. Protein AF has several subtypes found in the various dystrophies. These noncollagenous proteins can be deposited in the cornea and conjunctiva and in intraocular or adnexal structures. At least 14 genes are responsible for amyloid proteins.

CLINICAL FINDINGS. A useful classification of amyloidosis considers four types. Each type will be considered separately:

□ Primary localized amyloidosis

□ Primary systemic amyloidosis

□ Secondary localized amyloidosis

□ Secondary systemic amyloidosis

322

TABLE XVI-6

AMYLOID IN THE EYE

TYPE	HEREDITY	OCULAR DISTRIBUTION	ASSOCIATED CONDITIONS	GENETIC LINKAGE
Primary localized amyloidosis	Nonfamilial	Conjunctival plaque Polymorphic amyloid degeneration	None	
	Familial	Lattice corneal dystrophy types I and II		5q 31 (keratoepithelin gene)
		Avellino and granular dystrophy		
		Gelatinous droplike dystrophy		(?)1q12–q23 (SAP gene)
Primary systemic amyloidosis	Nonfamilial	Skin and conjunctiva (very rare)	Occult plasma cell dyscrasias	
	Familial	Ophthalmoplegia (orbital and muscle infiltrates), ptosis, vitreous veils, dry eye, pupil abnormalities	Cardiomyopathy Peripheral neuropathy Gastrointestinal disease Skin involvement	18q11.2–q12.1 (transthyretin gene) Many others
		Lattice corneal dystrophy type II, cranial neuropathies	Meretoja syndrome, (facial palsies, skin nodules, rarely renal involvement)	9q34 (gelsolin gene)
Secondary localized amyloidosis	Nonfamilial	Conjunctiva Skin Cornea	Trachoma, psoriasis, trauma, phlyctenulosis, retinopathy of prematurity, keratoconus, bullous keratopathy, interstitial keratitis, leprosy, contact lens wear, trichiasis, tertiary syphilis, uveitis, climatic droplet keratopathy	
	Familial	None		
Secondary systemic amyloidosis	Nonfamilial	Rarely vitreous body (corneal deposits are not amyloid)	Multiple myeloma	
		Conjunctiva, skin (rare)	Infectious diseases (tuberculosis, leprosy, syphilis)	
			Inflammatory diseases (rheumatoid arthritis, other connective tissue disorders)	
			Hodgkin disease	
	Familial	(Corneal nerve enlargement is not amyloid)	MEN type IIa	10q11.2 (RET oncogene)

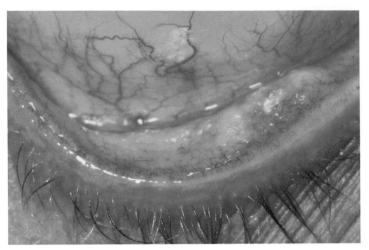

FIG XVI-25—Conjunctival amyloidosis.

Ocular amyloidosis is classified as either primary (idiopathic) or secondary (to some chronic disease) and either localized or systemic.

Primary localized amyloidosis. This form of ocular amyloidosis is the most common. Conjunctival amyloid plaques occur in the absence of systemic involvement (Fig XVI-25). Primary familial amyloidosis of the cornea (gelatinous droplike dystrophy), in which puddinglike translucent nodules occur as cobblestone masses on the central corneal surface (see Figure XVI-8), is discussed on p 298. Lattice corneal dystrophy is a special form of primary localized amyloidosis discussed on pp 296–297. Polymorphic amyloid degeneration is discussed on p 343.

Primary systemic amyloidosis. In this heterogenous group of diseases waxy ecchymotic eyelid papules occur in association with vitreous veils and opacities as well as pupillary anomalies such as light–near dissociation. Orbital involvement, including extraocular muscle involvement with ophthalmoplegia, has been reported. The most common form of primary systemic amyloidosis is an autosomal dominant group of diseases linked to 18q11.2–q12.1 with more than 40 different mutations of the transthyretin (TTR, prealbumin) gene described. Corneal involvement occurs in lattice dystrophy type II (Meretoja syndrome) as discussed on p 297.

Secondary localized amyloidosis. This form develops in eyes with long-standing chronic inflammatory disease such as trachoma, interstitial keratitis, tumors, or connective tissue disorders, usually rheumatoid arthritis. Corneal involvement may be seen in keratoconus, trachoma, phlyctenulosis, bullous keratopathy, interstitial keratitis, leprosy, contact lens wear, trichiasis, tertiary syphilis, uveitis, and climatic droplet keratopathy. Secondary deposition takes the form of a degenerative pannus, lamellar deposits in the deep stroma, or perivascular deposits. Deposits are typically yellowish pink or yellow-gray depending on the associated disease.

Secondary systemic amyloidosis. This form features amyloid AA and is seen in association with rheumatoid arthritis, Mediterranean fever, bronchiectasis, and Hansen disease (leprosy). The eyelids can be affected but less commonly than with primary systemic amyloidosis. Amyloid does not deposit in the cornea in secondary systemic amyloidosis.

Goodfriend AN, Ching SST. Corneal and conjunctival degenerations. In: Krachmer JH, Mannis MJ, Holland EJ, eds. *Cornea*. St Louis: Mosby; 1997;2:1119–1137.

Online Mendelian Inheritance in Man website (under OMIM Allied Resources) at http:www3.ncbi.nlm.nih.gov/omim/citations.html. Bethesda: National Center for Biotechnology Information, National Library of Medicine; 1996.

Disorders of Immunoglobulin Synthesis

The excess synthesis of immunoglobulins by plasma cells in multiple myeloma, Waldenström macroglobulinemia, and benign monoclonal gammopathy is rarely associated with crystalline corneal deposits.

PATHOGENESIS. Monoclonal proliferation of plasma cells (B lymphocytes) leads to overproduction of both light (κ or λ) chains and heavy (α, γ, ε, δ, or μ) chains (together M proteins), overproduction of light chains with or without production of heavy chains (Bence Jones protein), or overproduction of heavy chains without light chains (heavy chain disease). Pathogenesis is related to either direct tissue invasion, particularly of the bone marrow, or to hyperviscosity syndrome. Secondary hypercalcemia may occur. Deposition of paraproteins in the cornea is very rare and related to diffusion of the proteins, probably from the limbal vessels or alternately from the tears or aqueous humor, followed by precipitation perhaps related to corneal temperature or local tissue factors.

CLINICAL FINDINGS. Ophthalmic findings include the following:

- Crystalline deposition in all layers of the cornea or in the conjunctiva
- Copper deposition in the cornea
- Sludging of blood flow in the conjunctiva and retina
- Pars plana proteinaceous cysts
- Infiltration of the sclera
- Orbital bony invasion with proptosis

Corneal deposits are numerous, scintillating, and polychromatic. They are typical of IgG-κ chain deposition and possibly related to the size of the paraprotein and the chronicity of the disease.

Waldenström macroglobulinemia is characterized by malignant proliferation of plasma cells generating IgM, causing hyperviscosity syndrome principally in older men. It has been associated with needlelike crystals and amorphous deposits subepithelially and in deep stroma.

Benign monoclonal gammopathy is a frequent finding in people over age 60 (up to 6%). The systemic evaluation in these cases is negative, but a mild increase in paraprotein is detected (<3 g/dl). Slit-lamp findings of iridescent crystals resemble myeloma and are also very infrequent (about 1%–2% of affected patients).

Cryoglobulins are proteins that precipitate on exposure to cold. They occur nonspecifically in autoimmune disorders, immunoproliferative disorders, or hepatitis B infection. Ophthalmic findings include retinal hyperviscosity signs, occasional crystalline corneal deposits, amorphous limbal masses, and signs of autoimmune disease.

LABORATORY EVALUATION. Corneal crystalline deposits have many causes, and evaluation depends on appearance and location in the cornea (see Table XVI-5). Serum protein electrophoresis, CBC, and general screen for albumin/globulin and calcium level are used for testing when clinical suspicion of immunoglobulin excess arises. Further evaluation for systemic evaluation depends on clinical suspicion and the initial findings.

MANAGEMENT. No ophthalmic treatment is needed unless the amorphous depositions interfere with vision and need to be removed with lamellar keratoplasty. Crystals will resolve slowly after successful treatment of an underlying malignancy.

Noninflammatory Disorders of Connective Tissue

Table XVI-7 on pp 328–329 summarizes the connective tissue disorders associated with corneal changes.

Ehlers-Danlos syndrome This heterogenous group of diseases is characterized by hyperextensibility of joints and skin, easy bruisability, and formation of "cigarette paper" scars. It has been discussed briefly in chapter XIV in connection with blue sclera.

PATHOGENESIS. The 11 known types of Ehlers-Danlos syndrome are classified as autosomal dominant and recessive and X-linked recessive forms confirmed with specific defects in collagen type I and III synthesis and lysyl hydroxylase deficiency.

CLINICAL FINDINGS. Ehlers-Danlos syndrome VI, or the ocular-scoliotic type, is autosomal recessive and associated with only moderate joint and skin extensibility, brittle cornea easily ruptured on minor trauma, blue sclerae, keratoconus and keratoglobus, and severe scoliosis. Type VI-A has lysyl hydroxylase deficiency, but type VI-B has normal production of lysyl hydroxylase.

LABORATORY EVALUATION. Traditionally, the clinical diagnosis is confirmed by an insufficiency of hydroxylysine on analysis of hydrolyzed dermis and/or reduced enzyme activity in cultured skin fibroblasts. But it can also be confirmed by the altered urinary ratio of lysyl pyridinoline to hydroxylysyl pyridinoline that is characteristic for EDS VI.

MANAGEMENT. Recognition of the syndrome and awareness of its association with mitral valve prolapse, spontaneous bowel rupture, complications of strabismus surgery, and potential confusion of the brittle cornea with child abuse are key. Scleral patch grafts for ruptures have been successful. Genetic counseling should be considered.

Marfan syndrome This common autosomal dominant disorder is associated with disorders of the eye (ectopia lentis), heart (dilation of the aortic root and aneurysms of the aorta), and skeletal system (arachnodactyly, pectus excavatum, and kyphoscoliosis). It maps to chromosome 15 q21.1 (fibrillin gene).

PATHOGENESIS. Fibrillin and glycoprotein make up the microfibrillar system of the extracellular matrix. Fibrillin is found in corneal basement membrane, zonular fibers of the lens and capsule, and sclera. Defects in fibrillin synthesis lead to thinning of the sclera (blue sclera), lens subluxation, and flattening of the cornea. BCSC Section 11, *Lens and Cataract,* discusses and illustrates the lens subluxation caused by Marfan syndrome.

CLINICAL FINDINGS. Megalocornea and keratoconus are uncommon, but excessive flattening (35 D range) occurs in up to 20% of patients.

MANAGEMENT. Cardiac evaluation should be completed, as premature mortality is associated with aortic complications. Open-angle glaucoma and cataract occur at a higher rate and earlier age than normal population and require attention as usually dictated by those conditions.

Disorders of Nucleotide Metabolism

Gout   *Hyperuricemia* is a heterogenous group of disorders of purine metabolism that result in increased uric acid. Discrete deposits of urate crystals into the joints or kidney is called *gout.*

PATHOGENESIS. Hyperuricemia may be familial, as a result of an enzyme deficiency (e.g., hypoxanthine phosphoribosyltransferase in Lesch-Nyhan syndrome). More commonly, it is polygenic or secondary to obesity, cytotoxic chemotherapy, myeloproliferative disease, diuretic therapy, or excessive alcohol consumption.

CLINICAL FINDINGS. Acute inflammation of the sclera, episclera, or conjunctiva can occur. Fine corneal epithelial and stromal deposits may appear in the absence of inflammation. See Table XVI-5 for differential diagnosis of corneal deposits. An orange-brown band keratopathy or a typical whitish band keratopathy is seen rarely.

LABORATORY EVALUATION. Serum uric acid level is typically elevated, although it may be normal even in the presence of keratopathy if not inflamed.

MANAGEMENT. Acute treatment is with indomethacin, colchicine, or phenylbutazone; but long-term reduction in uric acid levels should be pursued with drugs such as allopurinol. Superficial deposits can be removed mechanically with scraping or keratectomy.

Porphyria   The porphyrias are a group of disorders characterized by excess production and excretion of porphyrins—pigments involved in the synthesis of heme.

PATHOGENESIS. *Porphyria cutanea tarda,* the form most commonly associated with ocular surface problems, is either sporadically or autosomal dominantly inherited (chromosome 1p34). The enzyme uroporphyrinogen decarboxylase is deficient, resulting in an accumulation of porphyrins in the liver and in the circulation. Typically, a second insult to the liver such as alcoholism or drug metabolism brings on the condition in late middle age.

The pathogenesis is related to porphyrin accumulation in the skin and mucous membranes and to significant iron overload. A severe form of porphyria, hepatoerythropoietic porphyria (HEP), is a homozygous presentation of the same enzymatic defect that results in onset of the disease in infancy.

CLINICAL FINDINGS. Sun-exposed surfaces develop hyperpigmentation, erythema, scleroderma-like changes, increased fragility, and vesicular and ulcerative lesions. Interpalpebral injection occurs, and the conjunctiva may develop vesicles, necrosis, scarring, and symblepharon mimicking bullous pemphigoid. The cornea may be affected by exposure or by thinning and perforation at the limbus. Skin and ocular lesions may fluoresce.

TABLE XVI-7

CONNECTIVE TISSUE DISORDERS ASSOCIATED WITH CORNEAL CHANGES

NAME AND MIM NO*	CORNEAL FINDINGS	OTHER OCULAR FINDINGS	GENETICS/MAP/OTHER INFORMATION
Apert syndrome (176943)	Exposure keratitis with severe proptosis Keratoconus (very rare) Megalocornea (very rare)	Strabismus (exotropia with V pattern) Absence of extraocular muscles, proptosis, ocular hypopigmentation, optic atrophy Rare: nystagmus, ptosis, cataract, ectopia lentis, coloboma of iris	AD Gene maps to 10q26 Mutations in fibroblast growth factor receptor–2
Carpenter syndrome Acrocephalo-polysyndactyly type II (201000)	Exposure keratitis secondary to severe proptosis Microcornea (rare) Corneal leukoma (rare)	Epicanthal folds, antimongoloid slant, hypertelorism or hypotelorism, optic atrophy, strabismus	AR
Crouzon syndrome (123500)	Exposure keratitis with severe proptosis Keratoconus (very rare) Microcornea (very rare)	Strabismus (exotropia with V pattern) Exophthalmos, hypertelorism, optic atrophy in 30% Rare: nystagmus, glaucoma, cataract, ectopia lentis, aniridia, anisocoria, myelinated nerve fibers	AD Gene maps to 10q26 Mutations in fibroblast growth factor receptor–2
Ehlers-Danlos syndrome (11 known types)	Brittle cornea, keratoglobus in type VI Keratoconus in types I and VI	Epicanthal folds, blue sclerae, retinal detachment, ectopia lentis, glaucoma, angioid streaks (rare)	Inheritance varies by type Type VI is AR and maps to 1p36.3–1p36.2 Mutations in lysine hydroxylase
Hallerman-Streiff-François syndrome Oculomandibulo-dyscephaly (234100)	Sclerocornea	Congenital cataracts, spontaneous resorption of lens cortex with secondary membranous cataract formation, glaucoma, uveitis, retinal folds, optic nerve dysplasia, microphthalmos	Sporadic Rarely AD Increased anesthetic risk secondary to tracheomalacia
Marfan syndrome (154700)	Megalocornea Flat cornea Keratoconus (uncommon)	Ectopia lentis, strabismus, cataracts, myopia, retinal detachment, glaucoma	AD 15q21.1 Mutations in fibrillin-1
Oculodentoosseous dysplasia (164200)	Microcornea	Hypotelorism, convergent strabismus, anterior segment dysgenesis, glaucoma, cataracts, remnants of the hyaloid system	AD Rarely AR

328

TABLE XVI-7 (Continued)

CONNECTIVE TISSUE DISORDERS ASSOCIATED WITH CORNEAL CHANGES

NAME AND MIM NO*	CORNEAL FINDINGS	OTHER OCULAR FINDINGS	GENETICS/MAP/OTHER INFORMATION
Osteogenesis imperfecta Type I (259400) Type II (166200) Type III (259420) Type IV (166220)	Decreased central corneal thickness Keratoconus Megalocornea (rare) Posterior embryotoxon (rare)	Blue sclerae Rare: congenital glaucoma, cataract, choroidal sclerosis, subhyaloid hemorrhage, hyperopia, ectopia lentis	AD in types I–IV 7q22.1 Mutations in COL1A2 Collagen type I, α-2 polypeptide; COL1A1 Collagen I, α-1 polypeptide
Pierre Robin malformation (261800)	Megalocornea (rare)	Congenital glaucoma, high myopia, vitreoretinal degeneration, retinal detachment, esotropia, congenital cataracts, microphthalmos	Sporadic Stickler syndrome in one third of cases Other syndromes NB: Increased anesthetic risk secondary to glossoptosis
Rothmund-Thomson syndrome (268400)	Degenerative lesions of cornea	Cataracts	AR 70% female Gene maps to chromosome 8
Treacher Collins syndrome Mandibulofacial dysotosis (154500)	Microcornea	Coloboma of lower eyelids, dysplasia of bony orbit, absent lower eyelid cilia, absent lower eyelid lacrimal punctae, iris colcboma, microphthalmos, strabismus, antimongoloid slant	AD Gene maps to 5q32–q33.1
Onychoosteodysplasia (Nail-patella syndrome) (161200)	Microcornea	Cataracts, microphthalmos	AD Gene maps to 9q34.1

Modified from Traboulsi EI, Kattan HM. Skeletal and connective tissue disorders with anterior segment manifestations. In: Krachmer JH, Mannis MJ, Holland EJ, eds. *Cornea.* St Louis: Mosby; 1997;2:927–928.

* From *Online Mendelian Inheritance in Man.* Baltimore: Center for Medical Genetics, Johns Hopkins University; and Bethesda: National Center for Biotechnology Information, National Library of Medicine; 1996. http:www3.ncbi.nlm.nih.gov/omim/citation.html

LABORATORY EVALUATION. Urine turns dark on standing. Reduced liver and red cell uroporphyrinogen decarboxylase is confirmatory, and hepatic biopsy shows liver parenchyma cells filled with porphyrins that fluoresce bright red in ultraviolet light.

MANAGEMENT. Protection from ultraviolet light and reduction of iron by phlebotomy are the principal treatments. No specific ocular treatment is available, and thinning and perforation are treated in standard ways.

Disorders of Mineral Metabolism

Wilson disease Inherited as an autosomal recessive metabolic defect linked to chromosome 13q14.3–q21.1, Wilson disease, or *hepatolenticular degeneration,* is caused by multiple allelic substitutions or deletions in DNA coding for an ATPase, Cu^{2+}–transporting, β-polypeptide.

PATHOGENESIS. Copper is deposited in the liver, then in the kidneys, and eventually in the brain and the cornea at Descemet's membrane.

CLINICAL FINDINGS. Muscular rigidity increases, and tremor and involuntary movement gradually occur in a fluctuating course resembling parkinsonism. Unintelligible speech and mild dementia usually occur concomitantly. Equal numbers of patients (40%) present with hepatic or nervous system symptoms. In the cornea a golden brown, ruby red, or green pigment ring (Kayser-Fleischer ring) appears in peripheral Descemet's membrane (Fig XVI-26). Not all patients with bona fide Wilson disease will manifest a Kayser-Fleischer ring, which appears first superiorly, gradually spreading and widening to meet deposits inferiorly. It consists of deposits of copper in the posterior lamella of Descemet's membrane. Gonioscopy may assist in visualization of the ring.

Differential diagnosis includes primary biliary cirrhosis, chronic active hepatitis, exogenous chalcosis, and progressive intrahepatic cholestasis of childhood. These and other non-Wilsonian hepatic disorders can also be associated with Kayser-Fleischer rings, but only Wilson disease has decreased serum ceruloplasmin and neurologic symptoms.

LABORATORY EVALUATION. Patients with Wilson disease can be differentiated from others with Kayser-Fleischer rings by their inability to incorporate radioactive copper into ceruloplasmin. Low serum ceruloplasmin, high nonceruloplasmin-bound serum copper, and high urinary copper suggest the diagnosis, which can be established with liver biopsy. Nonspecific findings of proteinuria, aminoaciduria, glycosuria, uricaciduria, hyperphosphaturia, and hypercalciuria are seen.

MANAGEMENT. Wilson disease can be treated with penicillamine. The Kayser-Fleischer ring disappears gradually with therapy, including liver transplantation, and the disappearance of the rings can be used to help monitor therapy.

Hypercalcemia Disorders of calcium and phosphate metabolism are associated with formation of *band keratopathy* (see also discussion on pp 345–346).

PATHOGENESIS. The cornea is a favored site for deposition of calcium because tear evaporation leads to local increased concentration, absence of the stabilizing effect of serum pH, and local increased pH secondary to loss of carbon dioxide from the surface. Calcium precipitates when its solubility product with phosphate is increased.

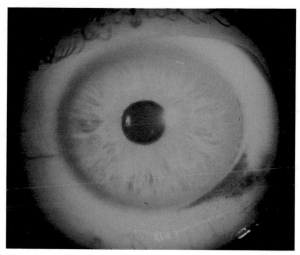

FIG XVI-26—Kayser-Fleischer ring of Wilson hepatolenticular degeneration; deposits of copper in Descemet's membrane.

CLINICAL FINDINGS. Calcific band keratopathy begins as fine, dustlike, basophilic deposits in Bowman's layer. These changes are usually first seen peripherally. A peripheral clear zone representing a lucid interval is seen between the limbus and the peripheral edge of the keratopathy. Eventually, the deposits may coalesce to form a horizontal band of dense calcitic plaques across the interpalpebral zone of the cornea (Fig XVI-27). Many systemic syndromes are associated with band keratopathy including

- Hypercalcemia from any cause such as myeloma or idiopathic infantile hypercalcemia
- Hyperparathyroidism
- Hypervitaminosis D
- Hypophosphatasia (Rathbun syndrome)
- Renal failure
- Mercury exposure
- Milk-alkali syndrome
- Discoid lupus erythematosus
- Paget disease
- Sarcoidosis
- Tuberous sclerosis
- Ichthysis
- Progressive facial hemiatrophy (Parry-Romberg syndrome)
- Rothmund-Thomson syndrome (bilateral cataract, skin pigmentation and telangiectasia)

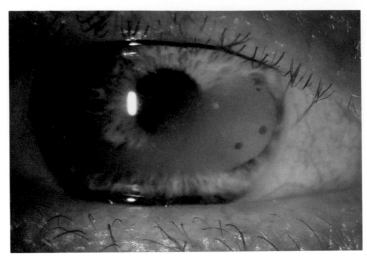

FIG XVI-27—Band keratopathy.

LABORATORY EVALUATION. Local causes of chronic inflammation such as intraocular silicone injection or treatment with mercury-containing or phosphate-containing eye medications may not be apparent. If review of systems does not direct specific testing, serum calcium, phosphate, alkaline phosphatase, and creatinine should be obtained.

MANAGEMENT. Underlying conditions such as keratoconjunctivitis sicca or renal failure should be treated or controlled as much as possible. This treatment may reduce or control the deposition of calcium or at least help reduce the recurrence of band keratopathy. The calcium can usually be removed from Bowman's layer by chelating it with a neutral solution of disodium ethylenediaminetetraacetic acid.

Hemochromatosis Systemic iron overload is not associated with corneal deposits or changes. Rarely, congenital spherocytosis has been associated with deep intra-epithelial reddish brown deposits in an oval shape of unknown pathogenesis. Iron depositions are discussed further in chapter XVIII.

Corneal and External Disease Signs of Systemic Neoplasia

Chapter XII discusses neoplastic disorders in greater depth. See pp 225–257. See also BCSC Section 7, *Orbit, Eyelids, and Lacrimal System.*

Enlarged corneal nerves Several conditions feature enlarged corneal nerves. The most important is multiple endocrine neoplasia (MEN) type IIB (Sipple-Gorlin syndrome). This autosomal dominant (chromosome 10q11.2) disease is characterized by medullary carcinoma of the thyroid gland, pheochromocytoma, and mucosal neuromas in patients who frequently have a marfanoid habitus. Besides the thickened corneal nerves, conjunctival and eyelid neuromas and keratoconjunctivitis sicca may occur. Recently, patients with MEN type IIA and type III have also been noted to have enlarged corneal nerves. Other causes of prominent corneal nerves from either true enlargement or increased visibility are listed in Table XVI-8.

TABLE XVI-8

PROMINENT CORNEAL NERVES

ENLARGED CORNEAL NERVES	MORE VISIBLE CORNEAL NERVES
Multiple endocrine neoplasia type IIB (Sipple-Gorlin syndrome)	Keratoconus
	Ichthyosis
Phytanic acid storage disease (Refsum syndrome)	Fuchs corneal dystrophy
Hansen disease (leprosy, beading of nerves)	Corneal edema
Familial dysautonomia (Riley-Day syndrome)	Congenital glaucoma
Neurofibromatosis	
Acanthamoeba perineuritis	

PART 8

DEGENERATIVE DISORDERS OF THE CONJUNCTIVA, CORNEA, AND SCLERA

CHAPTER XVII

Degenerative and Aging Processes of the Conjunctiva, Cornea, and Sclera

Degenerations of the ocular surface may occur from the physiologic changes associated with aging, or they may follow an environmental insult to the eye such as exposure to ultraviolet light.

Degeneration of a tissue is a physiologic decomposition of tissue elements and deterioration of tissue functions. Table XVII-1 summarizes the differences between degenerations and corneal dystrophies.

Aging of the Conjunctiva

The conjunctiva loses transparency as an individual ages. The epithelium thickens and may become keratinized in exposed zones. The substantia propria becomes thinner and less elastic. These changes are not necessarily uniform and tend to be more pronounced in the interpalpebral fissure zone. Increased laxity is often apparent in the lower bulbar conjunctiva where redundant conjunctiva wrinkles onto the lower eyelid margin, a condition sometimes referred to as *conjunctivochalasis*. The conjunctival vessels develop fusiform and saccular dilations in older persons.

TABLE XVII-1

DIFFERENCES BETWEEN CORNEAL DEGENERATIONS AND CORNEAL DYSTROPHIES

DEGENERATION	DYSTROPHY
Opacity often peripherally located	Centrally located
May be asymmetric	Bilateral and symmetric
Presents later in life, associated with aging	Presents early in life, hereditary
Progression can be very slow or rapid	Progression usually slow

Aging of the Cornea

The cornea gradually becomes flatter, thinner, and slightly less transparent. Its refractive index increases, and Descemet's membrane becomes thicker, increasing from 3 μm at birth to 10 μm in adults as a result of the increased thickness of its posterior nonbanded zones. Occasional peripheral guttatae, formerly known as Hassall-Henle bodies, can form with age. Age-related attrition of corneal endothelial cells results in a loss of about 100,000 cells during the first 50 years of life, from a cell density of about 4000 cells/mm^2 at birth to a density of 2500–3000 cells/mm^2 in adults.

Johnson DH, Bourne WM, Campbell RJ. The ultrastructure of Descemet's membrane. I. Changes with age in normal corneas. *Arch Ophthalmol.* 1982;100:1942.

Laule A, Cable MK, Hoffman CE, et al. Endothelial cell population changes of human cornea during life. *Arch Ophthalmol.* 1978;96:2031–2035.

Degenerative Changes in the Cornea

The cornea of the aging eye is more susceptible to degenerative changes, and these occur most often near the limbus. Peripheral corneal degeneration can be divided into two general categories:

□ Deposition of lipid or other substances

□ Connective tissue changes with thinning

The peripheral cornea differs from the central cornea in several unique anatomical and physiologic features. Contiguity with the limbal vasculatures is the most important difference. Unlike the central cornea, the peripheral cornea can be adversely affected by the pathologies associated with blood vessels, such as inflammatory infiltrations and depositions of serum proteins or other substances. Because of its proximity to limbal vessels, the peripheral cornea is inevitably involved in the early stage of any condition causing corneal vascularization.

The peripheral cornea is also close to the surrounding conjunctiva, episclera, and sclera, and it is secondarily affected by the primary diseases of these adjacent tissues. Conjunctival inflammatory conditions such as pterygium and trachoma often involve the peripheral cornea. Mechanical disruption of normal corneal wetting by the adjacent swollen conjunctiva can lead to drying of the peripheral cornea and dellen formation.

Corneal epithelial stem cells are located in the limbal basal epithelium. These cells are the proliferative source of corneal epithelium and are responsible for the renewal of the corneal surface. Disruption of this important corneal physiologic barrier may lead to conjunctival invasion, resulting in surface irregularity and vascularization, as in pterygium and keratinization of the eyelid margin.

Aging of the Sclera

Age-related changes in the sclera involve connective tissue changes and atrophy of scleral fibrocytes. The most common alteration is lipid deposition in the deeper layers that can give the anterior sclera a yellowish color. A gradual loss of elasticity can result in increased rigidity that can affect estimation of the intraocular pressure.

CHAPTER XVIII

Clinical Approach to Depositions And Degenerations of the Conjunctiva, Cornea, and Sclera

Conjunctival Degenerations

Pinguecula

This very common conjunctival condition occurs typically at the nasal and temporal anterior bulbar conjunctiva.

PATHOGENESIS. This degenerative lesion of the bulbar conjunctiva occurs as a result of the effects of ultraviolet light (actinic exposure), but it may also be related to other insults such as welding. The epithelium overlying a pinguecula may be normal, thick, or thin. Calcification occurs occasionally.

CLINICAL FINDINGS. Pingueculae appear adjacent to the limbus in the interpalpebral zone, more often nasally, and have the appearance of yellow white, amorphous subepithelial deposits. They may enlarge gradually over long periods of time. Recurrent inflammation and ocular irritation may be encountered.

LABORATORY EVALUATION. The subepithelial collagen fibers become fragmented, curled, and more basophilic with hematoxylin-eosin stain. The fibers also stain with elastic tissue stains but are not elastic tissue. These fibers are insensitive to treatment with elastase, which does not prevent positive staining for elastin. This particular kind of degeneration of collagen, in which it takes on staining characteristics of elastic tissue, is referred to as *elastoid* or *elastotic degeneration* or, simply, *elastosis*.

MANAGEMENT. Lubricant therapy to alleviate ocular irritations is often used clinically. Excision is indicated only when pingueculae constitute cosmetic problems or in the rare instances in which they become chronically inflamed or interfere with successful contact lens wear. The inflammation of a pinguecula should be distinguished from nodular scleritis or episcleritis. Judicious use of topical steroids can be considered in patients with chronic inflammation.

Jaros PA, DeLuise VP. Pingueculae and pterygia. *Surv Ophthalmol.* 1988;33:41–49.

Pterygium

PATHOGENESIS. Strong correlation with UV exposure has been documented, although dryness, inflammation, and exposure to wind and dust or other irritants may also be factors. The pathologic changes consist of elastoid degeneration of collagen and the appearance of subepithelial fibrovascular tissue. The cornea shows destruction of Bowman's layer by fibrovascular ingrowth, frequently with mild inflammatory changes. The epithelium may be normal, thick, or thin, and it occasionally shows dysplasia.

CLINICAL FINDINGS. A pterygium is a wing-shaped fold of conjunctiva and fibrovascular tissue that has invaded the superficial cornea. Pterygia are nearly always preceded and accompanied by pingueculae. It is not known why some patients develop pterygia while others have only pingueculae, but the prevalence of pterygia increases steadily with proximity to the equator. Astigmatism is often associated with fibrovascular contraction of the cornea. A pigmented iron line *(Stocker's line)* may be seen in advance of a pterygium on the cornea (Fig XVIII-1).

MANAGEMENT. Excision is indicated if the visual axis is threatened or in cases of extreme irritation, but surgery should not be undertaken casually. The recurrence rate is significant, and recurrent pterygia are often more serious than primary ones. Although the recurrence rate is estimated at 40%, conjunctival transplantation following excision can effectively reduce this rate to about 5%. Ipsilateral bulbar conjunctiva from the superotemporal quadrant (if the pterygium is nasal) is removed and free-grafted into the episcleral bed of the excised pterygium. Beta-irradiation with strontium 90 also reduces the recurrence rate but not as well as conjunctival transplantation. Complications of beta-irradiation include aseptic necrosis of the sclera and cornea as well as cataract. This technique has fallen into disfavor because of these complications.

The object of surgery is to remove the pterygium in such a way that regrowth, which occurs from the conjunctival aspect, does not occur. Except in children, local anesthesia is satisfactory. The corneal and conjunctival portions of the pterygium are dissected from the underlying tissues, and the lesion is removed from the eye by snipping the remaining attachments at the limbus. A roughly semicircular area of exposed sclera adjacent to the limbus is then covered by mobilization of adjacent conjunctiva or by a rotational flap. Closure by rotational flap is generally the preferred method, although a bare sclera technique can also be used. The cornea and

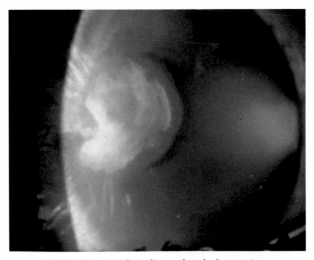

FIG XVIII-1—Stocker's line at head of pterygium.

limbus should be left as smooth as possible at the close of surgery. Care should be taken to avoid deep dissection in the cornea, since the lesion does not usually extend deeper than Bowman's layer.

Free conjunctival autografting and limbal-conjunctival autografting techniques have shown excellent results and are especially recommended for a recurrent pterygium. Some believe these conjunctival grafting procedures should be used for all cases of pterygium surgery. Intraoperative or postoperative use of mitomycin-C 0.2 mg/ml (0.02%) has been shown to significantly reduce recurrence, but complications such as scleral necrosis, cataract, persistent epithelial defects, and visual loss have also been reported. Extreme caution should be exercised in using topical mitomycin-C in patients with uncomplicated pterygium. See discussion on page 394.

Gans LA. Surgical treatment of pterygium. In: *Focal Points: Clinical Modules for Ophthalmologists.* San Francisco: American Academy of Ophthalmology; 1996;14:2.

Conjunctival Concretions

Concretions appear histopathologically to be epithelial inclusion cysts filled with epithelial and keratin debris. Yellow-white deposits are sometimes found in the palpebral conjunctiva of patients who are elderly or who have had chronic conjunctivitis. Secondary calcification occurs occasionally, in which case the lesions are sometimes referred to as *conjunctival lithiasis.* The subconjunctival deposition of tetracycline mimics concretions. Concretions are almost always asymptomatic but may erode the overlying epithelium to cause foreign body sensation. If symptomatic, concretions can be easily removed under topical anesthesia.

Elastofibroma Oculi

Elastofibroma is a rare pseudotumorous lesion composed of thick collagen bundles, linear elastinophilic material, and adipose tissue. These lesions occur on the temporal epibulbar surface where they may imitate a pterygium, hamartoma, or choristoma. The etiology is uncertain, but the lesion may be either a response to inciting trauma or, because adipose tissue is present, a hamartomatous lesion. The collagen and elastic fibers are probably produced by activated fibroblasts. Treatment is complete excision.

Corneal Degenerations

Epithelial and Subepithelial Degenerations

Coats white ring   A small (1 mm or less in diameter) circle of discrete gray-white dots is sometimes seen in the superficial stroma. Referred to as *Coats white ring,* it represents iron-containing fibrotic remnants of a metallic foreign body. These rings probably develop when a rust ring from an iron foreign body is not entirely removed. No treatment is required.

Spheroidal degeneration   This common degeneration is often bilateral and more common in males. It is characterized by the appearance in the cornea, and sometimes in the conjunctiva, of translucent, golden brown, spheroidlike deposits in the superficial stroma. The condition has been reported under different names, including corneal elastosis, keratinoid degeneration, climatic droplet keratopathy, Bietti nodular dystrophy, proteinaceous degeneration, and Labrador keratopathy. In *primary spheroidal degeneration* the deposits are bilateral and initially located in the nasal and temporal cornea; they can extend onto the conjunctiva. The spheroidal deposits sometimes extend across the interpalpebral zone of the cornea, producing a noncalcific band keratopathy.

Secondary spheroidal degeneration is associated with ocular injury or inflammation. The deposits aggregate near the area of corneal scarring or vascularization. All cases show extracellular proteinaceous deposits with characteristics of elastotic degeneration, which are thought to be secondary to the combined effects of genetic predisposition, actinic exposure, age, and perhaps various kinds of environmental trauma other than sunlight. The pattern is similar to other ultraviolet light–associated degenerations such as pingueculae. No medical therapy is of value. Superficial keratectomy or excimer excision may be useful for this condition.

Stromal Degenerations: Age-Related (Involutional) Changes

White limbal girdle   Two forms of the white limbal girdle of Vogt have been described. *Type I* is a narrow, concentric, whitish superficial band running along the limbus in the palpebral fissure. A lucid interval appears between the limbus and the girdle. This girdle is a degenerative change of the anterior limiting membrane, with chalklike opacities and small clear areas like Swiss cheese. *Type II* consists of small white flecklike and needlelike deposits that are often seen at the nasal and temporal limbus in older patients. No clear interval separates this girdle from the limbus. The histopathologic picture represents epithelial elastotic degeneration of collagen, sometimes with particles of calcium.

Corneal arcus (arcus senilis)   PATHOGENESIS. Arcus senilis is most often an involutional change modified by genetic factors. However, arcus is sometimes indicative of a hyperlipoproteinemia (low-density lipoprotein) with elevated serum cholesterol, especially in patients under 40 years of age (see chapter XVI). It is also a prognostic factor for coronary artery disease in this age group. Arcus occurs occasionally as a congenital anomaly *(arcus juvenilis)*, usually involving only a sector of the peripheral cornea and not associated with abnormalities of serum lipid.

CLINICAL FINDINGS. Arcus is a deposition of lipid in the peripheral corneal stroma. It starts at the inferior and superior poles of the cornea and encircles the entire circumference in the late stages. Incidence is 60% in individuals between the ages of 50 and 60 and approaches 100% of persons over 80. Frequency is higher in the black population. The arcus has a hazy white appearance, a sharp outer border, and an indistinct central border and is denser superiorly and inferiorly. A lucid interval is usually present between the peripheral edge of the arcus and the limbus. Unilateral arcus is a rare condition associated with contralateral carotid artery disease or ocular hypotony. Arcus is also seen in Schnyder central crystalline dystrophy.

LABORATORY EVALUATION. The lipid can be demonstrated histopathologically only by the use of fat stains of frozen sections, because standard fixation techniques dissolve it. The lipid is found to be concentrated mainly in two areas of the peripheral cornea stroma: one adjacent to Bowman's layer and another near Descemet's membrane.

Crocodile shagreen   Anterior crocodile shagreen, or *mosaic degeneration*, is a central corneal opacity at the level of Bowman's layer characterized by mosaic, polygonal, gray opacities separated by clear zones. Histologically, Bowman's layer is thrown into ridges and may be calcified. Posterior crocodile shagreen shows similar changes in the deep stroma near Descemet's membrane. The posterior variety of crocodile shagreen may be related to central cloudy dystrophy of François (see Figure XIV-4).

Cornea farinata   This involutional change is probably dependent on a dominantly transmitted genetic predisposition. The deep corneal stroma shows many opacities in the shapes of dots and commas. They are very nebulous and subtle and often can be seen with retroillumination. The condition does not affect vision and has no clinical significance, except that it is sometimes mistaken for a progressive dystrophy. The deposits may consist of lipofuscin, a degenerative pigment that appears in some aged cells. Pre-Descemet's dystrophy is probably a morphological variant of cornea farinata. Although these conditions are probably related, it is unclear whether they are degenerations or dystrophies.

Polymorphic amyloid degeneration   This bilaterally symmetric, slowly progressive corneal degeneration appears late in life. The corneal opacities emerge as either stellate flecks in mid- to deep stroma or irregular filaments. Both forms may occur together, but usually one predominates. These deposits are usually axial, polymorphic, and filamentous. The opacities are gray to white and somewhat refractile but appear translucent in retroillumination. The intervening stroma appears clear. Visual acuity is usually normal. The corneal deposits consist of amyloid and can resemble some of the deposits seen in early lattice corneal dystrophy.

Stromal Degenerations: Peripheral Cornea

Senile furrow degeneration   This condition is an appearance of thinning that is seen in older people in the lucid interval of a corneal arcus. There is no inflammation, vascularization, or tendency to perforate. Vision is rarely affected, unless astigmatism occurs because of the thinning. Although slight thinning is occasionally present, it is usually more apparent than real. The epithelium is intact. No treatment is required.

> Mondino BJ. Inflammatory diseases of the peripheral cornea. *Ophthalmology.* 1988; 95:463–472.

Terrien marginal degeneration   PATHOGENESIS. The cause is unknown, although association with vernal keratoconjunctivitis has been reported.

CLINICAL FINDINGS. This condition is a quiet, essentially noninflammatory, unilateral or asymmetrically bilateral, slowly progressive thinning of the peripheral cornea. Sex prevalence is roughly equal, and cases usually occur in the second or third decade of life. The corneal thinning can be localized or involve extensive portions of the peripheral cornea.

Terrien marginal degeneration begins superiorly, spreads circumferentially, and rarely involves the inferior limbus. The central wall is steep, and the peripheral wall slopes gradually. The epithelium remains intact, and a fine vascular pannus traverses the area of stromal thinning. A line of lipid deposits appears at the leading edge of the pannus (central edge of the furrow). Spontaneous perforation is rare, although perforation can easily occur with minor trauma. Corneal topography reveals flattening of the peripheral thinned cornea, with steepening of the corneal surface approximately 90° away from the midpoint of the thinned area. This pattern usually results in high against-the-rule or oblique astigmatism. Spontaneous ruptures in Descemet's membrane can result in interlamellar fluid or even a corneal cyst.

An inflammatory condition of the peripheral cornea very rarely occurs in children and young adults that may resemble Terrien marginal degeneration. Also known as *Fuchs superficial marginal keratitis,* progressive thinning without epithelial ulceration occurs that can lead to perforation.

LABORATORY EVALUATION AND MANAGEMENT. Electron microscopic studies have revealed histiocytes that may be responsible for phagocytosis of corneal collagen. Resection of the adjacent conjunctiva may halt the progression of peripheral keratolysis. Crescentic full-thickness or lamellar corneoscleral patch grafts may eventually be required.

Stromal Degenerations: Postinflammatory Changes

Salzmann nodular degeneration   This noninflammatory corneal degeneration sometimes occurs as a late sequel to old, long-standing keratitis, or it may be idiopathic. Causes include phlyctenulosis, trachoma, and interstitial keratitis. The degeneration may not appear until years after the active keratitis has subsided. It can be bilateral and is more common in middle-aged and older women. The nodules are gray-white or blue-white and elevated, and they may be associated with recurrent erosion. They often develop in a roughly circular configuration in the central or paracentral cornea and at the ends of vessels of a pannus. Histopathologic examination reveals localized replacement of Bowman's layer by hyaline and fibrillar material, probably representing basement membrane and material similar to that found in spheroidal degeneration. Treatment is with superficial keratectomy or lamellar or even penetrating keratoplasty. This degeneration may recur after keratoplasty. Excimer laser may prove valuable for this condition.

Amyloid degeneration   Acquired (secondary localized) corneal amyloidosis may be associated with corneal inflammation (such as trachoma, keratoconus, Hansen disease, or phlyctenulosis) or intraocular disease (such as uveitis, retinopathy of prematurity, or glaucoma) or secondary to trauma. Clinically, amyloid deposits usually occur as raised, yellow-pink, nodular masses in the cornea. Less commonly, they may appear as perivascular deposits. In most cases corneal vascularization is associated with the amyloid. The deposits may be refractile with retroillumination. See discussion on amyloidosis in chapter XVI.

Corneal keloid   These white, sometimes protuberant, glistening corneal masses often resemble dermoids and can involve the entire corneal surface. They are thought to be secondary to a vigorous fibrocytic response to corneal perforation or injury. The resemblance to corneal dermoids can make diagnosis difficult. Subtle differences between corneal keloids and dermoids include the glistening and jellylike quality of the keloids. Definitive diagnosis can be made by performing corneal biopsy. Study of enucleation specimens has revealed associated findings including cataract, anterior staphyloma, ruptured lens capsule with lens fragments in the wound, buphthalmos, chronic glaucoma, and angle-closure glaucoma. Proper diagnosis may result in the use of appropriate procedures other than enucleation to treat this condition.

Lipid keratopathy Yellow or cream-colored lipids containing cholesterol, neutral fats, and glycoproteins are deposited in the superficial or deeper cornea, usually in areas of vascularized corneal scars. The epithelium is involved secondarily, after prolonged corneal inflammation with corneal vascularization (e.g., herpes simplex or herpes zoster keratitis or trachoma). This form would best be described as *secondary lipid keratopathy*. Lipid keratopathy has been rarely reported with no evidence of an antecedent infection, inflammatory process, or corneal damage. These cases would best be described as *primary lipid keratopathy*.

Calcific band keratopathy (calcium hydroxyapatite deposition) PATHOGENESIS. This calcific degeneration of the superficial cornea involves mainly Bowman's layer. There are six main causes:

- Chronic ocular disease (usually inflammatory) such as uveitis in children, interstitial keratitis, severe superficial keratitis, and phthisis bulbi
- Hypercalcemia caused by hyperparathyroidism, vitamin D toxicity, milk-alkali syndrome, sarcoidosis, and other systemic disorders
- Hereditary transmission (primary hereditary band keratopathy, with or without other anomalies)
- Elevated serum phosphorus with normal serum calcium, which sometimes occurs in patients with renal failure
- Chronic exposure to mercurial vapors or to mercurial preservatives (phenylmercuric nitrate or acetate) in ophthalmic medications (the mercury causes changes in corneal collagen that result in the deposition of calcium)
- Silicone oil instillation in an aphakic eye

Other rare associated disorders have been reported including iris melanoma. Band keratopathy may also result from the deposition in the cornea of urates, which appear brown, unlike the gray-white calcific deposits, and may be associated with gout or hyperuricemia.

CLINICAL PRESENTATION. Calcific band keratopathy begins as fine, dustlike, basophilic deposits in Bowman's layer. These changes are usually first seen peripherally. A peripheral clear zone representing a lucid interval is seen between the limbus and the peripheral edge of the keratopathy. Eventually, the deposits may coalesce to form a horizontal band of dense calcific plaques across the interpalpebral zone of the cornea.

MANAGEMENT. Underlying conditions such as keratoconjunctivitis sicca or renal failure should be treated or controlled as much as possible, which may reduce or control the deposition of calcium or at least help reduce the recurrence of band keratopathy. The calcium can usually be removed from Bowman's layer by chelation with a neutral solution of disodium ethylenediaminetetraacetic acid (EDTA) 150 mg/ml (Endrate, 20 ml per vial). A proper concentration can be made by mixing one 20-ml vial with 100 ml of sterile ophthalmic irrigation solution, and this mixture can be warmed to speed up the chemical chelation of calcium. The epithelium overlying the calcium must be removed. Warmed EDTA solution is then dropped onto the cornea or held in contact with the surface of the cornea by a syringe or soaked cellulose sponge. The calcium is usually removed within 5–30 minutes. If used at all, scraping should be gentle so as to prevent damage to Bowman's layer. A fibrous pannus may develop along with extensive calcific band keratopathy, especially if silicone oil is responsible, and neither EDTA nor scraping will remove such fibrous tissue. A soft contact lens or collagen shield can be helpful postoperatively until the epithelium has healed. The problem can recur but may not do so for years, at which time the treatment may be repeated. Phototherapeutic keratectomy using excimer laser has also been used to manage band keratopathy.

Endothelial Degenerations

Hassall-Henle bodies (peripheral corneal guttatae)   These small, wartlike excrescences appear in the peripheral portion of Descemet's membrane as a normal aging change. They occur on the posterior aspect of the membrane and protrude toward the anterior chamber. With the slit lamp, Hassall-Henle bodies have the appearance of small, dark dimples within the endothelial mosaic, and they are best seen by specular reflection. Rarely seen before age 20, they then increase steadily in number with age. They are pathologic when they appear in the central cornea and are then referred as *cornea guttatae.* Central cornea guttatae associated with progressive stromal and eventually epithelial edema represent Fuchs endothelial-epithelial dystrophy (see chapter XVI). They are the result of localized overproduction of basement membrane by endothelial cells and so have the same collagenous structure as does normal Descemet's membrane.

Melanin pigmentation   Deposits of melanin on the corneal endothelium can be observed in patients with glaucoma associated with pigment dispersion syndrome. Typically, the cluster of vertically oriented pigments is known as *Krukenberg spindle,* (see Table XVIII-2).

Drug-Induced Deposition and Pigmentation

Rarely, ophthalmic ointment preparation can become entrapped in the epithelium after corneal abrasions have healed. Clear globules appear within the epithelium. These deposits are usually well tolerated; however, some vascular ingrowth may occur if they are located near the limbus. Subepithelial deposits of tetracycline ointment in the fornix sometimes may simulate amyloid deposition.

Corneal Epithelial Deposits

Cornea verticillata   Amiodarone, a coronary artery dilator, produces lysosomal deposits in the basal epithelial layer, creating a whorl-like pattern resembling that seen in Fabry disease with accumulation of sphingolipid. Such a distinctive pattern of deposits can also be seen with long-term chloroquine, chlorpromazine, or indomethacin therapy. It is unusual for these deposits to result in reduction of visual acuity or ocular symptoms, although this has occurred in some patients.

The development of deposits is not necessarily an indication to stop these medications, although the deposits will resolve with discontinuation of the responsible agents. Chronic administration of chloroquine can lead to a retinopathy that has

TABLE XVIII-1

DRUGS ASSOCIATED WITH CORNEAL DEPOSITS

EPITHELIAL DEPOSITS	STROMAL DEPOSITS
Aminoquinolones	Antacids
Amodiaquine	Gold
Chloroquine	Indomethacin
Hydroxychloroquine	Phenothiazines
Clofazimine	Phenylbutazone
Indomethacin	Practolol
Naproxen	Retinoids
Perhexiline	Silver
Suramin	
Tamoxifen	
Thioxanthines	
Chlorprothixine	
Thiothixine	
Tilorone	

Reproduced by permission from Arffa RC, Eve FR. Systemic associations of corneal deposits. *Int Ophthalmol Clin.* 1991;31:89–110.

no specific relationship with the corneal deposits. Drugs associated with corneal deposits are summarized in Table XVIII-1. Toxic ulcerative keratopathy related to topical ophthalmic medications, or frequently the preservatives within them, is a significant cause of ocular morbidity as a result of exogenously administered ophthalmic medications. See also discussion of persistent epithelial defect in chapter VI and material on toxic medication reaction in chapter X.

Ciprofloxacin deposits Topical ciprofloxacin therapy can result in the deposition of a chalky white precipitate within an epithelial defect. The precipitate is composed of ciprofloxacin crystals. Although white plaques predominate, a crystalline pattern may be also observed.

Pigmentation

Corneal pigmentation may result from deposits of melanin, blood or blood products, or a variety of metallic compounds. Table XVIII-2 lists pigments that may be of diagnostic importance with their locations and associated conditions. See also Table XVI-5.

Argyriasis Silver compounds (particularly Argyrol) were commonly used in the preantibiotic era for the treatment of external infections. Their chronic use can result in a condition known as *argyriasis,* consisting of a slate gray or silver discoloration involving the bulbar and palpebral conjunctiva. This condition can be permanent.

TABLE XVIII-2

CORNEAL PIGMENTATIONS

PIGMENT	CLINICAL CONDITION	LOCATION IN CORNEA
Melanin	Krukenberg spindle	Endothelium, in a vertically oriented ellipse; sometimes associated with pigmentary glaucoma
Melanin-like pigment (oxidized epinephrine)	Adrenochrome deposition	Between basement membrane and Bowman's layer or in conjunctival cysts; occurs in patients using topical epinephrine compounds for glaucoma
Melanin-like pigment (alkapton)	Ochronosis	Epithelium and superficial stroma, peripherally; occurs in the metabolic disease alkaptonuria
Iron	Blood staining	Chiefly stroma; epithelium in some cases; occurs in some cases of hyphema
Iron (foreign body)	Siderosis	Chiefly stroma; epithelium in some cases
Iron	Ferry's line	Corneal epithelium anterior to filtering bleb
Iron	Fleischer ring (or line) (Fig XVI-18)	Corneal epithelium surrounding base of cone in keratoconus
Iron	Hudson-Stähli line	Corneal epithelium at junction of upper two thirds with lower one third of the aging cornea
Iron	Stocker's line (Fig XVIII-1)	Corneal epithelium anterior to head of pterygium
Copper	Kayser-Fleischer ring (Fig XVI-26)	Descemet's membrane peripherally, in patients with Wilson hepatolenticular degeneration
Copper	Chalcosis	Descemet's membrane
Silver	Argyriasis	Deep stroma and Descemet's membrane
Gold	Chrysiasis	Deep stroma (more in periphery)
Gold, platinum, India ink	Corneal tattoo	Stroma

Adrenochrome   Long-standing administration of epinephrine compounds may lead to black or very dark brown deposits in the conjunctiva and cornea. Composed of adrenochrome, an oxidation product of the basic epinephrine compound, these melanin-like deposits can accumulate in conjunctival cysts and concretions in the conjunctiva (Fig XVIII-2). They may discolor the cornea or contact lens as well. The deposits are harmless, although they are occasionally misdiagnosed as conjunctival melanoma or other conditions.

Arffa RC. *Grayson's Diseases of the Cornea.* 4th ed. St Louis: Mosby; 1997.

Kaiser PK, Pineda R, Albert DM, et al. "Black cornea" after long-term epinephrine use. *Arch Ophthalmol.* 1992;110:1273–1275.

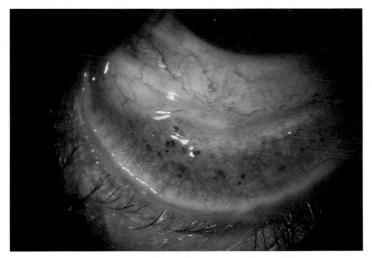

FIG XVIII-2—Adrenochrome deposits in inferior cul-de-sac.

Iron deposits Iron deposition in the corneal stroma can occur as a result of retained metallic foreign body or corneal blood staining from prolonged hyphema with secondary glaucoma. A Fleischer ring, representing iron deposition in keratoconus, is one of many corneal iron lines associated with epithelial irregularities (see Figure XVI-18). This sign is exceedingly useful in the diagnosis of mild or early cases of keratoconus. Many times, it can only be seen using red-free or cobalt blue illumination prior to the instillation of fluorescein. The Hudson-Stähli line, generally located at the junction of the upper two thirds and lower third of the cornea, is ubiquitous. Most iron lines are related to abnormalities of tear pooling related to surface irregularities. An iron line has recently been associated with keratorefractive procedures. Common conditions associated with corneal iron lines are listed in Table XVIII-2.

Scleral Degenerations

Senile Plaques

Scleral rigidity increases in elderly persons along with a relative decrease in scleral hydration and the amount of mucopolysaccharide. These changes are accompanied by subconjunctival deposition of fat, which gives the sclera a yellowish appearance. Calcium may also be deposited either diffusely among the scleral collagen fibers in granular or crystalline form or focally in a plaque anterior to the horizontal rectus

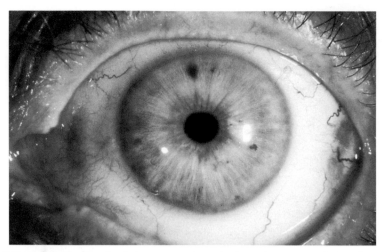

FIG XVIII-3—Senile scleral plaques anterior to horizontal rectus muscle insertions.

muscle insertions. The plaques are visible as ovoid or rectangular zones of grayish translucency (Fig XVIII-3). Histologically, the midportion of the involved sclera contains a focal calcified plaque surrounded by relatively acellular collagen. The plaques do not elicit inflammation and rarely extrude.

PART 9

TOXIC AND TRAUMATIC INJURIES
OF THE ANTERIOR SEGMENT

CHAPTER XIX

Wound Healing of the Conjunctiva, Cornea, and Sclera

Wound Healing of the Conjunctiva

The conjunctival epithelium heals like other mucous membranes. Abrasions stimulate sliding and proliferation, and conjunctival epithelial defects often heal within a day or so. The substantia propria heals with revascularization of the wound, with budding of nonfenestrated capillaries. The superficial layer of loose tissue may not regenerate, and the deeper, fibrous layer can predominate in a healed conjunctival wound, making the conjunctiva more adherent to the sclera.

Wound Healing of the Cornea

Corneal healing is generally avascular. Corneal reepithelialization is similar to other mucous membranes, with epithelial migration and proliferation. Corneal wound healing is also discussed on page 390.

Stromal Wound Healing

Unlike other tissues, the cornea heals through fibrosis rather than fibrovascular proliferation. After penetrating injury of the stroma, keratocytes immediatedly adjacent to the wound margin are killed, and the deficiency soon fills with a fibrin clot. Neutrophils arrive, carried by the tears, within 2–6 hours and engage in proteolytic debridement of necrotic cellular and extracellular debris. Healing factors derived from vessels are not present.

The fibroblasts of the stroma become activated, eventually migrating across the wound, laying down collagen and fibronectin. The direction of the fibroblasts and collagen is not parallel to the stromal lamellae. Hence, cells are directed anteriorly and posteriorly across a wound that is always visible microscopically as an irregularity in the stroma and clinically as an opacity. If the wound edges are separated, the gap is not completely filled by proliferating fibroblasts, and a partially filled crater results.

If the epithelium does not cover the wound within days, the subjacent stromal healing is limited and the wound is weak. Growth factors from the epithelium stimulate and sustain healing. The endothelial cells adjacent to the wound slide across the posterior cornea, and the endothelium lays down a new thin layer of Descemet's membrane. If the internal margin of the wound is not covered by Descemet's membrane, the stromal fibroblasts may continue to proliferate into the anterior chamber as a fibrous ingrowth. In the late months of healing, the initial fibrillar collagen is replaced by stronger collagen. Bowman's layer does not regenerate when incised or destroyed. With an ulcer, epithelium covers the surface, but little of the lost stromal volume is replaced by fibrous tissue.

Endothelial Wound Healing

Since maintenance of a continuous endothelial cell monolayer is critical to stromal deturgescence and hence optical clarity, endothelial repair processes are of great clinical concern. A variety of inflammatory and mechanical insults can incite these repair responses.

Successful endothelial healing Immediately after a posterior corneal wound, the cut edges of Descemet's membrane retract and curl anteriorly toward the stroma. Adjacent endothelial cells are lost, and a fibrin clot is formed in the wound. Within hours, adjoining endothelial cells attenuate with extensive cytoplasmic processes and migrate into the wound. In the adult human almost the entire healing effort occurs by means of cellular reorganization, enlargement, and migration to reconstitute an intact monolayer.

Once Descemet's membrane has been resurfaced by a continuous endothelial monolayer, the cells become contact-inhibited and form contiguous cellular junctions. The cells that have been involved in the healing process are now much larger than those in uninvolved areas. Once the integrity of the endothelial cell layer has been restored, its pump and barrier functions soon begin to stabilize, as shown by stromal deturgescence, thinning, and increasing clarity. As a nonspecific response to any form of endothelial trauma, the regenerating endothelium deposits new layers of Descemet's membrane material.

Where the wound is well apposed, a single endothelial layer appears and functions normally. Where wound apposition is poor, endothelial cells are multilayered and undergo a fibroblastic transformation resulting in posterior collagen layers comprising fibrillar banded collagen, basement membrane material, and fine filaments. Although these cells also appear capable of eventually reverting to a more normal endothelial morphology, months to years may be required for transformation into endothelium with new Descemet's membrane of normal morphology and thickness.

Pathophysiology of Corneal Edema: The Sequelae of Endothelial Dysfunction

The endothelium functions as a permeability barrier between the aqueous humor and the corneal stroma and as a pump to maintain the cornea in a partially dehydrated state. Water is pumped across the endothelial apical plasma membrane into the aqueous humor in an energy-dependent process. The endothelium derives oxygen from the aqueous humor to maintain normal pump function. Two forces allow the corneal stroma to naturally imbibe water:

□ The glycosaminoglycans exert an osmotic pressure that pulls water into the stroma

□ The pump function osmotically draws water out of the stroma

The endothelial barrier is leaky, and the leak rate normally equals the metabolic pump rate, so that the endothelium maintains a stromal water content of 78% and an average corneal thickness of 0.52 mm.

If endothelial function fails, water diffuses into the stroma, disrupting the orderly structure of the collagen fibrils, and light scattering and corneal opacification result. The water may also pass through the stroma to accumulate as microcysts and bullae beneath and within the epithelium, which forms a virtually impermeable barrier with its zonula occludens junctions.

Wound Healing of the Sclera

When stimulated by wounding, the episclera migrates down the scleral wound, supplying vessels, fibroblasts, and activated macrophages. The sclera differs from the cornea in that the collagen fibers are randomly distributed, not laid down in orderly lamellae, and the glycosaminoglycan is dermatan sulfate, not the keratan sulfate and chondroitin sulfate present in the cornea. The sclera is avascular and acellular. If the uvea is damaged, uveal fibrovascular tissue may enter the wound. The end result is a scar with a dense adhesion between uvea and sclera.

> BCSC Section 4, *Ophthalmic Pathology and Intraocular Tumors,* discusses ophthalmic wound healing in depth with several illustrations.

CHAPTER XX

Clinical Aspects of Toxic and Traumatic Injuries of the Anterior Segment

Injuries Caused by Temperature and Radiation

Thermal Burns

Heat   The rapid-reflex eyelid closure and Bell's phenomenon usually limit damage to the globe from flames. Contact burns from molten metal that stays in contact with the eye are more likely to cause corneal injuries that result in permanent scarring. The major objectives of therapy for burns caused by heat are the following:

□ Relieve discomfort

□ Prevent secondary corneal inflammation, ulceration, and perforation from infection and exposure

□ Minimize eyelid scarring and resultant malfunction

A cycloplegic agent can help relieve discomfort from secondary ciliary spasm or iridocyclitis. Topical antibiotics may prevent infection of burned eyelids and/or reduce the chances of infectious corneal ulceration. Limited debridement of devitalized tissues and granulation tissue, used with full-thickness skin grafts and tarsorrhaphy, help minimize eyelid scarring and ectropion formation. Burned ocular tissue can be protected temporarily by covering the eye with a lubricant and a piece of sterile plastic wrap. Topical corticosteroids help suppress any associated iridocyclitis, but they can also inhibit corneal wound healing and must be used cautiously.

Curling irons for the hair have recently emerged as a cause of corneal burns. Fortunately, burns caused by curling irons are usually limited to the epithelium and generally require only a brief period of pressure patching and cycloplegia to resolve.

Freezing   Transient corneal stromal edema induced by cold has been reported in a variety of settings, including individuals with Raynaud disease. Associated conjunctival vascular changes consistent with Raynaud's phenomenon have been documented under cold stress. Transient cold-induced corneal edema has also been reported in several patients with cranial nerve V (trigeminal) dysfunction. Research suggests that sensory denervation of the eye influences ocular temperature regulation as well as altering the morphological characteristics of the corneal endothelial cell. At least one case report has documented the regular recurrence of reversible corneal edema after cold stress in an individual without evidence of either trigeminal neuropathy or Raynaud disease.

Ultraviolet (UV) Radiation

The corneal epithelium is highly susceptible to injury from UV radiation. Symptoms usually occur a few hours after exposure, when the injured epithelial cells are shed. The condition, although painful, is generally self-limited, and the epithelium heals within 24 hours.

The most common causes of ocular UV injuries are unprotected exposure to sunlamps or arc welding and prolonged outdoor exposure to reflected sunlight. An example of the latter appears in skiers and is called *snow blindness,* caused by UV light reflected from the snow. Appropriate protection with UV-filtering eyewear can prevent such injuries. Treatment consists of pressure patching to minimize discomfort from eyelid movement and cycloplegia. If discomfort is severe, patients may require systemic analgesics.

Ionizing Radiation

Exposure to ionizing radiation may be associated with nuclear explosions, x-rays, and radioisotopes. The amount of exposure is related to the amount of energy, the type of rays being emitted, and the proximity of the ionizing source. Tissue destruction may be the result of direct killing of cells, cellular DNA changes that produce lethal or other abnormal mutations, or radiation damage to blood vessels with secondary ischemic necrosis. Longer wavelengths penetrate less deeply, causing a more intense reaction in superficial layers. Shorter wavelengths penetrate to deeper tissues and may not cause extensive damage to superficial tissues.

Most cases of ocular exposure to ionizing radiation involve both the conjunctiva and the cornea. Conjunctival edema and chemosis occur acutely, often followed by scarring, shrinkage, loss of tear production, and alterations in conjunctival blood vessels with telangiectasia. Necrosis of the conjunctiva and underlying sclera can occur if radioactive material is embedded in the conjunctiva. Acute corneal changes are typified by punctate epithelial erosions. Explosions involving ionizing radiation may lead to perforation of ocular tissues with immediate radiation necrosis.

Management of acute problems includes removal of all foreign bodies. Depending on the severity of the injury, a bandage soft contact lens, tissue adhesive, or penetrating keratoplasty may be necessary. Poor wound healing is a hallmark of ionizing radiation injuries. Late complications are related to lack of tears, loss of corneal sensation, loss of corneal epithelium and its failure to heal, secondary microbial keratitis, vascularization, and keratitis. Management of these sequelae includes the use of artificial tears and tarsorrhaphy. Late changes in the conjunctiva preclude its use for a conjunctival flap. If the opposite eye has not been injured, a contralateral autologous conjunctival flap may be helpful. The prognosis for penetrating keratoplasty in these situations is poor.

Miller D, ed. *Clinical Light Damage to the Eye.* New York: Springer-Verlag; 1987.

Chemical Injuries

Chemical trauma to the external eye is a common problem that may vary in severity from mild irritation to complete destruction of the ocular surface epithelium, corneal opacification, loss of vision, and rarely loss of the eye. The offending chemical may be in the form of a solid, liquid, powder, mist, or vapor. Chemical injuries can occur in the home, most commonly from detergents, disinfectants, solvents, cosmetics, drain cleaners, oven cleaners, ammonia, bleach, and other common household alkaline agents. Fertilizers and pesticides are common offending agents in agriculturally related chemical injuries. Chemical injuries occurring in industry are usually caused by caustic chemicals and solvents. Some of the worst ocular chemical injuries result when strong alkalis (lye) or acids are used as assaultive weapons.

Whenever possible, the offending chemical agent should be identified, because the severity of a chemical injury is dependent on the pH, the volume and duration of contact, and the inherent toxicity of the chemical. The most severe chemical injuries are caused by strong alkalis and acids. The damaging effects of these solutions results from their ability to drastically change the concentration of highly reactive hydrogen and hydroxyl ions in affected tissues.

Alkali Burns (Figs XX-1, XX-2)

Strong alkalis raise the pH of tissues and cause saponification of fatty acids in cell membranes and ultimately cellular disruption. Once the surface epithelium is damaged, alkaline solutions readily penetrate the corneal stroma, where they rapidly destroy the proteoglycan ground substance and collagen fibers. Strong alkaline substances may also penetrate into the anterior chamber and produce tissue damage and intense inflammation (Fig XX-3).

The visual prognosis is determined by the extent of ocular surface epithelial injury, the presence and degree of skin burns, and the eyelid function. The most unfavorable visual prognosis is associated with extensive limbal epithelial damage and intraocular chemical penetration. The limbus contains the putative corneal epithelial stem cells; when these are damaged, the denuded surface of the cornea is often resurfaced by the neighboring conjunctival epithelium. If left unattended, the process of conjunctivalization of the cornea is accompanied by vascularization, chronic inflammation, and persistent and recurrent epithelial defects. Intraocular chemical penetration is often accompanied by cataract formation and secondary glaucoma. In the most severe cases, phthisis of the globe may occur.

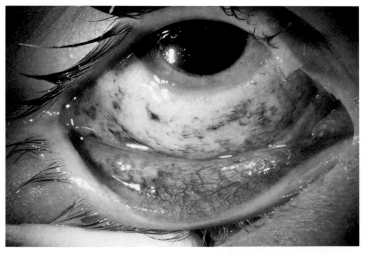

FIG XX-1—Mild alkali burn. Note inferior scleral ischemia.

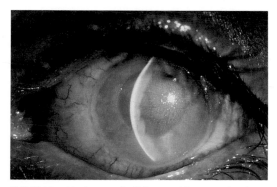

FIG XX-2—Moderate alkali burn with corneal edema and haze.

Acid Burns

Acids denature and precipitate proteins in tissues they contact. Acidic solutions tend to cause less severe tissue damage than alkaline solutions, because of the buffering capacity of tissues, as well as the barrier to penetration formed by precipitated protein. Acids do not cause loss of the proteoglycan ground substance in the cornea.

Therapy of Chemical Injuries to the Eye

No consensus currently exists regarding the optimal management of chemical injuries. Few clinical trials have been performed in humans, and many of the current

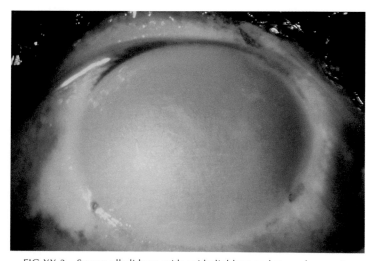

FIG XX-3—Severe alkali burn with epithelial loss and stromal necrosis.

recommendations for management are based on animal models of acute alkaline injury. The most important step in the management of chemical injuries is generally thought to be *immediate and copious irrigation* of the ocular surface with water or normal saline solution. If possible, this irrigation should be initiated at the site of the chemical injury and continued until the patient is evaluated by an ophthalmologist. The eyelid should be immobilized with a retractor or eyelid speculum, and topical anesthetic should be instilled. Irrigation may be accomplished using a handheld intravenous tubing, irrigating eyelid speculum, or Medi-flow lens (a special scleral contact lens that connects to IV tubing). It should be continued until the pH of the conjunctival sac normalizes. The conjunctival pH can be checked easily with a urinary pH strip.

Particulate chemicals should be removed from the ocular surface with cotton-tipped applicators and forceps. Double eversion of the upper eyelid should be performed to search for material in the upper fornix (see Figure XX-9). Severe chemical injuries can be approached by performing a paracentesis of the anterior chamber, removing 0.1–0.2 ml of aqueous humor, and re-forming the chamber with balanced salt solution to try to normalize the anterior chamber pH. *Debridement* of necrotic epithelium and debris on the ocular surface has been recommended by some authorities.

The next phase of therapy should be directed toward *decreasing inflammation, controlling IOP, limiting sterile keratolysis,* and *promoting reepithelialization* of the cornea. An intense polymorphonuclear (PMN) leukocyte infiltration of the corneal stroma has been noted in histologic sections of corneas subjected to acute alkali burns. PMNs may be a major source of enzymes capable of dissolving corneal stromal collagen and ground substance. Corticosteroids are excellent inhibitors of PMN function, and intensive topical steroid administration is recommended for the first 2 weeks following chemical injuries. The dosage should be markedly reduced after 2 weeks, because of the ability of steroids to inhibit wound healing and potentiate infection.

A deficiency of calcium in the plasma membrane of PMNs inhibits their ability to degranulate, and both tetracycline and citric acid are potent chelators of extracellular calcium. Therefore, oral tetracycline has theoretical benefits for inhibiting PMN-induced collagenolysis.

Topical cycloplegics are recommended for patients with significant anterior chamber reaction. IOP is best controlled by using oral carbonic anhydrase inhibitors, in order to prevent toxicity from topical glaucoma medications. BCSC Section 10, *Glaucoma,* discusses medications for IOP control in depth.

Measures to promote wound healing and inhibit collagenolytic activity may help prevent stromal ulceration. Severe alkali burns in rabbit eyes have been found to reduce aqueous humor ascorbate levels to one third of normal levels, and reduced aqueous humor ascorbate has been correlated with corneal stromal ulceration and perforation. Systemic administration of ascorbic acid to rabbits with acute corneal alkaline injuries has restored the aqueous humor ascorbate level to normal and significantly reduced the incidence of ulceration. Ascorbic acid is believed to promote collagen synthesis in the alkali-burned eye, because ascorbic acid is required as a cofactor for this synthesis. It is currently recommended that patients with chemical injuries receive 2 grams of oral ascorbic acid (vitamin C) per day.

Another strategy that has been effective clinically for inhibiting stromal ulceration is gluing a hard contact lens onto the denuded corneal stroma using cyanoacrylate adhesive. The seal created over the corneal stroma prevents influx of ocular surface and tear neutrophils. In some cases, epithelium will eventually grow underneath the contact lens and dislodge it.

There are several strategies for promoting epithelial healing in acute chemical injury. Patients should be treated initially with intensive nonpreserved lubricants. A bandage contact lens or tarsorrhaphy may be beneficial for protecting ocular surface epithelium once it has begun to move onto the peripheral cornea. Autologous conjunctival or limbal transplants from the uninvolved fellow eyes of patients with chemical injuries may restore the integrity of the corneal epithelium. Limbal stem cell transplantation may be performed as soon as 2 weeks after chemical injury if no signs of corneal epithelialization have appeared by that time. Corneal transplantation has a poor prognosis and is often delayed for years after a severe alkali injury.

Fogle JA, Kenyon KR, Foster CS. Tissue adhesive arrests stromal melting in the human cornea. *Am J Ophthalmol.* 1980;89:795–802.

Kenyon KR, Tseng SC. Limbal autograft transplantation for ocular surface disorders. *Ophthalmology.* 1989;96:709–723.

Pfister RR. Chemical corneal burns. *Int Ophthalmol Clin.* 1984;24:157–168.

Wagoner MD. Chemical injuries of the eye: current concepts in pathophysiology and therapy. *Surv Ophthalmol.* 1997;41:275–313.

Animal and Plant Substances

A variety of other external agents have been reported to result in trauma to the cornea.

Insect injuries   Bee and wasp stings to the cornea are rare but among the more frequently encountered traumas caused by insects. Acutely, conjunctival hyperemia and chemosis usually occur, sometimes associated with severe pain, corneal edema, and infiltrate with subsequent decreased vision. The variability of the acute response is thought to reflect differences in the quantity of the venom injected and whether the reaction to the venom is toxic or immunologic. Rarely, more serious sequelae have been documented, including linear keratitis, hyphema, lenticular opacities, iritis, secondary glaucoma, and heterochromia.

Initial therapy with cycloplegics and topical and, occasionally, systemic steroids has been beneficial. Removal of externalized stingers may be attempted. After the acute episode, retained stingers may remain inert in the cornea for years. Tarantula hairs have also become embedded in the cornea, and these may elicit a focal inflammatory response, remain inert, or migrate.

Vegetation injuries   Ocular contact with the sap (latex) from a variety of trees has caused toxic reactions manifested by acute keratoconjunctivitis, epithelial defects, and stromal infiltration. The pencil tree and the manchineel tree, widely distributed in tropical regions, are known offenders. The dieffenbachia plant is known to cause keratoconjunctivitis associated with calcium oxalate corneal crystals. Corneal foreign bodies associated with a coconut shell, sunflower stalk, and ornamental cactus have all been documented.

Initial management for all these plant materials should include irrigation, removal of foreign bodies when possible, and administration of topical cycloplegics and corticosteroids with prophylactic antibiotic coverage as indicated by the clinical situation. Surgical removal of foreign bodies may be required in the setting of uncontrolled inflammatory response or associated secondary microbial infections.

Toxic Keratoconjunctivitis Resulting from Medications

A commonly encountered and frequently unrecognized clinical problem is that of epithelial keratopathy secondary to ocular medications and their preservatives. Topical *anesthetics* have repeatedly been shown to be toxic if given for prolonged administration. Even a single application of topical anesthetic may cause transient epithelial irregularities and edema, while prolonged use can lead to frank epithelial loss, stromal edema, infiltration, and corneal opacities. Medical personnel with easy access to anesthetics are especially susceptible to this factitious disorder.

One of the most toxic portions of these preparations is the *preservative*. The corneal epithelium and conjunctiva act as depots for these preservatives with residual amounts of preservative detected in the epithelium days after a single topical application. Benzalkonium chloride is a common preservative that has been studied extensively. Corneal application can cause severe epithelial changes with loss of microvillae, plasma membrane disruption, and subsequent cell death. Chapter X discusses toxic reactions to ophthalmic medications and other substances in greater depth.

Grant WM. *Toxicology of the Eye.* 3rd ed. Springfield, IL: Thomas; 1986.

Concussive Trauma

Conjunctival Hemorrhage

Blood under the conjunctiva creates a dramatic appearance that can alarm the patient. Most frequently, patients present with intraconjunctival or subconjunctival hemorrhage without a history of antecedent trauma. When trauma has occurred, damage to deeper structures of the eye must be ruled out. Subconjunctival hemorrhage is usually not associated with an underlying systemic disease and rarely has an identifiable cause. Occasionally, a history of vomiting, coughing, or other forms of the Valsalva maneuver can be elicited.

Most patients simply require the reassurance that things are not as bad as they appear to be. However, if a patient suffers from repeated episodes of subconjunctival hemorrhage or indicates the presence of a possible bleeding diathesis (easy bruising, frequent bloody noses) a careful medical evaluation may be warranted. Recurrent subconjunctival hemorrhages can be seen in association with systemic illness such as uncontrolled hypertension, diabetes mellitus, or a bleeding diathesis. No therapy is necessary, as the hemorrhage usually resolves spontaneously in 7–12 days. Patients should be warned that the hemorrhage may spread around the circumference of the globe before it resolves and that it may change in color from red to yellow to green during its dissolution.

Corneal Changes

Blunt trauma to the cornea can result in abrasions, edema, tears in Descemet's membrane, and corneoscleral lacerations, usually located at the limbus. Traumatic posterior annular keratopathy or traumatic corneal endothelial rings have also been described. The rings, composed of disrupted and swollen endothelial cells, are whitish gray in appearance and occur directly posterior to the traumatic impact. The last rings appear within several hours of a contusive injury and usually disappear within a few days.

Traumatic Mydriasis and Miosis

Blunt injury to the globe may result in traumatic mydriasis or, less commonly, miosis. Traumatic mydriasis is often associated with iris sphincter tears that can result in a permanent alteration of pupillary shape. Miosis tends to be associated with anterior chamber inflammation. Pupillary reactivity may be sluggish in both situations. Cycloplegia is essential to prevent formation of posterior synechiae.

Traumatic Iritis

Photophobia, tearing, and ocular pain may occur within the first 24 hours after injury. The inflammation of traumatic iritis is often associated with diminished vision and perilimbal conjunctival injection. The anterior chamber reaction can be surprisingly minimal but is usually present if carefully searched for. IOP is characteristically reduced, but it may be elevated if associated trabecular meshwork dysfunction occurs.

Treatment should consist of, at the very least, a topical cycloplegic agent to relieve patient discomfort. Prepresbyopic patients are counseled to expect a loss of near vision as a result of the paralysis of accommodation. Topical corticosteroids may be used if significant inflammation is present and compliance can be expected. Once the iritis has diminished, cycloplegia may be discontinued, and topical corticosteroids should be tapered slowly over a number of weeks to prevent a rebound iritis. Long-acting agents such as atropine 1%, homatropine 5%, or scopolamine 0.25% are administered in the office when the potential for noncompliance is significant. Rarely, traumatic iritis may be the trigger for a chronic or bilateral uveitis. See BCSC Section 9, *Intraocular Inflammation and Uveitis,* for a more detailed discussion of uveitis.

Rosenbaum JT, Tammaro J, Robertson JE Jr. Uveitis precipitated by nonpenetrating ocular trauma. *Am J Ophthalmol.* 1991;112:392–395.

Iridodialysis and Cyclodialysis

Iridodialysis　Blunt trauma may cause traumatic separation of the iris root from the ciliary body. Frequently, anterior segment hemorrhage ensues, and the iridodialysis may not be recognized until the hyphema has cleared. A small iridodialysis requires no treatment. A large dialysis may cause polycoria and monocular diplopia, necessitating later surgical repair.

Cyclodialysis　A traumatic cyclodialysis is characterized by a separation of the ciliary body from its attachment to the scleral spur, resulting in a cleft. Gonioscopically, this cleft appears at the junction of the scleral spur and the ciliary body band. Sclera may be visible through the disrupted tissue. A cyclodialysis cleft can cause increased uveoscleral outflow and aqueous hyposecretion, leading to chronic hypotony and macular edema. If treatment with topical cycloplegics does not suffice, closure may be attempted by using argon laser, diathermy, cryotherapy, or direct suturing. If repair is necessary, it should be done at the time of resolution of the hyphema.

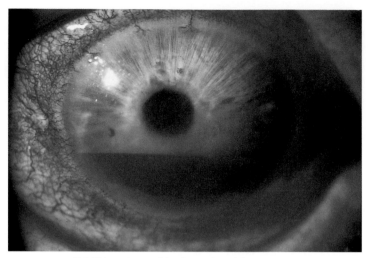
FIG XX-4—Layered hyphema from blunt trauma.

Traumatic Hyphema

Traumatic hyphema occurs most commonly in young males. It results from injury to the vessels of the peripheral iris or anterior ciliary body. Trauma causes posterior displacement of the lens–iris diaphragm and scleral expansion in the equatorial zone, which leads to disruption of the major iris arterial circle, arterial branches of the ciliary body, and/or recurrent choroidal arteries and veins. Histopathologic studies of gross hyphemas reveal a red blood cell aggregate surrounded by a pseudocapsule of fibrin/platelet coagulum.

Anterior segment bleeding can often be seen on penlight examination as a layering of blood inferiorly in the anterior chamber (Fig XX-4). At other times the bleeding is so subtle that it can be detected only as a few circulating red blood cells on slit-lamp examination (microscopic hyphema). At presentation more than 50% of hyphemas occupy less than one third of the height of the anterior chamber; fewer than 10% fill the whole chamber. The prognosis is good in patients who do not develop complications, but it is not dependent on the size of the hyphema itself. Even "eight-ball," or total, hyphemas can resolve without sequelae, unless secondary complications result (Fig XX-5). Hyphema is frequently associated with corneal abrasion, iritis, and mydriasis, as well as significant injuries to the angle structures, lens, posterior segment, and orbit.

Spontaneous hyphema is much less common and should alert the examiner to the possibility of clotting abnormalities, herpetic disease, or rubeosis iridis in adults. Juvenile xanthogranuloma, retinoblastoma, and leukemia are associated with spontaneous hyphema in children.

Rebleeding The major concern after a traumatic hyphema is rebleeding. Complications associated with secondary hemorrhage include glaucoma, optic atrophy, and corneal blood staining (Fig XX-6). The rate of rebleeding varies from 3% to 30%.

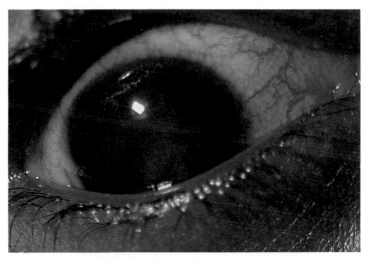

FIG XX-5—Total, or "eight-ball," hyphema.

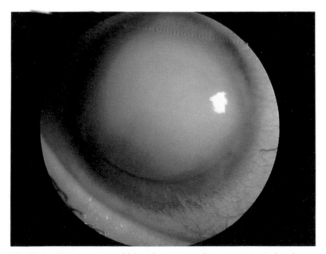

FIG XX-6—Dense corneal blood staining after a traumatic hyphema.

Rebleeding may complicate any hyphema, regardless of size, and occurs most frequently between 2 and 5 days after injury. The timing of the rebleeding may be related to the lysis and clot retraction that occurs during this period. Numerous studies have documented the importance of rebleeding as a prognostic factor for poor visual outcome.

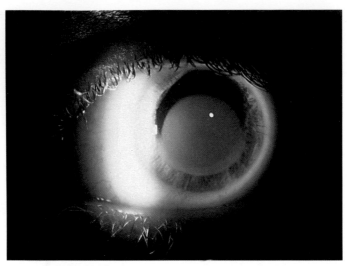

FIG XX-7—Blood staining of the cornea. Opacity consists of free hemo-globin and small amounts of hemosiderin and develops in association with large or protracted hyphemas, especially in the presence of endo-thelial dysfunction or increased intraocular pressure.

Approximately 50% of patients with rebleeding develop elevated IOP. The combination of elevated IOP, endothelial dysfunction, and anterior chamber blood predisposes the eye to corneal blood staining, which is difficult to detect when blood is in apposition to the endothelium. On slit-lamp examination, early blood staining is detected by yellow granular changes and reduced fibrillar definition to the posterior corneal stroma. Blood staining leads to a reduction in corneal transparency that may persist for years and can lead to the development of amblyopia in children. Histologically, red blood cells and their breakdown products can be seen within the corneal stroma (Fig XX-7). Corneal blood staining slowly clears in a centripetal pattern starting in the periphery.

Medical management   The overall treatment plan for traumatic hyphema should be directed at minimizing the possibility of secondary hemorrhage. Elevated IOP may require treatment in order to reduce the chances of corneal blood staining and optic atrophy. Specifics of medical management remain controversial; however, most patients are treated with the following:

□ A protective shield to the injured eye

□ Moderate restriction of physical activity

□ Elevation of the head of the bed

□ Frequent observation

Non–aspirin-containing analgesics should be used for pain relief, because aspirin has been demonstrated to increase the risk of rebleeding. Hospitalization often facilitates daily examination and is required if satisfactory home care and outpatient observation cannot be ensured.

Most ophthalmologists administer long-acting topical cycloplegic agents initially for comfort, to facilitate posterior segment evaluation, and to eliminate iris movement. Others, however, think these agents should be instituted only after the hyphema has cleared. Miotics are rarely used, because they may increase inflammation. Topical corticosteroids are of benefit in cases with significant anterior chamber inflammation. Topical β-adrenergic antagonists and carbonic anhydrase inhibitors are the mainstays of IOP control but should be used only after the patient has been checked for sickle cell trait or disease. Intravenous and oral hyperosmotic agents may be required. The administration of systemic corticosteroids has been advocated as a means of reducing the rate of rebleeding.

Prospective studies have supported the efficacy of antifibrinolytic agents in reducing the incidence of rebleeding. It is postulated that these agents act to inhibit fibrinolysis at the site of the injured blood vessel. However, the side effects of antifibrinolytic agents include nausea, vomiting, postural hypotension, muscle cramps, conjunctival suffusion, nasal stuffiness, headache, rash, pruritus, dyspnea, toxic confusional states, and arrhythmias.

Hospitalized patients may be treated with aminocaproic acid (Amicar), an oral or intravenous antifibrinolytic agent that has been recommended at an oral dose of 50 mg/kg every 4 hours for 5 days (up to 30 g/day). A recent randomized clinical trial has demonstrated a rebleeding rate of 7.1% with the use of aminocaproic acid or systemic prednisone in a series of 112 patients. Rebleeding rates in untreated patients have ranged from 20% to 33% in various studies. In predominantly white populations a significantly lower incidence of secondary hemorrhage (4.1%–5.4%) has been noted. Tranexamic acid is an antifibrinolytic agent similar to aminocaproic acid that has been used successfully to reduce the rate of rebleeding in studies performed outside the United States.

Surgery Surgery may be required to prevent corneal blood staining and optic atrophy from persistently elevated IOP. The timing of surgery is controversial, but immediate surgery is indicated at the earliest detection of blood staining. Some authors suggest that surgery may be indicated if the IOP averages greater than 25 mm Hg for 6 days when the blood is in direct apposition to the endothelium. In healthy individuals surgical intervention should be considered when the IOP is greater than 50 mm Hg despite maximal medical management. Patients with preexisting optic nerve damage or hemoglobinopathies may require earlier intervention.

Surgical techniques are multiple and varied. The simplest technique is paracentesis and anterior chamber irrigation with balanced salt solution. The goal is to remove circulated red blood cells that may be obstructing the trabecular meshwork; removal of the entire clot is neither necessary nor wise. This procedure can be repeated. Large limbal incision techniques with clot expression, if necessary, are best performed 4–7 days following initial injury when clot consolidation is at its peak. Automated cutting/aspiration instruments can be used to remove blood and clots through quite small incisions. Intraocular diathermy may also be employed to control active intraoperative bleeding. Iris damage, lens injury, and creation of additional bleeding are the major complications of surgical intervention.

Sickle cell complications When an African American patient develops a traumatic hyphema, a sickle cell work-up or, when indicated, a hemoglobin electrophoresis should be performed to evaluate the patient for the possibility of sickle cell hemoglobinopathy. Sickle cell patients and carriers of the sickle cell trait are predisposed to sickling of red blood cells in the anterior chamber. Rigid sickled cells are restricted in their outflow through the trabecular meshwork and may raise the IOP dramatically. In addition, the optic nerve appears to be at greater risk for damage in sickle cell patients, even with modest IOP elevation.

All efforts must be made to normalize IOP in these patients. Carbonic anhydrase inhibitors and osmotic agents must be used with caution, because of their tendency to reduce pH and lead to hemoconcentration, both of which may exacerbate sickling of red blood cells. Surgical intervention has been recommended if the average IOP remains 25 mm Hg or more after the first 24 hours or increases transiently and repeatedly over 30 mm Hg, despite medical intervention.

Crouch ER Jr, Williams PB, Gray MK, et al. Topical aminocaproic acid in the treatment of traumatic hyphema. *Arch Ophthalmol.* 1997;115:1106–1112.

Deutsch TA, Weinreb RN, Goldberg MF. Indications for surgical management of hyphema in patients with sickle cell trait. *Arch Ophthalmol.* 1984;102:566–569.

Fong LP. Secondary hemorrhage in traumatic hyphema. Predictive factors for selective prophylaxis. *Ophthalmology.* 1994;101:1583–1588.

Kaufman HE, Barron BA, McDonald MB, et al, eds. *The Cornea.* 2nd ed. Boston: Butterworth-Heinemann; 1997.

Kearns P. Traumatic hyphema. A retrospective study of 314 cases. *Br J Ophthalmol.* 1991;75:137–141.

Teboul BK, Jacob JL, Barsoum-Homsy M, et al. Clinical evaluation of aminocaproic acid for managing traumatic hyphema in children. *Ophthalmology.* 1995;102:1646–1653.

Volpe NJ, Larrison WI, Hersh PS, et al. Secondary hemorrhage in traumatic hyphema. *Am J Ophthalmol.* 1991;112:507–513.

Nonperforating Mechanical Trauma

Conjunctival Laceration

In managing conjunctival lacerations associated with trauma, the physician must be certain that the deeper structures of the eye have not been damaged and that no foreign body is present. It is often useful to explore the limits of a conjunctival laceration using sterile forceps or cotton-tipped applicators. The slit lamp is used following the instillation of a topical anesthetic. If any question remains as to whether the globe has been penetrated, consideration must be given to performing a peritomy in the operating room to better explore and examine the injured area. In general, conjunctival lacerations do not need to be sutured.

Conjunctival Foreign Body

Foreign bodies on the conjunctival surface are best recognized with slit-lamp examination. Foreign bodies can lodge in the inferior cul-de-sac or can be located on the conjunctival surface under the upper eyelid (Fig XX-8). It is imperative to evert the upper eyelid to examine the superior tarsal plate and eyelid margin in all patients with a history that suggests a foreign body. If several foreign bodies are suspected or particulate matter is present, double eversion of the eyelid with a Desmarres retractor or a bent paper clip is advised to allow the examiner to effectively search the entire arc of the superior cul-de-sac (Fig XX-9).

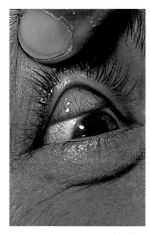

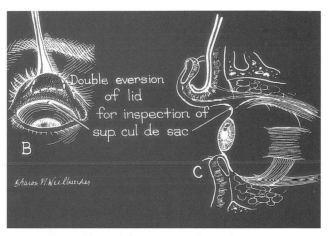

FIG XX-8—Foreign bodies seen on the everted surface of the upper eyelid.

FIG XX-9—Double eyelid eversion with a Desmarres retractor. (Reproduced with permission from Deutsch TA, Fellen DB. *Paton and Goldberg's Management of Ocular Injuries.* 2nd ed. Philadelphia: Saunders; 1985.)

Following eversion of the upper eyelid, copious irrigation should be used to cleanse the fornix. This procedure should then be repeated using a Desmarres retractor for the upper and lower eyelids. Glass particles, cactus spines, or insect hairs are often difficult to see, but a careful search of the cul-de-sac with high magnification aids in isolation and removal. Using slit-lamp magnification, the clinician can use a moistened cotton-tipped applicator to gently remove superficial foreign material. Occasionally, saline lavage of the cornea or cul-de-sac washes out debris that is not embedded in tissue.

When a patient complains of foreign body sensation, topical fluorescein should be instilled to check for the fine, linear vertical corneal abrasions that are characteristic of retained foreign bodies on the eyelid margin or superior tarsal plate. If such vertical lines are noted, their source must be identified, as these lines are a fairly specific localizing sign. Foreign matter embedded in tissue is removed with a sterile, disposable hypodermic needle. Glass or particulate matter may be removed with a fine-tipped jeweler's forceps or blunt spatula. If a foreign body is suspected but not seen, the cul-de-sac should be irrigated and wiped with a moistened cotton-tipped applicator.

Corneal Foreign Body

Corneal foreign bodies are identified most effectively during slit-lamp examination. Prior to removing the corneal foreign body, the clinician should assess the depth of corneal penetration. If anterior chamber extension is present or suspected, the foreign body should be removed in a sterile, operating-room environment with sufficient microscopic magnification and coaxial illumination, adequate anesthesia, and appropriate instruments. Overly aggressive attempts to remove deeply embedded foreign bodies at the slit lamp may be rewarded with the leakage of aqueous humor.

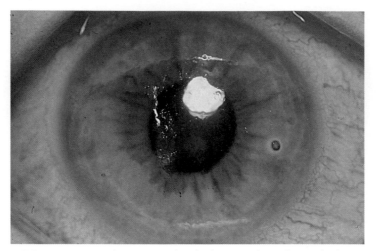

FIG XX-10—Corneal rust ring and multiple retained iron foreign bodies.

If such a leak occurs and cannot be adequately tamponaded with a therapeutic bandage contact lens, tissue adhesive and/or urgent surgical repair is required.

If several glass foreign bodies are present, all of the exposed fragments should be removed. Fragments that are deeply embedded in the cornea are often inert and can be left in place. Careful gonioscopic evaluation of the anterior chamber is essential to ensure that the iris and the angle are free of any retained glass particles.

When an iron foreign body has been embedded in the cornea for more than a few hours, an orange-brown "rust ring" results (Fig XX-10). Corneal iron foreign bodies can usually be removed at the slit lamp under topical anesthesia with a disposable hypodermic needle. The rust ring can be removed with a battery-powered dental burr inserted with a sterile tip. It is advisable to remove as much metallic material as possible, as material left in the cornea may lead to persistent epithelial defects and poor healing secondary to chronic, smoldering inflammation. Corneal perforation is a rare complication of foreign body removal.

Therapy following the removal of a corneal foreign body includes topical antibiotics, cycloplegia, and the application of a firm pressure patch. Reexamination the following day is usually indicated. If the residual corneal abrasion does not heal or if additional curettage is needed to remove a rust ring, cycloplegic and antibiotic drops are again instilled prior to reapplication of a new pressure patch.

Corneal Abrasion

Corneal abrasions are usually associated with immediate pain, foreign body sensation, tearing, and discomfort with blinking. Abrasions may be caused by contact with a finger, fingernail, fist, or even the edge of a piece of paper. The abrasion can also be caused by a propelled foreign body or by contact lens wear, either because of improper fit or excessive wear. On occasion a patient may not recall a definite history of trauma but still presents with signs and symptoms suggestive of a corneal abrasion. Herpes simplex virus keratitis must be excluded as a possible diagnosis in such cases.

A slit-lamp examination is essential to determine the presence, extent, and depth of the corneal defect. It is very important to make a distinction between a "clean" corneal abrasion, which generally has sharply defined edges and little to no associated inflammation (when seen acutely), versus a true corneal ulcer. Foreign body sensation is an exceedingly specific localizing symptom for a corneal epithelial defect.

Patching may not be necessary for small, superficial abrasions, as the primary indication for pressure patching is to relieve discomfort, but patches prevent eyelid movement from continually abrading the denuded surface. Many patients find patches uncomfortable, and a decision as to whether a given patient will be more uncomfortable from the abrasion or from the patch must be made by the clinician. Many small abrasions can be managed with antibiotic drops or ointment alone. Extensive corneal abrasions usually require topical antibiotics, cycloplegics, and pressure patching. Abrasions caused by organic material require closer follow-up to monitor for infection.

As shown in Figure XX-9, it is essential to evert the upper eyelid and examine the superior cul-de-sac to rule out a retained foreign body. In some cases therapeutic bandage soft contact lenses can be used in lieu of pressure patching. However, the decision to use these lenses must be weighed against the possibility of other related complications, such as secondary infection or tight lens syndrome. The use of collagen shields has been advocated for this purpose, as they dissolve over a 12–72 hour period, but many abrasion patients find these lenses too uncomfortable to tolerate. Patients with contact lens–associated epithelial defects should never be patched, because of the possibility of promoting a secondary infection. These patients should be treated with topical antibiotic drops or ointment.

Posttraumatic Recurrent Corneal Erosion

A corneal abrasion can precipitate future recurrent corneal erosions. Chapter VI discusses the treatment of recurrent corneal erosions in detail. This condition may present with symptoms of foreign body sensation with intense pain, tearing, and discomfort, most frequently in the early morning hours or upon awakening. Corneal erosions can occur weeks, months, or years after the initial injury. They develop when the corneal epithelium fails to bind adequately to the basement membrane during the healing process. The loose epithelial cells are dislodged when the patient opens the eyelids upon awakening. These patients show corneal epithelial pooling in the area of the previous corneal abrasion on examination. Occasionally, only subtle epithelial irregularities are present in the involved area. When precipitated by injury, the disease is usually unilateral and occurs in the same corneal area.

Perforating Trauma

It is important to differentiate a *penetrating* wound from a *perforating* wound. A penetrating wound passes *into* a structure; a perforating wound passes *through* a structure. For example, an object that passes through the cornea and lodges in the anterior chamber perforates the cornea but penetrates the eye.

Evaluation

History   If a patient presents with both eye and systemic trauma, diagnosis and treatment of any life-threatening injury takes precedence over evaluation and management of the ophthalmic injury. Once the patient is medically stable, the ophthalmologist should then elicit a complete presurgical history (Table XX-1). Even though the diagnosis of perforating injury in many cases may be obvious from casual eye examination, a detailed history of the nature of the injury should include questions about factors known to predispose to ocular penetration, so that this diagnosis will not be overlooked in more subtle cases. Such factors include

- Metal on metal strike
- High-velocity projectile
- High-energy impact on globe
- Sharp injuring object
- Lack of eye protection

Examination   Evaluation of the patient with suspected perforating injury to the eye should include a complete general and ophthalmologic examination. As soon as possible, the examiner should make a determination of visual acuity, which is the

TABLE XX-1

PENETRATING OCULAR INJURY HISTORY

Nature of injury
  Concomitant life-threatening injury
  Time and circumstances of injury
  Suspected composition of intraocular foreign body
  (brass, copper, iron, vegetable, soil-contaminated)
  Use of eye protection
  Prior treatment of injury

Past ocular history
  Refractive history
  Eye diseases
  Current eye medications
  Previous surgery

Medical history
  Diagnoses
  Current medications
  Drug allergies
  Risk factors for HIV/hepatitis
  Currency of tetanus prophylaxis
  Previous surgery
  Recent food ingestion

TABLE XX-2

OCULAR SIGNS OF PENETRATING TRAUMA

SUGGESTIVE	DIAGNOSTIC
Deep eyelid laceration	Exposed uvea, vitreous, retina
Orbital chemosis	Positive Seidel test
Conjunctival laceration/hemorrhage	Visualization of intraocular foreign body
Focal iris–corneal adhesion	Intraocular foreign body seen on x-ray
Shallow anterior chamber	or ultrasonography
Iris defect	
Hypotony	
Lens capsule defect	
Acute lens opacity	
Retinal tear/hemorrhage	

most reliable predictor of final visual acuity in traumatized eyes. Unfortunately, this part of the examination may be omitted by busy emergency room staff, so the ophthalmologist must both check the visual acuity and help educate nonophthalmic practitioners about its importance. The ophthalmologist should then look for key signs that are suggestive or diagnostic of perforating ocular injury (Table XX-2).

If a significant perforating injury is suspected, forced duction testing, gonioscopy, tonometry, and scleral depression should be avoided. Ancillary tests that may be useful in this setting are summarized in Table XX-3. Regardless of the results of laboratory tests, all cases should be managed with safeguards appropriate for patients known to have HIV infection or hepatitis (universal precautions).

TABLE XX-3

ANCILLARY TESTS IN PENETRATING EYE TRAUMA

Useful in many cases
    CT scan
    Plain-film x-rays
    CBC, differential, platelets
    Electrolytes, blood urea nitrogen, creatinine
    Test for HIV status, hepatitis

Useful in selected cases
    MRI (especially in cases of suspected organic foreign objects in the eye or orbit; but this should never be used if a metallic foreign object is suspected)
    Prothrombin time, partial thromboplastin time, bleeding time
    Sickle cell
    Drug and/or ethanol levels

Management

Preoperative management   If surgical repair is required, the timing of the operation is crucial. While studies have not documented any disadvantage in delaying the repair of an open globe for up to 36 hours, intervention ideally should occur as soon as possible. Prompt repair can help minimize numerous complications:

□ Pain

□ Prolapse of intraocular structures

□ Microbial contamination of the wound

□ Proliferation of the microbes projected into the eye

□ Migration of epithelium into the wound

□ Intraocular inflammation

□ Lens opacity

In a late-night or weekend injury these concerns must be balanced against the benefits of keeping the patient NPO, having a well-rested surgeon, and using experienced ophthalmic operating room staff during regular hours.

The deleterious effects of a small delay in repair can be offset by many steps that can be taken during the preoperative period (Table XX-4). Injuries with soil-contaminated, retained intraocular foreign bodies require attention to the risk of *Bacillus* endophthalmitis. Because this organism can destroy the eye within 24 hours, intravenous and/or intravitreal therapy should be considered with an antibiotic effective against *Bacillus* species, usually clindamycin or vancomycin. Surgical repair should be undertaken with minimal delay in cases at risk for contamination with this organism.

Nonsurgical options   Some penetrating injuries are so minimal that they spontaneously seal prior to ophthalmic examination, with no intraocular damage, prolapse, or adherence. These cases may require only systemic and/or topical antibiotic therapy along with close observation. If a corneal wound is leaking (Fig XX-11),

TABLE XX-4

PREOPERATIVE MANAGEMENT OF PENETRATING EYE TRAUMA

Protective shield
Avoid topical medications
NPO
Sedation
Pain control
Antiemesis
Facial nerve block to reduce eyelid squeezing
External eye cultures
Intravenous antibiotics (such as tobramycin with either clindamycin or vancomycin)
Tetanus prophylaxis
Anesthesia consultation

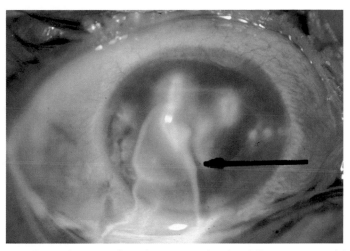

FIG XX-11—Leakage of aqueous from the anterior chamber following a corneal laceration. Concentrated fluorescein on the edge of the aqueous rivulet (Seidel test) indicates an active flow of fluid from a leaking anterior chamber.

but the chamber remains formed, the clinician can attempt to seal the leak with pharmacologic suppression of aqueous production (topical or systemic), patching, and/or a therapeutic contact lens. Generally, if these measures fail to seal the wound in 3 days, closure with cyanoacrylate glue or sutures is recommended. Although cyanoacrylate tissue adhesives are not approved by the Food and Drug Administration (FDA) for use in the eye, they have been used extensively over the past two decades to seal perforations. Several glues are available, such as Histocryl and Bucrylate. A therapeutic contact lens must be used after application of glue, since polymerization of the glue produces a rough surface that abrades the palpebral conjunctiva.

Surgical repair Obviously, great internal damage to the eye can occur with even a small, seemingly insignificant wound. The management of a typical corneoscleral laceration with uveal prolapse generally requires surgery (Fig XX-12). The primary goal of initial surgical repair of a corneoscleral laceration is to restore the integrity of the globe. The secondary goal, which may be accomplished at the time of the primary repair or during subsequent procedures, is to restore vision through repair of both external and internal damage to the eye.

If the prognosis for vision in the injured eye is hopeless and the patient is at risk for sympathetic ophthalmia, enucleation must be considered. Primary enucleation should be used only in a devastating injury so severe that restoration of the anatomy is impossible, when it may spare the patient another procedure. In the overwhelming majority of cases, however, the advantages of delaying enucleation for a few days far outweigh any advantage of primary enucleation. This delay, which should not

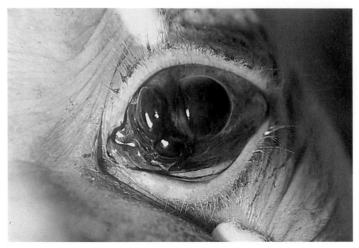

FIG XX-12—Rupture of globe secondary to blunt trauma.

exceed the 14 days thought necessary for an injured eye to incite sympathetic ophthalmia, allows for assessment of postoperative visual function, vitreoretinal or ophthalmic plastic consultation, and stabilization of the patient's medical condition. Most important, delay in enucleation following unsuccessful repair and loss of light perception allows the patient time to acknowledge that loss and accompanying disfigurement and to consider enucleation in a nonemergency setting.

Anesthesia. General anesthesia is almost always required for repair of an open globe, because retrobulbar or peribulbar anesthetic injection increases orbital pressure, which may cause or exacerbate the extrusion of intraocular contents. A nondepolarizing muscle relaxant is preferred, because of the theoretical possibility that cocontraction of the extraocular contents may occur. After the surgical repair is complete, a periocular anesthetic injection may be used to control postoperative pain.

Steps in the repair of a corneoscleral laceration. All attempts at repair of a corneoscleral laceration should be performed in the operating room with use of the operating microscope and trained ophthalmic personnel. Table XX-5 summarizes the basic steps to restore the integrity of the globe with a corneoscleral laceration. No attempt should be made to fixate an open globe with rectus muscle sutures. Because eyelid surgery may put pressure on an open globe and because certain eyelid lacerations may actually improve globe exposure, repair of adnexal injury should follow repair of the globe itself.

The corneal component of the injury is approached first. If vitreous or lens fragments have prolapsed through the wound, these should be cut flush with the cornea, taking care not to exert traction on the vitreous or zonular fibers. If uvea or retina (seen as translucent, tan tissue with extremely fine vessels) protrudes, it should be reposited using a gentle sweeping technique through a separate limbal incision, with

TABLE XX-5

ESSENTIAL STEPS IN THE SURGICAL REPAIR
OF A CORNEOSCLERAL LACERATION

General anesthesia

Excision of anteriorly prolapsed vitreous, lens fragments, transcorneal foreign bodies

Reposition of anteriorly prolapsed uvea, retina

Closure of corneal component of laceration at limbus, landmarks

Completion of watertight corneal closure (10-0 nylon)

Peritomy as necessary for exposure of scleral component

Stepwise excision of posteriorly prolapsed vitreous

Stepwise reposition of posteriorly prolapsed uvea, retina

Stepwise closure of scleral component (9-0 nylon or 8-0 silk)

Conjunctival closure

Subconjunctival antibiotics, steroids

the assistance of viscoelastic injection to temporarily re-form the anterior chamber (Fig XX-13). If epithelium has obviously migrated onto a uveal surface or into the wound, an effort should be made to peel this tissue off. Only in cases of frankly necrotic uveal prolapse should uveal tissue be excised.

Points at which the laceration crosses landmarks such as the limbus are then closed with 10–0 nylon suture, followed by closure of the remaining corneal components of the laceration. It may be necessary to reposit iris tissue repeatedly after each suture is placed to avoid entrapment of iris in the wound. Despite these efforts, uvea may still remain apposed to the posterior corneal surface. Many surgeons place very shallow sutures at this stage of the closure, in order to avoid impaling uvea with the suture needle. Then, after the closure is watertight, the uvea can be definitively separated from the cornea with viscoelastic injection, followed by replacement of shallow sutures with new ones of ideal, near-full-thickness depth (Fig XX-14). Suture knots should be buried in the corneal stroma, not in the wound.

When watertight closure of the wound proves difficult to obtain, because of unusual laceration configuration or loss of tissue, X-shaped sutures or other customized (ad hoc) techniques may suffice. Cyanoacrylate glue or even primary penetrating keratoplasty may be required in extremely difficult cases. A conjunctival flap should not be used to treat a wound leak.

The scleral component of the laceration is then approached with gentle peritomy and conjunctival separation only as necessary to expose the wound. Prolapsed vitreous is excised, and prolapsed nonnecrotic uvea and retina are reposited with a spatula or similar instrument. The scleral wound is closed with 9-0 nylon or 8-0 silk suture. Often, dissection of Tenon's capsule and management of prolapsed tissue must be repeated incrementally after each suture is placed.

Some posterior wounds are more easily approached with loupes and a headlight, since the open globe does not need to be rotated as far. If the laceration extends under an extraocular muscle, the muscle may be resected at its insertion and

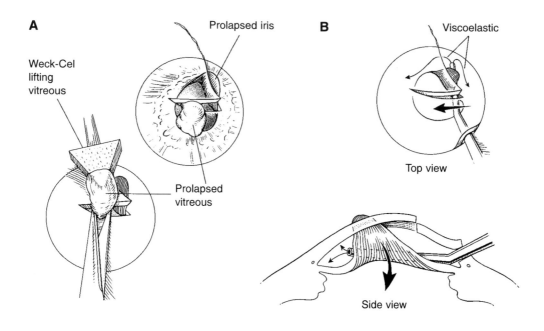

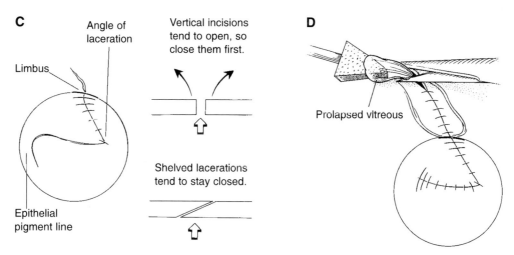

FIG XX-13—Restoring anatomic relationships in corneoscleral laceration repair. *A*, Prolapsed vitreous or lens fragments are excised. *B*, Iris is reposited by means of viscoelastic and a cannula inserted through a separate paracentesis. *C*, Landmarks such as limbus, laceration angles, or epithelial pigment lines are closed. Vertical lacerations are closed first to create a watertight globe more quickly, followed by shelved lacerations. *D*, The scleral part of the wound is exposed, prolapsed vitreous is severed, and the wound is closed from the limbus, working posteriorly. (Reproduced with permission from Hamill MB. Repair of the traumatized anterior segment. In: *Focal Points: Clinical Modules for Ophthalmologists.* San Francisco: American Academy of Ophthalmology; 1992;10:1. Illustrations by Christine Gralapp.)

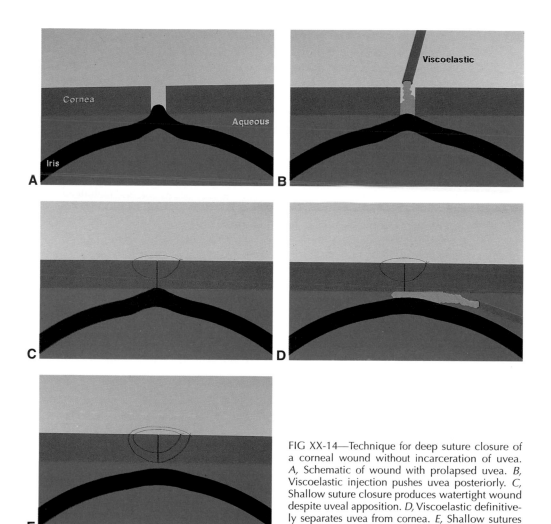

FIG XX-14—Technique for deep suture closure of a corneal wound without incarceration of uvea. *A*, Schematic of wound with prolapsed uvea. *B*, Viscoelastic injection pushes uvea posteriorly. *C*, Shallow suture closure produces watertight wound despite uveal apposition. *D*, Viscoelastic definitively separates uvea from cornea. *E*, Shallow sutures are replaced with deep ones.

reinserted following repair. Closure of the laceration should continue posteriorly only to the point at which it becomes technically difficult or requires undue pressure on the globe. Very posterior lacerations benefit from effective physiologic tamponade by orbital tissue and are best left alone.

Once the globe is watertight, a decision must be made as to whether intraocular surgery (if necessary) should be attempted immediately or postponed. Subconjunctival injections of antibiotics to cover both gram-positive and -negative organisms are given prophylactically at the conclusion of primary repair. Intravitreal antibiotics such as vancomycin 1 mg and amikacin 200 μg may be used after contaminated wounds involving the vitreous.

Secondary repair of intraocular trauma. Following primary repair of a corneoscleral laceration the following secondary measures may be indicated:

☐ Removal of intraocular foreign bodies

☐ Iris repair

☐ Cataract extraction

☐ Mechanical vitrectomy

☐ Intraocular lens (IOL) insertion

☐ Cryotherapy of retinal tears

Deciding whether to pursue such intervention at the time of initial repair is a complex process. The expertise of the surgeon; the adequacy of the facility, technical equipment, and instruments; the adequacy of the view of the anterior segment structures; and issues of informed consent should be considered.

For example, the average anterior segment surgeon should not attempt automated vitrectomy with retina present in the anterior chamber, and even the most expert cataract surgeon may not attempt a lens extraction with no view of the lens. On the other hand, opacity of a damaged lens may increase, intraocular inflammation may worsen, opportunity for placement of an IOL in the capsular bag may be lost, and the patient may experience increased pain and expense if these procedures are delayed.

As always, the welfare of the patient should determine the proper course. In general, if a foreign body is visible in the anterior segment and can be grasped, it is reasonable to remove it, either through the wound or through a separate limbal incision. If removal of opacified lens material is attempted, it is helpful to know if the posterior capsule has been violated and lens–vitreous admixture has occurred. BCSC Section 11, *Lens and Cataract,* also discusses the issues of cataract surgery and IOL placement following trauma to the eye.

Sometimes the leaflets of a damaged anterior capsule can be manipulated to form a partial or complete circular capsulorrhexis, which will facilitate placement of an IOL in the bag. If the posterior capsule is ruptured, a capsulorrhexis allows more stable ciliary sulcus fixation of an IOL. In the older patient a firm nucleus may be extracted with a lens loop or emulsified, but it probably should not be extracted with pressure on the globe. However, the soft lens material of the average young eye trauma patient is most easily removed using a mechanical vitrector in the aspiration mode, cutting only when vitreous is encountered.

The primary surgical goal is to remove all lens cortical and nuclear material as well as vitreous in the anterior segment, preserving as much lens capsule and zonular support as possible, all without causing additional vitreous traction. If a reasonable refractive history has indicated similarity between the two eyes, and the axial length and keratometry of the fellow eye are known, primary placement of an IOL should be considered. If adequate capsular support is present, placement within the capsular bag is preferred to sulcus fixation. Most surgeons prefer not to place an anterior chamber IOL in these typically young patients.

Iris repair can be undertaken either primarily or secondarily. Closure of iris lacerations not only may restore iris function and improve vision, but it also tends to keep the iris in its proper plane, decreasing the formation of anterior or posterior synechiae. The McCannel technique using 10-0 polypropylene suture requires only

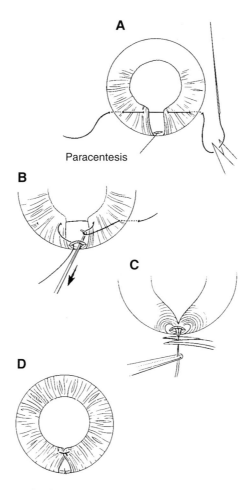

Paracentesis

FIG XX-15—The McCannel technique for repairing iris lacerations. With large lacerations, multiple sutures may be used. *A,* A limbal paracentesis is made over the iris discontinuity. Then a long Drews needle with 10-0 polypropylene is passed through the peripheral cornea, the edges of the iris, and the peripheral cornea opposite, and the suture is cut. *B,* A Sinskey hook, introduced through the paracentesis and around the suture peripherally, is drawn back out through the paracentesis. *C,* The suture is securely tied. *D,* After the suture is secure, it is cut, and the iris is allowed to retract. (Reproduced with permission from Hamill MB. Repair of the traumatized anterior segment. In: *Focal Points: Clinical Modules for Ophthalmologists.* San Francisco: American Academy of Ophthalmology; 1992;10:1. Illustrations by Christine Gralapp.)

a small additional limbal incision to be made (Fig XX-15). Iridodialysis, usually resulting from blunt trauma, may cause monocular diplopia and an eccentric pupil if left untreated. The McCannel technique can also be used to repair iridodialysis (Fig XX-16). In the event that corneal opacity prevents safe repair of internal ocular injury, repairs can be combined later with penetrating keratoplasty or with placement of a temporary keratoprosthesis, if posterior segment repair is planned.

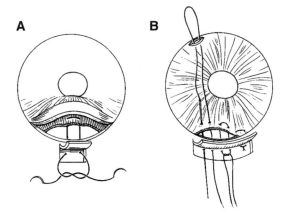

FIG XX-16—Repair of iridodialysis. *A*, A cataract surgery–type incision is made at the site of iridodialysis or iris disinsertion. A double-armed, 10-0 polypropylene suture is passed through the iris root, out through the angle, and tied on the surface of the globe under a partial-thickness scleral flap. The corneoscleral wound is then closed with 10-0 nylon sutures. *B*, In an alternative technique, multiple 10-0 Prolene sutures on double-armed Drews needles are passed through a paracentesis opposite the site of iris disinsertion to avoid the need to create a large corneoscleral entry wound. (Reproduced with permission from Hamill MB. Repair of the traumatized anterior segment. In: *Focal Points: Clinical Modules for Ophthalmologists.* San Francisco: American Academy of Ophthalmology; 1992;10:1. Illustrations by Christine Gralapp.)

Postoperative management   After repair of penetrating anterior segment trauma, therapy is directed at prevention of infection, suppression of inflammation, control of IOP, and relief of pain. Intravenous antibiotics are usually continued for 3–5 days, and topical antibiotics are generally used for about 7 days. Topical corticosteroids and cycloplegics are tapered off, depending on the degree of inflammation. A massive fibrinous response may respond well to a short course of systemic prednisone.

Corneal sutures that do not loosen spontaneously are generally left in place for at least 3 months and then removed incrementally over the next few months. Fibrosis and vascularization are indicators that enough healing has occurred to render suture removal safe.

These traumatized eyes are at increased risk of retinal detachment, so frequent examination of the posterior segment is mandatory. If media opacity precludes an adequate fundus examination, evaluation for an afferent pupillary defect and B-scan ultrasonography are helpful in monitoring retinal status.

Refraction and correction with contact lenses or spectacles can proceed when the ocular surface and media permit. Because of the risk of amblyopia in a child or loss of fusion in an adult, visual rehabilitation should not be unnecessarily delayed.

Barr CC. Prognostic factors in corneoscleral lacerations. *Arch Ophthalmol.* 1983;101: 919–924.

Catalana RA, ed. *Ocular Emergencies*. Philadelphia: Saunders; 1992.

Hamill MB. Repair of the traumatized anterior segment. In: *Focal Points: Clinical Modules for Ophthalmologists*. San Francisco: American Academy of Ophthalmology; 1992;10:1.

Kenyon KR, Starck T, Hersh PS. Anterior segment reconstruction after trauma. In: Brightbill FS, ed. *Corneal Surgery: Theory, Technique, and Tissue*. 2nd ed. St Louis: Mosby; 1993:352–359.

Lin DT, Webster RG Jr, Abbott RL. Repair of corneal lacerations and perforations. *Int Ophthalmol Clin*. 1988;28:69–75.

Shingleton BJ, Hersh PS, Kenyon KR, eds. *Eye Trauma*. St Louis: Mosby; 1991.

Spoor TC. *An Atlas of Ophthalmic Trauma*. London: Martin Dunitz; 1997.

Surgical Trauma

Epithelial Changes from Intraocular Surgery

The corneal epithelium functions as a barrier to corneal absorption of fluid from tears, including medication instilled topically, and pathogens residing on the ocular surface. A breakdown of the epithelial barrier function, resulting in epithelial edema and stromal swelling, can follow any of these surgical missteps:

- Inadvertent intraoperative trauma to the epithelium by the surgical instruments
- Dessication of the epithelium through inadequate intraoperative hydration
- Toxic keratopathy resulting from excessive preoperative instillation of topical ophthalmic preparations (and their preservatives)
- Accidental instillation of preoperative periocular facial scrub detergents

While epithelial damage permits fluid to reach the stroma, it is resisted by the intraocular pressure and pumped out by the endothelium. Therefore, endothelial damage has a far greater effect on corneal edema than does epithelial damage. Intraoperative damage to the corneal endothelium and/or Descemet's membrane can result in a positive stromal fluid pressure and subsequent epithelial edema. Epithelial edema begins in the basal cell layers of the epithelium, then spreads through the epithelium, occasionally resulting in subepithelial bullae.

The transparency of the corneal epithelium is a result of the homogeneity of the refractive index throughout the epithelium. When epithelial edema occurs, this layer loses its homogeneity and the corneal surface becomes irregular. This surface irregularity causes symptoms of glare, photophobia, and haloes around lights from light scattering. Vision is often reduced. In bright light edematous epithelium causes more light scattering and can have a marked effect on vision. Surface irregularities caused by epithelial edema are more damaging to vision than stromal edema or scarring. Often the influence of epithelial surface irregularities on visual acuity is underestimated, whereas the role of stromal scarring and edema is overestimated.

Descemet's Membrane Changes During Intraocular Surgery

The distensibility of Descemet's membrane permits stretching, or distortion, followed by return to its original shape. When the stroma imbibes fluid and thickens, the increased volume is distributed posteriorly, producing bowing and folding of

Descemet's membrane (striate keratopathy). Detachment of Descemet's membrane can occur when an instrument or intraocular lens is introduced through the surgical incision or when fluid is inadvertently injected between Descemet's membrane and the corneal stroma, resulting in stromal swelling and epithelial bullae localized in the area of detachment. Detachments can be reattached with air tamponade or nonexpansile concentrations of sulfur hexafluoride (SF_6) in the anterior chamber. Recurrence may require suturing after replacement of Descemet's membrane.

Endothelial Changes from Intraocular Surgery

Aphakic and pseudophakic corneal edema   Corneal hydration involves the following factors:

- Stromal swelling pressure
- Barrier function of the epithelium and endothelium
- The endothelial pump
- Evaporation from the corneal surface
- Intraocular pressure

Causes of corneal edema following surgical procedures are often multifactorial—related to the health of the patient's endothelium as well as to iatrogenic factors such as surgical technique, duration of surgery, and intraocular irrigating solutions.

Any decompression operation may result in corneal edema. Patients with underlying corneal endothelial dysfunction such as Fuchs corneal dystrophy are at risk to develop postoperative corneal edema, even after smooth, atraumatic surgery.

Manipulation of instuments in the eye through a limbal or clear corneal incision during cataract surgery can compromise the functional reserve of an already partially compromised endothelium, leading to localized edema at the site. During phacoemulsification, heat transferred from the probe to the cornea can result in stromal shrinkage. A wound that is too tight to allow adequate irrigation fluid flow through the probe or the occlusion of irrigation or aspiration tubing can cause such heat transfer. A phaco tip held too close to corneal endothelium during surgery allows the ultrasonic energy to injure and cause loss of endothelial cells. Corneal edema in these cases may appear on the first postoperative day or months to years after surgery.

Uncomplicated intracapsular cataract extraction or complicated extracapsular cataract extraction may result in vitreous touch to the corneal endothelium. Persistent corneal edema can occur in the region of vitreocorneal adherence either early or late. Early recognition and treatment with anterior vitrectomy as soon as corneal edema develops can help prevent irreversible corneal edema. More advanced cases with prolonged corneal edema may require a penetrating keratoplasty combined with vitrectomy.

Current irrigating solutions are superior to those used in the past. They are pH balanced with bicarbonate buffers, have no epinephrine, and contain glutathione. Endothelial cell loss rates of 8% or less have been reported in multiple series. Preserved solutions either irrigated into or inadvertently injected into the anterior chamber can be toxic to the corneal endothelium and cause temporary or permanent corneal edema. Subconjunctival antibiotic injections have been reported to enter the anterior chamber through scleral tunnel incisions acting as one-way valves.

The presence of IOLs such as iris-fixated or closed-loop flexible anterior chamber lenses has historically been associated with significant chronic corneal edema and development of pseudophakic bullous keratopathy. Reduced visual acuity, foreign body sensation, photophobia, epiphora, and occasional infectious keratitis are usually associated.

Laser burns Endothelial damage occurs following argon laser procedures. Endothelial burns are usually dense white with sharp margins and result from the thermal effects of iris photocoagulation. They may result in focal endothelial cell loss. An increase in mean endothelial cell size and endothelial cell loss associated with the use of greater laser power has also been reported. In follow-up periods of up to 1 year the endothelial cell loss following laser iridectomy has not been found to be statistically significant, however.

PART 10

SURGERY OF THE OCULAR SURFACE

CHAPTER XXI

Introduction to Surgery of the Ocular Surface

The term *ocular surface* describes the entire epithelial surface of the external eye, encompassing the corneal epithelium as well as the bulbar and palpebral conjunctival epithelium. Initially, the ocular surface was considered solely an anatomic classification that recognized the physical continuity of the stratified nonkeratinizing epithelium of the conjunctiva, limbus, and cornea. More recently, clinical and research insights have offered compelling evidence of important functional relationships within this anatomic entity. This rethinking of the ocular surface as a functional unit has stimulated a complete reorganization of the current approach to the management of ocular surface disease (Table XXI-1).

TABLE XXI-1

INDICATIONS FOR OCULAR SURFACE RECONSTRUCTION

CONJUNCTIVAL AUTOGRAFT	LIMBAL AUTOGRAFT OR ALLOGRAFT*	MUCOUS MEMBRANE OR AMNIOTIC MEMBRANE† TRANSPLANTATION
Recurrent pterygium	Chemical injury (acute and chronic)	Fornix reconstruction (bilateral)
Cicatricial strabismus (bilateral)	Thermal burn (acute and chronic)	Chemical injury‡
Fornix reconstruction (unilateral)	Contact lens keratopathy	
Postexcision of conjunctival tumor	Persistent epithelial defect (various etiologies)	
	Post–multiple surgery limbal depletion	
	Chronic medication toxicity	
	Stevens-Johnson syndrome	
	Ocular cicatricial pemphigoid	
	Aniridia	
	Atopy	

*Limbal autograft preferable in unilateral or asymmetric cases; limbal allograft reserved for bilateral cases.
†May be used in conjunction with limbal autograft or allograft.
‡Indicated for fornix reconstruction after cicatricization.

Corneal and Conjunctival Epithelial Wound Healing

The mechanisms of wound healing of the corneal stroma and sclera have been covered in chapter XIX. Observations of the normal replacement process of corneal epithelium provide valuable insights into the rationale for various ocular surface replacement techniques. Numerous studies have demonstrated that central corneal epithelial mass is maintained by continued centripetal movement of peripheral corneal epithelium toward the visual axis, as well as by anterior movement from the basal epithelial cells.

Role of Stem Cells

Since the corneal epithelium is a highly differentiated cell type with rapid self-renewal, its stem cells are essential for epithelial replacement and migration. The limbal basal layer contains the stem cells of the corneal epithelium that are the most qualified cells to repopulate and differentiate into normal corneal epithelium after severe injuries (e.g., chemical) accompanied by extensive loss of corneal epithelium. These are the cells that must be available and responsive to the need for epithelial replacement and migration.

Conjunctival Epithelium

Healthy conjunctival epithelium also has the ability to replace directly damaged corneal epithelium and possibly to maintain normal corneal epithelium. Following complete traumatic loss of corneal and limbal epithelium, the remaining conjunctival epithelium resurfaces corneal epithelium by an advancing wave of adjacent conjunctiva. *Conjunctival transdifferentiation* is the process by which the normal phenotype of conjunctival epithelium—columnar epithelium with numerous goblet cells—transforms to normal stratified squamous corneal epithelium without goblet cells. This process implies that the normal conjunctival epithelium retains the capability of phenotypic change to that of corneal epithelium. Such epithelial differentiation involves not only morphological change but the acquisition of the biochemical and physiologic properties of corneal epithelium as well.

Maintenance of the Ocular Surface and its Response to Wound Healing

In the mechanically abraded cornea (e.g., total epithelial debridement during vitrectomy surgery) reepithelialization and restoration of a relatively normal corneal surface usually occur. In chemically injured eyes, however, the new corneal epithelium often maintains conjunctival characteristics, with goblet cells and neovascularization, suggesting that the regulatory processes controlling proper differentiation are abnormal. Based on these observations, autologous conjunctival transplantation has been used for resurfacing the unilateral or asymmetrically chemically injured eye. The success of this procedure is contingent on the ability of the transplanted conjunctival epithelium to migrate across the stromal tissue of the recipient eye, to adhere firmly, and to assume and maintain the biochemical and morphological features of normal corneal epithelium (conjunctival transdifferentiation).

If the goal of surgery is the restoration of a more functional conjunctival mucosal surface, as in bilateral conjunctival cicatricial disorders, a buccal mucosal graft or amniotic membrane may be employed. This procedure is used to restore more normal forniceal architecture and to diminish ocular surface inflammation and corneal damage resulting from abnormal eyelid–globe relationships (e.g., entropion, trichiasis), chronic exposure (lagophthalmos), and direct corneal trauma (palpebral conjunctival keratinization). In advanced cases complications caused by recurrent corneal epithelial breakdown, secondary infectious keratitis, vascularization, and scarring may lead to corneal blindness.

Mucosal membrane grafting is not, however, effective in repopulating the cornea with normal stem cells directly and normalizing a better corneal epithelial surface. Rather, it improves ocular surface wetting by narrowing the palpebral fissure, thereby reducing exposure and evaporation, and by enhancing eyelid movement and distribution of the tear film over the cornea. Preserved amniotic membrane is another tissue that can be used for ocular surface reconstruction. It can be used alone to prevent further stromal degradation or in conjunction with limbal autograft or allograft to repopulate the corneal stem cells. Grafting also provides favorable extracellular matrix substrate for better epithelial migration and adhesion.

CHAPTER XXII

Surgical Procedures of the Ocular Surface

This chapter covers many of the surgeries performed on the ocular surface and non-surgical techniques such as the use of bandage contact lenses and cyanoacrylate adhesives. Part 11 of this volume discusses corneal transplantation, and Part 12 covers keratorefractive surgery.

Conjunctival Biopsy

Indications

A conjunctival biopsy can be helpful in the evaluation of chronic conjunctivitis and unusual ocular surface diseases, including the following:

- Parinaud oculoglandular syndrome
- Superior limbic keratoconjunctivitis
- Conjunctival lymphoid tumors
- Cicatricial pemphigoid

Surgical Technique

After a topical anesthetic agent is administered, a pledget wet with proparacaine or similar agent is applied to the lesion or site for 2–3 minutes. Subconjunctival anesthesia can also be given but is usually not necessary. A drop of topical phenylephrine can blanch the conjunctival vessels and reduce bleeding. The surgeon uses forceps and scissors to snip a conjunctival specimen. Lesions are completely excised if possible. A wedge or block is excised for a subepithelial lesion. Tissue crushing must be minimized by grasping only the edge of the biopsy. Gentle cauterization can be used to facilitate hemostasis.

Tissue Processing

The sample is placed on a carrier template and inserted into appropriate fixative, such as formalin (for histology), glutaraldehyde (for electron microscopy), or saline (for frozen-section or immunopathologic processing).

Preferred Practice Patterns Committee, Cornea Panel. *Conjunctivitis.* San Francisco: American Academy of Ophthalmology; in press.

Tarsorrhaphy

Tarsorrhaphy is the surgical fusion of the upper and lower eyelid margins. It is most commonly performed to protect the cornea from exposure caused by proptosis or to aid the healing of indolent corneal ulceration caused by cranial nerve VII (facial) palsy, neuroparalytic keratopathy, tear film deficiency, and eyelid dysfunction. Tarsorrhaphies may be temporary or permanent, in which case raw tarsal edges are created to form a lasting adhesion. They may be total or partial, depending on whether all or only a portion of the palpebral fissure is occluded. Finally, they are classified as lateral, medial, or central, according to the position in the palpebral fissure.

The eyelid margin is composed of an *anterior lamella* consisting of the skin and orbicularis muscle and a *posterior lamella* consisting of the tarsus and conjunctiva. Tissue excision is confined exclusively to the posterior lamella, preserving the anterior lamella and lash line. This approach results in an excellent cosmetic result if the tarsorrhaphy is opened later. It may also prevent complications from irregular eyelid margins, entropion, and trichiasis that may prove more damaging to the cornea than the initial exposure. BCSC Section 7, *Orbit, Eyelids, and Lacrimal System,* discusses eyelid anatomy and surgical procedures in detail.

Lateral Tarsorrhaphy

The degree of effective closure that can be surgically achieved can be estimated by lightly squeezing the upper and lower eyelids together laterally and noting the extent of closure. A satisfactory result should ensure covering of the cornea during active closure.

The surgeon slits the gray line of the upper and lower eyelids from the point of minimum closure to the lateral canthal angle. The two lamellae of each eyelid are then separated inferiorly and superiorly for a distance of approximately 3–4 mm vertically. Two parallel cuts are made in the posterior lamella of each eyelid, one at the extreme medial edge of the gray line slit and one at the extreme lateral edge. The mucocutaneous junction at the margin of the upper and lower eyelids is then removed. Excision should be minimal and the edges should be even. The surgeon makes a fourth cut in the upper eyelid to excise a rectangular piece of tarsoconjunctiva from the posterior lamella and then excises a 1-mm strip from the posterior margin of the lower eyelid.

Thus, a "tongue-and-groove" is created: the "tongue" of tissue in the lower eyelid is slid into the "groove" created in the upper eyelid. A double-armed 6-0 chromic suture is passed through the superior aspect of the tongue from the lower eyelid and sutured into the superior aspect of the lateral superior upper eyelid groove. Although the anterior lamella is left untouched in most cases, when it appears to be under tension after the tarsus has been sutured, or when a previous tarsorrhaphy has broken down, the tarsal bites should be reinforced with anterior lamellar sutures.

Medial Tarsorrhaphy and Canthoplasty

A nasal ectropion or persistent medial ectropion following a lateral tarsorrhaphy is corrected by a medial tarsorrhaphy and canthoplasty. The adherence is created on the nasal side of the inferior and superior limbs of the anterior portions of the medial canthal tendons. With lacrimal probes in place in the canaliculi, the surgeon makes slits at the gray line, beginning 1–3 mm medial to the punctum and carried as far medially as possible. Rectangles of tissue approximately 2 mm wide are excised anterior to the inferior and superior slits. The marginal epithelium of the upper and lower eyelids is excised, and a layered closure of posterior and anterior lamellae is completed.

Postoperative Care

Antibiotic ointment is usually applied to the wound twice a day for the first 5 days. If anterior lamellar sutures over a pledget are used, ointment is applied until they are removed 2 weeks later. Ointment containing corticosteroids should be avoided, because it may impair a rapid healing. The clinician should use slit-lamp examination of the cornea to guide administration of lubricants.

A tarsorrhaphy can be released under local anesthesia. A muscle hook is placed under the tissue and a blade is used to incise the tarsorrhaphy adhesion parallel to the upper and lower eyelid margins. Iris scissors can also be used to cut along the margin. If the status of the corneal exposure is uncertain, the tarsorrhaphy can be taken down in stages, a few millimeters at a time. If the tarsorrhaphy has been performed properly, eyelid margin deformity will be minimal.

Alternatives to Tarsorrhaphy

Other therapeutic modalities can protect the integrity of the ocular surface. Periorbital injection of botulinum toxin type A (Botox) to paralyze the orbicularis and levator muscles can lead to pharmacologic ptosis and provide temporary protective effects. Application of cyanoacrylate tissue adhesive (see pp 406–407) to the eyelid margins may also provide temporary closure of the eyelids for therapeutic purposes. Implantation of gold weights in the upper eyelid can also mechanically close the eyelids for patients with exposure keratopathy.

Pterygium Excision

A pterygium is an abnormal overgrowth of conjunctiva onto the cornea, almost always in the palpebral fissure (see pp 339–341). Indications for pterygium excision include persistent discomfort, vision distortion, and restricted ocular motility.

Microsurgical excision of a pterygium aims to achieve a normal, topographically smooth ocular surface. The role of carbon dioxide and excimer lasers in pterygium surgery remains uncertain. Also, the relative benefits and risks of physiochemical methods to prevent recurrence, such as mitomycin-C and irradiation, are unclear.

A common surgical technique is to remove the pterygium from both the corneal and scleral surfaces using a flat blade to dissect a smooth plane toward the limbus. The bulky fibrous tissue is removed, and the limbus is scraped or polished. Light thermal cautery is usually applied to the sclera. Options for wound closure include (Fig XXII-1)

- Bare sclera: no sutures or fine, absorbable sutures are used to appose the conjunctiva to the superficial sclera in front of the rectus tendon insertion, leaving an area of exposed sclera.
- Simple closure: the free edges of the conjunctiva are secured together.
- Sliding flap: an L-shaped incision adjacent to the wound is made to allow a conjunctival flap to slide into place.

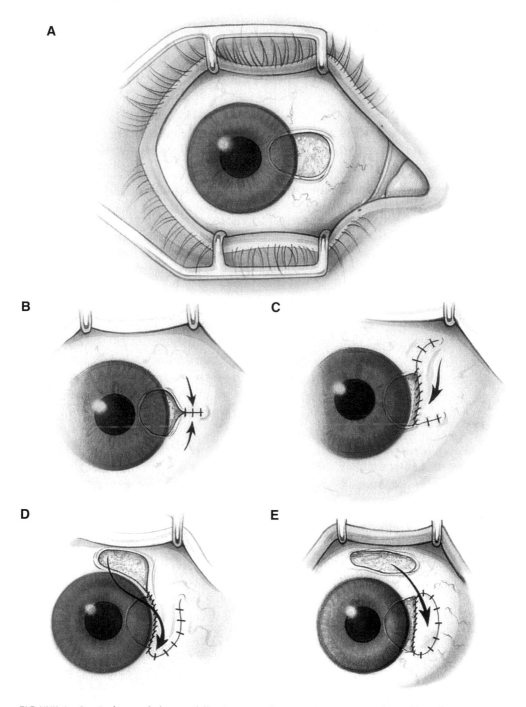

FIG XXII-1—Surgical wound closures following pterygium excision. *A,* Bare sclera, although sutures can be placed to tack down conjunctival wound edges. *B,* Simple closure with fine, absorbable sutures. *C,* Sliding flap that is closed with interrupted and/or running suture. *D,* Rotational flap from the superior bulbar conjunctiva. *E,* Conjunctival autograft that is secured with interrupted and/or running suture. (Reproduced with permission from Gans LA. Surgical treatment of pterygium. In: *Focal Points: Clinical Modules for Ophthalmologists.* San Francisco: American Academy of Ophthalmology; 1996;14:12. Illustration by Christine Gralapp.)

- Rotational flap: a U-shaped incision adjacent to the wound is made to form a tongue of conjunctiva that is rotated into place.
- Conjunctival graft: a free graft, usually from the superior bulbar conjunctiva, is excised to correspond to the size of the wound that is then moved and sutured into place. This technique is described in more detail below.

Conjunctival Transplantation

Only those situations in which abnormalities of conjunctival inflammation, scarring, or loss are not complicated by extensive damage or destruction of the limbal epithelial stem cells are appropriate for conjunctival autograft transplantation (see Table XXI-1). This technique is essentially an ocular surface patch graft designed to

- Replace either a focal or localized defect in the conjunctiva (such as after pterygium excision)
- Relieve the restriction of extraocular muscle movement caused by scarring of conjunctival and Tenon's tissue (after pterygium removal, strabismus surgery, or bulbar tumor excision)
- Eliminate problems of conjunctival fornix scarring

The most common indication for conjunctival transplantation is the management of advanced primary and recurrent pterygium. This technique reduces the risk of pterygium recurrence to approximately 5% and ameliorates the frequently encountered restriction of extraocular muscle function after pterygium excision. Since the superior bulbar conjunctiva is usually normal and undamaged, conjunctival autograft can be obtained from this area in the same eye.

Various techniques of conjunctival transplantation have been used to manage pterygium surgically. The procedure is performed on an outpatient basis, using topical plus peribulbar or retrobulbar anesthesia, especially in recurrent cases complicated by scarring. Traction sutures at the 12 o'clock and 6 o'clock positions facilitate maximal exposure of the pterygium. Multiple focal cautery spots or conjunctival markings with a pen delineate the area of conjunctiva to be excised. Beginning at the head of the pterygium, the surgeon uses a disposable scarifier to excise superficially the corneal portion of the pterygium to the limbus, followed by complete excision of the conjunctiva to the marks. Blunt dissection is used to free conjunctiva and Tenon's capsule from the horizontal rectus muscles. Care should be taken to identify and dissect the extraocular muscles involved, especially when they are enmeshed in the scar tissue of recurrent cases. Then complete resection of involved conjunctiva, Tenon's capsule, and fibrovascular scar is performed, leaving the bare sclera and rectus muscle exposed. The adjacent limbus and cornea are polished by scraping with the scarifier blade.

The size of the conjunctival graft is determined by measuring the area of exposed bare sclera with calipers. The eye is then turned down and in to expose the superior bulbar conjunctiva, the area of corresponding size is measured, and the exact dimensions are marked with several cautery spots. These marks are included within the graft tissue margins during the excision of the donor tissue to facilitate its reorientation in the recipient site. The conjunctival graft is thinly dissected, avoiding Tenon's capsule and episclera. After the graft is freed, it is transferred to the recipient bed and secured to adjacent conjunctiva and episclera with absorbable sutures. The donor site is usually left bare or closed with a single suture. Postoperatively, topical antibiotic-corticosteroid ointment is administered frequently for approximately 4–6 weeks until inflammation subsides.

Complications

Intraoperative or postoperative topical mitomycin-C is toxic and may cause visually significant complications such as aseptic scleral necrosis and infectious keratoscleritis. While short-term, low-dosage therapy (0.2–0.4 mg/ml TID for 3–5 days) with mitomycin-C has less hazardous potential for serious complications, even lower dosages in patients with ocular surface disorders must be evaluated further before this adjunctive pharmacotherapy can be considered superior to the relatively complication free conjunctival autograft.

The risk of recurrent pterygium following conjunctival autografting is between 2% and 7%. Self-limited problems include conjunctival graft edema, corneoscleral dellen, and epithelial cysts. Cases of recurrent pterygium after conjunctival autograft transplantation may be substantially improved by either repeated conjunctival autograft or modified limbal autografts.

Other Indications

Conjunctival autografts can also be used for fornix reconstruction when conjunctival fibrosis and cicatrization lead to fornix foreshortening, symblepharon formation, cicatricial entropion, trichiasis, and ocular surface keratinization and vascularization. Occasionally, unilateral fornix foreshortening occurs after localized disease, retinal detachment surgery, or excision of ocular surface tumors. It can be remedied by placement of a conjunctival autograft from the opposite eye. Usually, however, conditions associated with fornix obliteration (cicatricial pemphigoid, Stevens-Johnson syndrome) are bilateral, so that uninvolved conjunctiva is not available as a source for replacement tissue. Mucous membrane grafting using buccal mucosa or amniotic membrane has become the preferred ocular surface replacement technique in such instances.

For rehabilitation of an eye that has sustained a severe chemical or thermal injury, the replacement of fibrotic conjunctiva and superficial corneal pannus with healthy conjunctival tissue and a relatively stable corneal surface may be achieved with conjunctival autografting. However, limbal transplantation is often favored over conjunctival autografts for this indication. Although in some cases conjunctiva-derived epithelium may adequately transform into normal corneal epithelium, in most instances the corneal surface, lacking stem cells, eventually resumes a conjunctival character.

Limbal Transplantation

When stem cells are destroyed by disease or injury, the corneal surface becomes covered with conjunctival epithelium, which is less transparent, more irregular, and more prone to erosion and vascularization than normal corneal epithelium. This condition can be diagnosed clinically by the absence of the limbal palisades of Vogt or cytologically with impression cytology or biopsy of the limbal region to show goblet cells. Loss of limbal stem cells is seen most often in chemical injury, but it can occur after contact lens overwear, multiple surgical procedures, large ocular surface abrasions, repeated infections, or subconjunctival injection of 5-fluorouracil.

If total loss of limbal stem cells occurs unilaterally, an autograft of limbal epithelium from the fellow eye can repopulate the diseased cornea with normal corneal epithelium (Fig XXII-2). In this procedure corneal epithelium, conjunctiva, and

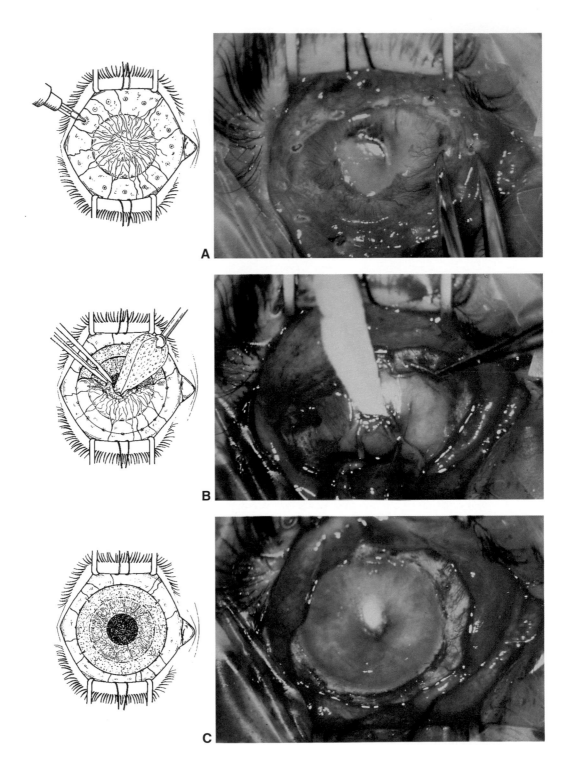

A

B

C

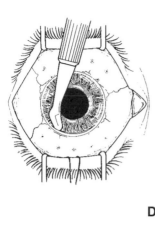

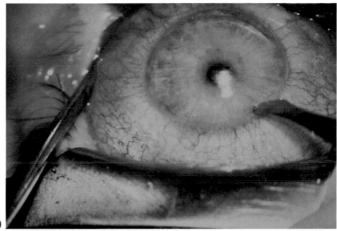

D

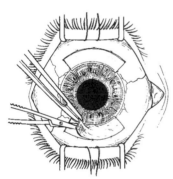

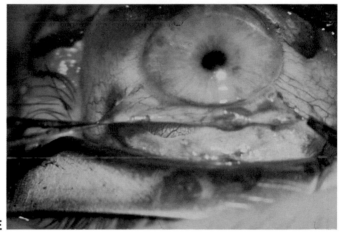

E

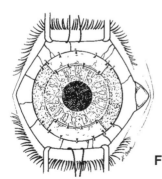

F

FIG XXII-2—Limbal autograft procedure. *A,* With disposable cautery, the area of bulbar conjunctiva to be resected is marked approximately 2 mm posterior to the limbus. *B,* After conjunctival resection, abnormal corneal epithelium and fibrovascular pannus are stripped by blunt dissection using cellulose sponges and tissue forceps. *C,* Additional surface polishing smooths the stromal surface and improves clarity. *D,* Superior and inferior limbal grafts are delineated in the donor eye with focal applications of cautery approximately 2 mm posterior to the limbus. The initial incision is made superficially within clear cornea using a disposable knife. *E,* The bulbar conjunctival portion of the graft is undermined and thinly dissected from its limbal attachment. *F,* The limbal grafts are transferred to their corresponding sites in the recipient eye and are secured with interrupted sutures, 10-0 nylon at the corneal edge and 8-0 vicryl at the conjunctival margin. (Reproduced by permission from Kenyon KR, Tseng SC. Limbal autograft transplantation for ocular surface disorders. *Ophthalmology.* 1989;96:709–723.)

superficial pannus are removed from within 2 mm outside the limbus of the recipient eye, then two thin limbal autografts from the fellow eye are attached to the limbus and allowed to regenerate and proliferate.

If total loss of limbal stem cells occurs bilaterally, the options for ocular surface transplantation are more limited. The appropriate selection of procedures depends on the relative health of the stem-cell population in the prospective donor eye. A limbal stem-cell allograft from a living related donor may be considered. A similar procedure, *keratoepithelioplasty,* uses peripheral cornea or corneolimbal rims from an eye bank donor eye. Even though host cells eventually reject or replace such a tissue, good long-term results have been reported. Although technical difficulties, poor epithelial viability, and rejection problems necessitating systemic immunosuppression have limited the usefulness of this modality, dramatic success has been observed in selected desperate cases. In contrast, the use of cultured limbal epithelium, while technically feasible, is largely investigational, and its practicality remains to be proven. For cases involving bilateral stem-cell loss, the most promising technique for transferring donor stem cells is limbal allograft transplantation.

Dua HS, Forrester JV. The corneoscleral limbus in human corneal epithelial wound healing. *Am J Ophthalmol.* 1990;110:646–656.

Kenyon KR, Tseng SC. Limbal autograft transplantation for ocular surface disorders. *Ophthalmology.* 1989;96:709–723.

Thoft RA. Keratoepithelioplasty. *Am J Ophthalmol.* 1984;97:1–6.

Conjunctival Flap

Indications

The conjunctival flap procedure covers an unstable or painful corneal surface with a hinged flap of more durable conjunctiva. Conjunctival flap surgery is performed less frequently now than in the past, because of broadened indications for penetrating keratoplasty (see chapters XXIII and XXIV), more effective antimicrobial agents, availability of therapeutic soft contact lenses, and improved management of corneal inflammatory diseases. However, this procedure remains an effective method of managing inflammatory and structural corneal disorders when restoration of vision is not an immediate concern. It should not be used for active microbial keratitis or corneal perforation since residual infectious organisms may proliferate under a flap if an ulcer is not sterilized first. A corneal perforation must first be sealed, because otherwise it would continue to leak under the flap. The principal indications for this procedure are

□ Chronic, sterile epithelial and stromal ulcerations (stromal herpes simplex virus keratitis, chemical and thermal burns, sicca, postinfectious ulcers, neurotrophic keratopathy)

□ Closed but unstable corneal wounds

□ Painful bullous keratopathy

□ A phthisical eye being prepared for a prosthetic shell

Reduction of visualization of the anterior chamber and creation of a potential barrier against drug penetration are among the disadvantages of conjunctival flap surgery.

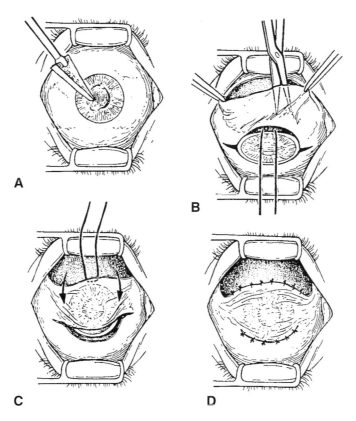

FIG XXII-3—Surgical steps for the Gundersen conjunctival flap. *A,* Removal of the corneal epithelium. *B,* A 360° peritomy with relaxing incisions, placement of superior limbal traction suture, superior forniceal incision, and dissection of a thin flap. *C,* Positioning of flap. *D,* Suturing of flap into position with multiple interrupted sutures. (Reproduced by permission from Mannis MJ. Conjunctival flaps. *Int Ophthalmol.* 1988;28:165–168.)

Surgical Technique

A thin hood, or *Gundersen flap* (Fig XXII-3), is highly successful if attention is paid to several fundamental principles:

□ Complete removal of the corneal epithelium and debridement of necrotic tissue

□ Creation of a mobile, thin conjunctival flap that contains minimal Tenon's capsule

□ Absence of any conjunctival buttonhole that may lead to flap retraction

□ Absence of any traction on the flap at its margins

Retrobulbar, peribulbar, or general anesthesia may be used. The corneal epithelium and all necrotic tissue are removed, and the eye is retracted inferiorly with an intracorneal traction suture at the superior limbus. Elevation of the flap with subconjunctival injection of lidocaine with epinephrine enhances anesthesia, facilitates dissection, and reduces bleeding. The needle for this injection should not pierce the conjunctiva in the area to be used for the flap.

The dissection may start from either the limbus or superior fornix. Dissection of conjunctiva from underlying Tenon's fascia must be performed carefully under direct visualization to prevent conjunctival perforation, especially in eyes with previous conjunctival surgery. Once the flap has been dissected, a 360° peritomy is performed, followed by scraping of all remaining limbal epithelium. Additional undermining of the flap allows it to cover the entire cornea and to rest there without traction. Any residual tension may foster later retraction of the flap. After the flap is positioned over the prepared cornea, it is sutured to the sclera just posterior to the limbus superiorly and inferiorly.

Partial conjunctival flap A partial, or *bridge,* flap may be used for temporary coverage of a peripheral wound or area of ulceration. Retraction is common despite adequate relaxation of the base. The flap should be well undermined to relieve tension and decrease the chance of retraction.

Bipedicle flap This partial, or *bucket handle,* flap has been used for small central or paracentral corneal lesions that do not require complete corneal coverage. The advantage is that the anterior chamber and the remaining uninvolved cornea are not obstructed to view. The flap is fashioned similar to the Gundersen flap with only enough dissection required to cover the lesion. The width of the flap should be 1.3–1.5 times the width of the lesion. Anesthesia is given, and the epithelium beneath the site of the flap is removed. After marking the bulbar conjunctiva with methylene blue, the surgeon can create the flap and mobilize it into position for suturing with interrupted nylon suture.

Advancement flap Peripheral limbal or paralimbal corneal lesions can be covered with a simple advancement conjunctival flap. A limbal incision is created with relaxing components, and the conjunctiva is simply advanced onto the cornea covering the defect. Scleral patch grafts and onlay grafts may also be used in conjunction with this technique. The disadvantage of this type of flap is a tendency to retract with time. *Single-pedicle flaps* (also known as *racquet flaps*) can be used for peripheral corneal lesions that are not large enough to require a total flap. The flap is more difficult to dissect than an advancement type flap yet is less prone to retraction.

Postoperative Care and Complications

Perforation, or buttonholing, of the flap is a major complication. Substitution of nasal, temporal, or inferior conjunctiva is one possible remedy, as is closure of the perforation with 10-0 nylon sutures. Inability to cover the cornea can be avoided by construction of a thin flap with adequate dissection to the limit of the superior fornix. Mobilization of an inferior flap is sometimes required, despite the desirability of avoiding a suture line on the cornea.

Retraction of the flap is the most common complication, occurring in about 10% of cases. Other complications include hemorrhage beneath the flap and epithelial cysts. Sometimes inclusion cysts enlarge to the point that they require excision or marsupialization. Ptosis may also occur postoperatively, usually of the levator-dehiscence type. Unsatisfactory cosmetic appearance can be improved with a painted contact lens. Progressive corneal disease under the flap is a concern with infective and autoimmune conditions.

Considerations in Removal of the Flap

If penetrating keratoplasty is to be performed in an eye that has had a conjunctival flap, the flap may be removed as a separate procedure or at the time of the graft. Simple removal of the flap (without keratoplasty) is usually unsatisfactory in restoring vision, as the underlying cornea is nearly always scarred. Because the conjunctival flap procedure tends to destroy or displace most limbal stem cells, a limbal autograft procedure after removal of the flap may be necessary to provide a permanent source of normal epithelium prior to an optical corneal transplant.

Abbott RL, Beebe WE. Corneal edema. In: Abbott RL, ed. *Surgical Intervention in Corneal and External Diseases.* Orlando: Grune & Stratton; 1987:81–84.

Mannis MJ. Conjunctival flaps. *Int Ophthalmol Clin.* 1988;28:165–168.

Mucous Membrane Grafting

Indications

The goal of surgery is to reconstruct a more functional conjunctival mucosal surface to ameliorate the fornix obliteration or the eyelid margin keratinization that usually occurs in relation to bilateral cicatricial conjunctival disorders such as Stevens-Johnson syndrome or ocular cicatricial pemphigoid (see Table XXI-1). Buccal mucosa or preserved amniotic membrane can be employed. Mucous membrane grafting has rarely been used as a treatment for unilateral chemical injury and is used only in desperate cases of bilateral injury where advancement of Tenon's capsule is not possible and allograft limbal tissue is not available. Nonetheless, this technique has long been a popular method of correcting eyelid position abnormalities caused by cicatrizing conjunctival disorders. Although good results have been reported in inactive cicatricial disorders such as late-stage, nonprogressive Stevens-Johnson syndrome, there has been some reluctance to apply this technique to advanced (stage III or IV) ocular cicatricial pemphigoid for fear of exacerbating this relentlessly progressive inflammatory disorder. Advances in immunosuppressive treatment, however, have brought promise that mucous membrane grafting for the eyelid abnormalities associated with late-stage ocular cicatricial pemphigoid can achieve substantial success.

The purpose of grafting mucosal membranes is to improve ocular surface wetting by improving eyelid movement and distribution of the tear film over the cornea, thereby reducing exposure and evaporation, as well as by providing favorable extracellular matrix substrate for better epithelial migration and adhesion. However, such a procedure is not effective in replacing the normal stem cells. In a small series of patients with advanced ocular cicatricial pemphigoid and Stevens-Johnson syndrome, combinations of allograft limbal transplantation, amniotic membrane transplantation, and tarsorrhaphy, followed by the use of serum-derived tears and systemic immunosuppression, were shown to reconstruct the ocular surface. Such therapeutic modalities appear to provide an alternative to other difficult procedures such as keratoprosthesis for treating patients with desperate cicatricial keratoconjunctivitis (see chapter XXIV).

Surgical Technique

After the eyelid has been split at the gray line, the posterior lamella is recessed and secured to the anterior lamella with interrupted 4-0 silk sutures. A diamond burr is used to smooth the margin and the posterior tarsal surface, and the entire conjunctiva is removed from the tarsal conjunctival surface. A full-thickness lip mucosal graft is hydraulically dissected and excised with freehand dissection at least 1 cm posterior to the vermilion border. Care is taken not to buttonhole the graft as the posterior surface of it is trimmed with sharp scissors. The graft is draped over the margin of the eyelid and sutured in position with a running, double-armed 8-0 nylon suture tied externally over silicone foam pledgets. Suture tarsorrhaphy placed through the centers of the grafts hold them in position and prevent graft movement caused by blinking during the first postoperative week. A conformer can be used to maintain the fornix and prevent the adhesion of bulbar and tarsal mucosal membranes. Complications include buttonholing, retraction, trichiasis, surface keratinization of the graft, ptosis, phimosis, depressed eyelid blink, incomplete eyelid closure, submucosal abscess formation, and persistent nonhealing epithelial defects of the cornea.

Shore JW, Foster CS, Westfall CT, et al. Results of buccal mucosal grafting for patients with medically controlled ocular cicatricial pemphigoid. *Ophthalmology.* 1992;99: 383–395.

Tsubota K, Satake Y, Ohyama M, et al. Surgical reconstruction of the ocular surface in advanced ocular cicatricial pemphigoid and Stevens-Johnson syndrome. *Am J Ophthalmol.* 1996;122:38–52.

Superficial Keratectomy and Corneal Biopsy

Indications

This procedure consists of excision of the superficial layers of cornea (epithelium, Bowman's layer, or superficial stroma) without replacement of tissue. The primary indications are

□ Removal of hyperplastic or necrotic tissue (e.g., corneal dermoid, pterygium, Salzmann degeneration, epithelial basement membrane reduplication)

□ Excision of retained corneal foreign material

□ Need for tissue for diagnosis (histopathology or microbiology)

□ Excision of scarring or superficial corneal dystrophic tissue

If corneal biopsy is performed for histopathology, preservation of tissue integrity and anatomical orientation is crucial. A small specimen can be placed on a filter or thin card to maintain the tissue orientation prior to fixation or cryosection. For microbiology work-up the biopsied specimens can be minced or homogenized prior to innoculation of the culture media or tissue smearing for histochemical stainings.

Surgical Techniques

Mechanical keratectomy If the corneal lesion is superficial enough, sometimes it can be scraped or peeled free without sharp dissection. When a deeper dissection is required, the surgeon can mark the area freehand with an adjustable-depth blade or use a trephine to mark the area superficially. Care must be taken to maintain the surgical plane and to avoid inadvertent perforation. A lamellar keratectomy can also be performed using a microkeratome, a diamond burr on a surgical drill, or phototherapeutic keratectomy with the excimer laser.

Phototherapeutic keratectomy The excimer laser can remove tissue with much greater precision than the mechanical techniques. One problem with its use is that scar tissue may ablate at a different rate from normal tissue, which results in an uneven surface even if the original surface was smooth. Conversely, if the corneal surface is irregular and ablates homogeneously, the irregularity will persist. Frequent application of viscous liquid to the corneal surface fills in the gaps during ablation, so that a smooth surface results. Most patients experience a hyperopic shift after photokeratectomy from the corneal flattening effect of the procedure. Nevertheless, phototherapeutic keratectomy may produce marked improvement in vision in selected patients with superficial stromal scarring or dystrophies, obviating the need for corneal transplant surgery.

> Campos M, Nielsen S, Szerenyi K, et al. Clinical follow-up of phototherapeutic keratectomy for treatment of corneal opacities. *Am J Ophthalmol.* 1993;115:433–440.

Management of Descemetocele, Corneal Perforation, and Corneal Edema

Bandage Contact Lens

The application of an ultrathin, continuous-wear soft contact lens as a therapeutic bandage can protect the loosely adherent remaining or regenerating epithelium from the windshield wiper action of the blinking eyelids. Use of bandage contact lenses has significantly improved and simplified the management of recurrent erosions and persistent epithelial defect. Continuous bandaging can reduce the stromal leukocyte infiltration and ensure the regeneration of basement membrane and restoration of tight epithelial–stromal adhesion without compromising the patient's vision and comfort.

Frequent irrigation and lubrication with unpreserved saline, prophylaxis with antibiotics, and close follow-up are crucial, especially in patients with decreased corneal sensitivity or dry eye. The choice of a soft contact lens for patients with severe dry eye can be difficult. In general, patients with dry eye run a high risk of infection with soft contact lenses. High-water-content lenses usually are not appropriate because rapid water evaporation further compounds the hypertonicity-induced surface damage in dry eyes. The use of a nonhydrophilic, acrylic scleral lens may circumvent the problems encountered with the hydrogel lens.

Even though the hydrogel lens can actually cause corneal hypoxia and increase corneal edema, continuous wear of this type of lens can provide symptomatic relief of painful bullous keratopathy. Mild corneal edema can often be managed with hypertonic saline solution or ointment and judicious use of topical steroids if indicated. Chronic use of the bandage contact lens can often lead to corneal pannus and compromise the success of future penetrating keratoplasty for visual rehabilitation.

However, extensive pannus formation may eliminate the bullous changes and associated pain, eliminating the need for bandage lenses in many patients.

Cyanoacrylate Adhesive

Tissue adhesives, particularly butylcyanoacrylate, have been used widely as an adjunct in the management of corneal ulceration and perforation. Early application of tissue adhesives in the management of stromal melting has greatly reduced the need for major surgical interventions such as therapeutic keratoplasty and conjunctival flap. Although cyanoacrylate tissue adhesives are not approved by the FDA for use on the eye, they have been used extensively over the past two decades to seal perforations.

Some perforations are so minimal that they seal spontaneously prior to any ophthalmologic examination, with no intraocular damage, prolapse, or adherence. These cases may require only treatment with systemic and/or topical antibiotic therapy, along with close observation. If a corneal wound is leaking but the chamber remains formed, sealing of the leak can be encouraged with pharmacologic suppression of aqueous production (topical or systemic), patching, and/or a therapeutic contact lens. Generally, if these measures fail to seal the wound in 3 days, closure with cyanoacrylate glue or sutures is recommended. Perforations greater than 2–3 mm are usually not amenable to tissue adhesive.

Cyanoacrylate tissue adhesive applied to thinned or ulcerated corneal tissue may prevent further thinning and support the stroma through the period of vascularization and repair. The adhesive plug is also thought to retard the entry of inflammatory cells and epithelium to the area, thus decreasing the rate of corneal melting. New stromal tissue may be laid down, and accompanying corneal vascularization may help to ensure the integrity of the area by providing nutrients and antiproteases. Tissue adhesives may be useful whether or not infection is present, since they are also bacteriostatic. Antimicrobial therapy must be continued, however.

Surgical technique Tissue adhesive can usually be applied on an outpatient basis for sterile ulcerations. However, when adherent or prolapsed uvea in the leakage site or flat chamber is encountered, the procedure should be performed in the operating room using air or hyaluronate to re-form the anterior chamber. The adhesive is applied under slit-lamp or microscopic observation using a topical anesthetic (0.5% proparacaine hydrochloride). An eyelid speculum is useful. Before the adhesive is applied, any necrotic tissue and corneal epithelium should be removed from the involved area and a 2-mm surrounding zone. The area is then dried using a cellulose sponge, and a small drop of the fluid adhesive is applied. The glue polymerizes completely within 5–10 minutes and usually adheres well to the de-epithelialized surface.

The glue does not polymerize on plastic, so a simple way to handle it is to spread a small amount on a surface such as the inside of the sterile plastic wrapping of any medical product cut to a size slightly larger than the perforation. It should then be applied to the surface of the cornea in as thin a layer as possible using the plastic handle of a cellulose sponge or the wooden stick of a cotton-tipped applicator. The adhesive plug has a rough surface and can be irritative, so a therapeutic contact lens is used to protect the upper tarsal conjunctiva and to prevent mechanical dislodgment of the plug by eyelid blinking.

Cases of poor epithelialization, such as following severe chemical burns, may be helped with a "glued-on" lens used as a barrier to corneal vascularization or further stromolysis. A small mount of the adhesive is applied around the corneal periphery, and a bandage contact lens is then quickly applied before the glue has polymerized. The adhesive plaque should remain in place for 6–8 weeks to allow healing. If it becomes dislodged prematurely, it can be reapplied. It often sloughs spontaneously, but it can be removed at any time using fine forceps. Topical cycloplegics, lubricants, and steroids are often useful adjuncts in addition to antimicrobials.

Reconstructive Lamellar and Patch Grafts

Chapter XXIV discusses these procedures in greater detail.

Lamellar keratoplasty Patch grafts with either lamellar or full-thickness corneal tissues can be used for tectonic or reconstructive purposes. Lamellar keratoplasty is the application of fresh or preserved corneal tissue onto a recipient corneal bed. It is generally performed using allograft tissue in a carefully dissected recipient bed. This procedure is useful in cases of corneal thinning because it provides immediate tissue substance to prevent frank perforation and exposure of the ocular contents.

Certain modifications in technique should be considered when lamellar keratoplasty is performed on a cornea with marked thinning or impending perforation. Infected or necrotic tissue should be removed as thoroughly as possible without penetrating the eye. In cases of possible infection the tissue removed should include a 1-mm clear zone outside the affected area. Great care should be taken to prevent perforation. In central lesions, dissection should be performed from the thinned area toward the periphery to minimize perforation risk. Establishing a perfect plane without interface irregularity is of less concern when the structural integrity of the eye is at stake.

Penetrating keratoplasty PK is the definitive method of treating a cornea that has suffered progressive thinning and faces impending perforation. Therapeutic keratoplasty can sometimes be employed to debulk or eradicate recalcitrant infectious keratitis. It provides a visual result superior to that of lamellar keratoplasty since there is no interface opacification. However, entering the eye should be avoided, if at all possible, in cases with active infection or inflammation. Instead, PK should be postponed until the inflammation has abated and the corneal disease process has stabilized. In cases of impending perforation with significant inflammation, tissue adhesives or a lamellar keratoplasty should be used. PK may be used in cases of corneal thinning without significant inflammation or after tissue adhesive or lamellar keratoplasty has been employed as a temporizing measure.

As in other cases of penetrating keratoplasty, inflammation should be controlled as much as possible before the procedure is performed. Trephination of a cornea with irregular thinning may be difficult, and the sharpest trephines available should be used to make a complete groove. If possible, a 1-mm zone of normal cornea should be removed along with the abnormal tissue. Another useful precaution is to avoid running sutures (see chapter XXIV).

Corneal Tattoo

Indications and Options

Corneal tattooing has been used for centuries to improve the cosmetic appearance of a blind eye with an unsightly leukoma. Occasionally, it has also been used in seeing eyes to reduce the glare from scars and to eliminate monocular diplopia in patients with large iridectomies or traumatic loss of iris. Congenital iris coloboma is another indication. Modern technology allows these conditions to be managed adequately with anterior segment reconstruction, tinted contact lenses, or thin scleral shells. However, corneal tattooing may still be a reasonable alternative in high-risk cases of leukoma or leukocoria where corneal transplantation would lead to rejection and graft failure or in eyes without visual potential. The most common complications of corneal tattooing have been ocular discomfort, conjunctival injection, and mild keratitis. Corneal ulceration, iridocyclitis, and even endophthalmitis have also been reported. Suggested contraindications are adherent leukoma, keratoectasia, anterior staphyloma, neurotrophic cornea, phthisis bulbi, and glaucoma because of the inherent risk of iridocyclitis.

Surgical Technique

Both eyes are prepared in sterile fashion and draped so that the color of the normal iris can be used for comparison. Topical and retrobulbar or peribulbar anesthesia is established and the corneal epithelium in the area to be tattooed is removed. A paste is made by mixing sterile saline or water with dry powder pigments that have been sterilized with ethylene oxide. India ink is the most commonly used material, but other staining pigments are available in various colors that can be combined and diluted. Colors available for mixing to match the iris of the normal eye include black (iron oxide), brown (iron oxide), white (titanium dioxide), and blue (titanium dioxide and phthalocyanide). Staining solutions must be sterilized before use.

The conventional method of corneal tattooing is similar to dermatographic methods. A trephine of 3–4 mm is centered on the central optical zone to mark the pupil, and multiple beveled stabs with a surgical blade are made to embed the pigments into the anterior stroma. Pigment can also be placed under a lamellar flap or into a lamellar dissection. In lamellar intrastromal keratography the staining pigment is spread in a dissected pocket.

The color of pigment is tested by first working in an area of the superior part of the cornea that will be covered by the eyelid. The color is compared with that of the iris of the opposite eye and modified until a satisfactory match is obtained. Because the pigment can become embedded into conjunctival openings, care is taken not to break the conjunctival surface in exposed areas. Postoperatively, the eye is patched with antibiotic ointment and checked daily until the epithelial surface is intact, usually within 3–5 days.

Anastas CN, McGhee CN, Webber SK, et al. Corneal tattooing revisited: excimer laser in the treatment of unsightly leucomata. *Aust NZ J Ophthalmol.* 1995;23:227–230.

Reed JW. Corneal tattooing to reduce glare in cases of traumatic iris loss. *Cornea.* 1994;13:401–405.

PART 11

CORNEAL TRANSPLANTATION

CHAPTER XXIII

Basic Concepts of Corneal Transplantation

Transplantation Immunobiology

Histocompatibility and Other Antigens

Antigens found within the host are known as *endogenous antigens*. The most important group of endogenous antigens are the *homologous antigens,* which are genetically controlled determinants specific to a given species. Histocompatibility antigens, homologous antigens found on the surfaces of most cells, are an expression of genetic material on human chromosome 6 in a region referred to as the *major histocompatibility complex (MHC)*. In humans the MHC is known as the *human leukocyte antigen (HLA) system.*

HLA antigens are found on the surface of all nucleated cells. They are determined by a series of four gene loci located on chromosome 6 known as *HLA-A, HLA-B, HLA-C,* and *HLA-D.* Each zone controls several different antigenic specificities, over 95% of which can be recognized by serologic methods. The histocompatibility antigens are important clinically because they form the basis for graft rejection in organ transplantation and for sensitization to most antigens. It is possible that HLA antigens are genetic markers rather than real transplantation antigens, and that strong transplantation antigens are closely linked with the HLA markers on the genetic material.

Some grafts are rejected even when donor–recipient pairs are HLA-compatible. Although minor histocompatibility antigens such as ABO and Lewis antigens are less potent than major histocompatibility antigens, they nonetheless add to the overall antigenicity of a graft. Little is known about the number of minor histocompatibility antigens or their importance in transplantation immunology.

Immune Privilege

The cornea was the first successfully transplanted solid tissue. After other tissues had also been transplanted, it was soon observed that corneas were rejected less frequently than other transplanted tissues. The concept emerged that the cornea was the site of "immunologic privilege" and that corneal grafts were somehow protected from immunologic destruction. It is now evident that corneal grafts are not different from other tissue grafts and that the so-called immunologic privilege accorded corneal grafts is simply the result of their relative isolation from recipient lymphatic channels. The fact that vascularized recipients reject corneal grafts more frequently than nonvascularized recipients supports this finding.

Tolerance to a corneal graft may also be a result of anterior chamber–associated immune deviation (ACAID) that involves the development of suppressor T cells.

ACAID is a downregulation of delayed type cellular immunity. Antigens released into the aqueous humor are, presumably, recognized by dendritic cells of the iris and ciliary body. These antigen-presenting cells can then enter the venous circulation and induce regulatory T cells in the spleen, bypassing the lymphatic system.

For an immune response to occur, an antigenic substance is introduced and "recognized" (afferent limb), producing the synthesis of specific antibody molecules and the appearance of "effector" lymphocytes that react specifically with the immunizing antigen (efferent limb). Although antibodies to foreign tissues are formed during graft rejection, they are not believed to be important in the usual type of rejection of allografts. Rather, extensive evidence indicates that cellular immune mechanisms are associated with allograft rejection. The term *delayed hypersensitivity,* or *Type IV, reactions* is used to describe these T lymphocyte–mediated responses. Other mechanisms are also probably involved.

See also discussion of immune-mediated disorders in Part 4 of this volume. BCSC Section 9, *Intraocular Inflammation and Uveitis,* covers the principles of immunology in greater detail with illustrations.

Pepose JS, Holland GN, Wilhelmus KR, eds. *Ocular Infection and Immunity.* St Louis: Mosby; 1996:435–445.

Eye Banking and Donor Selection

Before reliable storage or preservation methods were available, it was imperative that corneas be transplanted immediately from donor to recipient. The McCarey-Kaufman tissue transport medium developed in the early 1970s significantly reduced endothelial cell attrition, allowing safe transplantation of corneal buttons for up to 4 days at 4° C. Improvements in storage media over the past two decades have extended the viable storage period to as long as 2 weeks, not only enhancing the availability of donor corneas, but also allowing PK to be done on a less exigent basis. Currently under investigation is the addition of insulin, epidermal growth factor, broader spectrum antibiotics, and other components to storage media. These changes may further improve endothelial cell viability and function and enhance sterility in the future.

Although previous smaller studies have shown benefit from HLA matching, a recent multicenter study of high-risk grafts found no reduction in the incidence of rejection with the use of HLA-matched or cross-matched tissue. The effect of ABO blood type matching remains uncertain.

The Eye Bank Association of America (EBAA) has developed extensive criteria for screening donor corneas prior to distribution to avoid transmissible infections and other conditions (Table XXIII-1). Criteria contraindicating donor corneal use include

□ Death of unknown cause

□ Unknown central nervous system disease or certain infectious diseases of the central nervous system (e.g., Creutzfeldt-Jakob disease, subacute sclerosing panencephalitis, progressive multifocal leukoencephalopathy, congenital rubella, Reye syndrome, rabies, viral encephalitis)

□ Systemic infections (e.g., septicemia, endocarditis, AIDS, viral hepatitis)

□ Social, clinical, or laboratory evidence suggestive of HIV infection, syphilis, or viral hepatitis

□ Active leukemia and disseminated lymphomas

- Intrinsic eye disease (e.g., anterior segment malignancies, conjunctivitis, scleritis, uveitis, retinitis, choroiditis); however, eyes with posterior choroidal melanoma are considered acceptable
- Congenital or acquired eye disorders that would preclude successful surgical outcome (e.g., keratoconus, scars, pterygia, Fuchs dystrophy)
- Prior intraocular or anterior segment surgery, except when endothelial adequacy is documented by specular microscopy

Even with these standards, the ultimate responsibility for accepting donor materials rests with the surgeon. Other factors that may be considered include the following:

- Slit-lamp appearance of donor tissue
- Specular microscopic data (endothelial cell counts <2000 cells/mm^2 not used)
- Death-to-preservation time (optimal range <12–18 hours)
- Tissue storage time prior to keratoplasty
- Donor age

Most surgeons do not use corneas from donors younger than 6–12 months, as these corneas are extremely flaccid and can result in high corneal astigmatism and myopia postoperatively. Most eye banks establish an upper age limit of 70 years, as older corneas tend to have lower endothelial cell counts. The age of acceptance of tissue for transplantation is up to the individual surgeon.

TABLE XXIII-1

DISEASES THAT HAVE BEEN TRANSMITTED OR PRODUCED BY THE DONOR CORNEA

Infections
    Bacterial or fungal endophthalmitis
    Bacterial or fungal keratitis
    Rabies
    Creutzfeldt-Jakob disease
    Hepatitis B
    Herpes simplex virus epithelial keratitis (?)

Other
    Primary endothelial failure
    Stromal dystrophy
    Corneal opacity
    Iris neoplasm

CHAPTER XXIV

Clinical Approach to Corneal Transplantation

Penetrating Keratoplasty: Corneal Allograft

Indications

The term *penetrating keratoplasty (PK)* commonly refers to surgical replacement of a portion of the host cornea with that of a donor eye. If the donor is another person, the procedure is called an *allograft;* use of donor tissue from the same or fellow eye is called an *autograft* (see p 429). Advances in microsurgery, suture materials, storage media, and postoperative medical management have allowed corneal transplant surgery to progress from the novelty it was in the mid–twentieth century to an accepted procedure performed almost 50,000 times annually in the United States alone. Indications for penetrating keratoplasty have also expanded considerably (Table XXIV-1).

Today the most common indication for PK is decreased visual acuity secondary to corneal opacity. Other objectives include correction of abnormal corneal contour, treatment of corneal thinning or perforation, relief of pain, removal of infectious or neoplastic foci, or cosmesis. Even though some ophthalmologists do not perform corneal transplants, all should be familiar with its postoperative complications, because patients do not always return to their surgeons when problems arise, and many of these problems require immediate intervention to save the graft.

TABLE XXIV-1

INDICATIONS FOR PENETRATING KERATOPLASTY
(IN APPROXIMATE ORDER OF PREVALENCE)

Pseudophakic or aphakic corneal edema

Fuchs endothelial dystrophy

Keratoconus

Failed previous corneal transplant

Stromal corneal dystrophies

Corneal opacification following infection (viral keratitis, microbial keratitis, syphilitic keratopathy)

Immune-mediated corneal diseases and perforation

Corneal degenerations

Mechanical and chemical trauma

Congenital opacity

Preferred Practice Patterns, Cornea Panel. *Corneal Opacification.* San Francisco: American Academy of Ophthalmology; 1995.

Soong HK. Penetrating keratoplasty. In: *Focal Points: Clinical Modules for Ophthalmologists.* San Francisco: American Academy of Ophthalmology; 1992;10:6.

Preoperative Evaluation and Preparation

A complete eye examination is necessary prior to keratoplasty, and a detailed social history helps predict whether the patient will be compliant with the postoperative regimen and report quickly if problems arise. Simple clinical tests, such as those for color recognition or an afferent pupillary defect, can be enormously important in the evaluation of patients with media opacity. Ocular surface problems, such as dry eye, trichiasis, exposure, blepharitis, and rosacea, must be recognized and treated prior to PK.

The preoperative evaluation addresses any neurologic or intraocular factors that could compromise the final visual result, such as other media opacity, uncontrolled glaucoma, amblyopia, macular abnormalities, retinal disease, or optic nerve damage. Preexisting glaucoma or ocular inflammation must be kept under control before PK is considered. Active keratitis or uveitis is treated medically if possible, and the eye should ideally remain quiet for several months before PK. An inflamed eye at the time of surgery is associated with a higher incidence of postoperative complications, such as graft rejection and failure, glaucoma, and cystoid macular edema. As an example, corneal perforations in an acutely inflamed eye should, if possible, be closed either with cyanoacrylate tissue adhesive or by means of a lamellar corneal graft, thus restoring the integrity of the globe and allowing the eye a chance to become quiet. A vision-restoring penetrating keratoplasty may then be undertaken at a later date. A lamellar graft should at least be considered in any case with normal endothelium.

Fluorescein angiography can be helpful in detecting retinal problems, such as cystoid macular edema and age-related macular degeneration, through less-than-ideal media. If the media are completely opaque, ultrasonography will detect some problems that affect the visual prognosis after PK. The potential visual acuity meter, laser interferometer, blue-field entoptic phenomenon testing, visual fields, and visually evoked cortical potentials may also help in preoperative assessment of the afferent system.

In general, deep corneal vascularization, ocular surface disease, active anterior segment inflammation, peripheral corneal thinning, and increased IOP worsen the prognosis for PK and therefore influence the appropriateness of recommending the procedure to the patient.

Surgical Technique

Penetrating keratoplasty *Preparation of the donor cornea.* Donor tissue is prepared by trephining the previously excised corneoscleral donor tissue endothelial side up in a concave nonstick block. The remaining donor rim and media fluid are then submitted for culture. Several devices designed for cutting donor corneal buttons aim the trephine blade precisely and vertically onto the button along a guiding shaft. Trephination of the donor button with the excimer and other lasers is under investigation.

Most surgeons size the donor button 0.25–0.50 mm larger than the diameter of the host corneal opening (e.g., an 8.0-mm diameter corneal button into a 7.5-mm wound). This size disparity may reduce postoperative glaucoma, enhance watertight wound closure, prevent peripheral anterior synechiae formation and excessive postoperative corneal flattening, and provide the recipient eye with more endothelial cells. In keratoconus, especially in eyes with high axial length, sizing the donor tissue to match the exact size of the wound may flatten the corneal contour and thereby reduce postoperative myopia. However, a watertight wound closure is more difficult to achieve in same-sized grafts.

Preparation of the recipient eye. Prior to trephination of the recipient eye, additional scleral support may be needed, especially in aphakic, pseudophakic, and pediatric corneal transplants. This support is commonly obtained by suturing a Flieringa ring to the episclera. By structurally bracing the anterior globe, the ring reduces scleral infolding, distortion of the wound opening, and forward bulging of the iris, lens, and/or vitreous. A scleral support ring combined with an eyelid speculum (McNeill-Goldmann blepharostat) is also available.

For cutting the recipient cornea, the surgeon has three options:

□ A simple manual trephine

□ A motorized trephine that allows wobble-free circular cutting

□ A vacuum trephine that adheres to the recipient cornea and reduces slippage during trephination

The anterior chamber may be entered directly with the trephine or with a microsurgical knife after partial-thickness trephination. The former method may create more vertical wound edges, whereas the latter method may reduce damage to the lens and iris. Excimer laser recipient trephination is under investigation.

The donor corneal button is placed endothelial side down into the recipient opening. Use of viscoelastic material helps protect the donor endothelium during surgical manipulation, keeps the anterior chamber formed, and shields the iris while the donor button is being sutured into the wound.

Combined procedures   PK may be combined with other procedures such as cataract extraction, primary or secondary IOL implantation, IOL removal or exchange, glaucoma surgery, vitrectomy, and retinal procedures. A temporary intraoperative keratoprosthesis may or may not be used with these procedures. Synechiolysis can be performed with caution, avoiding excessive bleeding, tearing, or tissue and inflammatory exudation. Iris defects may be repaired with 10-0 polypropylene sutures to achieve pupil constriction, eliminate monocular diplopia, improve spectacle acuity, reduce glare, and minimize chances of iridocorneal adhesion. In eyes at risk for postoperative uveitis (e.g., those with herpes simplex or interstitial keratitis), a peripheral iridectomy will reduce the change of postoperative pupillary-block glaucoma.

Suturing techniques   The donor button is secured with at least four interrupted cardinal sutures. Complete wound closure is achieved with either interrupted sutures, one or two continuous sutures, or a combination (see below). Although intraoperative keratometry may help control corneal astigmatism, astigmatism management falls primarily within the scope of postoperative care, which is discussed below.

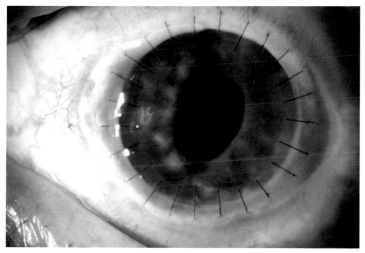

FIG XXIV-1—PK for syphilitic interstitial keratopathy, with 24 interrupted 10-0 nylon sutures in place.

The suture knots may be positioned in either donor or host tissue and are buried in the corneal stroma, not left in the wound. Most surgeons prefer partial-thickness corneal suture bites over full-thickness bites, since the latter may be associated with a higher chance of leakage along the suture tracks and serve as a portal of entry for microorganisms or epithelial ingrowth. Following suture placement, the wound is tested for aqueous leakage using either a methylcellulose spear to blot the wound or a Seidel test with fluorescein paper strips.

Interrupted sutures. Vascularized, inflamed, or thinned corneas tend to heal unevenly and unpredictably. Interrupted sutures, usually 16–24 in number, are the technique of choice in such corneas because they may be removed selectively if they attract blood vessels or if they loosen because of wound contraction (Fig XXIV-1). Astigmatism may be reduced postoperatively by selective removal of sutures in the steep corneal meridian, although such removal risks wound dehiscence if it is done too early.

Continuous sutures. In the absence of vascularization, focal inflammation, or thinning, single or double continuous sutures can be used to close the PK (Figs XXIV-2, XXIV-3). Continuous sutures allow even distribution of tension and healing around the wound, and they are less time-consuming to place and remove post-operatively. A continuous suture, however, may be compromised in its entirety by sectorial loosening, or cheese wiring. Double continuous sutures give an added measure of wound protection should one running suture break or loosen. Moreover, the second running suture can be placed in a manner that counteracts the torque induced by the first. The tension on a single, continuous suture may be adjusted intraoperatively or at the slit lamp to reduce astigmatism in the first few postoperative weeks.

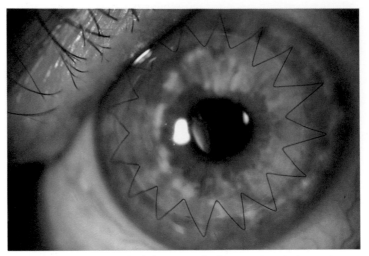

FIG XXIV-2—PK for pseudophakic corneal edema, with a single continuous 10-0 nylon suture in place.

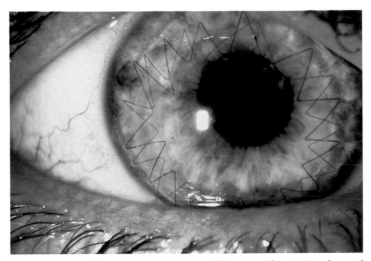

FIG XXIV-3—Double continuous suturing technique employs 10-0 nylon and 11-0 nylon running sutures, in this case with keratoconus.

Combined sutures. The combined interrupted and continuous suture technique offers several of the advantages of both methods (Fig XXIV-4). The interrupted sutures may be removed as early as 1 week after PK in order to reduce corneal astigmatism, while the continuous suture remains to protect against wound dehiscence.

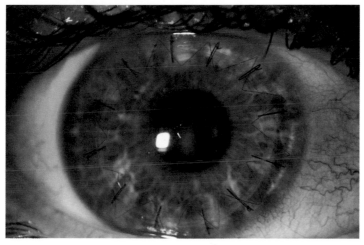

FIG XXIV-4—Combined suturing technique employs both interrupted 10-0 nylon and continuous 11-0 nylon sutures, in this case with Fuchs endothelial dystrophy.

Intraoperative Complications

Complications that can occur intraoperatively include the following:

- Damage to the lens and/or iris from the trephine, scissors, or other instruments
- Irregular trephination
- Inadequate vitrectomy resulting in vitreous contact with graft endothelium
- Poor graft centration onto the host bed
- Excessive bleeding from the iris and wound edge (in vascularized host corneas)
- Choroidal hemorrhage and effusion
- Iris incarceration into the wound
- Damage to the donor epithelium during trephination and handling

In aphakic eyes with large pupils or sector iris defects, the graft may drop back into the vitreous prior to suture fixation, especially if vitrectomy has previously been performed on the eye.

In severely edematous corneas, recipient Descemet's membrane may be inadvertently left behind after corneal excision, as it is easily stripped completely from the stroma. The recipient eye must be carefully examined for retained Descemet's membrane; otherwise, donor endothelium resting against host Descemet's membrane may severely compromise the graft.

Postoperative Care and Complications

The postoperative care of a corneal transplant is far more complex than the care that follows cataract surgery. The long-term success of a PK is probably more dependent on the quality of the postoperative care than on the expertise of the operative technique. Routine postsurgical care—use of topical antibiotics and tapering topical steroids and frequent office visits—is directed at prevention and early recognition of the myriad complications that can occur after PK. This section covers some of the more common postsurgical complications. Astigmatism and graft rejection are discussed separately.

Wound leak   The wound is always checked carefully for leakage at the end of surgery. Small wound leaks that do not cause anterior chamber shallowing frequently close spontaneously. Patching, therapeutic contact lenses, and use of inhibitors of aqueous production may hasten wound closure. Resuturing is advised for leaks lasting longer than 3 days.

Flat chamber/iris incarceration in the wound   Both of these problems imply either poor wound integrity or excessive posterior pressure, and early surgical intervention is advised.

Glaucoma   High IOP may occur at any time after PK. Often, the first clinical sign is the loss of folds in Descemet's membrane, usually seen in the early postoperative period. Glaucoma should be treated aggressively with medical, laser, or surgical intervention as indicated.

Endophthalmitis   After PK, endophthalmitis may arise from intraoperative contamination, donor button contamination, or postoperative invasion by organisms. Extremely aggressive intervention can save the eye in some cases.

Primary endothelial failure   When the graft is edematous from the first postoperative day and remains so without inflammatory signs, a deficiency of donor endothelium is presumed (Fig XXIV-5). Most surgeons allow several weeks for spontaneous resolution of edema and then consider a regraft.

Persistent epithelial defect   Large epithelial defects are common after PK, but they should heal within 14 days. After this time irreversible scarring and ulceration may occur. Ocular surface disease (such as dry eye, exposure, rosacea, blepharitis, or trichiasis) should be ruled out or treated. Lubrication, patching, therapeutic contact lenses, and tarsorrhaphy may be helpful in difficult cases.

Recurrence of primary disease   Bacterial, fungal, viral, and amoebic keratitis, as well as stromal dystrophies, can recur in a graft (Fig XXIV-6). Treatment is directed at the causative agent in recurrent infections; regraft may be required for recurrent dystrophy.

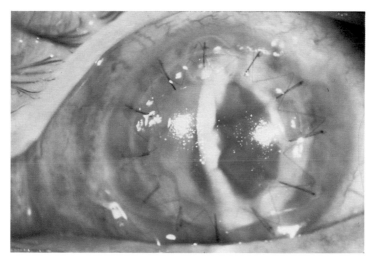

FIG XXIV-5—Primary endothelial failure after PK.

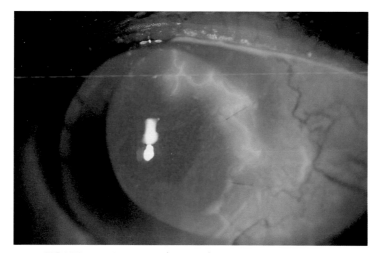

FIG XXIV-6—Herpes simplex virus keratitis recurrent in a graft.

Suture-related problems Postoperative problems related to sutures include the following:

□ Excessive tightness

□ Loosening (usually as a result of wound contraction, suture breakage, or suture cheese wiring)

□ Infectious abscesses (usually localized around loose, broken, or exposed sutures, Figs XXIV-7, XXIV-8)

□ Noninfectious (toxic) suture infiltrates (Fig XXIV-9)

□ Giant papillary conjunctivitis from exposed knots

□ Vascularization along suture tracks

Loose and broken sutures do not contribute to wound stability and, therefore, are removed as soon as possible. Totally buried interrupted suture fragments may be left. Vascularization along the suture indicates that the wound is adequately healed in the vicinity and that sutures may be removed safely. Vascularized sutures are prone to loosen and may increase the chance of graft rejection.

Microbial keratitis The use of topical steroids, the presence of epithelial defects or edema, and exposed sutures predispose the PK patient to infectious keratitis, sometimes with unusual organisms. Decreased corneal sensation and topical steroid use may also delay presentation. Lesions must be scraped immediately for diagnosis, followed by broad-spectrum antibiotic therapy, in order to preserve the graft. A peculiar form of keratitis, *infectious crystalline keratopathy,* is seen in grafts and other

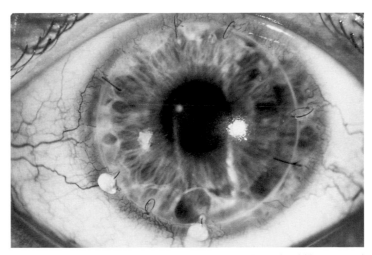

FIG XXIV-7—Broken and exposed sutures after PK. These should be removed immediately, because of the risk of infection and rejection.

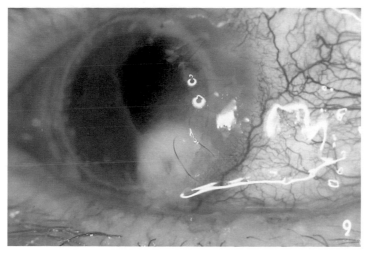

FIG XXIV-8—Suture abscess caused by *S pneumoniae,* 2 years after PK.

immunocompromised corneas (Fig XXIV-10). Branching colonies of organisms proliferate in the deep corneal stroma with no visible inflammatory response. Many organisms have been implicated, but streptococci are seen most frequently.

Late nonimmune endothelial failure When a graft becomes edematous after months to years without inflammatory signs, two causes are possible. First, the tissue may have originally possessed a marginal number of endothelial cells, and the normal spreading of these cells has resulted in inability to maintain graft clarity.

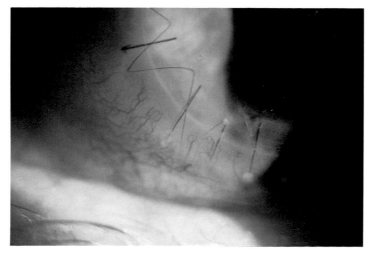

FIG XXIV-9—Deep, noninfectious toxic suture infiltrates after PK.

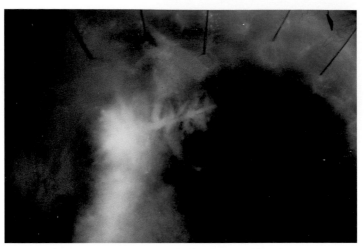

FIG XXIV-10—Infectious crystalline keratopathy after PK.

Alternatively, partial loss of endothelial cells may have occurred later in the postoperative period; possible causes include successfully treated rejection episodes or retention of an intraocular lens that causes endothelial damage.

Control of Postoperative Corneal Astigmatism

A corneal transplant was once considered successful merely if the graft remained clear. Only later in the refinement of surgical procedures was the vexing and relatively common problem of high corneal astigmatism after surgery seriously addressed. Severe astigmatism may be associated with decreased visual acuity, anisometropia, aniseikonia, image distortion, and monocular diplopia, thus rendering an otherwise successful operation ineffective.

Astigmatism is the most frequent complication of PK. It may result in anisometropic asthenopic symptoms or in the inability to wear contact lenses. Many methods have been used to reduce the occurrence:

◻ Varying suture techniques

◻ Making intraoperative and postoperative adjustments

◻ Improving trephines to better match donor and host

◻ Matching donor 12 o'clock position to host 12 o'clock position

◻ Using computerized videokeratography for postoperative management

Use of *relaxing incisions* is the prinicipal measure taken to reduce astigmatism. Incisions are placed inside the graft–host junction at the steep (plus cylinder) meridian in an arcuate manner for maximum effect. Placement in the wound is complicated by varying thickness and the possibility of perforation, and placement in the host is less predictable because the ring scar at the wound interferes with normal deflection of the cornea. The proper axis and length of incision are choosen based on evaluation of the peripheral cornea with Placido disk image or videokeratography.

Overcorrections can be treated by opening the wound, removing the epithelial plug, and resuturing. *Compression sutures* placed across the graft–host junction can be added in the opposite meridian from the relaxing incisions to increase the incisional wound gape and enhance the effect. The surgical goal is a 50% overcorrection early. Permanent sutures of 10-0 nylon or Mersilene are placed with a slip knot and adjusted to give the desired effect prior to burying the knots. Compression sutures can be removed to titrate the effect.

Wedge resection in the flat meridian is reserved for high degrees of astigmatism (≥8 D) associated with marked flattening (<35 D) and hyperopic spherical equivalent. Wedge resection effectively shortens the radius of curvature in its axis, adding power to the cornea (Fig XXIV-11). The length (70°–90° of arc) and width (maximum

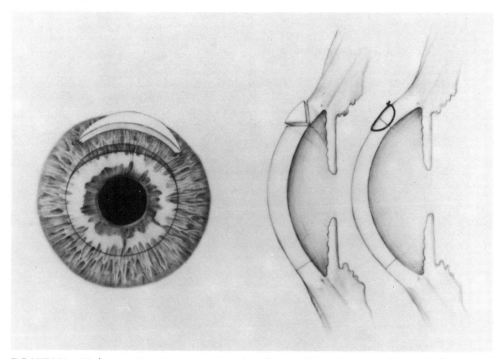

FIG XXIV-11—Wedge resection. A crescentic wedge of corneal tissue is removed from the flat corneal meridian to reduce postoperative astigmatism. (Reproduced by permission from Schwab IR, ed. *Refractive Keratoplasty.* New York: Churchill Livingstone; 1987.)

of 1.5 mm) of resection determine the final results, but the operation is more complex and less predictable than use of relaxing incisions.

All of these procedures are associated with potential for micro- or macroperforation, infection, rejection, under- and overcorrections, chronic epithelial defects, and worsening of irregular astigmatism.

Krachmer JH, Mannis MJ, Holland EJ, eds. *Cornea*. St Louis: Mosby; 1997;3:chap 137.

Tasman W, Jaeger EA, eds. *Duane's Clinical Ophthalmology*. Philadelphia: Lippincott; 1994;6:chap 26.

Diagnosis and Management of Graft Rejection

Corneal allograft rejection rarely occurs within 2 weeks, and it may occur as late as 20 years after PK. Fortunately, most episodes of graft rejection do not result in irreversible graft failure if recognized early and treated aggressively with corticosteroids. Early recognition of rejection is the key to survival of an affected corneal graft. Corneal transplant rejection takes three clinical forms, which may occur either singly or in combination.

Epithelial rejection   The immune response may be directed purely toward the donor epithelium (Fig XXIV-12). Lymphocytes cause an elevated, linear epithelial ridge that advances centripetally. Since host cells replace lost donor epithelium, this form of rejection is problematic only in that it may herald the onset of endothelial rejection. Epithelial rejection has been reported at a rate of 10% of those patients experiencing rejection, and it is usually seen early in the postoperative period (1–13 months).

Subepithelial rejection   Corneal transplant rejection may also take the form of subepithelial infiltrates (Fig XXIV-13). When seen alone, these may cause no symptoms. It is not known if these lymphocytic cells are directed at donor keratocytes or

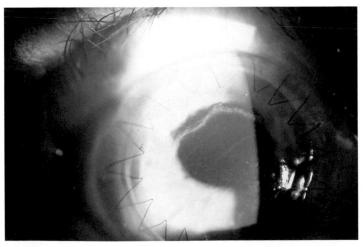

FIG XXIV-12—An epithelial rejection line after PK.

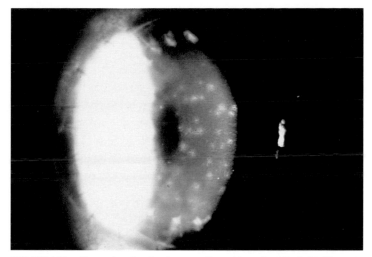

FIG XXIV-13—Corneal graft rejection manifested by subepithelial infiltrates.

at donor epithelial cells. A cellular anterior chamber reaction may also accompany this form of rejection. Easily missed on cursory examination, subepithelial infiltrates can best be seen with broad, tangential light. They resemble infiltrates of adenovirus keratitis. Subepithelial graft rejection leaves no sequelae if treated, but it may pre-date the more severe endothelial graft rejection.

Isolated stromal rejection is not common but can be seen as stromal infiltrates and neovascularization. In very aggressive severe or prolonged bouts of graft rejection, the stroma can become necrotic.

Endothelial rejection The most common form of graft rejection is endothelial rejection with reported rates of 8%–37%. It is also the most serious form of corneal transplant rejection, because endothelial cells destroyed by the host response can be replaced only by a regraft. Inflammatory precipitates are seen on the endothelial surface in fine precipitates, in random clumps, or in linear form (Khodadoust line, Fig XXIV-14). Inflammatory cells are usually seen in the anterior chamber as well. As endothelial function is lost, the corneal stroma thickens and the epithelium becomes edematous. Patients have symptoms related to inflammation and corneal edema such as photophobia, redness, halos around lights, and fogginess of vision.

Treatment Frequent administration of corticosteroid eyedrops is the mainstay of therapy for corneal allograft rejection. Either dexamethasone 0.1% or prednisolone 1.0% eyedrops are used as often as every 15 minutes to 2 hours, depending on the severity of the episode. Although topical corticosteroid ointments may be used on occasion, their bioavailability is not as good as frequently applied eyedrops.

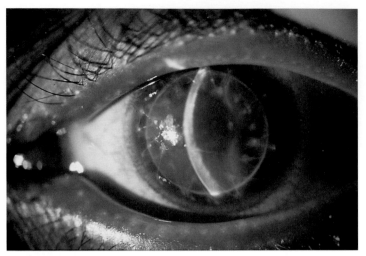

FIG XXIV-14—Endothelial graft rejection with stromal and epithelial edema on the trailing aspect of the migrating Khodadoust line.

Corticosteroids may be given by periocular injection for severe rejection episodes or noncompliant patients. In particularly fulminant cases systemic corticosteroids may be administered either orally or intravenously (80–120 mg methylprednisolone as a one-time dose). Oral or topical cyclosporine (2% in corn oil) has been used prophylactically in high-risk grafts and may help reverse an ongoing graft-rejection episode.

Brightbill FS, ed. *Corneal Surgery: Theory, Technique, and Tissue*. 2nd ed. St Louis: Mosby; 1993.

The Collaborative Corneal Transplantation Studies Research Group. Effectiveness of histocompatibility matching in high-risk corneal transplantation. *Arch Ophthalmol*. 1992;110:1392–1403.

Donnenfeld ED, Ingraham HJ, Perry HD, et al. Soemmering's ring support for posterior chamber intraocular lens implantation during penetrating keratoplasty. Changing trends in bullous keratopathy. *Ophthalmology*. 1992;99:1229–1233.

Litoff D, Krachmer JH. Complications of corneal surgery. *Int Ophthalmol Clin*. 1992; 32:79–96.

Mamalis N, Anderson CW, Kreisler KR, et al. Changing trends in the indications for penetrating keratoplasty. *Arch Ophthalmol*. 1992;110:1409–1411.

Pediatric Corneal Transplants

Corneal transplantation in infants and children presents special problems. Development of amblyopia and the presence of concomitant ocular abnormalities often result in poor vision despite a technically successful graft. Improvements in pediatric anesthesia and the recognition that development of amblyopia following congenital and childhood diseases of the anterior segment is a major impediment to useful vision have led to PK being performed in neonates as early as 2 weeks after birth. Increased understanding of the special problems associated with pediatric grafts and advances in surgical methods have improved the outlook for corneal transplants and have permitted earlier and more frequent surgical intervention. The best chance for a successful outcome in these cases comes with comanagement by the cornea specialist and the pediatric ophthalmologist.

Corneal grafting in children under the age of 2 is associated with rapid neovascularization, especially along the sutures, which necessitates suture removal as early as 2 weeks after PK. The eye wall is extremely flaccid at this age and collapses readily during surgery when the diseased cornea is excised. Other common problems include anterior bulging of the lens–iris diaphragm (sometimes resulting in spontaneous delivery of the lens) and the propensity to develop large zones of iridocorneal adhesions.

A scleral ring is crucial for providing additional support in most pediatric grafts, particularly in neonates. Intravitreal pressure may be reduced by preoperative massage, ocular compression, or systemic hyperosmotic agents. Using a small-sized corneal opening may reduce the degree of anterior lens–iris bulge and the chance of peripheral synechiae formation. Preplaced mattress sutures in the recipient tissue can be brought up quickly over the donor tissue and secured, allowing for quicker re-formation of the anterior chamber and placement of definitive 10-0 nylon sutures. Early fitting with a contact lens (as early as the time of PK) and ocular occlusive therapy are necessary to stem the development of amblyopia in children with monocular aphakia.

Postoperative glaucoma, self-induced trauma, and immune rejection are extremely common, and pediatric patients should be examined very frequently and closely after surgery. Sedation or general anesthesia is usually necessary for detailed postoperative examination and suture removal.

Corneal Autograft Procedures

The great advantage of a corneal autograft is the elimination of the risk of allograft rejection. Although cases with clinical circumstances appropriate for autograft are uncommon, an astute ophthalmologist who recognizes the possibility of a successful autograft can spare a patient the risk of long-term topical steroid use and the necessity of lifelong vigilance against rejection.

Rotational Autograft

A rotating autograft can be used to reposition a localized corneal scar that involves the pupillary axis. By making an eccentric trephination and rotating the host button prior to resuturing, the surgeon can place a paracentral zone of clear cornea in the pupillary axis. The procedure is particularly useful in children, who have a poorer prognosis for PK. Graft edema can still be a problem, since both the preexisting disease/scar and the rotating keratoplasty procedure usually cause endothelial cell loss. Residual postoperative astigmatism is also a problem because of the eccentric location of the graft.

Bourne WM, Brubaker RF. A method for ipsilateral rotational autokeratoplasty. *Ophthalmology.* 1978;85:1312–1316.

Contralateral Autograft

A contralateral autograft is reserved for patients who have in one eye a corneal opacity with a favorable prognosis for visual recovery and in the other eye both a clear cornea and severe dysfunction of the afferent system (e.g., retinal detachment, severe amblyopia). The clear cornea is transplanted to the first eye, and the cornea in the second eye is replaced either with the diseased cornea from the first eye or with an allograft, or the eye is eviscerated/enucleated. Such bilateral grafting carries the risk of bilateral endophthalmitis.

Lamellar Keratoplasty

Lamellar keratoplasty is a partial-thickness corneal allograft procedure. The high success rate of PK has reduced the need for lamellar keratoplasty in treating corneal disease. Antimicrobial agents, corticosteroids, bandage lenses, and tissue adhesives now control many disorders that were previously managed by this technique. Despite these advances, the cornea surgeon should be familiar with the special indications and limitations of lamellar keratoplasty.

Indications

Lamellar corneal grafting may be indicated in patients who present with opacities or loss of tissue that, for the most part, does not involve the full thickness of the cornea (Fig XXIV-15). These conditions include

- Superficial stromal dystrophies and degenerations (e.g., Reis-Bücklers dystrophy, Salzmann nodular degeneration, band keratopathy)
- Superficial corneal scars
- Recurrent pterygium in the presence of secondary stromal thinning
- Corneal thinning (e.g., Terrien marginal degeneration, descemetocele formation, pellucid marginal degeneration)
- Superficial corneal tumors
- Congenital lesions (e.g., dermoid)
- Corneal perforations that are not amenable to resuturing or that occur in patients with ocular surface disease (e.g., keratitis sicca)
- Keratoconus

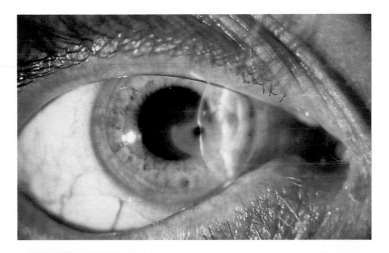

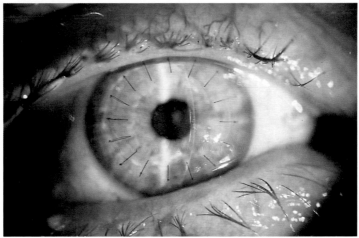

FIG XXIV-15—Descemetocele in a patient with rheumatoid arthritis *(top)*. Same patient after lamellar keratoplasty *(bottom)*.

Advantages   Lamellar keratoplasty has the following advantages over penetrating keratoplasty:

- Minimal requirements for donor material (as preservation of endothelium is not mandatory)
- Avoidance of entrance into the anterior chamber
- Shorter wound healing and convalescence
- Reduced incidence of allograft rejection and, consequently, decreased need for topical steroids

Lamellar keratoplasty is less risky than PK in patients who have ocular surface disease, show poor compliance with medical instructions, or experience difficulty in obtaining frequent follow-up.

Disadvantages Lamellar keratoplasty does not replace damaged endothelium, and this obvious restriction is the major determinant of the indications. The procedure is technically more difficult, and it may cause opacification and vascularization of the interface, which may limit visual function. Some authors consider herpes simplex virus keratitis to be a contraindication for lamellar keratoplasty.

Surgical Technique

Penetration into the anterior chamber remains the major operative complication, and it may at times require conversion to a PK. A few basic principles apply to the lamellar graft technique. The recipient cornea is dissected first, because a full-thickness graft may be necessary if the cornea sustains a large perforation during the lamellar dissection and to allow for accurate sizing of donor tissue. The donor lamellar graft may be taken from the whole globe. If possible, more than one donor eye should be available because of the difficulty of the lamellar dissection. In addition, preground stromal buttons for lamellar grafting are now available.

A microkeratome is capable of making both the recipient lamellar dissection and the donor dissection. The precision of this instrument has greatly reduced the opacification at the host–donor interface. The donor button can also be prepared by resecting Descemet's membrane from a corneal button using fine (Vannas) scissors.

Postoperative Care and Complications

Opacification and vascularization of the interface Meticulous irrigation and cleaning of the lamellar bed at surgery may reduce opacification and vascularization, which may occur despite corticosteroid therapy. Postoperatively, best-corrected visual acuity is usually limited to 20/40 or worse.

Allograft rejection Since the endothelium is not transplanted, endothelial rejection cannot take place. Epithelial rejection, subepithelial infiltrates, and stromal rejection occasionally occur, but they respond to corticosteroid therapy. If graft edema occurs, another cause must be found for endothelial dysfunction.

Inflammatory necrosis of the graft Although inflammatory necrosis of the graft has previously been described as an allograft reaction, no immunohistopathologic evidence has confirmed this, and recent series have not demonstrated this phenomenon. The mechanism probably relates to the preexisting corneal disease. Prognosis for retention of a clear graft is poor despite corticosteroid therapy.

Future Developments

Studies are under way to evaluate the feasibility of using intrastromal lasers to assist in the creation of the lamellar bed and to remove Descemet's membrane from the donor button. The donor–host interface could be made much more smoothly with lasers than with manual techniques, perhaps in turn reducing postoperative opacity at this level. One concern under investigation is whether shock waves from deep lamellar ablation may damage host endothelium. By facilitating the more technically difficult components of a lamellar keratoplasty, the laser may increase the frequency with which this procedure is recommended.

Arentsen JJ. Lamellar grafting. In: Brightbill FS, ed. *Corneal Surgery: Theory, Technique, and Tissue.* 2nd ed. St Louis: Mosby; 1992:360–368.

Ehrlich MI, Phinney RB, Mondino BJ, et al. Techniques of lamellar keratoplasty. *Int Ophthalmol Clin.* 1988;28:24–29.

Keratoprosthesis

In the presence of severe cicatricial changes with total loss of the fornices and deep corneal vascularization, PK has little, if any, chance for success. In those patients with bilateral disease, keratoprosthesis surgery may afford the only hope for useful vision. Many types of keratoprosthesis have been tried, but in all systems an artificial cornea must both focus light and serve as an interface between biological tissue and the environment. Because the best results are obtained when keratoprosthesis is the initial procedure, patients should be spared massive anterior segment reconstruction when the prognosis for visual improvement is hopeless.

Although keratoprosthesis has had acceptable short-term success, long-term results have been discouraging. Common and serious complications include sterile vitritis, the formation of a retroprosthetic membrane that effectively obscures vision, glaucoma, endophthalmitis, and extrusion of the prosthesis. Because of the occurrence and severity of postoperative problems and the poor visual outcome, a keratoprosthesis is indicated only in a bilaterally blind patient whose prognosis with other reconstructive surgery is extremely poor. It should not be considered when a reasonable prognosis for some visual restoration with penetrating keratoplasty exists or when some useful vision remains in the fellow eye.

Hicks CR, Fitton JH, Chivila TV, et al. Keratoprosthesis: advancing toward a true artificial cornea. *Surv Ophthalmol.* 1997;42:175–189.

Scleral Grafting

Surgical therapy for defects in the sclera is rarely necessary. Scleral thinning or ectasia can be seen following trauma, infection, or scleritis, while staphylomas are more likely to develop in the setting of associated chronic elevated IOP. Adequate medical therapy often allows the base of small scleral defects to be covered by newly formed collagen.

Chapter X discusses scleritis and episcleritis in the context of immune-related disorders. Scleritis and scleromalacia perforans are sometimes associated with significant and progressive thinning of the sclera. Although even very large scleral defects generally do not perforate spontaneously, such eyes are more susceptible to trauma and may warrant coverage with a scleral patch graft. Eye bank sclera in full or split thickness or corneal tissue is used in the size necessary to encompass the area of pathology. When these grafts can be covered by conjunctiva, they usually remain viable.

Scleral grafts do not prevent progressive disease such as necrotizing scleritis in the host tissue, where it will also destroy the scleral patch graft if uncontrolled. Scleral grafts are commonly used in reconstructive eyelid procedures and in association with setons for management of glaucoma.

PART 12

KERATOREFRACTIVE SURGERY

CHAPTER XXV

Basic Science of Keratorefractive Surgery

Refractive surgery encompasses a broad range of procedures to change the refraction of the eye. BCSC Section 3, *Optics, Refraction, and Contact Lenses,* discusses the optical considerations for these procedures. Such procedures include techniques to alter the basic shape of the cornea or its ability to refract light. A classification of terms used in "keratospeak" is summarized in Table XXV-1.

Currently, the most prevalent refractive surgery is cataract removal with intraocular lens implantation, which is covered in BCSC Section 11, *Lens and Cataract.* Other related techniques include removal of the natural lens to treat myopia (clear lens extraction), removal and replacement of the natural lens with IOLs to treat both hyperopia or myopia, or insertion of an artificial lens without natural lens removal (phakic IOL). All are effective methods for correcting refractive errors, but safety has not been established; the rate of complications including retinal detachment and loss of corneal endothelial cells is undetermined.

Refractive surgery involving the cornea is rapidly changing with advances in technology. Chapter XXVI discusses the clinical aspects of keratorefractive surgery, and chapter XXVII covers laser techniques. Schematic illustrations of the more frequent procedures are shown later in this chapter.

Corneal Optics

Zones of the Cornea

For more than 100 years the *corneal shape* has been recognized as aspheric. Typically, the central cornea is about 3 D steeper than the periphery, a positive shape factor. Clinically, the cornea is divided into zones that surround fixation and blend into each other. The *central zone* of 1–2 mm closely fits a spherical surface. Adjacent to the central zone is a 3–4 mm doughnut with an outer diameter of 7–8 mm. Termed the *paracentral zone,* this doughnut represents an area of progressive flattening from the center. Adjacent to the paracentral zone is the *peripheral zone* with an outer diameter of approximately 11 mm, and adjoining this is the *limbus* with an outer diameter on average of 12 mm. The central and paracentral zones are primarily responsible for the refractive power of the cornea (Fig XXV-1, see p 442).

Together, the paracentral and central zones constitute the *apical zone* as used in contact lens fitting. The peripheral zone is also known as the *transitional zone,* as this is the area of greatest flattening and asphericity of the normal cornea. The limbal zone sits adjacent to the sclera and represents an area of steepening of the cornea prior to joining the sclera at the limbal sulcus.

TABLE XXV-1
CLASSIFICATION OF CORNEAL REFRACTIVE SURGERY

TYPE OF REFRACTIVE KERATOPLASTY	BASIC SURGICAL TECHNIQUE	VARIATIONS OF SURGICAL TECHNIQUE OR MATERIAL	REFRACTIVE ERROR TREATED	COMMENT
Lamellar	Keratomileusis (KM, cutting corneal disc with microkeratome)	Microkeratome techniques ■ Manual or mechanical advance ■ Oscillating or rotating blade Methods of making refractive stromal cut ■ Barraquer's cryolathe	Myopia (MKM) hyperopia, aphakia	Suture techniques: Appositional, overlay, no suture Computerized calculations and control
		■ Nonfreeze—microkeratome with suction mold (BKS)	Myopia, hyperopia, aphakia	
		■ Excimer laser (ArF, 193 nm)	Myopia	Early clinical trials
		Source of tissue for disc ■ Patient (autoplastic) ■ Donor (homoplastic)		
	KM in situ (carving corneal bed)	Microkeratome (plano excision)	Myopia	
		Keratokyphosis (refractive mold in microkeratome)	Myopia	In laboratory development
		Excimer laser (ArF, 193 nm) ■ Complete disc ■ Flap disc (LASIK)	Myopia, astigmatism Hyperopia	Phase III FDA trials in U.S. Early clinical trials
		Autokeratophakia (same as KM in situ, except stromal button is cut smaller with trephine and left in place)	Hyperopia	In development in Moscow
	Epikeratoplasty (Epi)	Human donor lenticule ■ Cryolathe ■ Suction mold (BKS) ■ Excimer laser ■ Lyophilized	Aphakia, hyperopia Myopia	If contact lens and IOL contraindicated, e.g., infant aphakia FDA core study; in laboratory development
		Synthetic (e.g., collagen and coated hydrogel)		
		Plano lenticule	Astigmatism and myopia in keratoconus	If penetrating keratoplasty contraindicated

Procedure	Technique/Subtype	Indication	Status/Comments
Intracorneal lens or ring (ICL, ICR, keratophakia)	Microkeratome (lamellar bed)		
	▪ Hydrogel lenticule	Aphakia, myopia	Early clinical trials
	▪ Human donor lenticule	Aphakia, myopia	Seldom used
	Lamellar pocket		
	▪ High index of refraction (e.g., fenestrated polysulfone)	Aphakia	In laboratory development
	▪ Fresnel hydrogel	Aphakia	In laboratory development
	Annular lamellar dissection		
	▪ Intracorneal ring		
	— Fixed volume: PMMA, silicone	Myopia	Phase III trials in U.S.
	▪ Gel injection adjustable (volume) keratoplasty	Myopia	In laboratory development
	Autokeratophakia; folded corneal flap	Aphakia	Under development in Russia
Lamellar keratotomy	Single deep microkeratome pass	Hyperopia	Early clinical trials
Lamellar keratoplasty	Central	Irregular astigmatism (e.g., keratoconus)	
	Crescentic	Astigmatism from marginal thinning (e.g., Terrien degeneration)	
Keratotomy (refractive keratotomy)			
Radial	Single nomogram	Myopia	
	Staged with repeated adjustments		
	Open and suture wounds		Reduce overcorrection
Transverse (TK, AK)	Isolated straight or arcuate (T cuts)	Astigmatism Primary (naturally occurring) Secondary (e.g. postoperative and posttraumatic)	Incision made transverse to steep corneal meridian (axis of plus refractive cylinder)
	Combined with radial	Compound myopic astigmatism	
	▪ Between radial		
	▪ Interrupted transverse		
	▪ Interrupted radial		
	▪ Trapezoidal (Ruiz, sem radial)		
	Modification of penetrating keratoplasty (relaxing incision)		
	▪ Wound separation or incision in wound	Postoperative astigmatism	Often staged under keratoscopic or keratometric control
	▪ Transverse incision in cone	Postoperative astigmatism	

Continued

KEY: KM, keratomileusis; MKM, myopic keratomileusis; BKS, Barraquer-Krumeich-Swinger; ArF, argon fluoride; PMMA, polymethylmethacrylate; Epi, epikeratoplasty; IOL, intraocular lens; ICL, intracorneal lens; ICR, intracorneal ring; TK, transverse keratotomy; AK, astigmatic keratotomy; PK, penetrating keratoplasty.

439

TABLE XXV-1. CLASSIFICATION OF CORNEAL REFRACTIVE SURGERY (Continued)

TYPE OF REFRACTIVE KERATOPLASTY	BASIC SURGICAL TECHNIQUE	VARIATIONS OF SURGICAL TECHNIQUE OR MATERIAL	REFRACTIVE ERROR TREATED	COMMENT
Keratotomy (refractive keratotomy) (cont)	Transverse (TK, AK) (cont)	Modification of cataract surgery ■ Intraoperative —Astigmatism neutral cataract incision —Manipulation of incision to reduce preexisting astigmatism, adjust wound size, center incision on steep meridian —Scleral flap recession or resection —Transverse keratotomy	Naturally occurring astigmatism	Limbal or corneal cataract incision acts like TK Length <5 mm Scleral tunnel Few or no sutures
		■ Postoperative —Transverse keratotomy —Wound revision	Postoperative astigmatism High against-the-rule astigmatism	
		Suture adjustment ■ Removal or cutting of interrupted ■ Distribution of tension on running ■ Placement of compression sutures	Postoperative astigmatism	
	Circumferential	Hexagonal —Nonconnected —With transverse (hex-T)	Hyperopia	Acts like keratotomy Seldom used Seldom used
		Circular, partial-thickness trephination with double running suture	Astigmatism	Acts like wedge resection
Keratectomy	Laser	Photorefractive keratectomy (PRK) (central sculpting, large area ablation, and multiple zone ablation) ■ Excimer laser (ArF, 193 nm) ■ 5th harmonic Nd:YAG laser (213 nm)	Myopia, astigmatism, hyperopia Primary (naturally occurring) Secondary (e.g., after radial, Epi, PK)	FDA approved for –1.00 to –10.00 D in U.S.
		Linear laser keratectomy (radial, transverse)	Myopia, astigmatism	–1.00 to –4.00 D of astigmatism in U.S. (hyperopia in FDA trial) Excimer laser (193 nm), seldom used
		Intrastromal photodisruption with Nd:YAG laser ■ Picosecond ND-YLF (1053 nm) ■ Nanosecond frequency—doubled Nd:YAG laser (532 nm)	Myopia	In laboratory development

Procedure	Technique	Indication (to be evaluated)	Status
Mechanical	■ Nanosecond Nd:YAG laser (1064 nm)	To be evaluated	In laboratory development
	Laser adjustable synthetic Epi	Astigmatism	
	Crescentic wedge ■ Wedge resection after PK ■ Wound repair during or after cataract extraction	Astigmatism	
	Crescentic lamellar corneal tuck or flap for Terrien or pellucid marginal degenerations		
	Mechanical central refractive superficial keratectomy ■ Rotating blades ■ Fine water stream	Astigmatism	In design phase
Thermokeratoplasty	Holmium YAG laser (2.06 μm) Radial or circular pattern, peripheral or paracentral	Hyperopia/myopia	In clinical trials
	Treatment in flat meridian with or without concurrent treatment for myopia and hyperopia	Astigmatism	
	Deep stromal hot needle thermocoagulation Peripheral, intrastromal, radial pattern	Hyperopia	Seldom used
	Arcuate in flat meridian	Astigmatism	
Penetrating keratoplasty (refractive aspects)	Donor–host size disparity Donor oversized	Hyperopia, aphakia	
	Donor undersized	Myopia, keratoconus	
	Suture adjustment during or after surgery Selective removal of interrupted sutures in steep meridian		
	Adjustment of running suture		
	Early opening of wound in steep meridian		
	Early placement of interrupted sutures in flat meridian		

KEY: KM, keratomileusis; MKM, myopic keratomileusis; BKS, Barraquer-Krumeich-Swinger; ArF, argon fluoride; PMMA, polymethylmethacrylate; Epi, epikeratoplasty; IOL, intraocular lens; ICL, intracorneal lens; ICR, intracorneal ring; TK, transverse keratotomy; AK, astigmatic keratotomy; PK, penetrating keratoplasty.

Modified from Waring GO III. Making sense of keratospeak IV: classification of refractive surgery, 1992. *Arch Ophthalmol.* 1992;110:1385–1391 For IOL implants, see BCSC Section 11, *Lens and Cataract.*

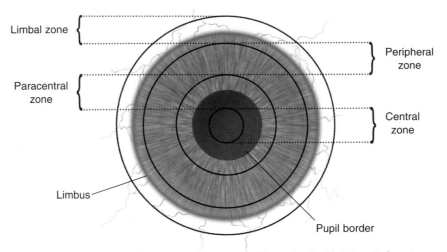

Limbal zone

Peripheral zone

Paracentral zone

Central zone

Limbus

Pupil border

FIG XXV-1—Topographic zones of the cornea. (Illustration by Christine Gralapp.)

The *optical zone* of the cornea is that portion that overlies the entrance pupil of the iris but is physiologically limited to approximately 5.4 mm because of the Stiles-Crawford effect. The *corneal apex* is the point of maximum curvature, typically temporal to the center of the pupil. The *corneal vertex* is the point located at the intersection of the patient's line of fixation and the corneal surface. It is represented by the corneal light reflex when the cornea is illuminated coaxially with fixation. The corneal vertex is the center of the keratoscopic image and does not necessarily correspond to the point of maximum curvature at the corneal apex (Fig XXV-2).

Shape, Curvature, and Power

Three topographic properties of the cornea are important to its optical function: the underlying *shape,* which determines its *curvature* and hence its refractive *power.* Shape and curvature are *geometric* properties of the cornea. Power is the *functional* property. Historically, power was the first parameter of the cornea described, and diopters representing the refractive power of the central cornea were accepted as the basic unit of measurement. The advent of contact lenses and refractive surgery has made knowing the overall shape and its related property of curvature more important. BCSC Section 3, *Optics, Refraction, and Contact Lenses,* covers these topics in greater depth.

The refractive power of the cornea is determined by *Snell's law,* or the *law of refraction.* The ophthalmometer (keratometer) empirically estimates corneal power by reading four points of the central 2.8–4.0 mm zone. These points do not represent the corneal apex or vertex but are a clinically useful estimation of central corneal power. The radius of curvature is calculated from the simple vergence formula using the known object size and measuring the distance with doubling prisms

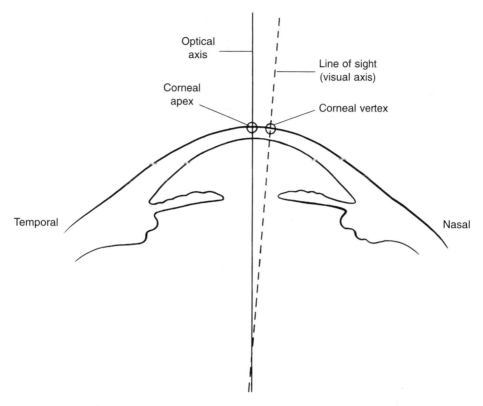

FIG XXV-2—Corneal vertex and apex. (Illustration by Christine Gralapp.)

to stabilize the image. The axial radius of curvature is then used in computing the corneal power in this region.

Snell's law requires a difference of two refractive indexes, that of the cornea and that of air divided by the radius of curvature. The anterior corneal power using air and corneal stromal refractive indices is higher than clinically useful because the negative contribution of the posterior cornea is not included. To accommodate this difference for most clinical purposes, a derived corneal refractive index of 1.3375 is used in calculating central corneal power. This value was chosen to allow 45 D to equate to a 7.5-mm radius of curvature. Average refractive power of the central cornea is about +43 D, which is the sum of the refractive power at the air–stroma interface of +49 D minus the endothelium–aqueous power of 6 D. The refractive index of air is 1.000, aqueous and tears is 1.336, and corneal stroma is 1.376. Although the cornea with its air–tear interface is responsible for most of the eye's refraction, the difference between total corneal power based on stroma alone and with tears is only –.06 D.

Corneal Topography

Snell's law indicates that the power is dependent on the angle of incidence of the light to the surface in question and the radius of curvature of the surface at that point. Keratometers and Placido disk–based computerized topographers assume the angle of incidence to be nearly perpendicular and the radius of curvature to be the distance from the surface to the intersection with the line of sight or visual axis of the patient *(axial distance)*.

These values *(axial curvature)* are a very close approximation to power in the central 1–2 mm of the cornea but fail to describe the true shape and power of the peripheral cornea. Ray tracing shows that the corneal power must increase in the periphery based on Snell's law in order to refract the light into the pupil. Ellipsoidal surfaces will show aspheric power that increases in the periphery *(spherical aberration)*. Conventionally, normal corneas show decreasing diopters toward the periphery as displayed by the Placido disk. This instrument gives an intuitive sense of the normal flattening of the cornea but does not represent the true refractive powers or the true curvature of the cornea as inspection moves away from the center.

A second method of describing the corneal curvature is to use the *instantaneous radius of curvature* at a certain point, also termed the *tangential power* by some manufacturers. This radius is determined by taking a perpendicular through the point in question from a plane that intersects the point and the visual axis but allowing the radius to be the length necessary to correspond to a sphere with the same curvature at that point. The instantaneous radius of curvature, with curvature given in diopters, is estimated by the difference between the corneal index of refraction and 1.000 divided by this tangentially determined radius. This map typically shows better sensitivity to peripheral changes with less "smoothing" of the curvature than the axial maps (Fig XXV-3). (Diopters in these maps are relative units of curvature and not the equivalent to diopters of corneal power.)

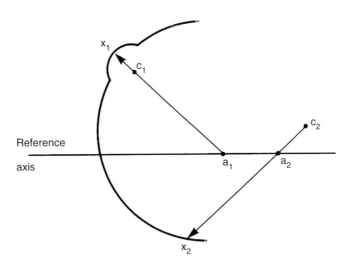

FIG XXV-3—Axial and instantaneous corneal power (two dimensional). Axial curvature at points x_1 and x_2 is based on axial distances x_1 to a_1 and x_2 to a_2. Instantaneous curvature at points x_1 and x_2 is based on radii of curvature from x_1 to c_1 and x_2 to c_2. (Illustration by Christine Gralapp.)

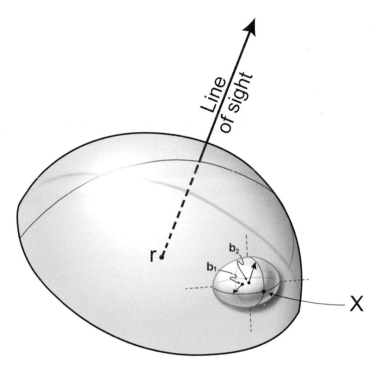

FIG XXV-4—Mean corneal power (three dimensional). Power at point x of this outpouching from the basic spheroid is calculated by averaging the minimum curvature represented by radius of curvature from b_1 to x and the maximum curvature from b_2 to x. These two lines do not necessarily cross the reference axis. r is the center of rotation of the large sphere; b_1 and b_2 are the centers of rotation of the minimum and the maximum best fit sphere. (Illustration by Christine Gralapp.)

A third map, the *mean curvature map,* does not require the perpendicular ray to cross the visual axis, allowing for an infinite number of spheres to fit the curvature at that point (Fig XXV-4). The algorithm determines a minimum and maximum size best fit sphere and from their radii determines an average curvature (arithmetic mean of principal curvatures) for that point, the *mean curvature.* These powers are then mapped using standard colors to represent diopter changes, allowing even more sensitivity to peripheral changes of curvature.

All of the maps described above are attempts to reflect the underlying shape of the cornea by scaling curvature through the familiar dioptric notation instead of the less familiar millimeters of radius. A more accurate way to describe curvature would be to use the true shape of the cornea. Other systems directly derive the shape of the cornea and then determine power from that shape.

In order to view shape directly, maps may display a *z-height* from an arbitrary plane (iris plane, limbal plane, or frontal plane) using color maps. Just as viewing the curvature of the earth in an appropriate scale fails to show details of mountains and basins, these "z" maps do not show clinically important variations. Geographic

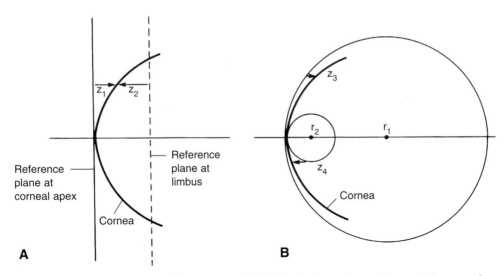

FIG XXV-5—Height maps (typically in microns). *A,* Height relative to plane surface. z_1 is below surface parallel to corneal apex. z_2 is above surface parallel to corneal limbus. *B,* Height relative to reference sphere. z_3 is below a flat sphere of radius r_1. z_4 is above a steep sphere of radius r_2. (Illustration by Christine Gralapp.)

maps show land elevation relative to sea level. Similarly, corneal surface maps are plotted to show differences from best fit spheres or other objects that closely mimic the normal corneal shape (Fig XXV-5).

Ideally, the corneal and lenticular shapes are detected for the anterior and posterior surfaces of each. Then ray tracing can develop an accurate refractive map of the eye to establish the normal effects of the cornea and lens surfaces on the wave front of light. Alterations of the shape of the eye structures can then be planned to maximize the refractive effect and minimize the aberrations of keratorefractive and other surgeries. The American National Standards Institute (ANSI) in the United States is currently developing standards for the corneal topography industry to make the comparison of maps more uniform and to clarify the confusion of terminology.

Indications Corneal topography detects irregular astigmatism from contact lens warpage, keratoconus and other thinning disorders, corneal surgery, trauma, and postinflammatory and degenerative conditions. Patients with corneal warpage (irregular astigmatism and/or peripheral steepening, distorted keratoscopic mires) should discontinue contact lens wear and allow the corneal map and refraction to stabilize prior to undergoing refractive surgery. Patients with keratoconus are not routinely considered for refractive surgery, as the thin cornea has an unpredictable response and reducing its thickness may lead to earlier corneal transplant. The form fruste, or subclinical, keratoconus recognized by Placido disk–based topography requires caution on the part of the ophthalmologist and is considered a contraindication to refractive surgery at this time, although studies are under way to determine suitability for keratorefractive procedures as an alternative to corneal transplant.

Corneal topography is needed in the management of congenital and postoperative astigmatism, particularly following PK. Complex peripheral patterns may result in a refractive axis of astigmatism that is not aligned with topographic axes. Failure to correct the underlying shape by removing appropriate sutures or operating on the appropriate axis (steep in incisional surgery and minus in ablative surgery) may lead to unexpected results.

Corneal topography is also used to determine the effects of keratorefractive procedures on the cornea. Pre- and postoperative maps may be algebraically subtracted to determine whether the desired effect was achieved. Corneal mapping may help to explain unexpected results including undercorrections, aberrations, induced astigmatism, or glare and haloes by detecting decentered surgery or inadequate surgery such as shallow incisions in radial keratotomy.

Corneal topography also confirms the expected physiologic effects of refractive surgery. In radial keratotomy peripheral incisions lead to flattening of the central cornea and would be predicted to lead to flattening in the periphery, even though the central effect is related to a relative peripheral steepening. Difference maps confirm an overall flattening of the entire corneal surface with a differential flattening centrally related to a relative steepening in the midperiphery (Fig XXV-6).

Limitations   In addition to the limitations of the algorithms and variation in terminology by manufacturer, corneal topography has several potential pitfalls summarized in Table XXV-2.

Roberts C. Principles of corneal topography. In: Elander R, Rich LF, Robin JB, eds. *Principles and Practice of Refractive Surgery.* Philadelphia: Saunders; 1997:475–497.

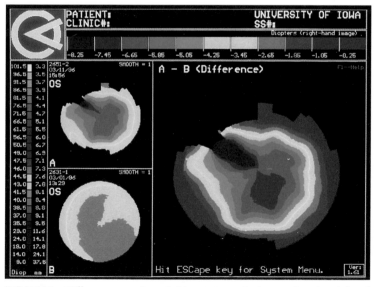

FIG XXV-6—Difference map in radial keratotomy. Both central and peripheral flattening are seen in the postoperative image *(A)* and in the difference map on the right. *B* is the preoperative image.

TABLE XXV-2

POTENTIAL PROBLEMS IN COMPUTERIZED VIDEOKERATOGRAPHY

Misalignment

Stability (test to test variation)

Sensitivity to focus errors

Tear film effects

Distortions

Area of coverage (central and limbal)

Nonstandardized data maps

Colors may be absolute or varied (normalized)

Biomechanics of the Cornea

The cornea is a composite material consisting of collagen fibrils that stretch from limbus to limbus packaged in lamellae that are arranged in parallel fashion and embedded in an extracellular matrix of glycosaminoglycans. The layers slide easily over each other, indicating a very low shear resistance, but the stroma itself is an inelastic, anisotropic structure that distributes tensile stress unequally throughout its thickness, depending on the corneal hydration (Fig XXV-7).

When the cornea is in a dehydrated state, stress is distributed either principally to the posterior layers or uniformly over the entire structure. When the cornea is healthy or edematous, the anterior lamellae take up the strain. Stress within the tissue is partly related to IOP but not in a linear manner under physiologic conditions (normal IOP range).

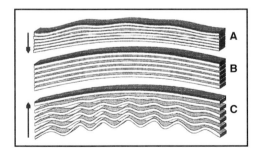
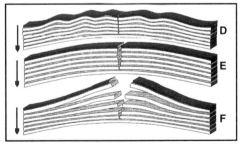

FIG XXV-7—Diagram of the corneal stress model. For nonoperated eyes, the anterior curvature is not affected by IOP or corneal hydration as a result of the inelasticity of the cornea. However, the stress in the cornea is displaced posteriorly (A) or uniformly (B) when dehydrated and is anteriorly displaced in a normal or hydrated cornea (C). After radial keratotomy the anterior curvature remains either unchanged or mildly affected when in dehydrated (D) or normally hydrated (E) states. The anterior lamellae remain closely packed, and the inelastic nature of the intact posterior lamellae prevents changes in the shape of the cornea. When hydration increases, the loose anterior stroma absorbs water (swells) and the stress attempts to move anteriorly. However, since these layers have been cut, the cornea flattens its curvature and the posterior lamellae retain their shape by holding the stresses (F). (Reproduced with permission from Simon G, Ren Q. Biomechanical behavior of the cornea and its response to radial keratotomy. *J Refract Corneal Surg* 1994;10;349.)

Effects of Keratorefractive Surgery

Keratorefractive surgery can alter the corneal biomechanics in several ways:

- Incisional effect
- Tissue addition or subtraction
- Alloplastic material addition
- Laser effect
- Collagen shrinkage

The *optical zone* in refractive surgery generally refers to the boundary between operated and nonoperated cornea.

Incisional effect Incisions perpendicular to the corneal surface will predictably alter the shape, depending on direction, depth, location, and number. All incisions will lead to a local flattening of the cornea. *Radial incisions* lead to flattening in both the meridian of the incision and 90° away. *Tangential incisions* (arcuate or linear, Fig XXV-8) lead to flattening in the meridian of the incision and steepening in the meridian 90° away that may be equal to or less than the magnitude of the decrease in the primary meridian, a phenomenon known as *coupling*.

The closer radial incisions approach the visual axis (i.e., the smaller the optical zone), the greater their effect, and the closer tangential incisions are placed to the visual axis, the greater the effect. The longer a radial incision, the greater the effect until approximately an 11-mm diameter is achieved, and then the effect reverses. The larger the angle severed by a tangential incision, the greater the effect.

For optimum effect the incision should be 85%–90% deep to allow an intact posterior lamellae and maximum anterior bowing of the other lamellae. Nomograms for numbers of incisions and optical zone size can be calculated based on finite element analysis, but they are typically generated empirically. The important variables for radial and astigmatic surgery include patient age, optical zone size, number of incisions, and length of incisions for astigmatic surgery. Intraocular pressure and preoperative corneal curvature are not significant predictors of effect.

The type of diamond knife and the direction of incision change the effect in radial keratotomy. Centripetal (Russian-style) incisions are deeper near the optical zone and have more effect than centrifugal (American style). Bidirectional knives

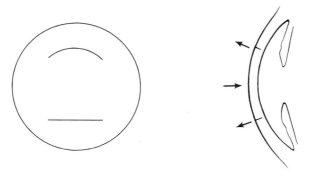

FIG XXV-8—Astigmatic keratotomy: schematic arcuate (above) and transverse (below) incision. The peripheral cornea bulges in axis perpendicular to keratotomy.

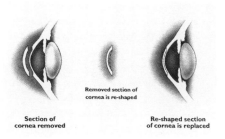

Removed section of
cornea is re-shaped

Section of
cornea removed

Re-shaped section
of cornea is replaced

FIG XXV-9—Keratomileusis.

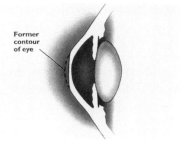

Former
contour
of eye

FIG XXV-10—Photorefractive keratectomy (PRK)
for myopia.

with a distal 200-μm front cutting tip and a full-length posterior blade allow for an initial centrifugal cut followed by centripetal to gain the paracentral, deep effect and decrease the risk of crossing the optical zone with each centripetal cut.

The effect of incisional surgery is dependent to a great deal on the hydration of the stroma and less on the IOP (see Figure XXV-7). A hyperopic shift of the refraction can occur in patients exposed to high altitude or low pO_2 following radial keratotomy as a result of swelling in the vicinity of the wound. Daily fluctuation in refraction (typically hyperopic in the morning) may also be related to stromal hydration effects in patients with radial keratotomy and not to diurnal variation in IOP.

Tissue addition or subtraction Lamellar surgery also alters the biomechanics of the cornea. *Keratomileusis* was initiated by Jose Barraquer as "carving of the anterior surface" of the cornea. It is defined as an intervention to modify the spherical or meridional surfaces of a healthy cornea by tissue subtraction (Fig XXV-9). Tissue subtraction may be performed on the surface (PRK, Fig XXV-10) or intrastromally (ALK and LASIK, Figs XXV-11, XXV-12). The critical uncut depth of the cornea necessary

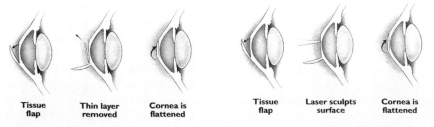

Tissue
flap

Thin layer
removed

Cornea is
flattened

Tissue
flap

Laser sculpts
surface

Cornea is
flattened

FIG XXV-11—Automated lamellar keratoplasty (ALK) for myopia.

FIG XXV-12—Laser in situ keratomileusis (LASIK).

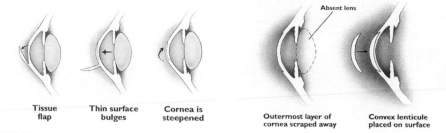

Tissue   Thin surface   Cornea is
flap   bulges   steepened

Absent lens

Outermost layer of   Convex lenticule
cornea scraped away   placed on surface

FIG XXV-13—Automated lamellar keratoplasty   FIG XXV-14—Epikeratophakia for hyperopia.
(ALK) for hyperopia.

to maintain normal integrity is not determined but is presumed to be at least 200–250 µm or 40% of the stromal depth, whichever is greater.

One method of hyperopic correction, *hyperopic automated lamellar keratoplasty,* uses a very deep lamellar pass (more than 70%) to allow the cornea to bow forward under physiologic conditions (Fig XXV-13). This procedure is unpredictable and may lead to progressive ectasia. It is not widely accepted.

Alloplastic material addition The biomechanics of the cornea can be altered by adding tissue or alloplastic material on the surface or into the corneal stroma to effect a change in the anterior shape or the refractive index of the cornea. *Epikeratoplasty* adds carved donor tissue to the surface to effect hyperopic (Fig XXV-14) or myopic changes. Hydrogel and other material is placed onto or into the cornea (Fig XXV-15). The *intrastromal corneal ring* is placed in two pockets of the stroma to directly alter the surface contour based on the profile of the individual rings (see Figure XXVI-2). These rings do not work by changing the circumferential measurement of the cornea (i.e., by spreading the peripheral cornea to flatten the center). The manufacturer suggests the rings work by stiffening or stretching the cornea much as a hammock spreader tightens and gives shape to the sagging mesh. Gel can be injected into the cornea in a similar manner to give an adjustable correction.

Laser effect *Photorefractive keratectomy (PRK)* of the anterior surface is limited in the depth that should be removed to avoid complications of forward bowing and scarring. The amount of tissue to remove centrally is estimated by *Munnerlyn's formula:*

> Ablation depth in microns (µm) equals diopters (D) of myopia
> divided by 3 times the square of the optical zone (mm)

Clinical experience has confirmed that the effective change is independent of the initial curvature of the cornea, although other formulas have been proposed that include preoperative curvature. Munnerlyn's formula also highlights some of the problems and limitations of PRK. The amount of ablation increases by the square of the optical zone, but the complications of glare, haloes, and regression increase when the optical zone decreases. To reduce these side effects the optical zone should be 6 mm or larger.

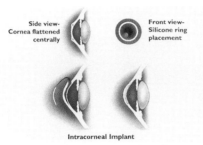

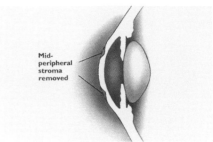

FIG XXV-15—Intracorneal implants.

FIG XXV-16—Hyperopic photorefractive keratectomy.

Efforts to use multiple-zone ablations are being evaluated. *Multizone keratectomies* use different optical zone sizes for part of the total refraction required. This method can generate a full correction centrally and a tapering peripheral zone, reducing symptoms and allowing higher degrees of myopia to be treated. For example, to treat 12 D, 6 D are treated with a 4.5-mm optical zone, 3 D with a 5.5-mm optical zone, and 3 D with a 6.5-mm optical zone. A total of 12 D correction is achieved in the center without using the same ablation depth that would be necessary for a single pass (103 μm instead of 169 μm).

Laser in situ keratomileusis (LASIK) combines a lamellar incision with ablation of the cornea, typically in the bed (see Figure XXV-12). The same theoretical limits for residual posterior cornea apply as with PRK, and the calculated effect is based on a modification of Munnerlyn's formula empirically. To reduce the complications of surface irregular astigmatism, the flap is typically cut 130–160 μm thick, but it is not made thicker to allow for the bending at Bowman's layer necessary for correcting the refractive error.

Hyperopic keratomileusis requires the addition of tissue (keratophakia) centrally. *Hyperopic PRK* uses a similar formula for determining the maximum ablation depth, but the optical zone is much larger. Consequently, the depth is much greater although located in the midperiphery (Fig XXV-16).

Collagen shrinkage Alteration in corneal biomechanics can also be achieved by shrinkage of collagen. Heating collagen to a critical temperature of 55°–60°C will cause it to shrink, inducing changes in the corneal curvature. *Thermokeratoplasty* is avoided in the central cornea because of scarring but used in the midperipheral cornea to induce peripheral flattening and central steepening to correct hyperopia (Fig XXV-17).

Shrinkage can also be done in a linear manner to induce central flattening and correct myopia, but no clinical trials have been conducted. If the source of heat is too high, local necrosis will occur, and if the source of heat is nonuniform or nonuniformly applied, irregular astigmatism will be induced.

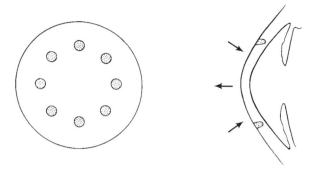

FIG XXV-17—Thermokeratoplasty: heat shrinks the peripheral cornea, causing central steepening.

Corneal Wound Healing

Chapter XIX has discussed the principles and mechanisms of corneal wound healing. All forms of keratorefractive surgery are exquisitely dependent on this process. Satisfactory results require either modifying or reducing wound healing or exploiting normal wound healing for the benefit of the patient. Radial keratotomy requires initial weakening followed by permanent healing with replacement of the epithelial plugs with collagen and remodeling of the collagen to ensure stability and avoid long term hyperopic drift. PRK requires the epithelium to heal quickly with minimal stimulation of the underlying keratocytes to avoid corneal scar and haze. Lamellar keratoplasty requires intact epithelium and healthy endothelium early postoperatively to seat the flap; later, the cornea must heal in the periphery to secure the cap in place and avoid late-term displacement yet minimize irregular astigmatism.

Understanding of corneal wound healing has advanced tremendously with recognition of the multiple factors responsible in a cascade of events initiated by corneal wounding. The cascade is somewhat dependent on the nature of the injury. Injury to the epithelium can lead to loss of underlying keratocytes from apoptosis. Remaining keratocytes respond by generating new glycosaminoglycans and collagen, to a degree dependent on the duration of the epithelial defect and the depth of the stromal injury. The tendency toward haze formation is greater with deeper ablations and prolonged absence of the epithelium. Despite losing Bowman's layer, normal or even enhanced numbers of hemidesmosomes and anchoring fibrils form to secure the epithelium to stroma.

Controversy persists over the value of different agents to modulate wound healing in PRK. Typically, clinicians in the United States use steroids in a tapering manner following surgery to reduce haze formation and stabilize surgical effect. Topical nonsteroidals have also been tried with no established effect. Other agents such as transforming growth factor–β (TGF-β) have been proposed, but no information on their value is available at this time.

The cycle of haze formation does not seem to occur following lamellar keratoplasties, which may be related to either lack of significant epithelial injury and subcellular signaling or the maintenance of some intact surface neurons. Lamellar surgery shows very little long-term evidence of healing between the disrupted lamellae and only typical stromal healing at the peripheral wound. The lamellae are initially held in position by negative stromal pressure generated by the endothelial cells aided by an intact epithelial surface. Even at 1 year, the lamellar interface can be broken and the flap lifted, indicating the minimal amount of healing that occurs. Aberrant healing can occur if the flap is placed with wrinkles or if epithelium grows into the interface.

Epithelium in the interface acts as a barrier to nutrient flow and must be removed with any sign of thinning, inflammation, or obstruction of visual axis. Interface debris can lead to inflammation or light scattering and should be minimized at the time of surgery. Hyperopic ALK also heals at the peripheral interface only, which may lead to late progressive effect. Epikeratoplasties from donor stroma will slowly repopulate with host keratocytes.

Laser Biophysics

Laser–Tissue Interactions

Three laser–tissue interactions are exploited for keratorefractive surgery. The first method is *photothermal* using a holmium:YAG laser focused into the anterior stroma with a wavelength of 2.13 μm that is absorbed by water, causing collagen shrinkage from heat. This technique has been used to treat low hyperopia in clinical trials in the United States.

The second laser–tissue interaction is *photodisruption.* Intrastromal ablations are performed with picosecond Nd:YAG laser or Nd:YSGG laser to produce optical breakdown within the corneal stroma and vaporization of tissue (Fig XXV-18). The laser–tissue interaction is entirely intrastromal and its refractive effect depends on collapse of the tissue above it. At this time there are no clinical trials using this technology.

Third, the most important laser–tissue interaction is *photoablation* with photochemical bond breakage using excimer (for *exci*ted di*mer*) lasers or other lasers of the appropriate wavelength. Laser energy of more than 4 eV per photon is sufficient to break carbon–nitrogen or carbon–carbon bonds of tissue. Argon-fluoride lasers are excimer lasers that use electrical energy to stimulate argon to form dimers with the caustic fluorine gas. They generate a wavelength of 193 nm with 6.4 eV per photon. The 193-nm light is in the ultraviolet C or high ultraviolet range, approaching the wavelength of x-rays. Light at this end of the electromagnetic spectrum, in addition to having high energy per photon, also has very low tissue penetrance and is

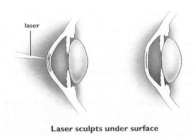

Laser sculpts under surface

FIG XXV-18—Intrastromal ablation.

454

suitable for operating on the surface of tissue. Not only is the laser energy capable of precision with little thermal spread in tissue, its lack of penetrance or lethality to cells makes the 193-nm laser nonmutagenic, enhancing its safety. DNA mutagenicity is in the range of 250 nm. Solid-state lasers can be designed to generate wavelengths of light near 193 nm without the need for toxic gas, possibly improving their reliability and decreasing their cost.

Types of Photoablating Lasers

Photoablating lasers can be divided into broad-beam lasers, scanning-slit lasers, and flying-spot lasers. *Broad-beam lasers* rely on internal optics to create a smooth and homogeneous multimode laser beam up to approximately 7 mm in diameter. They have very high energy per pulse and require a low number of pulses to ablate the cornea. *Scanning-slit lasers* use excimer technology to generate a smaller slit beam that is scanned over the surface to alter the lasing profile, improving the smoothness of the ablated cornea and allowing for larger-diameter ablation zones. *Flying-spot lasers* use the slightly longer wavelengths of solid-state lasers in fundamental mode, but they require a tracking mechanism because of the very high frequency and precise placement required for the 0.2–1.0 mm beam. Each solid-state laser spot contains approximately 1/1000 the amount of total energy of the wide-area beam at its maximum diameter. Wide-area beams and some scanning lasers require an iris or other masking to create the desired shape in the cornea. The flying spots and some of the scanning lasers use the pattern projected onto the surface to create the desired laser ablation profile without masking.

Surgical Guidelines

The following guidelines apply to all forms of refractive surgery and vary only by the specific refractive error to be achieved and the individual patient's special requirements (tolerance for risk, need for rapid rehabilitation, cost sensitivity, and perhaps wound-healing history). Until an ideal (i.e., safe, predictable, and reversible) refractive procedure is developed, disagreement will persist among ophthalmologists as to which eyes and which patients are appropriate for refractive surgery.

Patient Selection

Most patients who seek refractive surgery state they wish to see well without dependence on spectacles or contact lenses. Some patients seek the surgery for occupational or cosmetic reasons. Because the procedure is elective, the ophthalmologist must ensure that a prospective patient has a realistic understanding of the benefits and limitations of surgery.

Patients must understand that the outcome of surgery cannot be precisely predicted for an individual eye, that spectacles or contact lenses may still be required for best vision after surgery, and that contact lens wear may be more difficult because of changes in the shape of the cornea. Furthermore, patients must be informed that this surgery may necessitate the use of reading glasses at an age of 40–45 years.

Patients with specific occupational goals are encouraged to get prior assurance that surgical correction of refractive error will satisfy the employment requirements. Finally, the remote possibility of loss of vision or loss of the eye should be openly stated. The surgeon assumes responsibility for obtaining proper informed consent and is advised to do so well in advance of surgery.

Preoperative evaluation The candidate for refractive surgery should have a generally stable refractive error, and corneal structure should be normal, free of disorders such as keratoconus or unstable contact lens warpage. The patient should be old enough (18 years) for ocular stability and to understand and give consent for an elective procedure. The candidate should be psychologically stable, have reasonable goals, indicate understanding of the risks involved, and be available for follow-up care.

Contraindications Any ocular disorders likely to elevate IOP or to require chronic topical corticosteroids should be absent. Systemic conditions that may alter wound healing (collagen vascular diseases, chronic exogenous steroids, immunocompromised status, pregnancy or nursing) are relative contraindications to surgery. Unreasonable expectations, unstable refraction (changing more than 1 D in the last 2 years), or keratometry are contraindications along with active, recurrent, or residual external problems of the conjunctiva, cornea, and eyelids. Most surgeons obtain computerized corneal topography on all eyes prior to refractive surgery to rule out subclinical keratoconus and irregular astigmatism or contact lens warpage.

Patients should discontinue soft or gas-permeable contact lens wear 1–2 weeks before measurement for surgery. Hard contact lenses should be discontinued for 3–6 weeks with repeated measures of refraction and keratometry to ensure stability.

Surgical Instruments

The following instruments are the minimum requirements:

- ☐ Surgical microscope with fixation or centering light
- ☐ Appropriate eyelid speculum
- ☐ Means of two-point fixation to avoid torque on the globe during incisions (Thornton ring, Kremer fixation forceps, etc.)
- ☐ Marking devices for centration
- ☐ Optical zone size and incision pattern
- ☐ Guarded gemstone blade to set depth and achieve desired incisional direction

Lamellar techniques require knowledge of the specific device (microkeratome) to ensure proper assembly and avoid cutting inappropriately deep or inadequately shallow. Selection of laser depends on the surgeon's preference, desired goals of surgery, availability and maintenance support from manufacturer, and costs.

Centering Procedures

Placement of the refractive surgery is most critical. Misalignment leads to multiple problems of undertreatment, glare, haloes, induced astigmatism, and patient dissatisfaction. The pupil is the critical structure in the pathway of light to the retina and consequently the basis for centering refractive procedures. It is important to make sure the patient is fixing coaxially with the surgeon or fixation light of the specific device, and that the eye is not tilted with respect to this axis. The head and eye should be level.

CHAPTER XXVI

Incisional, Inlay, and Onlay Procedures

Surgical Correction of Myopia

Radial Keratotomy

Corneal incisions were first used to correct refractive errors in the late 1890s. Refractive keratotomy for myopia then underwent a long period of international development. Radial keratotomy (RK) has been the most common surgical procedure used to correct myopia since its modernization by Fyodorov in the 1970s (Fig XXVI-1).

Preoperative evaluation In addition to the patient selection criteria discussed in chapter XXV, refractive errors appropriate for RK limit patients to those with 1.00–4.00 D of myopia or less. Otherwise, complications include optical zones smaller than 3.0 mm and the need for more than eight incisions. Patients may chose RK over intracorneal ring placement (discussed below) or LASIK or PRK (see chapter XXVII) because of lower costs, reduced postoperative medications, and rapid rehabilitation. Surgeons may choose RK because of lower initial costs of equipment, reduced number of postoperative visits, and familiarity with incisional techniques. Disadvantages of RK are the limited range of refractive error, potential for long-term hyperopic drift, reduced ocular integrity, risk of intraoperative perforation, and risk of infectious keratitis or endophthalmitis.

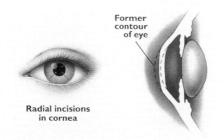

Former contour of eye

Radial incisions in cornea

FIG XXVI-1—Radial keratotomy for myopia.

Surgical techniques   Radial corneal incisions sever collagen fibrils in the corneal stroma. Stress becomes transferred to the posterior fibers, and relaxation in the anterior stromal fibers and hydration in the anterior layers then produce in these wounds a gape (see Figure XXV-7). This gape increases the radius of curvature in the central cornea, flattening it and decreasing its refractive power, hence decreasing myopia in the patient.

Currently, instrumentation and manual techniques employed by individual surgeons for RK vary considerably, as does the response in individual patients. As with many other types of ophthalmic surgery, the surgeon performing RK must develop individual skills to accommodate differences among patient responses, instruments, and patterns of incisions.

Most surgeons use a diamond-bladed micrometer knife. Blade design (angle and sharpness of cutting edge, width of blade) and footplate design influence both the depth and contour of incisions. The length of the knife blade is set based on the corneal thickness, which is usually measured with an ultrasonic pachymeter. Not all pachymeters with the same settings will read the same corneal thickness, so the surgeon must know the idiosyncrasies of individual instruments.

Furthermore, incision depth is not always the same as the length of the knife blade, since the blade displaces some tissue while cutting. A vertical blade that is pushed centripetally (Russian technique) will cut deeper than an angled blade pulled centrifugally through the tissue (American technique). Both techniques deliberately spare the limbus. An eye with high IOP during the surgery is likely to have a deeper, more uniform incision; pressure is affected by a fixation forceps or ring and by the amount of force exerted by the knife.

Variables affecting outcome   *Surgical variables.* Four variables controlled by the surgeon affect the outcome of surgery:

☐ *Centering.* Corneal surgical procedures are preferably centered around the pupil.

☐ *Clear zone diameter.* A central clear zone of 3.0–5.0 mm is used in most cases; smaller diameters produce a greater change in corneal curvature and refractive power. The availability of PRK has prompted many surgeons to increase the minimum clear zone to 3.5 mm.

☐ *Number of incisions.* Most surgeons use four or eight incisions. Since most central corneal flattening is achieved with the initial four incisions, many surgeons prefer to use four incisions on eyes with 4.00 D or less of myopia and perform a second operation later if necessary.

☐ *Depth of incisions.* The ideal depth of radial incisions is 80%–90% of the corneal thickness. Deeper incisions produce greater flattening but less stability. The effect of depth is not linear, however; incisions through only the anterior 50% of the cornea have little effect and cutting more than 90% through the stroma produces a proportionately greater effect. Inability to obtain an accurate and consistent depth from one end of an incision to another for all incisions is one of the major weaknesses of RK technique.

Patient variables. The greater the patient's age, the greater the effect achieved with the same surgical technique. The increase is approximately 0.50–1.00 D per decade, but it is not known if this increase is linear or proportionately greater in older patients.

No data have consistently demonstrated any meaningful effect of the following patient characteristics: corneal curvature, central corneal thickness, corneal diameter, ocular rigidity, axial length, or gender. Application of these surgical and patient factors to achieve an optimal result for an individual eye is an area of continuing study.

Adjustments of variables. Alternative approaches to surgery range from simple surgical plans using four to eight incisions at a fixed depth around a clear zone of 3.0–5.0 mm to complex nomograms and formulae incorporating many preoperative factors and adjusting all four surgical variables accordingly. Enhancement of an undercorrection by lengthening, deepening, or adding incisions is much easier than repair of an overcorrection. Thus, many surgeons use algorithms that accept a high (around 40%) undercorrection and reoperation rate in order to avoid overcorrection. Since any published guide to RK surgery is based on a specific technique, individual surgeons must therefore make modifications to suit their techniques.

Efficacy and predictability The ideal result after surgery is mild residual myopia, on the order of –0.50 to –1.00 D, for three reasons:

□ Individuals with residual myopia often see better without correction than unoperated patients with the same refractive error

□ Residual myopia delays the onset of symptomatic presbyopia

□ Residual myopia offsets the continued tendency after surgery toward hyperopia that occurs in some patients

As surgical techniques and experience in RK improve, so do surgical results. Unfortunately, there are no large-scale prospective studies of RK using contemporary techniques. Based on the simple indicator of percentage of eyes with final spherical equivalent refractive error within ±1.00 D, reported results range from 54% to 96%. Series that include reoperations for undercorrection generally show a higher percentage of eyes with the target refraction.

The best measure of the predictability of RK surgery is the *prediction interval* around the desired outcome for an individual eye. The Prospective Evaluation of Radial Keratotomy (PERK) Study used a 90% prediction interval to indicate the range of postsurgical refractive error that the eye has a 90% chance of achieving. A 90% prediction interval with a range of approximately 4.00 D has been reported in many studies, indicating that the surgery using those techniques is six to eight times less predictable than the fitting of spectacles or contact lenses.

The success rate of RK, however, cannot be fully evaluated on the basis of spherical equivalent refractive error. For example, a simple 2.00 D myope whose postoperative result is +1.00 –2.00 × 75 would not be considered a success, even though the spherical equivalent is zero. Following RK, a patient's uncorrected visual acuity may exceed that predicted by the spherical equivalent. Patients who are overcorrected and young enough to have good accommodation will have good uncorrected acuity. Additionally, the redistribution of flat and steep zones on the cornea after RK creates a multifocal cornea, allowing some apparently undercorrected patients to see well without spectacles.

The percentage of patients who do not wear optical correction represents a reasonable measure of the overall success of surgery. Among 310 patients with bilateral radial keratotomy in the PERK study, 70% reported not wearing spectacles or contact lenses for distance vision at 10 years and 42% reported no correction at all.

Postoperative refraction, visual acuity, and corneal topography RK changes not only the curvature of the central cornea but also its overall topography, creating a multifocal cornea. The result is a decrease in the direct correlation among refraction, central keratometry, and uncorrected visual acuity, presumably because the new corneal topography creates a more complex optical system, consisting of central flattening, paracentral steepening or flattening, and relative peripheral steepening. Thus, keratometric readings that sample only two points approximately 3.0 mm apart may indicate amounts of astigmatism different from those detected by refraction. Similarly, uncorrected visual acuity for a residual refractive error may vary, particularly depending on pupil diameter: the smaller the pupil, the smaller the multifocal effect of postoperative changes in the cornea. The study of corneal topography after RK is currently an area of active research.

Stability of refraction Almost all eyes show a decrease in myopia immediately following radial keratotomy. The vast majority lose some of this initial effect a few weeks after surgery, presumably because of changes induced by stromal edema and initial wound healing and remodeling. By 3 months after surgery most eyes are generally stable. However, two phenomena of postoperative refractive instability—fluctuation of vision and a continued effect of surgery—may persist for several years.

Diurnal fluctuation of vision. Diurnal fluctuation in vision can occur because the cornea is flatter upon awakening and gradually steepens during the patient's waking hours. In a subset of the PERK study at 10 years, the mean change in the spherical equivalent of refraction between the morning (waking) and evening examinations was 0.31 ±0.58–D increase in minus power in first eyes. Thirty-six eyes (51%) had an increase in minus power of the manifest refraction of 0.50–1.62 D; 22 (31%) had a change in refractive cylinder power of 0.50–1.25 D; 9 (13%) had a decrease in uncorrected visual acuity of two to seven Snellen lines; and 25 (35%) showed central corneal steepening measured by keratometry of 0.50–1.94 D.

Continued effect of surgery. The refractive error of 43% of eyes in the PERK study changed in the hyperopic direction by 1.00 D or more between 6 months and 10 years postoperatively. The hyperopic shift was statistically associated with the diameter of the clear zone. Duration of this ongoing effect is one of the major unknowns about RK.

Complications Probably the best measure of the safety of RK is the rate of loss of best spectacle-corrected visual acuity. From 1% to 3% of eyes lose two or more Snellen lines. The 97%–99% majority of patients can put on spectacles postoperatively and obtain their baseline visual acuity.

Mild to moderate irregular astigmatism can cause visual distortion and glare, especially in eyes that have had one of the following:

□ More than eight incisions

□ Incisions extending inside a 3.0-mm central clear zone

□ Intersecting radial and transverse incisions

□ Hypertrophic scarring

Many patients report seeing a starburst pattern around lights at night that presumably results from light scattering off the radial scars. While most individuals find the effect comparable to looking through dirty spectacles or contact lenses, some have had to stop driving at night because of this complication. No clinical trials have objectively demonstrated an increase in disabling glare after RK. Common side effects that do not reduce corrected visual acuity include

- Postoperative pain for about 24 hours
- Undercorrection and overcorrection
- An increase in astigmatism of 1.00–3.00 D in approximately 15% of eyes
- Inclusion cysts and vascularization of stromal scars
- Slight, nonprogressive endothelial disruption beneath the incisions at the time of surgery

Potentially blinding complications occur rarely after RK. These include

- Perforation of the cornea, which can lead to endophthalmitis, epithelial ingrowth, and traumatic cataract
- Bacterial keratitis immediately after surgery or delayed 1–3 years, presumably because the epithelium of the incision scars heals slowly and is constantly turning over, creating a site for bacterial adherence

Ocular surgery after radial keratotomy Eyes that have unacceptable residual myopia after RK can undergo repeated surgery by opening the incisions with a blunt instrument and deepening or extending them to a smaller clear zone, or by making additional incisions between the initial ones. Eyes that are unacceptably overcorrected can be managed by opening the wounds, removing the epithelial plug, and suturing the wounds closed with interrupted or purse-string sutures overlying the radial wounds to compress the peripheral "knee." In general, the results of repeated surgery are less predictable than the initial procedure.

Stevens SX, Young DA, Polack PJ, et al. Complications of radial keratotomy. In: Krachmer JH, Mannis MJ, Holland EJ, eds. *Cornea*. St Louis: Mosby; 1997;3:2101–2116.

Following RK, some eyes with marked irregular astigmatism and subjective glare must undergo penetrating keratoplasty. Since the keratotomy wounds may open during PK, sutures are placed to reinforce them prior to trephination. Both myopic keratomileusis and myopic epikeratoplasty have been performed following RK with overall technical success but variable refractive outcome. Cataract surgery may lead to temporary hyperopia following RK. Calculation of implant power for cataract surgery is done using standard formulas and determining keratometric power in one of three ways: direct measurement using computerized videography; knowledge of pre-RK keratometry minus the refractive change; or adjustment of the base curve of a plano contact lens by the overrefraction.

Future developments RK continues to evolve with improvements in technique and instrumentation. Gemstone knives continue to be improved: thinner multifaceted blades appear in different configurations, and more stable and highly finished footplates permit better visibility as keratotomy is performed. Also under development are knives with motorized blade advance, as well as guides to direct the knife in a radial direction, and suction rings to steady the eye and raise IOP. Technology that will permit real-time measurement of incision depth, perhaps coupled to the blade itself, is being investigated.

Steinert RF. Surgical correction of myopia: radial keratotomy and excimer laser photorefractive keratectomy. In: Smolin G, Thoft RA, eds. *The Cornea*. Boston: Little, Brown; 1993:673–696.

Waring GO III. Radial keratotomy for myopia. In: *Focal Points: Clinical Modules for Ophthalmologists.* San Francisco: American Academy of Ophthalmology; 1992;10:5.

Lamellar Procedures

Current techniques have evolved from the pioneering work of José Barraquer cutting with a microkeratome through the cornea in the plane perpendicular to the visual axis (see Figure XXV-9). In the group of procedures referred to as *keratomileusis* many variations now exist. The posterior aspect of the lenticule can be carved mechanically, either with or without freezing, or it can be modified with laser photoablation. Alternatively, the host bed can be modified with mechanical (ALK, automated lamellar keratectomy) or laser techniques (LASIK) to correct myopia.

Myopic keratomileusis   Originally, the lenticule was quick-frozen and carved on a cryolathe, thawed, and replaced on the patient's cornea. The resultant loss of keratocytes and epithelial cells required 6–8 months to clear the lenticule. The improved technique of Barraquer-Krumeich-Swinger (BKS), which reshapes the lenticule over a vacuum mold without freezing, addresses this problem.

Patient selection. BKS can correct up to 24.00 D of myopia in patients who are intolerant of spectacles and contact lenses.

Surgical techniques. A disk of 300 µm thickness is completely removed, reshaped on the lathe or vacuum mold, and sutured to the host cornea.

Instrumentation. Keratomileusis requires an expensive lathe or set of vacuum molds in addition to the automated microkeratome.

Variables affecting outcome. Refractive change was based on formulas derived by Barraquer and created by concave remodeling of the lenticular stroma.

Efficacy and predictability. Very little information is available, but one study reported a mean preoperative refraction of –11.16 and postoperatively +0.38 D ±2.54 standard deviation and range from –7.75 to +8.50 D.

Postoperative refraction, visual acuity, and corneal topography. Up to 67% of patients gain one line of vision, which may be a result of reduction of myopic minification. Up to 31% of patients lose one or more lines of best-corrected vision.

Stability of refraction. One study reported a 0.30-D increase in myopia per year over 5 years, which may be caused by lenticular or elongation changes.

Complications. Irregular astigmatism has been reported in 14% of eyes. Other problems include loss of lenticule, interface opacities, delayed epithelialization, corneal perforation, central ectasia, and loss of endothelial cells.

Ocular surgery after myopic keratomileusis. Many times secondary procedures such as homoplastic keratomileusis (with a donor lenticule), astigmatic relaxing incisions, or radial keratotomy have to be done. No information is available on success of subsequent PK or cataract surgery.

Future developments. Improvements in automated microkeratomes will benefit this procedure, but most of these patients will be treated by LASIK or intraocular surgery, which are more predictable procedures, although relative risks are not enumerated.

American Academy of Ophthalmology. Keratophakia and keratomileusis: safety and effectiveness. Ophthalmic Procedures Assessment. *Ophthalmology.* 1992;99:1334–1341.

Automated lamellar keratoplasty (ALK) In situ keratomileusis (now called ALK) uses a first pass with the keratome followed by a second, deeper pass to remove a lamellar (not lenticular) button of defined central thickness and diameter to correct higher degrees of myopia (see Figure XXV-11). Initially, a manual keratome was used, but the advent of the automated keratome along with the use of a hinged flap and the avoidance of suturing improved the predictability and reduced the complications. The popularity of this procedure has declined with the advent of LASIK.

Patient selection. Although theoretically able to correct up to 30.00 D of myopia, the procedure has been used on published ranges from –4.50 D to –22.75 D.

Surgical techniques. Two cuts are done with the automated keratome. The first is a minimum of 7.2 mm in diameter and 130–160 μm in thickness and is hinged at the nasal end (i.e., an incomplete pass). The second cut is the refractive cut, which varies in thickness and diameter according to the manufacturer's nomogram.

Instrumentation. The mainstay of this procedure is the automated keratome, which consists of a vacuum fixation ring with dovetail and adjustable height, the shaper head and oscillating blade, the motorized handle, and a system of calibrated plates. The vacuum ring allows the surgeon to maintain IOP near 65 mm Hg for optimum resistance and varies in height to allow the corneal dome to project above the cutting plane, determining the diameter of the cut. The calibrated depth plates determine the thickness to be resected. Instrument designs vary in the frequency of oscillation of the blade, speed of the lamellar dissection, angle of the blade in creating the lamellar cut, and the technique needed to vary thickness and shape of the second cut. A special centration marker is used to allow accurate replacement of the flap should it become detached.

Variables affecting outcome. Optical zone size (diameter of second lenticule) is varied from approximately 5.0 mm with thickness of 33 μm for a –2.50 D target to 3.5 mm and thickness of 126 μm for –30.00 D according to one nomogram. No other variables are used.

Efficacy and predictability. Lack of peer-reviewed published studies make definitive statements impossible. Two studies with 6- and 12-month minimal follow-up suggest reduction in myopia but do not report mean refraction or standard deviation. Reoperation rates were 59% and 77%, including RK, astigmatic keratotomy (AK), and repeat ALK.

Postoperative refraction, visual acuity, and corneal topography. At 1 month 38% of eyes were ±1.00 D and 67% were ±2.00 D. In a second study at 12 months with multiple surgeries, 76.2% of eyes were within 1.00 D of emmetropia, and 93.6% within 2.00 D. Uncorrected vision of 20/20 occurred in 19% of eyes and 20/40 in 75%. Topographic central islands occurred in 6 of 43 eyes in another study without effect on final vision.

Stability of refraction. Regression occurred from 1 to 6 months in approximately 5% of patients, with greater regression in the higher myopes.

Complications. In addition to the high reoperation rates, loss of best-corrected vision of two or more lines was reported in 6% of patients, usually secondary to irregular astigmatism. Other complications included loss of the cap, epithelial ingrowth into the interface (2%), overcorrection >1.00 D, infection, and decentration.

Ocular surgery after ALK. Experience is limited, but one report mentions a dislocated cap during retinal detachment surgery 5 months following hyperopic ALK. Incisional AK and RK are less predictable following ALK.

Future developments. Improvement in nomograms and design of the automated keratome to allow for larger optical zone sizes and smoother interfaces are likely, but LASIK and intraocular lenses are displacing this procedure in clinical trials.

American Academy of Ophthalmology. Automated lamellar keratoplasty. Preliminary procedure assessment. *Ophthalmology.* 1996;103:852–861.

Lyle WA, Jin GJ. Initial results of automated lamellar keratoplasty for correction of myopia: one year follow-up. *J Cataract Refract Surg.* 1996;22:31–43.

Ophthalmic Procedures Assessment Committee. *Automated Lamellar Keratoplasty.* San Francisco: American Academy of Ophthalmology; 1995.

Price FW Jr, Whitson WE, Gonzales JS, et al. Automated lamellar keratomileusis in situ for myopia. *J Refract Surg.* 1996;12:29–35.

Epikeratoplasty

Also called *epikeratophakia,* this procedure to correct adult and pediatric aphakia, myopia, or keratoconus involves rehydration and suturing of a preprocessed, freeze-dried lenticule of human corneal tissue onto bare Bowman's layer of the recipient cornea (see Figure XXV-14). Since no viable donor cells are involved, classic graft rejection is not possible. Host epithelium migrates over the surface of the graft.

This procedure found its greatest use in the correction of adult and pediatric aphakia in patients who were poor candidates for an IOL. Complications such as persistent epithelial defects, ulceration, interface scarring, sloughing of tissue, and refractive under- or overcorrection together with development of transscleral IOL placement techniques have reduced its use in recent years.

Epikeratoplasty never achieved predictable correction of myopia (reduction from −12.50 to −1.40 ±3.64 D in a nationwide study), although dramatic results have been seen in some patients. Its use in keratoconus is limited by its rather stringent indication: keratoconus without stromal scarring but so severe that correction with a contact lens is not possible. The lenticule used in keratoconus actually compresses and deforms the ectatic host cornea, which is not true in other indications for epikeratoplasty. The FDA considers epikeratoplasty an investigational procedure.

American Academy of Ophthalmology. Epikeratoplasty. Ophthalmic Procedure Assessment. *Ophthalmology.* 1996;103:983–991.

Alloplastic Intracorneal Implants

Materials used for keratorefractive surgery should correct a large range of spherical and cylindrical errors and be reversible. Alloplastic materials are desirable. Barraquer abandoned intracorneal methyl methacrylate discs in the 1960s because of necrosis anterior to the corneal implant. Other materials have been used including perfilicon A, hydroxy ethyl methacrylate (HEMA), and other copolymers (soft contact lens material), which require a lamellar keratotomy to allow Bowman's layer to de-form. None of these materials are currently available.

Polysulfone is a plastic with a high index of refraction (1.633) that can be placed in a stromal pocket without the lamellar keratotomy. But it is impermeable and requires microperforations, which degrade the optics, to allow nutrients to move anteriorly. Copolymers are also in preliminary trials in primates for use as an epikeratoplasty lenticule. Processed collagen molded onto the cornea and allowed to heal, followed by final adjustment with laser, has been proposed as well.

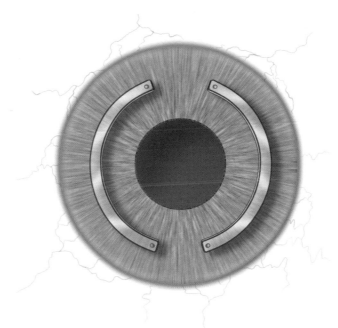

FIG XXVI-2—Intrastromal ring segments. (Illustration by Christine Gralapp.)

Intracorneal ring (ICR) Placement of a PMMA ring into the cornea has evolved to the placement of two segments of 150° arc for the correction of low myopia (Fig XXVI-2).

Patient selection. Ring segments of 0.25–0.45 mm thickness are used for –0.50 to –5.00 D corrections.

Surgical techniques. A vacuum centering guide is used to pass a special stromal separator at approximately two thirds of the stromal depth with an inner diameter of 7.0 mm in two 180° arcs (clockwise and counterclockwise from a small superior radial incision). The ring segments are placed in each arc.

Instrumentation. The procedure requires the vacuum-guided stromal separator to ensure the two parts are in the same plane of appropriate depth.

Variables affecting outcome. The thickness of the ring is the only nomogram variable.

Efficacy and predictability. FDA phase II studies of the split ring design show reduction in myopia, especially for less than 4.00 D.

Postoperative refraction, visual acuity, and corneal topography. At 3 months 73% of eyes were ±1.00 D, and 95% were ±2.00 D. In phase IIIa, uncorrected vision of 20/20 occurred in 75% and 20/40 in 97% of 244 eyes. Normal prolate asphericity of the peripheral cornea is maintained.

Stability of refraction. A Brazilian study of nine patients showed stability from day 1 to year 4.

Complications. Complications have included corneal perforation, induced irregular and regular astigmatism, peripheral corneal haze, stromal neovascularization, and superficial pannus. Ten of ninety patients in the first U.S. trial underwent explantation; half for undercorrection and half for incision-related complications. Five percent of the split ring group lost two or more lines of best-corrected vision.

Ocular surgery after ICR. Removal of the rings has resulted in return to baseline refraction and visual acuity.

Future developments. Applications for astigmatic correction are being evaluated and refinements in surgical technique are expected.

Krueger RR, Burris TE. Intrastromal corneal ring technology. *Int Ophthalmol Clin.* 1996;36:89–106.

Nose W, Neves RA, Burris TE, et al. Intrastromal corneal ring: 12-month sighted myopic eyes. *J Refract Surg.* 1996;12:20–28.

Surgical Correction of Hyperopia and Presbyopia

Epikeratoplasty for aphakia has been discussed under lamellar procedures. It can also be considered in select cases of unilateral pediatric and adult aphakia where contact lens wear is unsuccessful and IOL placement is contraindicated.

Hexagonal Keratotomy

Devised as an incisional correlate to radial keratotomy for the low hyperope, this procedure is not recommended because it induces an unstable cornea with significant irregular astigmatism and wound-healing complications.

Hyperopic Keratomileusis

This procedure is similar to myopic keratomileusis except that the lenticule is reshaped to correct for hyperopia. Complications are also similar and results show unpredictability (51% within 3.00 D of emetropia) and high complication rates (14%).

Keratophakia

This special form of keratomileusis uses a plus power donor corneal lenticule (up to 20.00 D) placed within a lamellar bed to increase the anterior curvature of the cornea. Initially, the lenticules were created on cryolathe and the lamellar dissection done with manual keratome. Advances in the creation of the lenticule by the BKS device and automation of the keratectomy did not enhance the predictability of the procedure, and it has been replaced first by epikeratoplasty and then by transsclerally sutured IOLs. At best 75% of patients are within 3.00 D of desired correction, and the complications are similar to other lamellar procedures.

Automated Lamellar Keratoplasty for Hyperopia

See the discussion of ALK under surgical correction for myopia. ALK for hyperopia creates a "controlled ectasia," which is similar to inducing keratoconus, to steepen the anterior curve of the cornea (see Figure XXV-13). Nomograms are used that predict what depth of lamellar cut will produce the desired anterior bowing of the cornea. Minimal peer-reviewed documentation is available (24 eyes followed for 6 months). A maximum depth of 70% is recommended, limiting correction of hyperopia to approximately +6.00 D. Stability cannot be assessed, but the procedure appears to produce less irregular astigmatism than ALK for myopia with none of the eyes losing two or more lines of best-corrected vision at 6 months.

Manche EE, Judge A, Maloney RK. Lamellar keratoplasty for hyperopia. *J Refract Surg.* 1996;12:42–49.

Presbyopia Correction

Intrastromal lens   High index of refraction, 2.0-mm intrastromal lenses are undergoing clinical trial for the treatment of presbyopia. The lenses are placed in the corneal pocket and create a multifocal effect. They can theoretically be adjusted or replaced. Patient acceptance is variable, and no peer-reviewed reports are available.

Scleral expansion   This newly described technique expands the ciliary ring to restore accommodation. It requires lengthy surgery and has few published results.

Surgical Correction of Astigmatism

Transverse Keratotomy

The cylindrical component of the cornea's refracting power can be altered by many different surgical maneuvers, such as modification of previous incisions, resection of tissue with resuturing, and application of heat to produce stromal shrinkage. However, simple incisional techniques at a depth similar to that of RK predominate in the correction of congenital and postoperative astigmatic refractive errors (see Figure XXV-8).

Although a single radial incision will induce flattening in that meridian, overall flattening will also occur, resulting in a hyperopic shift. Arcuate or transverse incisions, on the other hand, produce concomitant steepening in the opposite meridian (coupling), thus inducing cylindrical change with less effect on the spherical equivalent of refraction. Cylindrical change will be increased by the following:

□ Reducing the distance between the visual axis and a transverse keratotomy

□ Increasing the length or depth of the incision

□ Using multiple incisions

□ Making radial cuts in the same meridian

Some authors argue that *coupling ratios,* the ratio of desired flattening to induced steepening in the opposite meridian, can be modified by the type of incision (arcuate versus tangential) and the length and number of parallel incisions. Short, straight, or tangential incisions induce less steepening (higher ratio) in the opposite meridian than arcuate or longer incisions. Modified Ruiz procedures (combination of nonintersecting radial and tangential incisions) produce the highest coupling ratios.

Paradoxically, higher coupling ratios mean lower effect on the opposite meridian but more effect on the spherical equivalent. A coupling ratio of 1:1 means no net effect on spherical equivalent. Procedures that lead to a coupling ratio lower than 1:1 are inherently unstable (more effect in the nonoperated meridian, as with an arcuate cut greater than 100°) and should be avoided. Incisional surgeries can only reduce the power of the cornea and therefore correct plus cylinder. To date there is no reliable nomogram to predict coupling and, consequently, the effect of astigmatic surgery on the spherical equivalent refraction of the eye.

467

Patient selection   The decision to correct astigmatism depends on patient needs and symptoms, the level and axis of astigmatism, and anisometropia. Low amounts of against-the-rule astigmatism (plus axis at 180°) may aid uncorrected near vision in presbyopes. Nomograms cover 1.00–6.00 D for congenital astigmatism. Higher amounts can be corrected postsurgically (PK or cataract/IOL). Predictability for an individual eye is not ideal in any current system.

Surgical techniques   Astigmatic keratotomy can be performed alone or in combination with RK or cataract surgery. As with RK, numerous tables and nomograms, as well as a variety of surgical equipment, are in use for astigmatic keratotomy.

Instrumentation   The instruments used are similar to RK with different diamond blade designs for specific nomograms. Thin trapezoid-shaped blades work better for tangential incisions. Front-cutting diamond blades allow better visibility of corneal marks. The Hanna arcuate trephine is specifically designed for making smooth curvilinear incisions of specified optical zone and arc length. Key operative features are accurate assessment not only of the visual axis as in RK, but also of the plus cylinder axis. The axis should be identified preoperatively and verified intraoperatively. To avoid instability of the cornea 80% of pachymetry settings are used for depth on initial surgery.

Variables affecting outcome   As with RK, patient age and closeness to the visual axis increase the effect. Length, type (curvilinear versus straight), and number of incisions change the amount of flattening. Additional incisions are placed based on the quantity of astigmatism and the surgeon's skill in reading the topography. Tangential incisions may be used in pairs along the steep meridian (maximum of two pairs, one on each side of the visual axis), no closer than on the 4.0-mm optical zone and preferably farther away. Arcuate incisions are usually not placed inside the 5.0-mm optical zone, and conservative nomograms use a standard 7.0-mm optical zone to reduce glare and aberrations. Incisions to correct post-PK astigmatism may be placed in the graft, in the graft–host junction, or in the host, but this last provides minimal effect.

Efficacy and predictability   Few large prospective trials exist. The ARC-T study (see reference below) showed reduction in astigmatism using a 7.0-mm optical zone and varying arc lengths of 1.6 D ±1.1 D from the preoperative mean of 2.8 D ±1.2 D. Other studies suggest final uncorrected visual acuity of 20/20 in 20%–33% and 20/40 in 65%–80% for congenital astigmatism. Overcorrections occur in 4%–20% of patients.

Postoperative refraction, visual acuity, and corneal topography   Irregular astigmatism can occur or increase after astigmatic correction.

Stability of refraction   There are no reports longer than 6 months.

Complications   Complications parallel RK. Off-axis astigmatic keratotomy can lead to undercorrection or worsening of the preexisting astigmatism. Astigmatic incisions should not intersect other incisions (radial) to avoid creating an isolated block or edge of cornea that swells and cannot be epithelialized.

Ocular surgery after refractive surgery   AK can be combined with cataract, RK, or PRK surgery, but no long-term results have been reported. PK can be done after extensive AK, but the wounds may have to be closed as in RK.

Future developments   PRK will replace incisional surgery as predictability becomes higher (see chapter XXVII). Holmium:YAG thermoplasty and PRK are undergoing clinical trials for treatment of hyperopic astigmatism (to treat minus cylinder axis).

Price FW, Grene RB, Marks RG, et al. ARC-T Study Group. Astigmatism reduction clinical trial: a multicenter prospective evaluation of the predictability of arcuate keratotomy. *Arch Ophthalmol.* 1995;113:277–282.

Laser Procedures

Laser Procedures for Myopia

The overwhelming advantage of photoablation is the submicron precision with which it removes tissue. This potential was first recognized in 1983 by Trokel and exploited in clinical trials in the United States beginning in 1988. The FDA granted approval for use in treatment of low myopia without significant astigmatism in 1995, but excimer lasers had already been in widespread use in Canada, European nations, Australia, Japan, and other countries.

Excimer Laser for Photorefractive Keratectomy (PRK)

PRK is not yet a fully matured clinical procedure. Ongoing studies continue to determine the optimum patient selection process and preferred practice of the following aspects:

- Range of refractive error
- Intraoperative removal of epithelium
- Nomogram for ablation profiles including optimal optical zone diameter
- Most effective technique of correcting astigmatism
- Postoperative pharmacologic management

Patient selection Ophthalmologists should consult the specific FDA pre–market approval documentation for the manufacturer's guidelines of the instrument they will be using. General guidelines have been discussed in chapter XXV. Careful attention to correction of tear deficiency should be considered before PRK to reduce problems of haze and regression. Patients with significant connective tissue disease and certainly with any active corneal disease or condition should not have PRK. Female patients who are pregnant or nursing are likewise not good candidates.

Surgical techniques Patients should be educated about the surgery, including the sights, sounds, and odors to be anticipated during the procedure. The laser is verified to be working optimally, then the patient is aligned under the instrument. The optical zone (typically 7.0 mm centered around the pupil) is marked. Epithelium is carefully and completely removed in this zone by the following methods:

- Mechanically scraping with spatula or blade, preserving central epithelium until the end with or without topical 20% ethyl alcohol
- Using an automated brush
- Using the laser to reduce the thickness and then scrape the residual or to completely remove epithelium to Bowman's layer

Ablation takes typically 20–60 seconds for broad-beam excimer lasers and two to three times as long for scanning and flying-spot lasers. The patient fixates with verbal encouragement of the surgeon, aided by tracking devices in flying-spot lasers. Sometimes mechanical fixation is used. Ablation may require an ablatable masking material for some lasers to improve the smoothness of the postoperative surface (see Figure XXV-10). Postoperatively, topical nonsteroidal agents and antibiotics are used to reduce pain and combat potential infection. Bandage contact lenses or patching may be used, and the patient is followed until the epithelium heals. Some surgeons will use topical steroids for 1–6 months postoperatively.

Instrumentation Three types of photoablating lasers are available: broad-beam excimer, scanning excimer, and flying-spot solid-state or excimer.

Variables affecting outcome Surgical variables include method of epithelium removal, type of laser, size of optical zone, and depth of ablation. Patient variables include type of wound-healing response, age, attempted correction, and pregnancy (effect is decreased during pregnancy).

Efficacy and predictability Almost all patients show a reduction in myopia and an increase in uncorrected visual acuity. Predictability varies by degree of myopia; greatest accuracy occurs with a target of less than 3.00 D. Overall, refractive outcome is within 0.50 D in approximately 50%–60% of patients and within 1.00 D in 85% at 1 year. Uncorrected visual acuity is 20/20 in approximately 50%–70% and 20/40 in 90%–95% of patients in more recent studies of low myopia (up to 6.00 D). For patients with myopia greater than 6.00 D, 20%–60% are within 1.00 D of emmetropia. Choice of laser, size of optical zone, and use of multizone/multipass technique can affect these results. Uncorrected visual acuity is 20/40 or better in 60%–90% of higher myopes.

Corneal topography after PRK Topography has been used to estimate decentration of ablation and to study central islands. *Decentration* of 1.0 mm or more is associated with increased symptoms of ghosting, induction of astigmatism, and monocular diplopia.

    Central islands are defined as 1.00–3.00 D elevations of 1–3 mm diameter occurring at least 1 month postoperatively and associated with visual symptoms or refractive changes. Central islands occur in up to 17% of patients depending on the diligence of interpretation of the computerized videokeratography and choice of laser (they are not reported with scanning or flying-spot lasers). No consensus exists on the cause of the islands, but they may be related to epithelial hyperplasia or incomplete ablation secondary to the collection of stromal fluid from acoustic shock wave or ablation plume. Nonhomogenous laser beam may be a possible cause as well. Symptomatic central islands that do not spontaneously resolve after 6 months can be treated with a transepithelial approach.

Change in best-corrected visual acuity Gain or loss of one line of best-corrected visual acuity is within normal variation of Snellen testing. Loss of two lines or more occurs in 15%–20% of patients at 1 month but declines to 3%–4% at 1 year and 0%–3% at 2 years.

Stability of refraction In general, a 1-month low hyperopic response (planned overcorrection) is followed by regression of 0.50–1.00 D toward myopia over 6–12 months and then no significant change for up to 6 years. Absolute values should be verified for each laser. No reports of long-term hyperopic drift, as seen in RK, have been recorded.

Complications Complications may be related to deviations from planned correction, postoperative medication, wound healing, or mechanical factors. *Undercorrections* occur much more frequently at higher degrees of myopia: 10%–20% of myopes less than –5.00 D will be undercorrected (> –1.00 D myopic) at 1 year, in contrast to 65% of extreme myopes (> –10.00). Regression is associated with smaller optical zones and deeper ablations and is reduced by multizone treatment and zone sizes of 6.0 mm and larger. Undercorrections are associated with loss of best-corrected visual acuity and may respond temporarily to increased steroid use. They may require retreatment if symptomatic, as reported in 9%–15% of patients.

Overcorrections of more than +1.00 D at 1 year are much less frequent, occurring in 1.5% of low myopes and 4.9% of extreme myopes. They may be related to age (>40 years). Overcorrections are more difficult to treat and do not always respond to withdrawal of steroids. Bandage lenses have been used to induce chronic hypoxia and thereby induce regression.

More than 1.00 D of *induced astigmatism* occurs in 3%–5% of patients at 1 year, which can be treated with astigmatic keratotomy peripheral to the ablation zone. Severe regression is unusual and is anecdotally linked to discontinuation of steroids, exposure to ultraviolet light in the early postoperative period, and pregnancy or other hormonal imbalance.

Steroid-induced glaucoma occurs in 1.5%–3.0% of patients using fluoromethalone but in up to 25% using dexamethasone or stronger steroids. *Steroid-induced herpes simplex virus keratitis* is a rare event that requires withdrawal of steroid and antiherpetic treatment. Known ocular herpes is a relative contraindication to PRK, but it may be managed with prophylactic oral acyclovir in PTK. *Steroid-induced ptosis* usually resolves on discontinuation of the steroid. *Steroid-induced cataract* has been reported with steroids other than fluoromethalone used qid or greater for more than 3 months.

Therapeutic contact lenses used for epithelial healing are associated with *sterile infiltrates,* especially in patients using topical nonsteroidal anti-inflammatory drugs (NSAIDs) for longer than 24 hours without concomitant topical steroids. Incidence of infectious keratitis has been reported as 0.2% (6 of 3000 PRKs); all infiltrates must be suspected to be infectious and managed appropriately.

Complications related to wound healing include *regression, recurrent corneal erosion, haze formation,* and *late scarring.* Although PTK is shown to be an effective treatment for traumatic recurrent corneal erosions, a small number of patients have had onset of erosions following PRK without demonstrated underlying dystrophy or additional trauma. These patients respond to standard treatments for recurrent corneal erosions.

Wound-healing patterns after PRK can be separated into three groups:

□ Normal healers who have trace to 1+ haze and refraction of 0 to +1.00 D at 1 month

□ Inadequate healers with no haze and refraction > +1.00 D at 1 month

□ Aggressive healers with 1+ or greater haze that increases in months 2 and 3 as refraction becomes myopic (regresses)

In addition, a group of very late (after 12 months) scar formers has been described.

Normally, haze peaks between 6 and 12 weeks and declines thereafter. The exact etiology of the haze is unknown, but it does not appear to be collagen as in the rabbit, and it may be newly formed glycosaminoglycans. Grade 2 haze, a reticular pattern easily detected over the ablation zone that interferes with refraction, occurs in 0%–17% of patients in different series with increased frequency in deeper ablations. Treatment with steroids or reablation shows variable effect, and haze is known to resolve spontaneously with normal wound remodeling. Reablation should therefore be delayed for at least 6 months.

Mechanical complications include decentration of ablation zone, haloes, and central islands. Haloes are associated with pupils that dilate beyond the ablation zone. Incidence of nighttime glare and haloes decreased from 75%–80% with a 4.0-mm optical zone to 5% with a 6.0-mm optical zone and 0.5% with a 7.0-mm optical zone. Decentration averages 0.3–0.6 mm as determined from computerized topography and is associated with decrease in low-contrast visual acuity. Small amounts are asymptomatic, requiring no treatment.

Ocular surgery after PRK   Retreatment with PRK, RK, and AK has been done successfully. Cataract surgery and PK have been performed without unusual responses. Lens power for cataract surgery is calculated similarly to RK.

Future trends and developments   Standardization of postoperative management and pharmacologic control of wound healing may improve results and reduce complications from individual patient variability. LASIK (see below) may improve predictability and stability in patients with higher myopia. Scanning and flying-spot lasers are reporting improved accuracy and reduced side effects compared to early reports from broad-beam excimer lasers. Water-jet technology undergoing development may remove anterior corneal layers without generating heat or central islands. Intrastromal lasers are in early stages of development.

Currently, RK is still the most widely available refractive procedure for myopia. Approval by the FDA of the excimer laser did not result in a substantial increase in demand for elective refractive surgery until adoption of LASIK (see below).

Predictability is an issue with all procedures. Most series of PRK for myopia now show that 90%–95% of eyes obtain uncorrected acuity of 20/40 or better (better than RK) and that 85% of eyes are within ±1.00 D of emmetropia (slightly better than RK). Postoperative pain is equivalent in intensity, but its duration is longer in PRK, and visual recovery is quicker after RK. PRK probably shows better long-term stability of refractive effect, with no diurnal fluctuation of refractive error.

Late progression of effect and traumatic wound rupture are concerns after RK, whereas stromal scarring is a problem after PRK. Glare and decreased contrast sensitivity can be seen with both procedures, manifesting as starbursts after RK and haloes after PRK. Postoperative medical management is more complex after PRK than after RK, primarily involving increased and prolonged use of topical steroids both to modulate the refractive effect and to counteract haze in the visual axis.

Finally, the equipment to perform PRK is about 20 times more expensive than that for RK. This factor alone will require PRK to be shown as clearly more effective before it is completely accepted. LASIK has rapidly gained favor with patients because of the rapid visual recovery and reduced need for topical medications similar to RK combined with the precision and predictability of PRK.

Maguen E, Machat JJ, Salz JJ. Results and complications of photorefractive keratoplasty. In: Krachmer JH, Mannis MJ, Holland EJ, eds. *Cornea.* St Louis: Mosby; 1997; 3:2191–2210.

Schallhorn SC, McDonnell PJ. Refractive surgery: past, present and future. In: Krachmer JH, Mannis MJ, Holland EJ, eds. *Cornea.* St Louis: Mosby; 1997;3:173–175.

Excimer Laser In Situ Keratomileusis (LASIK)

Different spellings of the acronym *LASIK* include the terms *laser-assisted* or *stromal,* but the most common usage is simply *laser in situ keratomileusis* (see Figure XXV-12). Pallikaris described the basics of the current procedure in 1990, and the first clinical results appeared in 1994. This procedure combines the accuracy of PRK with the healing advantages of ALK, the maintenance of intact Bowman's layer–epithelial complex. Similarly, LASIK adds the complications of the complex automated keratectomy devices to the wound-healing complications of PRK. This procedure is in early development with minimal short-term follow-up and wide variance in outcomes based on keratectomy device and laser. Patient acceptance has been very high because of low perioperative discomfort, rapid return of vision, and reduced need for long-term topical medications.

Patient selection   Patients are selected for myopia greater than 3.00–8.00 D depending on surgeon and study protocols. The upper limit with a 6.0-mm optical zone is approximately 16.00 D, but multizone/multipass protocols may allow up to 30.00 D (in practice, about 15.00 D). Patients with excessive scarring from PRK may benefit from this alternative in the second eye, but the optimal indications have not been established.

Surgical techniques   Similar to ALK, a single large-diameter (9.0 mm or more) lamellar flap of 130–160 µm thickness is created in the standard manner. Again as in ALK, careful attention to the maintenance, assembly, and operation of the automated keratome is essential. The flap is hinged nasally or superiorly and folded back, and the stromal ablation is done. The flap is repositioned after irrigation of the interface, allowed to dry, and verified to be adherent. The eye is shielded (not patched) and treated with antibiotics.

Instrumentation   Similar to ALK and PRK.

Variables affecting outcome   The size of the optical zone and depth and profile of the laser ablation determine the theoretical correction. Some lasers overcorrect and some undercorrect using PRK nomograms. The effect of patient age or gender and the humidity of the laser room are being studied.

Efficacy and predictability   Few reports give longer than 3 months' follow-up. As with PRK, accuracy depends on the level of myopia. Data from 6 months suggest 40%–60% of patients are within 0.50 D of emmetropia, and 70% within 1.00 D. Uncorrected visual acuity of 20/20 occurs in 30%–40% and 20/40 in 80%–90%. Reoperation rate is 5%–10% for undercorrections with overcorrections very rare.

Postoperative refraction, visual acuity, and corneal topography   Loss of two lines of best-corrected visual acuity is reported in up to 9% at 6 months. Systematic analysis of corneal topography has not reported irregular astigmatism, but the reports are very few. Central islands are infrequent, but decentration does occur with outcomes similar to PRK.

Stability of refraction   Refraction shows myopic regression of magnitude similar to PRK up to 1 year.

Complications   Haze has not been reported in the absence of infection. Interface opacities do occur. Epithelial ingrowth and implantation in the interface is reported at a rate lower than 3%. Ingrowth may be related to type of keratome, angle of keratectomy blade, and surgeon experience. It can result in loosening of the flap, necrosis of the overlying flap, or significant opacity. Lost, miscut, or displaced flaps are reported at rates varying from 1% to 3%. Infections can occur at the flap interface. Retinal detachment and corneal edema have been reported.

An unusual syndrome, "sands of the Sahara (SOS)," with diffuse interface haze, may occur at postoperative day 1–3 with decrease in vision. After infection is ruled out, the interface is irrigated, and the eye treated with intense topical steroids. There is usually recovery of vision.

Ocular surgery after LASIK   Elevation of the flap within 12 months and retreatment with excimer has been successfully done.

Future developments   Key to the widespread adaptation of this technology are the following developments:

- Improved automated keratomes or alternative instruments with more consistent flap creation
- Refinement of nomograms
- Establishment of the baseline rate of flap complications
- Detailed corneal topographic analysis
- Long-term data collection on accuracy and stability

As with the adoption of phacoemulsification with a risk profile different from standard extracapsular cataract surgery, the adoption of LASIK will require clear delineation of its advantages and improvement in the technology of flap creation.

Whether LASIK will supplant RK and PRK is not known. At present its predictability is similar to PRK, but stability is undetermined. Potential complications of LASIK are more severe than with PRK, including potential for perforation and endophthalmitis. However, common problems of PRK are absent with LASIK (epithelial healing, topical steroids for months, haze formation) and reoperations may be more predictable. Cost of LASIK is 10%–15% greater than PRK with the addition of the keratome. Greater surgical skill is required, and recurring costs will also be larger than with PRK or RK. Ultimately, patients will decide based on their perception of the value, convenience, and risk of the procedures to them.

Pallikaris IG, Siganos DS. Excimer laser in situ keratomileusis and photorefractive keratectomy for correction of high myopia. *J Refract Corneal Surg.* 1994;10:498–510.

Salah T, Waring GO III, el Maghraby A, et al. Excimer laser in situ keratomileusis under a corneal flap for myopia of 2 to 20 diopters. *Am J Ophthalmol.* 1996;121:143–155.

Laser Procedures for Myopic Astigmatism

Photoastigmatic Refractive Keratectomy (PARK)

This procedure is evolving along several tracks. Surface ablation is done in two ways with moving shutters:

□ Sequentially, a cylinder is removed from the flat or minus axis using a slit shutter with a transition zone followed by the spherical ablation with the iris shutter (or vice versa)

□ Elliptically, simultaneous movement of the iris and the slit shutters corrects cylinder and sphere

Theoretical limits based on Munnerlyn's formula (see chapter XXV), the width of the ablation zone, and residual corneal thickness dictate the amount of astigmatism relative to the spherical equivalent that can be treated (Fig XXVII-1).

Ablation can also be achieved by using opaque masks with scanning slits, erodible masks, or patterns of flying spots. Handheld erodible masks have been supplanted by "in the rail" masks for more accurate and stable placement (Fig XXVII-2). No randomized prospective trials have compared these different technologies, many of which are proprietary and will be limited to certain lasers. Techniques to treat irregular astigmatism are likewise evolving.

Patient selection　Congenital astigmatism of 1.00–6.00 D and postoperative astigmatism (following PKP and cataract surgery) of up to 10.00 D have been treated. If the spherical equivalent is greater than 0 D, then hyperopic astigmatism techniques are required to avoid overcorrections.

Surgical techniques　Astigmatic correction is incorporated into the PRK program by the manufacturer. Accurate preoperative refraction and careful alignment on axis is key, since a 15° offset in the treating axis can decrease effective cylinder change by 50% and result in a significant refractive axis shift.

Instrumentation　The astigmatic axis (minus cylinder) is marked in addition to the standard setup.

Variables affecting outcome　PARK is probably similar to PRK, but no multivariate analysis is available.

Efficacy and predictability　PARK is similar to PRK in the few studies available. Low degrees of astigmatism are corrected less efficiently than moderate and high amounts. Uncorrected visual acuity tends to be lower than with spherical PRK, but loss of best-corrected visual acuity is the same.

Postoperative refraction, visual acuity, and corneal topography　PARK corrects from 43% to 47% of preoperative cylinder with the VISX laser.

Stability of refraction　The longest reported follow-up is 12 months, and the refractive astigmatism was unchanged from 15 days to 1 year.

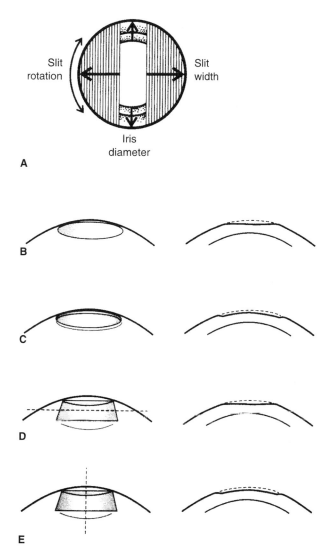

FIG XXVII-1—Photorefractive keratectomy for astigmatism (PARK). Schematic illustration *(A)* of the method of creating cylindrical ablations by progressively widening the separation between parallel blades during the ablation. Variables that can be controlled include depth of ablation, width of ablation zone, and orientation of the slit. With blades oriented as shown, the cornea would be flattened in the horizontal meridian to correct an against-the-rule astigmatism. Comparison of myopic ablation *(B)*, in which the greatest amount of tissue is removed centrally, with progressively less removed toward the periphery; a phototherapeutic keratectomy with small transition zone *(C)*, in which a uniform amount of tissue is ablated without intended refractive change; and cylindrical ablation *(D, E)* for correction of against-the-rule astigmatism. Cross section through the originally steep meridian after ablation *(D)* is identical to myopic ablation *(B)*, whereas a cross section through the originally flat meridian *(D)*, in which no refractive change is intended, is identical to phototherapeutic keratectomy *(C)*. (Reproduced with permission from Sietz B, McDonnell PJ. Astigmatism. In: Talamo JH, Krueger RR. *The Excimer Manual. A Clinician's Guide to Excimer Laser Surgery.* Boston: Little, Brown; 1997:94. Used by permission of Lippincott-Raven Publishers.)

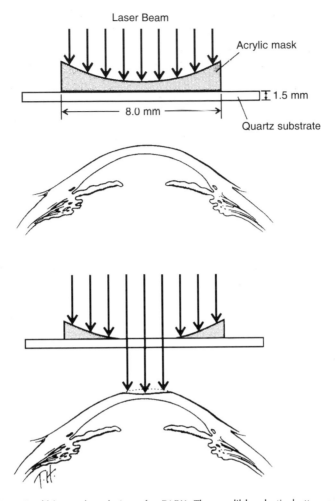

FIG XXVII-2—Erodible mask technique for PARK. The erodible plastic button adheres to a quartz substrate (transparent for 193-nm radiation). The shape of the mask is transferred by the wide-area laser beam inversely onto the cornea underneath the mask. When the mask is completely eroded, the greatest amount of tissue will have been ablated centrally, with progressively less tissue removed toward the periphery of the ablation zone, and more tissue ablated in the original steep meridian. (Reproduced with permission from Sietz B, McDonnell PJ. Astigmatism. In: Talamo JH, Krueger RR. *The Excimer Manual. A Clinician's Guide to Excimer Laser Surgery.* Boston: Little, Brown; 1997:95. Used by permission of Lippincott-Raven Publishers.)

Complications In addition to PRK complications, problems related to misalignment and the potential for inducing more irregular astigmatism also must be considered.

Ocular surgery after PARK No reported series of reoperations is available.

Future developments With the large number of astigmatic patients in the population, a need clearly exists. Improvements and comparisons of techniques among the various PARK machines and between incisional and photoablative approaches, and the timing of sequential procedures all require further study.

Sietz B, McDonnell PJ. Astigmatism. In: Talamo JH, Krueger RR. *The Excimer Manual. A Clinician's Guide to Excimer Laser Surgery.* Boston: Little, Brown; 1997:92–102.

Thermokeratoplasty

The holmium-YAG laser is being investigated for its ability to heat and shrink corneal stroma (laser thermokeratoplasty), producing corneal steepening and correction of hypermetropia or hyperopic astigmatism. Noncontact holmium-YAG continues in phase IIb trials for low degrees (1.00–2.00 D) of hyperopia and hyperopic astigmatism. The contact holmium-YAG laser has been withdrawn from the market because of regression and unpredictability of effect. Heated wire shrinkage of collagen is no longer done for refractive correction.

Laser Treatment of Hyperopia

As this volume goes to press, modified broad-beam excimer lasers and scanning spot lasers are in FDA trials for treatment of hyperopia and hyperopic astigmatism using either surface ablation or ablation under a stromal flap (LASIK). These ablation patterns are 9.0–10.0 mm in diameter and require more accurate centration than myopic ablations. Preliminary results are promising but show high rates of regression.

BASIC TEXTS

External Disease and Cornea

Arffa RC. *Grayson's Diseases of the Cornea.* 4th ed. St Louis: Mosby; 1997.

Chandler JW, Sugar J, Edelhauser HF, eds. *External Diseases: Cornea, Conjunctiva, Sclera, Eyelids, Lacrimal System.* St Louis: Mosby; 1994.

Dohlman CH, et al, section eds. Conjunctiva, cornea, and sclera. In: Albert DM, Jakobiec FA, eds. *Principles and Practice of Ophthalmology,* vol 1. Philadelphia: Saunders; 1994.

Duke-Elder S, Abrams D, eds. *System of Ophthalmology,* vols VII and VIII. St Louis: Mosby; 1970.

Friedlander MH, section ed. Ocular allergy and immunology; and Baum J, Liesegang TJ, section eds. Ocular microbiology. In: Tasman W, Jaeger EA, eds. *Duane's Foundations of Clinical Ophthalmology,* vol. 2. Philadelphia: Lippincott-Raven; 1997.

Kastl PR, ed. *Contact Lenses. The CLAO Guide to Basic Science and Clinical Practice.* Dubuque, Iowa: Kendall/Hunt; 1995.

Kaufman HE, Barron BA, McDonald MB, eds. *The Cornea.* 2nd ed. Boston: Butterworth-Heinemann; 1997.

Krachmer JH, Mannis MJ, Holland EJ, eds. *Cornea.* St Louis: Mosby; 1997.

Leibowitz HM, Waring GO III, eds. *Corneal Disorders: Clinical Diagnosis and Management.* 2nd ed. Philadelphia: Saunders; 1998.

Mannis MJ, Macsai MS, Huntley AC, eds. *Eye and Skin Disease.* Philadelphia: Lippincott-Raven; 1996.

Ostler HB, Ostler MW. *Diseases of the External Eye and Adnexa: A Text and Atlas.* Baltimore: Williams & Wilkins; 1993.

Pepose JS, Holland GN, Wilhelmus KR, eds. *Ocular Infection and Immunity.* St Louis: Mosby; 1996.

Smolin G, Thoft RA, eds. *The Cornea: Scientific Foundations and Clinical Practice.* 3rd ed. Boston: Little, Brown; 1994.

Tabbara KF, Hyndiuk RA, eds. *Infections of the Eye.* 2nd ed. Boston: Little, Brown; 1996.

Troutman RC. *Corneal Astigmatism: Etiology, Prevention & Management.* St Louis: Mosby; 1992.

Atlases

Abbott RL, ed. *Surgical Intervention in Corneal and External Diseases.* Orlando: Grune & Stratton; 1987.

Brightbill FS, ed. *Corneal Surgery: Theory, Technique, and Tissue.* 2nd ed. St Louis: Mosby; 1993.

Bruner WE, Stark WJ, Maumenee AG, eds. *Manual of Corneal Surgery.* New York: Churchill Livingstone; 1987.

Buratto L, ed. *Corneal Topography: The Clinical Atlas.* Thorofare, NJ: Slack; 1996.

Casey TA, Sharif KW. *A Colour Atlas of Corneal Dystrophies and Degenerations.* London: Wolfe; 1991.

Hersh PS, Wagoner MD. *Excimer Laser Surgery for Corneal Disorders.* New York: Thieme; 1997.

Kaufman HE, et al. Corneal and refractive surgery. In: Wright KW, ed. *Color Atlas of Ophthalmic Surgery.* Philadelphia: Lippincott; 1992.

Krachmer JH, Palay DA. *Cornea Color Atlas.* St Louis: Mosby; 1995.

Lindquist TD, Lindstrom RL, eds. *Ophthalmic Surgery.* St Louis: Mosby; 1996.

Mandel ER, Wagoner MD. *Atlas of Corneal Disease.* Philadelphia: Saunders; 1989.

Rabinowitz YS, Wilson SE, Klyce SD. *Color Atlas of Corneal Topography: Interpreting Videokeratography.* New York: Igaku-Shoin, 1993.

Sanders DR, Koch DD, eds. *An Atlas of Corneal Topography.* Thorofare, NJ: Slack; 1992.

Steele AD McG, Kirkness CM. *Manual of Systematic Corneal Surgery.* Edinburgh: Churchill Livingstone; 1992.

Waring GO III, ed. *Refractive Keratotomy for Myopia and Astigmatism.* St Louis: Mosby; 1992.

Watson P, Ortiz JM. *Color Atlas of Scleritis.* St Louis: Mosby; 1995.

RELATED ACADEMY MATERIALS

Focal Points: Clinical Modules for Ophthalmology

Belin MW. Optical and surgical correction of keratoconus (Module 11, 1988).

deLuise VP. Management of dry eyes (Module 3, 1985).

Dubord PJ. Scleritis and episcleritis (Module 9, 1995).

Gans LA. Surgical treatment of pterygium (Module 12, 1996).

Hamill MB. Repair of the traumatized anterior segment (Module 1, 1992).

Helm CJ. Melanoma and other pigmented lesions of the ocular surface (Module 11, 1996).

Hodge W, Hwang DJ. Antibiotic use in corneal and external disease (Module 10, 1997).

Kenyon KR, Wagoner MD. Therapy of recurrent erosion and persistent defects of the corneal epithelium (Module 9, 1991).

L'Esperance FA. Choosing the appropriate PRK patient (Module 9, 1998).

Liesegang TJ. Diagnosis and treatment of herpes zoster ophthalmicus (Member Benefit Module 2, 1984).

Maguire LJ. Computerized corneal analysis (Module 5, 1996).

Margo CE. Nonpigmented lesions of the ocular surface (Module 9, 1996).

Matoba AY. Infectious keratitis (Module 9, 1992).

Miller KN, Carlson AN, Foulks GN, et al. Associated glaucoma and corneal disorders (Module 4, 1989).

Parrish CM. Herpes simplex virus eye disease (Module 2, 1997).

Raizman MB. Update on ocular allergy (Module 5, 1994).

Rapoza PA, Chandler JW. Neonatal conjunctivitis: diagnosis and treatment (Module 1, 1988).

Schanzlin DJ. Herpes simplex eye infections (Module 1, 1983).

Sher NA. Postoperative management of the PRK patient (Module 10, 1998).

Soong HK. Penetrating keratoplasty (Module 6, 1992).

Stein RM, Stein HA. Corneal complications of contact lenses (Module 2, 1993).

Stern WH, O'Donnell FE Jr. Vitrectomy techniques for the anterior segment (Module 11, 1987).

Wagoner MD, Kenyon KR. Diagnosis and treatment of noninfectious corneal ulcers (Module 7, 1985).

Waring GO III. Radial keratotomy for myopia (Module 5, 1992).

Publications

Lane SS, Skuta GL, eds. *ProVision: Preferred Responses in Ophthalmology,* Series 3 (Self-Assessment Program, 1999).

Schwab L. *Eye Care in Developing Nations.* 3rd ed. (1999).

Skuta GL, ed. *ProVision: Preferred Responses in Ophthalmology,* Series 2 (Self-Assessment Program, 1996).

Wilson FM II, ed. *Practical Ophthalmology: A Manual for Beginning Residents* (1996).

Slide-Scripts

External Disease and Cornea: A Multimedia Collection (1994).

Fong DS. *Eye Care for the Elderly* (Eye Care Skills for the Primary Care Physician Series, 1999).

Mead MD, Shingleton BJ. *Eye Trauma and Emergencies* (Eye Care Skills for the Primary Care Physician Series, 1996).

Young SE. *Managing the Red Eye* (Eye Care Skills for the Primary Care Physician Series, 1994).

Continuing Ophthalmic Video Education

Abbott RL. *Surgical Intervention in Corneal and External Diseases* (1989).

Carlson A. *The Sixty-Minute Triple;* and Sajjadi H. *A Simple Technique for Centering the Recipient Trephine in Corneal Transplant* (1995).

Cohn H. *Indentation Gonioscopy;* Heyworth P, Morlet N, Dart J. *Contemporary Surgical Management of Pterygium;* and Langford J, Schwartz T, Linberg J. *A New Technique for Silicone Stent Intubation* (1996).

Farrell TA, Alward WLM, Verdick RE. *Fundamentals of Slit-Lamp Biomicroscopy* (1993).

Hannush SB. *Corneal Triple Procedure: Another Twist;* and Croasdale CR, Holland EJ. *Keratolimbal Allograft (KLAL) for Severe Ocular Surface Disease: Surgical Technique* (1998).

Gelender H, Mandelbaum SH. *Postoperative Astigmatism: Prevention and Management* (1987).

Wright KW. *Inferior Oblique Surgery;* John T. *Intraoperative Control of Corneal Astigmatism During Penetrating Keratoplasty;* and Goldberg RA. *The Transcaruncular Approach to the Medial Orbit* (1997).

Preferred Practice Patterns

Preferred Practice Patterns Committee, Cornea Panel. *Bacterial Keratitis* (1995).

Preferred Practice Patterns Committee, Cornea Panel. *Blepharitis* (1998).

Preferred Practice Patterns Committee, Cornea Panel. *Conjunctivitis* (1998).

Preferred Practice Patterns Committee, Cornea Panel. *Corneal Opacification* (1995).

Preferred Practice Patterns Committee, Cornea Panel. *Dry Eye Syndrome* (1998).

Ophthalmic Procedures Assessments

Ophthalmic Procedures Assessment Committee. *Automated Lamellar Keratoplasty* (1995).

Ophthalmic Procedures Assessment Committee. *Corneal Endothelial Photography* (1996).

Ophthalmic Procedures Assessment Committee. *Epikeratoplasty* (Revised) (1995).

Ophthalmic Procedures Assessment Committee. *Keratophakia and Keratomileusis: Safety and Effectiveness* (1992)

Ophthalmic Procedures Assessment Committee. *Punctal Occlusion for the Dry Eye* (1996).

Ophthalmic Procedures Assessment Committee. *Radial Keratotomy for Myopia* (1992).

LEO Clinical Topic Updates

Pflugfelder S. *Cornea, External Disease, and Anterior Segment Trauma* (1996).

To order any of these materials, please call the Academy's Customer Service number at (415) 561-8540.

CREDIT REPORTING FORM

BASIC AND CLINICAL SCIENCE COURSE
Section 8

1999–2000

CME Accreditation

The American Academy of Ophthalmology is accredited by the Accreditation Council for Continuing Medical Education to sponsor continuing medical education for physicians.

The American Academy of Ophthalmology designates this educational activity for a maximum of 40 hours in category 1 credit toward the AMA Physician's Recognition Award. Each physician should claim only those hours of credit that he/she has actually spent in the educational activity.

If you wish to claim continuing medical education credit for your study of this section, you must complete and return the study question answer sheet on the back of this page, along with the following signed statement, to the Academy office. This form must be received within 3 years of the date of purchase.

I hereby certify that I have spent _____ (up to 40) hours of study on the curriculum of this section, and that I have completed the study questions. (The Academy, *upon request,* will send you a transcript of the credits listed on this form.)

☐ *Please send credit verification now.*

Signature _____   _____
                                                                                                          Date

Name: _____

Address: _____

City and State: _____ Zip: _____

Telephone: (_____) _____   *Academy Member ID# _____
                    area code

* Your ID number is located following your name on any Academy mailing label, in your Membership Directory, and on your Monthly Statement of Account.

Section Evaluation

Please indicate your response to the statements listed below by placing the appropriate number to the left of each statement.

1 = agree strongly
2 = agree
3 = no opinion
4 = disagree
5 = disagree
   strongly

_____ This section covers topics in enough depth and detail.

_____ This section's illustrations are of sufficient number and quality.

_____ The references included in the text provide an appropriate amount of additional reading.

_____ The study questions at the end of the book are useful.

In addition, please attach a separate sheet of paper to this form if you wish to elaborate on any of the statements above or to comment on other aspects of this book.

Please return completed form to: **American Academy of Ophthalmology**
P.O. Box 7424
San Francisco, CA 94120-7424
ATTN: Clinical Education Division

BASIC AND CLINICAL SCIENCE COURSE

ANSWER SHEET FOR SECTION 8

Question	Answer	Question	Answer	Question	Answer
1	a b c d e	18	a b c d e	35	a b c d e
2	a b c d e	19	a b c d e	36	a b c d e
3	a b c d e	20	a b c d e	37	a b c d e
4	a b c d e	21	a b c d e	38	a b c d e
5	a b c d e	22	a b c d e	39	a b c d e
6	a b c d e	23	a b c d e	40	a b c d e
7	a b c d e	24	a b c d e	41	a b c d e
8	a b c d e	25	a b c d e	42	a b c d e
9	a b c d e	26	a b c d e	43	a b c d e
10	a b c d e	27	a b c d e	44	a b c d e
11	a b c d e	28	a b c d e	45	a b c d e
12	a b c d e	29	a b c d e	46	a b c d e
13	a b c d e	30	a b c d e	47	a b c d e
14	a b c d e	31	a b c d e	48	a b c d e
15	a b c d e	32	a b c d e	49	a b c d e
16	a b c d e	33	a b c d e	50	a b c d e
17	a b c d e	34	a b c d e		

STUDY QUESTIONS

STUDY QUESTIONS

The following multiple-choice questions are designed to be used after your course of study with this book. Record your responses on the answer sheet (the back side of the Credit Reporting Form) by circling the appropriate letter. For the most effective use of this exercise, *complete the entire test* before consulting the answers.

Although a concerted effort has been made to avoid ambiguity and redundancy in these questions, the authors recognize that differences of opinion may occur regarding the "best" answer. The discussions are provided to demonstrate the rationale used to derive the answer. They may also be helpful in confirming that your approach to the problem was correct or, if necessary, in fixing the principle in your memory.

1. The normal human cornea

   a. Has a refractive index less than air
   b. Is less than 1 mm thick
   c. Is innervated by terminal branches of the superorbital nerve from the first division of the trigeminal nerve (cranial nerve V)
   d. Receives most of its oxygen supply for aerobic metabolism from the limbal circulation
   e. Efficiently transmits ultraviolet C (190–290 nm) light

2. Which of the following statements regarding the normal adult cornea is NOT true?

   a. The extracellular matrix of the normal corneal stroma consists primarily of a glycosaminoglycan, keratan sulfate, attached to a core protein, lumican.
   b. The sum of the imbibition pressure and swelling pressure of the cornea equals the intraocular pressure.
   c. Keratocytes synthesize procollagen and collagen-degrading enzymes.
   d. Collagen fibrils are assembled into fibers that form about 300 lamellae.
   e. Keratocytes in one plane are prevented from contacting other cell layers by each lamella.

3. Which of the following does NOT usually accompany or follow corneal inflammation?

   a. Pannus
   b. Pseudoguttata
   c. Ghost vessels
   d. Lipid keratopathy
   e. Hassall-Henle bodies

4. Each of the following statements about specular photomicroscopy of the corneal endothelium is true EXCEPT:

   a. Posterior corneal rings remain in the same place regardless of the diurnal fluctuation of intraocular pressure.
   b. Donor corneas distributed for penetrating keratoplasty should have an endothelial density of at least 2000 cells/mm^2.
   c. The coefficient of variation indicates variability of cell sizes and is often abnormally high in iridocorneal endothelial syndrome.
   d. The percentage of normal endothelial cells with six apices should be about 50%.
   e. Because of the restricted depth of field of the specular photomicroscope, only a narrow band of endothelium is in focus at a given time.

5. Each of the following statements pertaining to corneal topography is true EXCEPT:

   a. Computerized videokeratoscopy of a perfectly smooth, spherical globe should show a simulated keratometry measurement of zero.
   b. The central portion of a normal cornea is steeper than the periphery.
   c. The orthogonal simulated K values are determined from more points reflected from the central cornea than are the values that are obtained by keratometry.
   d. With-the-rule astigmatism produces a vertical bow-tie topographic pattern.
   e. A color map is a result of computerized analysis of placido disk photo-keratoscopy.

6. Conjunctival follicles in the inferior fornix are often found in

   a. Neonatal conjunctivitis caused by *Chlamydia trachomatis*
   b. Adult conjunctivitis caused by *Chlamydia trachomatis*
   c. Ocular cicatricial pemphigoid
   d. Stevens-Johnson syndrome
   e. All of the above

7. Active childhood trachoma produces all the following conjunctival cytologic changes EXCEPT:

   a. Intranuclear inclusions within conjunctival epithelial cells
   b. Neutrophils
   c. Lymphocytes
   d. Plasma cells
   e. Leber cells

8. Recurrent corneal erosions

   a. Are almost always associated with subepithelial haze
   b. Are typically present within 1 month after a corneal abrasion
   c. May occur spontaneously
   d. Are uncommon over the age of 50 years
   e. Frequently require phototherapeutic keratectomy

9. Neurotrophic keratopathy

    a. Results from damage to cranial nerve VII
    b. Is rarely associated with bulbar conjunctival anesthesia
    c. May be associated with a persistent epithelial defect
    d. Is more likely with herpes simplex virus than with herpes zoster virus
    e. Produces decreased osmolarity of the tear film

10. Which of the following statements concerning conjunctival xerosis is INCORRECT?

    a. Bitôt spots are composed of keratin and saprophytic bacteria.
    b. Night blindness often precedes xerophthalmia.
    c. Conjunctival keratinization can occur as a result of an intestinal malab-sorption syndrome.
    d. Children with vitamin A deficiency have fewer viral infections because of immune hyperreactivity.
    e. Topical retinoic acid can affect conjunctival differentiation.

11. The diagnosis of Sjögren syndrome is suggested by each of the following EXCEPT:

    a. Punctate staining of the bulbar conjunctiva with rose bengal solution within the intrapalpebral area
    b. Prolonged tear breakup time using fluorescein
    c. Reduced wetting of the Schirmer strip after 5 minutes
    d. Reduced concentrations of tear lysozyme and tear lactoferrin
    e. Increased osmolarity of the tears

12. A 30-year-old woman with chronic irritation in both eyes is found to have mild papillary conjunctivitis, punctate staining of the superior cornea and conjunctiva of both eyes, and filaments attached to the upper limbus of one eye. Bulbar conjunctival biopsy of the involved area showed keratinization, acanthosis, and intracellular glycogen granules. Which of the following diagnostic tests would be most appropriate?

    a. Bacterial cultures of the eyelid margins
    b. Histamine level of the tear film
    c. Serum rheumatoid factor
    d. Thyroid function testing
    e. HLA typing

13. Limbal stem cell dysfunction may be a component of which of the following conditions?

    a. Aniridia
    b. Atopic keratoconjunctivitis
    c. Chronic contact lens wear
    d. Stevens-Johnson syndrome
    e. All of the above

14. Chronic follicular conjunctivitis is a feature of

    a. Behçet syndrome
    b. Herpes zoster
    c. Ligneous conjunctivitis
    d. Molluscum contagiosum
    e. Rosacea

15. Which therapy is LEAST appropriate for treating dendritic epithelial keratitis caused by herpes simplex virus?

    a. Vidarabine 3% ointment five times per day
    b. Irifluridine 1% solution eight times per day
    c. Oral acyclovir 2 g per day
    d. Rimexolone 1% solution four times per day
    e. Minimal wiping debridement with a dry cotton-tip applicator

16. All of the following are manifestations of herpes simplex virus ocular disease EXCEPT:

    a. Recurrent epithelial erosion
    b. Geographic epithelial defect
    c. Disciform corneal edema
    d. Lipid keratopathy
    e. Limbal follicles

17. Subepithelial infiltrates in adenovirus keratoconjunctivitis

    a. Typically develop 3 days after onset of conjunctival hyperemia
    b. Are associated with deep corneal stromal neovascularization
    c. May persist for months
    d. Are not responsive to topical corticosteroids
    e. Improve with oral antihistamines

18. Which of the following statements regarding disorders of the corneal epithelium is INCORRECT?

    a. Thygeson superficial punctate keratitis produces randomly distributed punctate epithelial changes in various stages of evolution.
    b. Sjögren syndrome produces punctate epithelial erosions of the 3 o'clock and 9 o'clock regions.
    c. Herpes simplex virus epithelial keratitis may be punctate or linear.
    d. Adenovirus epithelial keratitis is usually limited to the corneal periphery.
    e. Recurrent erosions are uncommon in Meesman corneal dystrophy.

19. Which of the following statements about the neonatal ocular surface is true?

    a. Subconjunctival hemorrhage usually indicates a subdural hematoma.
    b. Syphilis is usually transmitted during delivery.
    c. The most common causes of bacterial conjunctivitis are *Chlamydia trachomatis, Neisseria gonorrhoeae,* and *Staphylococcus aureus.*
    d. Hunter syndrome produces mucopolysaccharide deposition in one or both corneas.
    e. Rieger anomaly is a cause of breaks in Descemet's membrane.

20. The preferred treatment for gonococcal conjunctivitis in an otherwise healthy adult is

 a. Penicillin VK orally for 5 days
 b. Ceftriaxone intramuscularly in a single dose
 c. Azithromycin orally in a single dose
 d. a and b
 e. b and c

21. Bacterial keratitis resulting from methicillin-resistant *S aureus* has failed to respond to topical cefazolin and tobramycin eyedrops administered every 2 hours. An appropriate alternate therapy for this patient would be

 a. Erythromycin ointment
 b. Vancomycin solution
 c. Norfloxacin solution
 d. Bacitracin ointment
 e. Conjunctival flap

22. A 10-year-old child presents with acute, spontaneous onset of nonsuppurative stromal keratitis of the left eye. Which of the following statements would be most likely?

 a. Serological testing is not needed because stromal keratitis as a result of congenital syphilis occurs before 6 years of age.
 b. Mumps should be considered a likely diagnosis, and parotid gland enlargement is likely to occur within 1 week.
 c. The lack of a prior history does not exclude herpes simplex virus stromal keratitis.
 d. Vaccination against varicella-zoster virus should be provided to the patient and classmates.
 e. Testing for food allergy should be part of the initial evaluation.

23. A 12-year-old girl presents with a granulomatous nodule of the bulbar conjunctiva in the lower fornix of the left eye. A large, tender preauricular lymph node is also present as well as submandibular and cervical lymphadenopathy. Conjunctival biopsy shows lymphocytes and giant cells. Which of the following tests is most likely to be helpful in the diagnosis?

 a. Antibodies to *Bartonella*
 b. Antibodies to HTLV-I
 c. Heterophile antibody
 d. Angiotensin-converting enzyme level
 e. Anti-Ro and anti-La autoantibodies

24. A phlyctenule of the limbus

 a. Is composed of degenerated mast cells
 b. Occurs with staphylococcal blepharitis
 c. Differentiates erythema multiforme from toxic epidermal necrolysis
 d. Should lead to careful examination for Lisch nodules
 e. Is a complication of hereditary benign intraepithelial dyskeratosis

25. Which of the following statements regarding pigmentation of the cornea is the most accurate?

   a.   Iron lines associated with keratoconus run parallel with Vogt's striae.
   b.   A total hyphema associated with increased intraocular pressure produces yellow-green deposits within the cornea.
   c.   Corneal chrysiasis produces a vortex opacity of the central cornea.
   d.   Chloroquine and related drugs occasionally produce conjunctival and corneal argyriasis with pigmentation in peripheral endothelial cells.
   e.   The yellow deposits of ochronosis often resemble pinguecula.

26. All of the following statements about rosacea are true EXCEPT:

   a.   It is more commonly diagnosed in white populations.
   b.   It rarely occurs in childhood.
   c.   Reduced goblet cells contribute to tear-film instability.
   d.   Cellular hypersensitivity may be involved.
   e.   Oral doxycycline may be an effective treatment.

27. Ocular cicatricial pemphigoid

   a.   Results in a lipid tear deficiency
   b.   Is rarely associated with involvement of nonocular mucous membranes
   c.   Is clinically indistinguishable from linear IgA dermatosis
   d.   Results from abnormalities of immediate hypersensitivity (Type I)
   e.   Is usually responsive to topical corticosteroid treatment

28. Stevens-Johnson syndrome

   a.   Is also referred to as erythema multiforme minor
   b.   Rarely presents as an acute febrile episode
   c.   Is generally a disease of elderly patients
   d.   Is commonly associated with drug hypersensitivity
   e.   Is believed to be caused by a retrovirus

29. Nodular scleritis is most likely to be associated with

   a.   Relapsing polychondritis
   b.   Multiple sclerosis
   c.   Orbital pseudotumor
   d.   Graft-versus-host disease following bone marrow transplantation
   e.   Contact allergy

30. Which condition does not have malignant potential?

   a.   Pseudoepitheliomatis hyperplasia
   b.   Viral conjunctival papilloma
   c.   Congenital melanosis oculi
   d.   Xeroderma pigmentosum
   e.   Primary acquired melanosis

31. All of the following statements concerning sebaceous carcinoma of the eye-lid margin are true EXCEPT:

    a. It may arise from the glands of Zeis.
    b. It is generally unresponsive to radiotherapy.
    c. Both the upper and lower eyelids may be involved in a single patient.
    d. It may present as chronic conjunctivitis.
    e. Tumor cells containing lipid are best demonstrated by stains of frozen sections.

32. Sebaceous gland carcinoma of the eyelid is characterized by all of the following EXCEPT:

    a. Usually fixed to adjacent tissue
    b. Usually painful
    c. Usually arises from the meibomian gland
    d. 10-year mortality exceeds 10%
    e. Often spreads intraepithelially

33. A virus has been incriminated in the pathogenesis of each of the following neoplasias EXCEPT:

    a. Squamous cell papilloma
    b. Squamous cell carcinoma
    c. Basal cell nevus
    d. Kaposi sarcoma
    e. Molluscum

34. Malignancy of the ocular surface is most likely to develop with

    a. Eyelid lentigines
    b. Conjunctiva ephelis
    c. Primary acquired melanosis
    d. Kissing nevi
    e. Oncocytoma

35. The nevus of Ota is

    a. A congenital blue nevus
    b. More prevalent in Scandinavia than Africa
    c. Not bilateral
    d. A complication of psoralen therapy
    e. X-linked

36. A 59-year-old woman presents with the recent onset of a flat, darkly pigmented macule of the left lower palpebral conjunctiva. Of the following conditions, which would be most likely?

    a. Benign acquired melanosis
    b. Blue nevus
    c. Oculodermal melanosis
    d. Lentigo senilis
    e. Primary acquired melanosis

37. Select the correct statement concerning congenital anomalies of the eye.

    a. A capillary hemangioma is a choristoma that can cause amblyopia.
    b. An epibulbar dermoid may be associated with facial asymmetry and malformation of the cervical spine.
    c. Cryptophthalmus is usually a nonfamilial, spontaneous occurrence that is possibly related to a teratogen.
    d. Cornea plana is often associated with angle-closure glaucoma and high myopia.
    e. Peters anomaly is classified into types depending on whether optic nerve hypoplasia is present.

38. All of the following conditions concerning corneal opacification in infancy and childhood are true EXCEPT:

    a. Peters anomaly with lens involvement is rarely bilateral.
    b. Interstitial keratitis caused by congenital syphilis is more common after 2 years of age compared to infants less than 2 years of age.
    c. Congenital hereditary endothelial dystrophy should prompt examination of relatives for posterior polymorphous dystrophy.
    d. Arcus juvenilis is usually unilateral.
    e. Forceps injury at birth produces oblique tears in Descemet's membrane because babies are most commonly delivered in the left occiput–anterior position.

39. Each of the following has been associated with keratoconus EXCEPT:

    a. Down syndrome
    b. Retinitis pigmentosa
    c. Floppy eyelid syndrome
    d. Ehlers-Danlos syndrome
    e. Hansen disease (leprosy)

40. All of the following conditions may result in stromal amyloid, but which does NOT produce refractile lines in the cornea?

    a. Lattice corneal dystrophy
    b. Meretoja syndrome
    c. Avellino corneal dystrophy
    d. Secondary systemic amyloidosis
    e. Interstitial keratitis

41. Which of the following syndromes of corneal clouding is associated with autosomal recessive inheritance of dwarfism and a normal retina?

    a. Hunter syndrome
    b. Hurler syndrome
    c. Morquio syndrome
    d. Scheie syndrome
    e. Macular corneal dystrophy

42. Cystinosis

    a.   Causes crystalline deposition within the epithelium

    b.   Always presents in early childhood

    c.   Is caused by a metabolic defect transmitted in an X-linked recessive manner

    d.   Is associated with renal abnormalities that first present in adulthood

    e.   Is characterized by corneal crystalline deposition that may be responsive to topical therapy

43. Which of the following statements regarding the management of pterygium is correct?

    a.   Topical mitomycin-C 0.02% twice daily can cause regression within 6 weeks.

    b.   Limbal ischemia and bacterial scleritis have occurred following thiophosphoramide (thiotepa) but not following β-irradiation.

    c.   Topical interferon-α is a potentially useful adjunct to a bare sclera excision.

    d.   A conjunctival autograft is typically obtained from the same eye that the pterygium affects.

    e.   A corneal keloid occurs in up to 5% of pterygium excision procedures.

44. Which of the following statements concerning a corneal abrasion is most accurate?

    a.   A corneal abrasion can easily be differentiated from early bacterial keratitis during external examination in the emergency room by using fluorescein eyedrops.

    b.   A corneal abrasion should always be patched to limit pain and to prevent neovascularization.

    c.   Corneal trauma is best managed by a collagen shield to allow for administration of a topical corticosteroid.

    d.   Trauma often precipitates future corneal erosions.

    e.   When associated with contact lens wear, the eye should not be patched because of the possibility of promoting infection.

45. The most accurate statement concerning patients with a traumatic hyphema is which of the following?

    a.   All adult patients should receive an oral antifibrinolytic agent to speed resolution of the blood clot.

    b.   Ongoing bleeding can usually be detected by a penlight examination.

    c.   Hemoglobin electrophoresis should be performed on African American children.

    d.   Approximately 80% of patients with rebleeding develop elevated intra-ocular pressure.

    e.   Evacuation of a total, eight-ball hyphema should never be accompanied by an iridectomy or trabeculectomy.

46. The selection of corneal donor tissue for corneal transplantation often de-
    pends on all of the following EXCEPT:

    a. Death-to-preservation time
    b. Tissue storage time
    c. Donor-recipient HLA matching
    d. Endothelial cell density
    e. Cause of death

47. The surgical correction of astigmatism

    a. Does not change the spherical equivalent power of the cornea
    b. Was established as safe and effective by the PERK study
    c. Requires surgery on the steep axis of the astigmatism
    d. Is more predictable than operating on the spherical power
    e. Is based primarily on the manifest refraction

48. Laser in situ keratomileusis

    a. Is another name for automated lamellar keratectomy
    b. Shows wound healing similar to radial keratotomy
    c. Results in progressive hyperopia during the first few postoperative
        months
    d. Has the same complications as photorefractive keratectomy
    e. None of the above

49. Computerized corneal topography

    a. Determines corneal power from four points measured in the 3-mm
        central diameter
    b. Displays steeper corneal curvatures as blue or purple on a color map
    c. Is not useful for detecting irregular astigmatism
    d. Accurately determines corneal power at each point
    e. Can be altered with artificial tears

50. The most important complications after keratoprosthesis surgery include

    a. Wound necrosis
    b. Uveitis
    c. Endophthalmitis
    d. Glaucoma
    e. All of the above

ANSWERS

1. Answer—b. The normal cornea measures approximately 0.5 mm central-ly and 0.7 mm peripherally. The refractive index of the cornea is 1.336, compared to the 1.000 of air, although most keratometers and topographic instruments assume a combined refractive index for the corneal surface of 1.3375. The cornea, one of the most sensitive tissues in the body, receives its sensory nerve supply from the long ciliary nerves derived from the oph-thalmic gland to the trigeminal nerve. During waking hours, aerobic me-tabolism of the cornea is maintained by glucose supplied by the aqueous humor and oxygen from the air via the tear film. Sleeping with prolonged eyelid closure results in lower oxygen levels and a shift from aerobic to anaerobic metabolism. The cornea absorbs ultraviolet radiation for wave-lengths less than 290 nm (UVC). Ultraviolet photokeratopathy can result from exposure to a germicidal UVC lamp or to a welding arc.

2. Answer—e. Proteoglycans of the cornea are composed of glycosaminogly-cans attached to core proteins. Keratan sulfate is the major glycosamino-glycan in a normal adult cornea, although hyaluronan is present in the embryonic cornea and during wound healing. Keratan sulfate binds to lumi-can, keratocan, and osteoglycin. Interfibrillary expansion between negatively charged glycosaminoglycans produces a swelling pressure (SP) that is re-lated to the imbibition pressure (IP) and intraocular pressure (IOP) by the following formula: $IP = IOP - SP$. Keratocytes synthesize the extracellular matrix of the corneal stroma, including matrix metalloproteases that degrade collagen, resulting in slow collagen turnover. About 300 lamellae are stacked parallel to the corneal surface, running from limbus to limbus. Scattered between these lamellae, keratocytes contact one another to form a three-dimensional network throughout the stroma.

3. Answer—e. Corneal inflammation often produces transient endothelial dys-function, manifesting structurally as endothelial pseudoguttata and stromal edema. Neovascularization may lead to fibrovascular proliferation from the limbus, called a pannus. These vessels may deposit cholesterol, phospho-lipids, and neutral fats, resulting in lipid keratopathy. Resolution of disease often leaves faint ghost vessels. Hassall-Henle bodies are peripheral guttata that are more common with advancing age than with corneal inflammation.

4. Answer—d. Specular microscopy enables visualization of the corneal en-dothelium, a single layer of six-sided cells that are 5 μm thick and 20 μm wide, arranged in a mosaic pattern. Normally, the dimensions and shapes of endothelial cells are uniform, and the cell density is about 3500 cells/mm^2 in young adults. Morphometric parameters aid in judging the state of the corneal endothelium. Normally, about 70%–80% of the endothelial cells are hexagonal; pleomorphism is any deviation, usually a decrease, from this hexagonality value. Polymegethism is the increased variability in cell area. Specular microscopy can also reveal other changes within the cornea, includ-ing posterior corneal rings that, like fingerprints, uniquely identify individuals and are used as landmarks for comparing photomicrographs.

5. Answer—a. Topographic mapping of the cornea by a videokeratoscope is more efficient than keratometry because many more points are measured simultaneously. For example, regular astigmatism produces bow-tie patterns. Irregular astigmatism is more difficult to quantify. Topographic indices include the simulated keratometric (SIM K).

6. Answer—b. Common causes of acute follicular conjunctivitis include adenoviral eye disease and primary herpes simplex virus eye disease. Conjunctival disease caused by *Chlamydia trachomatis* may present as acute follicular conjunctivitis in adults. Because neonates do not have sufficient lymphoid tissue in their conjunctiva, hyperemia and pseudomembranes are the main clinical features, although the disease may become follicular if the duration is longer than 8 weeks. While drug-induced conjunctivitis can produce chronic follicular changes, ocular cicatricial pemphigoid and Stevens-Johnson syndrome do not. Typical features of these causes of cicatrizing conjunctivitis include conjunctival erosion and symblepharon.

7. Answer—a. Giemsa-stained smears of conjunctival scrapings can show a characteristic inflammatory pattern during active trachoma, including both acute and chronic inflammatory cells with plasma cells and large macrophages called Leber cells. The intracellular portion of the chlamydia life cycle produces basophilic intracytoplasmic inclusions within conjunctival epithelial cells. Intranuclear inclusions can occur in certain viral infections such as those caused by herpes simplex virus and varicella-zoster virus.

8. Answer—c. Corneal erosions may be a manifestation of corneal epithelial–based membrane dystrophy. It may be difficult to detect on slit lamp biomicroscopy. Recurrent erosions may also follow trauma, often several months or even years after the initial injury. Recurrent corneal erosion can occur at any age, but its prevalence is higher after the age of 50. An acute erosion responds to patching. Preventive therapy includes lubrication and hypertonic agents. Debridement or stromal micropuncture may be effective if more conservative management fails.

9. Answer—c. Neurotrophic keratopathy is frequently associated with a persistent corneal epithelial defect, usually located in the palpebral fissure just below midline. These neurotrophic epithelial defects are usually horizontally oval with rolled edges. When lubrication and more conservative measures fail, a tarsorrhaphy is often required. Damage to cranial nerve VII results in neuroparalytic keratopathy. Corneal anesthesia associated with cranial nerve V involvement is the principal cause of neurotrophic keratopathy, and damage to both nerves leads to serious ocular surface disease. Causes of neurotrophic keratopathy include ophthalmic zoster.

10. Answer—d. Approximately five million children, predominantly in developing nations, have xerophthalmia. Altered dietary intake, impaired intestinal absorption, or altered liver storage and metabolism are the most common reasons for conjunctival xerosis in the United States. Ingestion of vitamin A or carotenoids with provitamin activity, such as beta-carotene, results in the absorption of retinol that is combined in the liver with retinol-binding protein. Retinol is an essential component of rhodopsin in the rod photo-receptors and is required for maintenance of mucous membranes. Vitamin A deficiency results in suppression of cell-mediated immunity that can predispose to herpes simplex virus keratitis and measles. Conditions such as ocular cicatricial pemphigoid and Stevens-Johnson syndrome that result in conjunctival keratinization may respond to topical retinoic acid.

11. Answer—b. Diagnosing the ocular component of Sjögren syndrome is made by slit-lamp biomicroscopy and tear production test. The height of the tear meniscus can be judged. Fluorescein or rose bengal solutions are then instilled to identify the defined punctate staining of the conjunctiva that often begins in the intrapalpebral fissure. Tear breakup time, normally at least 10 seconds, is often reduced to a few seconds. The Schirmer test measures the amount of wetting on the paper strip. Patients with severe aqueous tear deficiency often have a measurement of 5 mm or less after 5 minutes. Lysozyme and lactoferrin, proteins produced by the lacrimal gland, are reduced during Sjögren syndrome. The reduced tear flow and increased tear evaporation also contribute to an increase in tear-film osmolarity.

12. Answer—d. Superior limbic keratoconjunctivitis (SLK) is characterized by chronic keratoconjunctivitis with inflammation of the superior bulbar conjunctiva and adjacent cornea. Filaments of the limbus and superior cornea occur in approximately one third of patients. Thyroid disease may be an associated condition.

13. Answer—e. The ocular surface is a functional unit that is maintained by stem cells for the conjunctival epithelium and by stem cells for the corneal epithelium. The function of stem cells for the corneal surface can be modulated by changes in their ecological niche. Abnormalities of limbal stem cells may occur from acute inflammation, chronic injury, or physiologic alterations at the limbus. Conditions with a clear pathogenic effect include chemical and thermal injuries, erythema multiforme, chronic medication toxicity, contact lens wear, and multiple surgical procedures at the limbal zone. Conditions such as atopic keratoconjunctivitis, aniridia, and neurotrophic keratopathy are associated with disrupted homeostasis of the microenvironment of the ocular surface that predisposes to conjunctivalization and neovascularization of the cornea.

14. Answer—d. Molluscum contagiosum typically forms a nodule on the eyelid. When the eyelid margin is involved, follicular conjunctivitis may also occur as well as corneal epithelial changes. Keratoconjunctivitis associated with contagiosum thus has many features mimicking chlamydial eye disease. The conjunctival changes of ophthalmic zoster are usually hypermia with a papillary reaction, although follicles can sometimes occur. Ligneous conjunctivitis is a rare type of pseudomembranous conjunctivitis with hyperemia. Rosacea is associated with meibomian gland dysfunction and chronic conjunctival injection. Behçet syndrome typically lacks conjunctivitis.

15. Answer—d. The least appropriate therapy for herpes simplex virus epithelial keratitis is a corticosteroid. Topical or oral antiviral agents are effective therapy. Debridement is also effective, although virus may remain in the non-removed epithelium and cause recrudescent epithelial keratitis several days later.

16. Answer—e. Herpes simplex virus may cause vesicular or erosive blepharitis, capillary or follicular conjunctivitis, dendritic or geographic epithelial keratitis, disciform corneal edema, necrotizing stromal keratitis, and iridocyclitis. Limbal follicles do not occur and are generally limited to keratoconjunctivitis caused by *Chlamydia trachomatis* and to toxic reactions caused by certain medications.

17. Answer—c. Subepithelial infiltrates in adenovirus keratoconjunctivitis typically develop approximately 2 weeks after the onset of conjunctivitis, are not associated with corneal neovascularization, and may persist for months. Topical corticosteroid therapy can suppress the symptoms and signs.

18. Answer—d. Adenovirus epithelial keratitis typically causes diffuse punctate epithelial changes that may evolve into scattered subepithelial infiltrates.

19. Answer—c. Infectious conjunctivitis in neonates is often caused by organisms that reside in the birth canal or are transmitted in the neonatal nursery. Prophylactic application of silver nitrate, erythromycin, or a similar agent can reduce the risk of infection. A chancre of the birth canal is infectious and can transmit primary syphilis to the neonate; however, congenital syphilis is almost always the result of transplacental dissemination from the mother to the fetus. Hunter syndrome, the only mucopolysaccharidosis that is inherited as an X-linked trait, is caused by deficiency of iduronate sulfatase that can lead to corneal clouding later in life. Rieger anomaly (Axenfeld-Rieger syndrome) includes iris abnormalities with strands extending to Schwalbe's ring and opacities, but not breaks, in Descemet's membrane.

20. Answer—e. More than a half million new cases of *Neisseria gonorrhoeae* infections occur each year in the United States. Gonococcal keratoconjunctivitis is uncommon, but most cases are the result of autoinoculation of the ocular surface from the genital tract. Several antibacterial regimens are effective against gonorrhea, but penicillin is no longer recommended because of the increase in penicillinase-producing *N gonorrhoeae* (PPNG). Single-dose treatments currently include intramuscular ceftriaxone or oral cefixime. Quinolone-resistant *N gonorrhoeae* (QRNG), although becoming widespread in Asia, remains uncommon in the United States, and oral ciprofloxacin or oral ofloxacin can also be used. Because patients infected with *N gonorrhoeae* are often also infected with *C trachomatis,* either testing for chlamydial coinfection or simultaneously treating with an antichlamydial agent such as azithromycin is indicated. Updated treatment recommendations for sexually transmitted diseases can be obtained from the U.S. Public Health Service (http://www.cdc.gov/nchstp/dstd/dstdp.html).

21. Answer—b. Vancomycin is a drug of choice for methicillin-resistant *Staphylococcus aureus.* While erythromycin and bacitracin may be effective in vitro, ointment formulations may not provide sufficient levels in the cornea.

22. Answer—c. Unilateral nonsuppurative stromal keratitis is most commonly caused by herpes simplex virus. Primary exposure to herpes simplex virus is typically subclinical, and recurrent disease can be manifested as blepharoconjunctivitis, epithelial keratitis, stromal keratitis, or iritis. Other causes of stromal keratitis include congenital and acquired syphilis. Mumps is a cause of disciform stromal keratitis but almost always has associated parotid gland inflammation.

23. Answer—a. Cat-scratch disease is a subacute bacterial infection caused by *Bartonella henselae* that can produce Parinaud oculoglandular syndrome. These small pleiomorphic rods can be detected by special silver stains of biopsy material. Medical treatment has included oral doxycycline, oral ciprofloxacin, and other antibiotics.

24. Answer—b. A phlyctenule of the conjunctiva or peripheral cornea is a focal cellular hypersensitivity reaction occurring in response to a variety of microbial agents such as staphylococci of the eyelid margin.

25. Answer—b. Gold (chrysiasis) and silver (argyriasis) deposits within the corneal stroma may occur from local or systemic use. A Fleischer ring associated with keratoconus is an iron line around the base of the cone. Other iron lines may be associated with a pterygium (Stocker line), filtering bleb (Ferry line), and other corneal surface irregularities. Corneal blood staining that complicates a hyphema with elevated intraocular pressure begins as small yellow granules within the posterior stroma, caused by hemoglobin and its metabolites, that can eventually produce a rust-colored opacity.

26. Answer—c. No cause has yet been identified for rosacea; however, a cell-mediated hypersensitivity mechanism may be involved. Rosacea is more prevalent (or at least is recognized more often) in fair-skin populations. Tear-film instability may occur as a result of meibomian gland dysfunction. Oral doxycycline can improve symptoms of blepharoconjunctivitis and reduce facial skin complications.

27. Answer—c. Ocular cicatricial pemphigoid cannot be reliably distinguished from linear IgA dermatosis on the basis of the eye examination. Features of the altered ocular surface include mucin and aqueous tear deficiency. Mucous membranes other than the eye can be involved such as the mouth, pharynx, genitalia, and anus. This condition probably represents an altered cytotoxic hypersensitivity reaction, in which cell injury results from autoantibodies directed against a cell-surface antigen. While systemic corticosteroids may provide limited success, immunosuppressive agents are usually more effective and should be considered in therapy.

28. Answer—d. Stevens-Johnson syndrome is commonly associated with a drug reaction. Patients often present with an acute febrile episode associated with skin eruption. The classical "target" lesion has a red center surrounded by a pale ring and an outer red circle.

29. Answer—a. Nodular anterior scleritis can be associated with a wide variety of systemic diseases, including relapsing polychondritis. Single or multiple inflammatory nodules result in severe ocular pain and recur in approximately one half of patients. Approximately 20% progress to necrotizing scleritis.

30. Answer—a. The prevalence of malignant transformation is highest in xeroderma pigmentosum and primary acquired melanosis. The less common malignant transformation can occur in association with viral conjunctival papilloma and congenital melanosis oculi. Pseudoepitheliomatis hyperplasia is not associated with the development of cancer.

31. Answer—b. This tumor often shows a good response to radiotherapy, which is fortunate since diffuse eyelid involvement is frequent. Nevertheless, complete surgical excision is generally preferred whenever possible. Extensive involvement may be related to a tendency to masquerade as chronic inflammation, although the tumor may arise at multifocal sites. Special stains of frozen sections aid in demonstrating the lipid-containing tumor cells.

32. Answer—b. Sebaceous gland carcinoma may masquerade as conjunctivitis, blepharitis, and chalazion, producing unilateral inflammation with minimal discomfort. Often originating from one or more meibomian glands, the tumor often shows pagetoid spread rather than focal growth. Diagnostic delay reduces survival, but more thorough surgical treatments have resulted in improved outcome.

33. Answer—c. Both host and environmental factors likely interact in the pathogenesis of neoplasia of the ocular surface. Human papilloma virus has been found in some cases of squamous cell papillomas and squamous cell carcinomas. A human herpes virus may be a cause of Kaposi sarcoma, especially in immunosuppressed individuals. *Molluscum contagiosum* is a poxvirus that produces molluscum lesions. The basal cell nevus syndrome is an autosomal dominant disorder.

34. Answer—c. Primary acquired melanosis is fairly common among middle-aged whites. Some cases have cellular atypia that can evolve to malignant melanoma.

35. Answer—a. Oculodermal melanocytosis (nevus of Ota) is a congenital blue-gray discoloration of the eyelids and sclera. The lesion may appear at birth or be recognized during adolescence.

36. Answer—e. The diagnosis of a pigmented conjunctival lesion depends on the patient's age, the configuration and pace of growth, and the level of involvement. The accompanying flow chart summarizes a decision-making scheme.

Pigmented Conjunctival Lesion

37. Answer—b. The Goldenhar syndrome results from dysmorphogenesis during the development of the first and second branchial arches. Most are unilateral. Clinical findings include maxillary hypoplasia, hearing loss, malformations of the external ear, epibulbar dermoids, vertebral hypoplasia, and abnormalities of the heart. Indications for surgical removal of an epibulbar dermoid include continued growth or irritation and cosmesis.

38. Answer—a. Peters anomaly is a type of anterior segment dysgenesis. This neurocristopathy likely occurs from maldevelopment of the anterior segment because of abnormal migration, proliferation, or differentiation of mesenchymal cells originating from the neural crest. A central corneal opacity with iris strands and a normal lens suggest an insult at approximately the fourth month of embryonic development and is usually unilateral. Peters anomaly with a central corneal opacity, iridocorneal synechiae, and an abnormal lens is most frequently bilateral and may be accompanied by other ocular or systemic abnormalities.

39. Answer—e. Several inherited connective tissue disorders such as Ehlers-Danlos syndrome, Morvan syndrome, and osteogenesis imperfecta have, rarely, been associated with keratoconus. Vernal conjunctivitis and floppy eyelid syndrome have also been linked, although the cause and effect is uncertain. Some patients with keratoconus have been found to also have retinitis pigmentosa. Hansen disease can produce corneal changes, including a corneal staphyloma, but not keratoconus.

40. Answer—d. Amyloid can take many forms in the eye. The most readily recognizable form is that produced by a lattice corneal dystrophy, where glassy, refractile, branching lines are visible in the corneal stroma. Avellino corneal dystrophy is a phenotype that localizes to the same gene as lattice corneal dystrophy. Any secondary corneal degenerations, such as corneal scarring following syphilitic interstitial keratitis, may result in depositions of amyloid throughout the stroma. Secondary systemic amyloidosis rarely involves the cornea, but when it does so, it appears in focal deposits.

41. Answer—c. Hunter syndrome is inherited in an X-linked recessive pattern. Hurler syndrome is associated with pigmentary retinopathy. Scheie syndrome is associated with normal stature. Macular corneal dystrophy does not have systemic features. Morquio syndrome is characterized by dwarfism, barrel chest, short neck, kyphoscoliosis, and aortic valve disease. Absence of pigmentary retinopathy leads to a good visual prognosis for penetrating keratoplasty in Morquio syndrome.

42. Answer—e. Cystinosis is an autosomal recessive metabolic disorder in which cystine accumulates within lysosomes. The disease may present in infantile, adolescent, and adult forms. Cystinosis is characterized by corneal crystalline deposits in the stroma that may be responsive to therapy with topical cysteamine eyedrops. Renal disease is more likely in the infantile form and much less likely in the older forms.

43. Answer—d. Many different surgical procedures have been described for the removal of a pterygium. A conjunctival autograft may be considered for a primary or recurrent lesion. Adjunctive therapies with antimetabolites and irradiation have been proposed but have rarely been complicated by late scleral necrosis.

44. Answer—e. A corneal abrasion is the traumatic removal of all or some of the epithelial layers of the cornea. Exclusion of microbial contamination can be difficult soon after the injury, especially when the abrasion is caused by a dirty foreign body or contact lens. A patch, collagen shield, or bandage contact lens can reduce discomfort but should be used cautiously when microbial keratitis is likely. Topical nonsteroidal anti-inflammatory agents can be useful to relieve discomfort.

45. Answer—c. Rebleeding and increased intraocular pressure are complications of traumatic hyphema, and medical and surgical therapy is directed at controlling these occurrences. Marked intraocular pressure is especially likely in patients with a sickle cell hemoglobinopathy, even with a small hyphema. These patients need to be identified, treated, and closely followed.

46. Answer—c. Tissue obtained for corneal transplantation may be preserved in short-term cold preservation medium or by intermediate-term organ-culture techniques. The cadaver time should be relatively short, and investigations into the cause of death must exclude potentially transmissible infectious diseases. Slit-lamp biomicroscopy and, for older donors, endothelial specular microscopy are routinely performed by U.S. eye banks. Antigen matching is not currently used for routine corneal transplantation.

47. Answer—e. The manifest refraction is used in planning astigmatism surgery, even though it may not equal the topographic power of the cornea. Surgically induced changes in the spherical power of the cornea will vary depending on the type of procedure performed and the coupling ratio. The Prospective Evaluation of Radial Keratotomy (PERK) study evaluated the spherical treatment of myopia. Incisional surgery for astigmatism is done on the steep axis of the astigmatism; ablative surgery is performed on the flat axis. Because of the complexity of combining offsetting cylinders, astigmatism is less predictably changed than the spherical power.

48. Answer—e. Automated lamellar keratectomy is a form of in situ keratomileusis performed with the mechanical microkeratome rather than the laser. Wound healing with laser in situ keratomileusis differs from radial keratotomy because of the depth and location of the incision. Like photorefractive keratectomy, this procedure generally shows mild regression in the first 6 postoperative months toward myopia. LASIK often reduces the need for postoperative pain relief and for corticosteroids.

49. Answer—e. The keratometer determines corneal power by assessing four points. Steeper corneal curvature is generally depicted as yellow-red colors. Computerized video topography is used in detecting and quantifying irregular astigmatism. Axial maps provide reasonable accuracy in the central part of the cornea, but most current systems become less accurate toward the periphery. Artificial tears can change the absolute value of the central corneal power by up to 1.00 D.

50. Answer—e. Keratoprosthesis surgery is rarely performed because of vision-threatening complications. Advances in keratoprosthesis design seek to prevent tissue necrosis around the keratoprosthesis and to improve wound healing. Postoperative uveitis contributes to vitreous opacities, cystoid macular edema, and retinal detachment. Postsurgical endophthalmitis is generally a complication of impaired wound healing with perforation. Glaucoma has been the most common complication leading to visual loss.

INDEX

Amoebic cyst, *Acanthamoeba* causing, 128, 129*i*

Amphotericin, for fungal keratitis, 176–177

Amphotericin B, 45

Amyloid degeneration, 344. *See also* Amyloidosis/amyloid deposits
polymorphic, 343

Amyloidosis/amyloid deposits, 322–325
conjunctival, 324, 324*i*
corneal
in gelatinous droplike dystrophy, 298, 299*i*, 324
in lattice dystrophy, 296–297, 296*i*, 324
primary localized, 323*t*, 324
primary systemic, 323*t*, 324
secondary localized, 323*t*, 324, 344
secondary systemic, 323*t*, 324–325

ANA. *See* Antinuclear antibody

Anaerobes, as normal ocular flora, 113*t*

Anaphylactic hypersensitivity (type I) reaction, 186–187, 186*i*, 187*t*

Anaplasia, definition of, 228

ANCA. *See* Antineutrophil cytoplasmic antibodies

Anesthetics
tear production affected by, 83*t*
topical
abuse of, conjunctivitis caused by, 103, 103*i*
toxic keratoconjunctivitis caused by, 362

Angioedema, 202*t*

Angiography, fluorescein
anterior segment, 35
before penetrating keratoplasty, 415

Angiokeratoma corporis diffusum (Fabry disease), 316–317

Anhidrotic ectodermal dysplasia, 77

Aniridia
gene linkage of, 289*t*
limbal stem-cell dysfunction and, 106, 106*t*
with Wilms tumor, chromosomal abnormalities in, 287*t*

Ankyloblepharon, 266

Anophthalmos, 267
chromosomal abnormalities in, 287*t*

Antazoline, 40, 41*t*

Anterior chamber, flat, after penetrating keratoplasty, 420

Anterior chamber–associated immune deviation, corneal graft tolerance and, 411–412

Anterior corneal dystrophies, 290–293

Anterior microphthalmos, 269

Anterior segment
development of, 7–9, 8*i*, 261–262, 262*t*, 263*i*
dysgenesis of, 272–278
echography of, 35–36
fluorescein angiography of, 35
photography of, 34–36
trauma to, 356–385
chemical, 357–362
concussive, 362–368
nonperforating mechanical, 368–371
perforating, 371–383
surgical, 383–385
temperature and radiation causing, 356–357

Anterior segment microsurgery, techniques of, 46–50

Anterior stromal micropuncture, for recurrent corneal erosions, 98, 99*i*

Anterior uveitis, in herpes zoster ophthalmicus, 153

Antiarrhythmic agents, tear production affected by, 83*t*

Antibiotics, 43–46. *See also specific agent*
for acute purulent conjunctivitis, 163
for bacterial keratitis, 173–174, 174*t*
with corticosteroids, 42, 42*t*
for gonococcal conjunctivitis, 163–164
for staphylococcal blepharoconjunctivitis, 159

Antidepressants, tear production affected by, 83*t*

Antifibrinolytic agents, for hyphema, 367

Antifibrotic agents, toxic medication reaction caused by, 212

Antihistamines, 40, 41*t*
for hay fever and perennial allergic conjunctivitis, 194
tear production affected by, 83*t*
with vasoconstrictors, 40, 41*t*
for vernal keratoconjunctivitis, 196

Anti-HIV antibody testing, 119, 120

Antihypertensive agents, tear production affected by, 83*t*

Anti-infective agents, 43–46. *See also* Antibiotics

Anti-inflammatory agents, 40–43, 41*t*, 42*t*
 nonsteroidal (NSAIDs), 40, 41*t*
Anti-La (SS-B) autoantibodies, in Sjögren
 syndrome, 82
Antineutrophil cytoplasmic antibodies,
 testing for, 180*t*
Antinuclear antibody
 in aqueous tear deficiency, 83
 testing for, 180*t*
Antiparkinson agents, tear production
 affected by, 83*t*
Antiulcer agents, tear production affected
 by, 83*t*
Antiviral therapy, 45
 for herpetic dendritic and geographic
  epithelial keratitis, 146
 for herpetic stromal keratitis, 148–149
 after penetrating keratoplasty
  for herpetic keratitis
  complications, 150
Apert syndrome, 328*t*
Aphakia, epikeratoplasty (epikeratophakia)
 for, 438*t*, 451, 451*i*, 452*i*
Apical zone, contact lens fitting and, 437
Apoptosis, definition of, 229*t*
Applanation tonometry, fluorescein for, 19
Aqueous layer of tear film, 54
 secretion of, 55
Aqueous tear deficiency, 54, 82–88. *See
 also* Keratoconjunctivitis, sicca
 medications causing, 83*t*
 in Sjögren syndrome, 82–83
 tests of, 60, 61
*Arachnia propionica. See
 Propionibacterium, propionicus*
Arcus (corneal)
 in hyperlipoproteinemia, 315, 315*t*
 juvenilis, 274, 342
  in hyperlipoproteinemia, 315
 senilis, 342
Argon-fluoride excimer laser
 for keratoconus, 308
 for photoablation, 454
Argon laser procedures, ocular damage
 after (laser burns), 385
Argyriasis, 347, 348*t*
Arlt's line, 165, 166*i*
Arthritis, rheumatoid. *See* Rheumatoid
 arthritis
Arthropods, ocular infection caused
 by, 130–131

Artificial tears. *See also* Lubricants
 for dry eye, 8/85, 85*t*
 for hay fever and perennial allergic
  conjunctivitis, 194
 for Stevens-Johnson syndrome, 202
Ascorbic acid, deficiency of, 91
Astigmatism
 cornea as source of, 11
 irregular, herpetic keratitis and, 149
 after penetrating keratoplasty, control of,
  424–426, 425*i*
 after photorefractive keratectomy, 472
 surgical correction of, 467–469
  laser procedures for, 476–479
Ataxia-telangiectasia (Louis-Bar syndrome),
 79, 250
ATD. *See* Aqueous tear deficiency
Atopic dermatitis, 193
Atopic hypersensitivity (type I) reaction,
 186–187, 186*i*, 187*t*
Atopic keratoconjunctivitis, 197, 198*i*
Atrophy, definition of, 229*t*
Attachment, as virulence factor, 113
Autoantibodies, in aqueous tear deficiency,
 82, 83
Autografts
 conjunctival, 396–397
  indications for, 389*t*
  for wound closure after pterygium
   excision, 395*i*, 396, 396–397
 corneal, 414, 429–430. *See also*
  Keratoplasty, penetrating
 limbal, 397–400, 398–399*i*
  indications for, 389*t*
Autoimmune disorders. *See also
 specific disorder*
 marginal keratolysis ("melting") in,
  214, 223
 peripheral keratitis in, 214–215, 215*i*
 scleritis in, 223
Automated lamellar keratoplasty
 for hyperopia, 451, 451*i*, 466–467
 for myopia, 450, 450*i*, 463–464
Avellino dystrophy, 295. *See also*
 Granular dystrophy
 gene linkage of, 289*t*
Axenfeld anomaly/syndrome. *See*
 Axenfeld-Rieger syndrome
Axenfeld-Rieger syndrome, 272, 273*i*
 chromosomal aberration in, 287*t*
 gene linkage of, 289*t*

Blepharitis
  herpes simplex virus causing, 116
  seborrheic, 71, 155, 156*t*
  staphylococcal, 155–160, 156*t*, 157*i*
    marginal infiltrates in, 214
Blepharoconjunctivitis
  herpes simplex virus causing, 143
  marginal corneal infiltrates associated
      with, 213–214
  Moraxella, 157
  staphylococcal, 156–157, 162
  vaccinia virus causing, 155
Blepharoptosis, mechanical, 22
Blindness
  trachoma causing, 165
  xerophthalmia causing, 89
Blinking (blink reflex), 9, 10*i*, 53
  in meibomian gland lipid release, 55
Blood, corneal staining by, 348*t*, 366, 366*i*
Blue sclera, 268–269
  in Ehlers-Danlos syndrome,
      268–269, 326
  in osteogenesis imperfecta,
      268–269, 329*t*
Borrelia burgdorferi, ocular infection
    caused by, 126
Botfly larvae, ocular infection caused
    by, 131
Botulinum toxin type A (Botox), 394
Bowman's layer, 12
bp. *See* Base pairs
Branhamella catarrhalis. See
    Moraxella, catarrhalis
Bridge flap, 402
Broad-beam lasers, for photoablation,
    455, 470
Bromhexine, tear secretion affected
    by, 85–86
Bucket handle (bipedicle) flap, 402
Bulbar conjunctiva, 10, 11
Bulla
  corneal, 22*t*
  of eyelid, 21*t*
Buttonholing, 402
Butylcyanoacrylate tissue adhesive,
    therapy with, 406–407. *See also*
    Cyanoacrylate adhesive

Calcific band keratopathy (calcium
    hydroxyapatite deposition), 345–346
Calcium, deposition of in hypercalcemia,
    330, 345
Calcium hydroxyapatite deposition
    (calcific band keratopathy), 345–346
Calcofluor white staining, 62, 63*t*
  in microbial keratitis, 172*t*
Calliphoria fly, ocular infection caused
    by, 131
Canaliculitis, actinomycetes causing, 125
Cancer, corneal and external disease signs
    of, 332–333
Candida
  albicans, 126
  ocular infection caused by, 126–128,
      127*i*, 176, 177
    keratitis, 176, 177
  parapsilosis, 126
  tropicalis, 126
Canthoplasty, with medial
    tarsorrhaphy, 393–394
Capnocytophaga, ocular infection caused
    by, 123
Capsulopalpebral fascia, involutional
    eyelid changes and, 94
Carbohydrate metabolism, disorders
    of, 312–314
Carcinoma
  definition of, 230
  of eyelid, 230
Carcinoma in situ, conjunctival, 238, 239*i*
Carpenter syndrome, 328*t*
Caruncle, 10
Cat-scratch disease, 121, 168–169
Cataract, steroid-induced, after
    photorefractive keratectomy, 472
Cataract surgery, after radial
    keratotomy, 461
Catarrhal infiltrates (marginal corneal
    infiltrates), blepharoconjunctivitis
    and, 213–214
CD4+ T lymphocytes. *See also* Helper
    T cells
  in HIV infection/AIDS, 119
CD8+ T lymphocytes. *See also* Cytotoxic
    T cells; Suppressor T cells
  in external eye, 184
Cefazolin, 44
  for bacterial keratitis, 173, 174, 174*t*

Cefotaxime, for gonococcal conjunctivitis
in neonates, 164
Ceftazidime, for bacterial keratitis,
174, 174*t*
Ceftriaxone, 44
for bacterial keratitis, 174*t*
for gonococcal conjunctivitis, 163
in neonates, 164
Cell turnover, 227–228
Cellular atypia, definition/implication
of, 229*t*
Cellular immunity, 184–185
Cellulitis, preseptal, *Haemophilus*
causing, 123
Centering procedures, for keratorefractive
surgery, 456
radial keratotomy outcome affected
by, 458
Centimorgans (cM), 284
Central cloudy dystrophy, 300, 301*i*
Central crystalline dystrophy, Schnyder,
289*t*, 298–300, 300*i*, 315
gene linkage of, 289*t*
Central islands, after photorefractive
keratectomy, 471
Central zone, 437, 442*i*
Cephalosporins, 44
Ceramide trihexoside accumulation, in
Fabry disease, 316
Chalazion, 71–73, 72*i*
Chalcosis, corneal pigmentation in, 348*t*
Chandler variant, of iridocorneal
endothelial syndrome, 280
CHED. *See* Congenital hereditary
endothelial dystrophy
Chelation therapy, for calcific band
keratopathy, 345–346
Chemical injury of eye, 357–362
acid burns, 359
alkali burns, 358, 358*i*, 359*i*
animal and plant substances
causing, 361–362
conjunctival autograft for, 397
limbal stem-cell dysfunction and, 107
medications causing, 361–362
therapy of, 359–361
Chemosis, 21*t*
Chickenpox (varicella), 117, 150–151
herpes simplex virus infection
differentiated from, 151*t*
Children, corneal transplantation in, 429

Chlamydia
cytoplasmic inclusions formed by,
66–67, 67*i*, 121
ocular infection caused by,
120–121, 165–169
agents for treatment of, 44, 166, 168
clinical aspects of, 165–169
isolation techniques for, 133
neonatal, 164–165
specimen collection for, 131*t*
psittaci, 165
trachomatis, 66 67, 120
conjunctivitis caused by
in adults, 167–168, 167*i*
in neonates, 164–165
isolation of, 133
trachoma caused by, 165–166,
166*i*, 167*i*
Chlorambucil, 42
Chloramphenicol, 43*t*, 44
with corticosteroids, 42*t*
Chlorhexidine, 45
Chloroquine, cornea verticillata caused
by, 346–347
Chlortetracycline, 43*t*
Choristoma, 254–257
complex, 257
definition of, 254
dermoid, 254–256, 255*i*, 256*i*
epibulbar, 254–255
neuroglial, 257
osseous, 257
phakomatous, 257
Chromosomes, 283–284
abnormalities of, corneal diseases
with, 287*t*
karyotyping of, 286
Chrysiasis, 348*t*
CHSD. *See* Congenital hereditary
stromal dystrophy
Cicatricial pemphigoid, ocular, 204–207,
205*i*, 206*i*, 207*i*
drug-induced (pseudopemphigoid),
204, 213
human leukocyte antigen (HLA)
association and, 184*t*, 204
mucous membrane grafting for, 403
Cilia (eyelashes), 9
CIN. *See* Conjunctival intraepithelial
neoplasia

Ciprofloxacin, 43*t*, 44
  for bacterial keratitis, 174
  corneal deposits caused by, 347
Circumferential keratotomy, 440*t*
Citrobacter, ocular infection caused
  by, 122
Clear zone diameter, radial keratotomy
  outcome affected by, 458
Climatotherapy, for vernal
  keratoconjunctivitis, 196
Clostridium, ocular infection caused
  by, 125
Clotrimazole, 45
cM. *See* Centimorgans
CMV. *See* Cytomegalovirus
Coats white ring, 341
Coccidioides immitis, ocular infection
  caused by, 128
Codon, 284
Coefficient of variation, specular
  photomicroscopy in evaluation of, 34
Cogan microcystic dystrophy, 291. *See*
  also Epithelial basement membrane
  dystrophy
Cogan-Reese (iris nevus) variant,
  of iridocorneal endothelial
  syndrome, 280
Cogan syndrome, 211–212
Collagen shrinkage, corneal biomechanics
  affected by, 452, 453*i*
Collagenases, in ocular infections, 114
Collarettes, in staphylococcal
  blepharitis, 157*i*
Combined sutures, for penetrating
  keratoplasty, 418, 419*i*
Complement, in tear film, 184
Complex choristoma, 257
Compression sutures, for corneal
  astigmatism after penetrating
  keratoplasty, 425
Concretions, conjunctival, 341
Concussive trauma, 362–368
Confocal microscopy, in anterior segment
  evaluation, 36
Congenital anomalies. *See also*
  specific type
  basic concepts of, 261–265
  causes of, 263–265
  clinical aspects of, 266–280
  diagnostic approach to, 265

Congenital hereditary endothelial
  dystrophy, 277, 277*i*
  gene linkage of, 289*t*
Congenital hereditary stromal
  dystrophy, 276
Conidiophores, 128
Conjunctiva. *See also* Ocular surface
  aging of, 337
  amyloid deposits in, 324, 324*i*
  biopsy of, 392
  blood under, 362
  blood vessels of, 57–58
  bulbar, 10, 11
  concretions of, 341
  in defense mechanisms of outer
    eye, 111–112
  degenerations of, 339–341
  development of, 261–262, 262*t*, 263*i*
  disorders of. *See also specific type and*
    Conjunctivitis; Keratoconjunctivitis
    immune-mediated, 188, 193–208
    neoplastic, 234–257
      human papillomaviruses causing,
        119, 236–237, 237*i*, 239
  epithelial tumors of, 236–241, 236*t*
  epithelium of, 57
    cysts of, 234–235, 235*i*
    cytologic identification of, 62, 63*i*
    healing of, 353
  follicles of, 21*t*, 25–26, 26*i*, 27*i*
  foreign body of, 368–369, 369*i*
  glandular tumors of, 241–243
  granuloma of, 23*t*
  hypersensitivity reactions of, 185–188
  immunologic features of, 183–185
  inclusion cysts of, 234–235, 235*i*
  infection of, 134–180. *See also*
    Conjunctivitis; Keratoconjunctivitis
  inflammation of, 21*t*, 23–26, 23*t*.
    See also Conjunctivitis;
    Keratoconjunctivitis
  intraepithelial neoplasia of, 238–239,
    238*i*, 239*i*
  laceration of, 368
  lithiasis of, 341
  lymphatic and lymphocytic tumors
    of, 252–254
  mechanical functions of, 58
  membrane of, 21*t*, 23*t*
  metastatic tumors of, 254

Deletion mapping, 287
Dellen, 104
Demodex
    brevis, 131
    folliculorum, 131
    as normal ocular flora, 113*t*
    ocular infection caused by, 131, 160
Demulcents, for dry eye, 85
Dendritic epithelial keratitis
    herpes simplex virus causing,
        144–146, 144*i*
    in herpes zoster ophthalmicus, 153
Deoxyribonucleic acid. *See* DNA
Dermal ridges (dermal papillae), 227, 228*i*
Dermatan sulfate
    in cornea, 12
    in mucopolysaccharidoses, 312, 313*i*
Dermatan sulfate–proteoglycan, macular
        dystrophy and, 297–298
Dermatitis herpetiformis, conjunctiva
        affected in, 208
Dermatoblepharitis
    contact, 191–193, 192*i*
    varicella-zoster virus causing, 150–154
Dermatoses, ocular surface, 69–77. *See*
        also specific type
Dermis, eyelid, 227
Dermoid choristoma, 254–256, 255*i*, 256*i*
    epibulbar, 254–255
        chromosomal abnormalities in, 287*t*
Dermoid cyst, 254, 255*i*
Dermolipoma, 256
Descemetocele, management of, 405–407
Descemet's membrane, 13
    changes in during intraocular
        surgery, 383–384
    retained, penetrating keratoplasty
        complicated by, 419
Desquamating skin conditions, ocular
        surface involved in, 76–77
Dexamethasone, 41*t*, 42
    with antibiotics, 42*t*
    for corneal graft rejection, 427–428
Diabetes mellitus, corneal changes in, 314
    persistent epithelial defect, 101
Diaminodiphenylsulfone. *See* Dapsone
Diclofenac, 41*t*
Didanosine, 45

Diffuse illumination, for slit-lamp
        biomicroscopy, 15
Dimorphic fungi. *See also* Fungi
    ocular infection caused by, 128
Disciform edema, in herpes zoster
        ophthalmicus, 153
Disciform keratitis, herpes simplex virus
        causing, 146–147, 147*i*
Disodium ethylenediaminetetraacetic acid
        (EDTA), for calcific band keratopathy,
        345–346
Distichiasis, 102
Diurnal fluctuation in vision, 460
DNA, 283–284
DNA viruses. *See also specific virus*
    ocular infection caused by, 116–119
Dominant trait, 285
Donor cornea
    preparation of for penetrating
        keratoplasty, 415–416
    selection of, 412–413
Double continuous sutures, for penetrating
        keratoplasty, 417, 418*i*
Doxycycline, 44
    for chlamydial conjunctivitis, 168
    for meibomian gland dysfunction, 70
    for rosacea, 75
Drug-induced cicatricial pemphigoid
        (pseudopemphigoid), 204, 213
Drugs, ocular
    delivery of, 39
    deposition and pigmentations caused by,
        346–349, 347*t*
    periocular, 39
    systemic administration and, 39
    topical, 39
Dry eye (keratoconjunctivitis sicca),
        79–81, 80*t. See also* Aqueous
        tear deficiency
    medications causing, 83*t*, 86
    rose bengal in diagnosis of, 59, 80, 81*i*
    in Sjögren syndrome, 82–83
    systemic diseases associated with, 84*t*
    tests for, 59–61
    treatment of, 85*t*
        medical, 85–86
        surgical, 86–88, 87*i*
Duplication mapping, 287

Dyskeratosis
    benign hereditary intraepithelial, 237
    definition/implication of, 229*t*
Dysmorphic sialidosis, 318
Dysplasia, definition of, 228, 229*t*
Dystrophies. *See also* Corneal dystrophies
    definition of, 290
    degenerations differentiated from, 337*t*

EBMD. *See* Epithelial basement membrane
    dystrophy
EBV. *See* Epstein-Barr virus
Echography, anterior segment, 35–36
Econazole, 45
Ectatic disorders, 305–311. *See also*
    specific type
Ectoderm, surface, external eye developed
    from, 261
Ectodermal dysplasia, 77
    anhidrotic, 77
    gene linkage of, 289*t*
Ectopic lacrimal gland, 257, 257*i*
Ectrodactyly–ectodermal dysplasial–
    clefting syndrome (EEC
    syndrome), 77
Ectropion
    involutional, 94
    medial tarsorrhaphy and canthoplasty
        for, 393–394
Eczema, of eyelid, 21*t*
Edema
    corneal, 32, 33*t*
        after intraocular surgery, 384
        pathophysiology of, 354–355
    epithelial
        central (Sattler's veil), 104
        in ocular inflammation, 22*t*
    stromal, 32
EDS. *See* Ehlers-Danlos syndrome
EDTA. *See* Disodium
    ethylenediaminetetraacetic acid
EEC syndrome. *See* Ectrodactyly–
    ectodermal dysplasial–clefting
    syndrome
Efavirenz, 45
EGF. *See* Epidermal growth factor
Ehlers-Danlos syndrome, 326, 328*t*
    blue sclera in, 268–269, 326
Eikenella corrodens, ocular infection
    caused by, 123

EKC. *See* Epidemic keratoconjunctivitis
Elastin, scleral, 13
Elastofibroma oculi, 341
Elastoid (elastic) degeneration/elastosis, 339
Elevated intraocular pressure
    in hyphema, 366
    after penetrating keratoplasty, 420
Embryotoxon, posterior, 272, 273*i*
    in Axenfeld-Rieger syndrome, 272
Encephalitozoon
    cuniculi, 169
    hellem, 169
    keratoconjunctivitis caused by, 169
Endemic syphilis (bejel), 125
Endonucleases, restriction, 288
Endophthalmitis
    bleb-associated, *Haemophilus*
        causing, 123
    after penetrating keratoplasty, 420
Endothelial cell density, specular
    photomicroscopy in evaluation of, 34
Endothelial degenerations, 346
Endothelial dystrophies, 301–305. *See also*
    specific type
    congenital hereditary, 277, 277*i*
    gene linkage of, 289*t*
    Fuchs, 301–303, 302*i*, 303*i*
Endothelial failure, after penetrating
    keratoplasty
    late nonimmune, 423–424
    primary, 420, 421*i*
Endothelial graft rejection, 427, 428*i*
Endothelial pump, corneal edema caused
    by inadequacy of, 32
Endothelium, corneal, 13
    dysfunction of, 354–355
    intraocular surgery causing changes
        in, 384–385
    wound healing of, 354–355
Enterobacter, ocular infection caused
    by, 122
    keratitis, 171*t*
Enterobacteriaceae, ocular infection
    caused by, 122
    keratitis, 171*t*
Enterococcus, ocular infection caused
    by, 124
Enterocytozoon hellem, ocular infection
    caused by, 129

Enteroviruses, ocular infection caused by, 119, 140
Entropion, involutional, 94
Enucleation, for corneoscleral laceration, sympathetic ophthalmia and, 375–376
Eosinophil chemotactic factor, 187*t*
Eosinophils
  cytologic identification of, 62*t*, 64, 65*i*
    in immune-mediated keratoconjunctivitis, 190*t*
  in external eye, 183*t*
Ephelis (freckle), conjunctival, 244, 247*t*
Epibulbar choristoma, 254–257. *See also* Choristoma
Epibulbar dermoids, 254–255
  chromosomal aberrations in, 287*t*
Epidemic keratoconjunctivitis, 119, 136–140, 137*i*
Epidermal growth factor, for persistent corneal defects, 101
Epidermal necrolysis, toxic, 201–204, 202*t*
Epidermis, eyelid, 9, 227, 228, 228*i*
  cell turnover and, 228
Epidermoid cyst, 254
Epidermolysis bullosa, conjunctiva affected in, 208
Epikeratoplasty (epikeratophakia), 438*t*, 451, 451*i*, 452*i*, 464
Epinephrine, adrenochrome deposition caused by, 348, 348*t*, 349*i*
Episcleritis, 22*t*, 31, 217–218, 218*i*
  mumps virus causing, 119
Epithelial basement membrane dystrophy, 290–292, 291*i*
Epithelial cells. *See also* Epithelium
  keratinized, cytologic identification of, 62*t*, 64, 64*i*
  in immune-mediated keratoconjunctivitis, 190*t*
Epithelial debridement, for recurrent corneal erosions, 99
Epithelial defects
  nonhealing trophic, herpetic keratitis and, 149
  in ocular inflammation, 21*t*, 22*t*
  persistent, 100–101
    after penetrating keratoplasty, 420
Epithelial degenerations, 341–342

Epithelial dystrophies
  basement membrane, 290–292, 291*i*
  juvenile (Meesmann), 292, 292*i*
    gene linkage of, 289*t*
Epithelial edema
  central (Sattler's veil), 104
  in ocular inflammation, 22*t*
Epithelial erosions
  herpetic keratitis and, 149
  punctate
    of conjunctiva, 21*t*
    of cornea, 22*t*, 27, 28*i*, 29*t*
      in vernal conjunctivitis, 195
Epithelial graft rejection, 426, 426*i*
Epithelial inclusion cysts, 234–235, 235*i*
Epithelioid cells (Leber cells), 65
Epitheliopathy
  microcystic, 104
  punctate or vortex, herpetic keratitis and, 149
Epithelium. *See also under Epithelial*
  conjunctival, 57, 227
    cytologic identification of, 62, 63*i*
    healing of, 353
  in contact lens overwear syndromes, 104
  corneal, 11–12, 12*i*, 56, 227
    cytologic identification of, 62
    intraocular surgery causing changes in, 383
  cysts of, 234–235, 235*i*
  immunologic and inflammatory cells in, 183*t*
  tumors of, 236–241, 236*t*. *See also specific type*
    benign, 236–237, 236*t*
    malignant, 236*t*, 240–241
    preinvasive, 236*t*, 238–240
Epstein-Barr virus, ocular infection caused by, 118, 154
Erodible masks, for photoastigmatic refractive keratectomy, 476, 478*i*
Erosions
  conjunctival, punctate epithelial, 21*t*
  corneal
    punctate epithelial, 22*t*, 27, 28*i*, 29*t*
    recurrent, 97–100, 371
  of eyelid, 21*t*

H$_1$-receptor blockers, 40
Haemophilus
  aphrophilus, 123
  haemolyticus, 123
  influenzae, 123
    acute purulent conjunctivitis caused
      by, 162
    biotype III (*H aegyptius*), 123, 162
    as normal ocular flora, 113*t*
    ocular infection caused by, 123
Halberstaedter-Prowazek inclusion bodies,
  66–67, 67*i*
Hallerman-Streiff-François syndrome, 328*t*
Haloes, after photorefractive
  keratectomy, 473
Hamartoma, 254
Hand washing, in infection control, 50
Hassall-Henle bodies (peripheral corneal
  guttatae), 346
Hay fever conjunctivitis, 193–194
Haze formation
  after keratorefractive surgery, 453–454
  after photorefractive keratectomy, 473
Healing (wound), 353–355
  keratorefractive surgery and, 453–454
Heat, anterior segment injuries caused
  by, 356
Helminths, ocular infection caused by, 130
Helper T cells. *See also* CD4+ T
  lymphocytes
  in external eye, 183*t*, 184
Hemangioma, 249–250
Hemizygous alleles, 285
Hemochromatosis, 332
Hemorrhage, subconjunctival, 78–79
  causes of, 78, 78*t*
Hemorrhagic conjunctivitis, viruses
  causing, 119
Henderson-Patterson bodies, 119
Heparan sulfate, in
  mucopolysaccharidoses, 312, 313*i*
Heparin, 187
Hepatolenticular degeneration (Wilson
  disease), 330, 331*i*
Herbert's pits, 165, 167*i*
Hereditary hemorrhagic telangiectasia
  (Rendu-Osler-Weber disease), 78–79

Herpes simplex virus, ocular infection
  caused by, 116, 117*t*, 141–150
  Acanthamoeba keratitis differentiated
    from, 179
  agents for treatment of, 45, 142, 143*t*,
    146, 148–149
  blepharoconjunctivitis, 143
  clinical aspects of, 141–150
  complications of, 149–150
  dendritic and geographic epithelial
    keratitis, 144–146, 144*i*, 145*i*
  in newborn, 141
  after photorefractive keratectomy, 472
  primary, 141–142, 142*i*, 143*t*
  recurrent, 116, 118*i*, 142–149
  stromal keratitis and uveitis, 146–149
  varicella-zoster virus infection
    differentiated from, 151*t*
Herpes zoster, 117–118
  ophthalmic manifestations in, 118,
    151–154, 152*i*
Herpes zoster ophthalmicus, 118,
  151–154, 152*i*
Heterozygous alleles, 285
Hexagonal cells, specular
  photomicroscopy in evaluation of
  percentage of, 34
Hexagonal keratotomy, 466
Hexamidine, 45
HHV8. *See* Human herpes virus 8
Hidden eye. *See* Cryptophthalmos
Histamine, 187
Histiocytes, cytologic identification of, 65
Histiocytoma, fibrous, 250
Histocompatibility antigens. *See* Human
  leukocyte antigens (HLA antigens)
Histoplasma capsulatum, ocular infection
  caused by, 128
HIV infection/AIDS, 119–120
  cytomegalovirus retinitis in, 118
  Kaposi sarcoma in, 250
  ocular infection caused by, 119–120
  varicella-zoster virus keratitis in, 153
HIV vaccine, 45
HLA antigens. *See* Human leukocyte
  antigens
Holmium:YAG laser, for
  thermokeratoplasty, 454, 479
Homozygous alleles, 285

Hordeolum, 73
  external (stye), 73, 160
  internal, 73, 160
  in staphylococcal
      blepharoconjunctivitis, 160
Horizontal shortening/tightening of eyelid
  for exposure keratopathy, 94
  for involutional ectropion, 94
  for involutional entropion, 94
  for involutional lower eyelid
      changes, 94
Horner-Trantas dots, 194–195
Host risk factors, in ocular infection,
    115–116
HPV. *See* Human papillomaviruses
HSV. *See* Herpes simplex virus
Hudson-Stähli line, 348*t*, 349
Human herpes virus 8, Kaposi sarcoma
    caused by, 118, 250
Human immunodeficiency virus infection.
    See HIV infection/AIDS
Human leukocyte antigens (HLA antigens),
    184, 411
  ocular disease associations and, 184*t*.
      See also specific disease
Human papillomaviruses, ocular infection
    caused by, 119, 236–237, 237*i*, 239
Human transforming growth factor–
    β–induced gene mutation
  in granular dystrophy, 294
  in Reis-Bücklers dystrophy, 293
Hunter syndrome, 313*t*
Hurler syndrome, 313*t*
  congenital corneal opacities in, 278
Hutchinson's sign, 92
Hydrocortisone, with antibiotics, 42*t*
Hydrops, in keratoconus, 306
  management of, 308
Hydroxyapatite deposition (calcific band
    keratopathy), 345–346
Hymenoptera (wasp) sting, ocular infection
    caused by, 131
Hypercalcemia, 330–332, 332*i*
Hyperemia, conjunctival, 21*t*
  causes of, 78
Hyperkeratosis, definition/implication
    of, 229*t*
Hyperlipoproteinemias, 314–315, 315*t*

Hyperopia, surgical correction
    of, 466–467
  laser procedures for, 479
Hyperopic automated lamellar
    keratoplasty, 451, 451*i*, 466–467
Hyperopic keratomileusis, 452, 466
Hyperopic photorefractive keratectomy,
    452, 452*i*
Hyperplasia, definition of, 229*t*
Hypersensitivity reactions, 185–188, 186*i*,
    186*t*. *See also specific type*
  anaphylactic or atopic (type I), 186–187,
      186*i*, 187*t*
  cytotoxic (type II), 186*i*, 187*t*, 188
  delayed (type IV), 186*i*, 187*t*, 188
  immune-complex (type III), 186*i*,
      187*t*, 188
Hypertrophy, definition of, 229*t*
Hyperuricemia, 327
Hyphae, 127
Hyphema
  spontaneous, 364
  traumatic, 364–368, 364*i*, 365*i*
    medical management of, 366–367
    rebleeding after, 364–366, 365*i*, 366*i*
    sickle cell complications of, 367–368
    surgery for, 367
Hypolipoproteinemias, 315–316
Hypovitaminosis A, 89–91, 90*i*

I-cell disease, 318
ICE. *See* Iridocorneal endothelial syndrome
Ichthyosis, 76
  gene linkage of, 289*t*
ICL/ICR. *See* Intracorneal lens/ring
Idoxuridine, contraindications to in
    Thygeson superficial punctate
    keratitis, 209
IgA, in tear film, 184
IgA bullous dermatosis, linear, conjunctiva
    affected in, 208
IK. *See* Interstitial keratitis
Illumination, for slit-lamp biomicroscopy
  direct, 15–17
  indirect, 17–18
Immediate hypersensitivity (type I)
    reaction, 186–187, 186*i*, 187*t*
Immune-complex hypersensitivity (type III)
    reaction, 188

Immune privilege, 411–412
Immunocompromised host, ocular
    infection and, 115–116
Immunoglobulins
    in conjunctiva, 183
    disorders of synthesis of, 325–326
    in tear film, 184
Immunology/immune response
    (ocular), 183–190
    disorders of. *See also specific type*
        clinical approach to, 191–224
        diagnostic approach to, 189–190
        patterns of, 188–189
    hypersensitivity reactions and, 185–188
    immunologic features of outer eye
        and, 183–185
Immunosuppressives, 42–43
    for scleritis, 224
Impression cytology, 61
    in limbal stem-cell dysfunction, 106–107
    in Sjögren syndrome diagnosis, 83
In situ hybridization, 287
Incisional biopsy, for neoplastic disorders
    of eyelid and ocular surface, 232
Inclusion cysts, epithelial, 234–235, 235*i*
Inclusions, cytoplasmic, cytologic
    identification of, 62*t*, 66–67, 67*i*
Index of refraction, 11
Indinavir, 45
Infants, corneal transplantation in, 429
Infection (ocular). *See also specific type*
    basic concepts of, 111–133
    clinical aspects of, 134–180
    defense mechanisms and, 111–112
    diagnostic laboratory techniques
        in, 131–133
    host risk factors and, 115–116
    inoculum size and, 114
    microbiology of, 116–131
    normal flora and, 112, 113*t*
    pathogenesis of, 113–116
    route of, 114–115
    virulence factors in, 113–114
Infection control, 49–50
Infectious crystalline keratopathy, after
    penetrating keratoplasty,
    422–423, 424*i*
Infectious mononucleosis, ocular
    involvement in, 154, 155*i*

Inferior tarsal muscle, involutional eyelid
    changes and, 94
Inflammation (ocular). *See also specific
    disorder causing*
    clinical evaluation of, 19–31
    of eyelid, 21*t*, 22
    signs of, 21–22*t*
    soluble mediators of, 185*t*
Inflammatory pseudoguttatae, 30
Influenza virus, ocular infection caused
    by, 119
Inoculum size, microorganism infective
    ability and, 114
Insect hairs, ocular injury/infection caused
    by, 131, 361
Insect stings, ocular injury/infection
    caused by, 131, 361
Instantaneous radius of curvature
    (tangential/instantaneous power; local
    curvature), 37, 444, 444*i*
Interferons, for viral infection, 45
Interleukins, T cells producing, 184
Internal hordeolum, 73, 160
    in staphylococcal
        blepharoconjunctivitis, 160
Interrupted sutures, for penetrating
    keratoplasty, 417, 417*i*
Interstitial keratitis
    syphilitic, 209–210, 211*i*
        intrauterine, corneal anomalies
            and, 278
    in systemic disease, 209–211
Interstitial keratopathy, neovascularization
    associated with contact lenses
    and, 105
Intracorneal implants, alloplastic, 451,
    452*i*, 464–466
Intracorneal lens/ring, 439*t*, 465–466, 465*i*
Intraepithelial dyskeratosis, benign
    hereditary, 237
Intraepithelial neoplasia
    conjunctival, 238–239, 238*i*, 239*i*
    corneal, 239–240, 240*i*
Intraocular pressure, elevated
    in hyphema, 366
    after penetrating keratoplasty, 420
Intraocular surgery. *See also* Surgery
    anterior segment trauma caused
        by, 383–385
Intrastromal ablation, laser, 454, 454*i*

Intrastromal corneal ring, 451, 465*i*
Intrastromal lens, for presbyopia
    correction, 467
Intrauterine keratitis, corneal anomalies
    and, 278
Invasion, as virulence factor, 114
Involutional ectropion, 94
Involutional entropion, 94
Ionizing radiation, anterior segment injury
    caused by exposure to, 357
Iridocorneal endothelial syndrome,
    279–280, 280*i*
Iridodialysis, 363
    McCannel technique for repair of,
        381, 382*i*
Iris, laceration of, repair of, 380–381, 382*i*
Iris atrophy variant, of iridocorneal
    endothelial syndrome, 280
Iris incarceration, after penetrating
    keratoplasty, 420
Iris nevus (Cogan-Reese) variant, of
    iridocorneal endothelial
    syndrome, 280
Iritis
    in Reiter syndrome, 211
    traumatic, 363
Iron foreign body, in cornea, 370, 370*i*
Iron lines, 348*t*, 349
    in pterygium, 340, 340*i*
Irregular astigmatism, herpetic keratitis
    and, 149
Irrigation, for chemical injuries, 360
Isolated stromal rejection, 427
Isolation techniques, in ocular
    microbiology, 133
Itraconazole, 45
Ivermectin, 45

Juvenile epithelial dystrophy (Meesmann
    dystrophy), 292, 292*i*
    gene linkage of, 289*t*
Juvenile xanthogranuloma, 250

Kaposi sarcoma, 250–251, 251*i*
    human herpes virus 8 causing, 118, 250
Karyotype/karyotyping, 286
Kayser-Fleischer ring, 330, 331*i*, 348*t*
KCS. *See* Keratoconjunctivitis, sicca
    (dry eye)

Keloids, corneal, 344–345
    congenital, 278
Keratan sulfate
    in cornea, 12
        macular dystrophy and, 297–298
    in mucopolysaccharidoses, 312, 313*i*
Keratectasia, 272
Keratectomy
    lamellar, 405
    mechanical, 405
    multizone, 452
    photorefractive, 440*t*, 451–452, 452*i*
        for astigmatism, 476–479, 477*i*, 478*i*
        excimer laser for, 470–474
        for hyperopia, 452, 452*i*
        for myopia, 470–474
    phototherapeutic, excimer laser, 405
        for recurrent corneal erosions, 100
    superficial, 404–405
Keratic precipitates, 30
Keratinized epithelial cells, cytologic
    identification of, 62*t*, 64, 64*i*
    in immune-mediated
        keratoconjunctivitis, 190*t*
Keratinocytes, in eyelid epidermis, 227
Keratitis, 27–31. *See also specific type*
    Acanthamoeba, 177–179, 178*i*
        agents for treatment of, 45, 179
        clinical aspects of, 177–179, 178*i*
        herpes simplex keratitis differentiated
            from, 179
        stains and culture media for
            identification of, 172*t*
    Acinetobacter causing, 122
    adenovirus, 136–140
        stages of, 138*i*, 138*t*, 139*i*
    bacterial, 169–176
        agents for treatment of, 173–175, 174*t*
        causes of, 171–173, 171*t*
        clinical presentation of, 170–171,
            170*i*, 171*i*
        contact lens wear and, 169
        intrauterine, corneal anomalies
            and, 278
        pathogenesis of, 170
        after penetrating keratoplasty,
            422–423, 424*i*
        after radial keratotomy, 461
        surgery for, 175

Candida, 126
in Cogan syndrome, 211–212
disciform, herpes simplex causing, 146–147, 147*i*
epithelial
  dendritic
    herpes simplex virus causing, 144–146, 144*i*
    in herpes zoster ophthalmicus, 153
  geographic, herpes simplex virus causing, 144–146, 145*i*
  punctate, 22*t*, 27, 28–29*i*, 29*t*
    measles virus causing, 119, 155
  varicella-zoster virus causing, 150–154
Epstein-Barr virus causing, 154, 155*i*
fungal, 176–177
Haemophilus causing, 123
herpes simplex virus, 116, 118*i*, 144–146
  Acanthamoeba keratitis differentiated from, 179
  complications of, 149–150
  after photorefractive keratectomy, 472
interstitial
  syphilitic, 209–210, 211*i*
  in systemic disease, 209–211
intrauterine, corneal anomalies and, 278
measles virus causing, 119, 155
peripheral, 29*t*
  Mooren ulcer and, 215–217, 216*i*, 217*i*
  in systemic immune-mediated diseases, 214–215, 215*i*
in Reiter syndrome, 211
in rosacea, 73, 74*i*
staphylococcal blepharoconjunctivitis and, 157–159
stromal
  acute, scleritis and, 222
  Epstein-Barr virus causing, 154, 155*i*
  herpes simplex virus causing, 146–149
  in herpes zoster ophthalmicus, 153
  measles virus causing, 119, 155
  microsporidial, 179
  mumps virus causing, 119
  necrotizing, herpes simplex causing, 147, 148*i*
  nonnecrotizing, herpes simplex virus causing, 146–147, 147*i*

nonsuppurative, 22*t*, 29, 29*t*, 30*i*
suppurative, 22*t*, 29, 29*t*, 30*i*
varicella-zoster virus causing, 150–154
syphilitic, 209–210, 211*i*
  intrauterine, corneal anomalies and, 278
Thygeson superficial punctate, 208–209, 208*i*
toxic, medications causing, 212–213
ulcerative
  Mooren ulcer and, 215–217, 216*i*, 217*i*
  in rosacea, 75
  in systemic immune-mediated diseases, 214–215, 215*i*
vaccinia, 119, 155
yeast, 176, 177
Keratoconjunctivitis
atopic, 197, 198*i*
epidemic (adenovirus), 119, 136–140, 137*i*
human leukocyte antigen (HLA) association and, 184*t*
immune-mediated, ocular surface cytology in, 190*t*
microsporidial, 169
sicca (dry eye), 79–81, 80*t*. *See also* Aqueous tear deficiency
  medications causing, 83*t*, 86
  rose bengal in diagnosis of, 59, 80, 81*i*
  in Sjögren syndrome, 82–83
  systemic diseases associated with, 84*t*
  tests for, 59–61
  treatment of, 85*t*
    medical, 85–86
    surgical, 86–88, 87*i*
superior limbic, 95–97, 96*i*
toxic, medications causing, 212–213, 362
vernal, 194–197, 195*i*, 196*i*
Keratoconus, 305–308, 306*i*, 307*i*, 308*i*, 309*t*, 310*i*
chromosomal aberrations in, 287*t*
in floppy eyelid syndrome, 94
posterior
  chromosomal abnormalities in, 287*t*
  circumscribed posterior, 274, 275*i*
  generalized, 271
in vernal conjunctivitis, 196

Leber cells (epithelioid cells), 65
Lecithin–cholesterol acyltransferase
  deficiency, 315–316
Lectin staining, in microbial keratitis, 172*t*
Leiomyosarcoma, 249
Leishmania, ocular infection caused
  by, 129–130
Lentigo, 244
Leukoma, in Peters anomaly, 274, 274*i*
Leukotrienes, 187*t*
Levocabastine, 40, 41*t*
Lice, ocular infection caused by, 130,
  130*i*, 160
Lichen planus, conjunctiva affected
  in, 208
Ligneous conjunctivitis, 199
Limbal autograft/allograft (limbal
  transplantation), 397–400, 398–399*i*
  indications for, 389*t*
Limbal stem-cell allograft, 400
Limbal stem-cell dysfunction,
  106–107, 106*t*
  limbal transplantation for, 397–400
Limbal vernal conjunctivitis,
  194–195, 195*i*
Limbal zone, 437, 442*i*
Limbus, 56, 437, 442*i*
  marginal corneal infiltrates in
    blepharoconjunctivitis and, 213
Linear IgA bullous dermatosis, conjunctiva
  affected in, 208
Linkage (gene), 283
  corneal conditions and, 289*t*
Linkage analysis, 288
Linkage disequilibrium, 287
Lipemia retinalis, 315*t*
Lipid keratopathy, 345
  in herpes zoster ophthalmicus, 153
  herpetic keratitis and, 150
Lipid layer of tear film, 54
  deficiency of, 88
    meibomian gland dysfunction and,
      54, 69
  secretion of, 55
Lipid metabolism and storage, disorders
  of, 314–319
Lipschütz bodies, 67
Lithiasis, conjunctival, 341
Loa loa (loiasis), ocular infection caused
  by, 130, 169

Local curvature (instantaneous radius of
  curvature; tangential/instantaneous
  power), 37, 444, 444*i*
Locus (gene), 284
LOD score, 288
Lodoxamide, 41*t*
  for hay fever and perennial allergic
    conjunctivitis, 194
  for vernal keratoconjunctivitis, 196
Loteprednol, 41*t*
Louis-Bar syndrome (ataxia-telangiectasia),
  79, 250
Lower eyelid, Involutional malposition
  of, 94
Lubricants, 40
Lumican, 12
Lyme disease, 126
Lymphangiectasia, 79, 252
Lymphangioma, 252
Lymphatic/lymphocytic tumors, 252–254.
  See also specific type
Lymphocytes
  cytologic identification of, 62*t*, 65, 66*i*
  in immune-mediated
    keratoconjunctivitis, 190*t*
  in external eye, 183*t*, 184
Lymphoid hyperplasia (reactive
  hyperplasia), 252, 253*i*
Lymphoid tissue, conjunctiva-
  associated, 57
Lymphoma, 252–254, 253*i*
Lysosomal metabolism disorders, 312–314.
  See also Mucopolysaccharidoses
Lysozyme, tear, 61

M cells, in conjunctiva-associated
  lymphoid tissue, 57
McCannel technique, for iris repair,
  380–381, 381*i*, 382*i*
McCarey-Kaufman tissue transport
  medium, 412
McNeill-Goldmann blepharostat, for
  penetrating keratoplasty, 416
Macroglobulinemia, Waldenström, corneal
  deposits in, 325–326
Macrophages, cytologic identification of,
  62*t*, 65
Macular dystrophy, 294*t*, 297–298, 298*i*
  gene linkage of, 289*t*
Macule, of eyelid, 21*t*

Major histocompatibility complex,
184, 411
Malassezia furfur, ocular infection caused
by, 126, 160
Mandibulofacial dysostosis, 329*t*
Mannosidosis, 318
Map-dot-fingerprint dystrophy (epithelial
basement membrane dystrophy),
290–292, 291*i*
Marfan syndrome, 326–327, 328*t*
Marginal corneal infiltrates,
blepharoconjunctivitis and, 213–214
Marginal degeneration, pellucid, 309*t*,
310–311, 310*i*, 311*i*
Marginal keratolysis ("melting")
scleritis and, 223
systemic immune-mediated diseases
and, 214, 223
Maroteau-Lamy syndrome, 313*t*
Masks, erodible, for photoastigmatic
refractive keratectomy, 476, 478*i*
Mast-cell inhibitors, for giant papillary
conjunctivitis, 201
Mast-cell stabilizers, 40, 41*t*
for hay fever and perennial allergic
conjunctivitis, 194
for vernal keratoconjunctivitis, 196
Mast cells
cytologic identification of, 62*t*, 65
in immune-mediated
keratoconjunctivitis, 190*t*
in external eye, 183*t*
Mean curvature map, 445, 445*i*
Measles virus (rubeola virus), ocular
infection caused by, 119, 155
Mechanical blepharoptosis, 22
Medications. *See* Drugs, ocular
Medrysone, 41*t*
for Thygeson superficial punctate
keratitis, 209
Meesmann dystrophy (juvenile epithelial
dystrophy), 292, 292*i*
gene linkage of, 289*t*
Megalocornea, 269–271, 270*i*
chromosomal aberrations in, 287*t*
gene linkage of, 289*t*
Meibomian glands, 9, 10*i*
dysfunction of, 54, 69–71, 70*i*,
155, 156*t*
lipid tears secreted by, 54, 55
obstruction of, chalazion caused by, 71

Melanin, corneal pigmentation caused by,
346, 348*t*
Melanin pigment granules, cytologic
identification of, 67, 67*i*
Melanocytes
in external eye, 227
tumors arising from, 243–249,
243*t*, 247*t*
Melanocytosis
ocular, 244, 245*i*, 247*t*
oculodermal, 244, 247*t*
Melanokeratosis, striate, 244
Melanoma, conjunctival, 247–248, 248*i*
Melanosis, 243
benign acquired, 244, 247*t*
congenital, 244, 245*i*, 247*t*
primary acquired, 246–247, 246*i*, 247*t*
MEN. *See* Multiple endocrine neoplasia
Meretoja syndrome, 297
Mesectoderm (neural crest), ocular
structures derived from, 7, 8*i*,
261, 263*i*
Mesenchymal tumors, 249–251
Messenger RNA (mRNA), 284
Metabolic disorders, 312–333. *See also*
specific type
clinical approach to, 312–333
corneal changes and, 312–333
diagnostic approach to, 285–288, 289*t*
molecular genetics of, 286–288, 289*t*
Metaplasia, definition of, 229*t*
Metastatic disease, conjunctival, 254
Methicillin, 44
Methotrexate, 42
for scleritis, 224
Methylprednisolone, for corneal graft
rejection, 428
Metrogel. *See* Metronidazole
Metronidazole, for rosacea, 75
MGD. *See* Meibomian glands,
dysfunction of
MHA-TP (microhemagglutination assay–
T pallidum) test, 126
Miconazole, for fungal keratitis, 176
Microbial transmission, host risk factors
and, 115
Microbiology (ocular), 116–131, 117*t. See
also specific organism*
bacteriology, 117*t*, 120–126

mycology, 117*t*, 126–128
parasitology, 117*t*, 128–131
virology, 116–120, 117*t*
Micrococcus
as normal ocular flora, 113*t*
ocular infection caused by, 124
Microcornea, 269
chromosomal aberrations in, 287*t*
cornea plana and, 271
Microcystic epitheliopathy, 104
Microhemagglutination assay–*T pallidum*
(MHA-TP) test, 126
Microorganisms, cytologic identification
of, 62, 68, 68*i*
Microphthalmos, 267–268, 267*i*
anterior, 269
Microscope
confocal, in anterior segment
evaluation, 36
for keratorefractive surgery, 456
operating, 48
slit-lamp. *See* Biomicroscopy, slit-lamp
specular, 34–35, 35*i*
Microsporida, ocular infection caused by,
129, 169, 179
stromal keratitis, 179
Microsurgery, anterior segment
instruments for, 48, 48*t*
techniques of, 46–50
Microsurgical needles, for corneal and
anterior segment surgery, 46–47,
47*i*, 47*t*
Microvilli, of corneal epithelium, 12
Mineral metabolism, disorders of, 330–332
Minocycline, 44
for meibomian gland dysfunction, 70
for rosacea, 75
Miosis, traumatic, 363
Mitomycin-C, 43
toxic medication reaction caused
by, 212
Mohs' surgery, for neoplastic disorders of
eyelid, 232
Molecular biologic techniques, 286–288
Moll, glands of, 9, 10*i*
Molluscum contagiosum, ocular infection
caused by, 119, 134–136, 135*i*
Monoclonal gammopathy, benign, corneal
deposits in, 325–326

Monocytes, cytologic identification of, 62*t*,
65, 66*i*
in immune-mediated
keratoconjunctivitis, 190*t*
Mononucleosis, infectious, ocular
involvement in, 154, 155*i*
Mooren ulcer, 215–217, 216*i*, 217*i*
Moraxella
blepharoconjunctivitis caused by, 157
catarrhalis, 122
lacunata (liquefaciens), 122, 157
nonliquefaciens, 122
as normal ocular flora, 113*t*
ocular infection caused by, 122
Morganella, ocular infection caused
by, 122
Morquio syndrome, 313*t*
Mosaic degeneration (anterior crocodile
shagreen), 343
MPS. *See* Mucopolysaccharidoses
mRNA. *See* Messenger RNA
Mucin layer of tear film, 54, 54*i*
deficiency of, 88
secretion of, 55
Mucoepidermoid carcinoma, 241
Mucolipidoses, 317–318
congenital opacities in, 278
Mucopolysaccharidoses, 312–314. *See*
also specific type
congenital opacities in, 278
differential features of, 313*t*
Mucor, ocular infection caused by, 128
Mucosal membrane grafting. *See* Mucous
membrane grafting (transplantation)
Mucous excess, in ocular inflammation, 21*t*
Mucous membrane grafting
(transplantation), 390–391, 403–404
indications for, 389*t*, 403–404
Mucus fishing syndrome, 102
Multinucleated cells, cytologic
identification of, 62*t*, 66, 67*i*
Multiple endocrine neoplasia
enlarged corneal nerves in, 332–333
limbal stem-cell dysfunction and,
106–107, 106*t*
Multiple sulfatase deficiency, 316–317
Multizone keratectomies, 452
Mumps virus, ocular infection caused by,
119, 155
Munnerlyn's formula, 451

Muscle spasm medications, tear
production affected by, 83*t*
Mutagens, congenital corneal anomalies
and, 265
Mycelium, 127
Mycobacterium
chelonei, 125
fortuitum, 125
leprae, 125
ocular infection caused by, 125
keratitis
agents for treatment of, 174*t*
stains and culture media for
identification of, 172*t*
tuberculosis, 125
Mycosis fungoides, herpetic keratitis
and, 149
Mydriasis, traumatic, 363
Myiasis, ocular, 131
Myopia
residual, after radial keratotomy, 459
surgical correction of, 457–466
alloplastic intracorneal implants
for, 464–466
automated lamellar keratoplasty for,
450, 450*i*, 463–464
epikeratoplasty (epikeratophakia)
for, 464
keratomileusis for, 462
lamellar procedures for, 462–464
laser procedures for, 470–475
radial keratotomy for, 457–462, 457*i*

Nail-patella syndrome
(onychoosteodysplasia), 329*t*
Nanophthalmos, 268
Naphazoline, 41*t*
Natamycin, 43*t*, 45
for fungal keratitis, 176
Natural killer cells, in external eye, 184
Nd:YAG laser, for intrastromal ablation,
454, 454*i*
ND:YSGG laser, for intrastromal ablation,
454, 454*i*
Necrosis, definition of, 229*t*
Needles (surgical), for corneal and anterior
segment surgery, 46–47, 47*i*, 47*t*
Negative staining (fluorescein), 19

Neisseria
gonorrhoeae, 121, 121*i*
conjunctivitis caused by, 121, 121*i*,
162–164, 163*i*
in neonates, 164
meningitidis, 121
ocular infection caused by, 121–122,
162–164
Nelfinavir, 45
Nematode infection, agents for treatment
of, 45
Neomycin, 43*t*, 45
with corticosteroids, 42*t*
Neonates
bacterial conjunctivitis in, 164–165
chlamydial, 164–165
gonococcal, 164
ocular herpes simplex virus in, 141
Neoplasia. *See also* Cancer;
Neoplastic disorders
definition of, 228, 229*t*
histopathologic features of, 229*t*
Neoplastic disorders. *See also specific type
and* Cancer
clinical approach to, 234–257
diagnostic approaches to,
231–233, 233*i*
epibulbar choristomas, 254–257
epithelial cysts, 234–235, 235*i*
epithelial tumors, 236–241
glandular conjunctival tumors, 241–243
histopathologic processes and
conditions and, 228–230, 229*t*
lymphatic and lymphocytic tumors,
252–254
management of, 233
neuroectodermal tumors, 243–249, 243*t*
tumor cell biology and, 227–231
vascular and mesenchymal tumors,
249–251, 250*t*
Neovascularization
corneal
contact lenses causing, 105
inflammation and, 31
stromal, contact lenses causing, 105
Neural crest (mesectoderm), ocular
structures derived from, 7, 8*i*, 261,
263*i*

Neuralgia, postherpetic, 154
Neurilemoma, 249, 249*i*
Neuroectoderm
    external eye derived from, 7, 8*i*, 261
    tumors arising in, 243–249, 243*t*
Neurofibroma, 249
Neurogenic tumors, 249
Neuroglial choristoma, 257
Neuroma, 249
Neurotrophic keratopathy, 91–93, 92*i*
Neurotrophic ulcers, 92, 92*i*
    herpetic keratitis and, 149
Neutrophil chemotactic factor, 187*t*
Neutrophils
    cytologic identification of, 62*t*, 64, 64*i*
        in immune-mediated
            keratoconjunctivitis, 190*t*
    in external eye, 183*t*
Nevirapine, 45
Nevus
    conjunctival, 244–246, 245*i*, 247*t*
    flammeus (port wine stain), 249–250
    of Ota, 244
Nevus cells
    in external eye, 227
    tumors arising from, 243–249,
        243*t*, 247*t*
Newborns. *See* Neonates
Newcastle disease virus, ocular infection
    caused by, 119
NK cells. *See* Natural killer cells
Nocardia, ocular infection caused by, 125
    asteroides, 125
Nodular fasciitis, 250
Nonhealing trophic epithelial defects,
    herpetic keratitis and, 149
Non-Hodgkin lymphoma, conjunctival,
    252–254, 253*i*
Nonpenetrant gene, 285
Nonseptate filamentous fungi. *See
    also* Fungi
    ocular infection caused by, 128
Nonsteroidal anti-inflammatory drugs
    (NSAIDs), 40, 41*t*
    for scleritis, 224
    for vernal keratoconjunctivitis, 196
Norfloxacin, 43*t*, 44
Normal ocular flora, 112, 113*t*
Nosema corneum, ocular infection
    caused by, 129
    stromal keratitis, 179

Nuclear inclusions, cytologic identification
    of, 67
Nucleotide metabolism, disorders
    of, 327–330
Nyctalopia, in hypovitaminosis A, 89

Ochronosis, 322
    corneal pigmentation in, 348*t*
Ocular bioavailability, 39–40
Ocular cytology, 61–68
    in immune-mediated
        keratoconjunctivitis, 190*t*
    interpretation of, 62–68, 62*t*
    specimen collection for, 61
    staining procedures in, 63*t*
Ocular immunology. *See*
    Immunology/immune response
Ocular infection. *See* Infection
Ocular inflammation. *See* Inflammation
Ocular melanocytosis, 244, 245*i*, 247*t*
Ocular pharmacology, 39–46. *See also
    specific agent and* Drugs, ocular
Ocular surface, 56–58. *See also*
    Conjunctiva; Cornea; Eyelids
    blood supply of, 57–58
    definition of, 389
    disorders of. *See also specific type*
        dermatoses, 69–77
        diagnostic approach to, 59–68
        limbal stem-cell dysfunction,
            106–107, 107*t*
        neoplastic
            diagnostic approaches to, 231–233
            histopathologic processes and
                conditions and, 228–230, 229*t*
            management of, 233
            neuroectodermal, 243–249, 243*t*
            oncogenesis and, 230–231, 230*t*
        noninflammatory vascular anomalies
            of conjunctiva, 78–79
        nutritional and physiologic, 89–93
        structural and exogenous, 93–105
        tear deficiency states, 79–88
    immunologic features of, 183–185
    maintenance of, 390–391
    mechanical functions of, 58
    microanatomy of, 227
    normal physiology of, 53–58
    response of to wound healing, 390–391

Pasteurella multocida, ocular infection
     caused by, 123
Patch grafts, 407
Patient selection, for keratorefractive
     surgery, 455–456. *See also specific
     procedure*
PAX6 gene, in Peters anomaly, 274
PCF. *See* Pharyngoconjunctival fever
PCR. *See* Polymerase chain reaction
Pediculosis (lice), ocular infection caused
     by, 130, 130*i*, 160
Pedigree analysis, 285–286, 286*i*
Pediococcus, ocular infection caused
     by, 124
Pellucid marginal degeneration, 309*t*,
     310–311, 310*i*, 311*i*
Pemphigoid
     immunosuppressive treatment for, 43
     ocular cicatricial, 204–207, 205*i*,
          206*i*, 207*i*
          drug-induced (pseudopemphigoid),
               204, 213
          human leukocyte antigen (HLA)
               association and, 184*t*, 204
          mucous membrane grafting for, 403
Pemphigus, conjunctiva affected in, 208
Penetrant gene, 285
Penetrating keratoplasty. *See* Keratoplasty,
     penetrating
Penetrating trauma. *See also* Perforating
     trauma
     definition of, 371
Penetration, as virulence factor, 114
Penicillin G, 44
Penicillinase, staphylococcal production
     of, 123–124
Penicillins, 44
Peptococcus, ocular infection caused
     by, 124
Peptostreptococcus, ocular infection
     caused by, 124
Perforating trauma, anterior segment,
     371–383
     ancillary tests in, 373*t*
     examination in, 372–373, 373*t*
     history in, 372, 372*t*
     management of, 374–383, 374*t*
          nonsurgical, 374–375, 375*i*
          preoperative, 374
          surgical, 375–383
     ocular signs of, 373*t*

Periocular drug administration, 39
Periodic acid–Schiff staining, 64
Peripheral corneal melt
     scleritis and, 223
     systemic immune-mediated diseases
          and, 214, 223
Peripheral keratitis, 29*t*
     ulcerative
          Mooren ulcer and, 215–217, 216*i*, 217*i*
          in systemic immune-mediated
               diseases, 214–215, 215*i*
Peripheral zone, 437, 442*i*
Persistence, as virulence factor, 114
Persistent epithelial defect, 100–101
     after penetrating keratoplasty, 420
Peters anomaly, 274, 274*i*
     chromosomal abnormalities in, 287*t*
     gene linkage of, 289*t*
Peters-plus syndrome, 274
Phakomatous choristoma, 257
Pharmacokinetics, of ocular drugs, 39
Pharmacology, ocular, 39–46. *See also
     specific agent and* Drugs, ocular
Pharyngoconjunctival fever, 136–140
Pheniramine, 40, 41*t*
Phenocopy, 285
Phenotype, 285
Phenylephrine, 41*t*
Phlyctenules, 21*t*
     in staphylococcal blepharoconjunctivitis,
          157–159, 158*i*
Photoablation, 454. *See also specific
     procedure*
     types of lasers for, 455
Photoastigmatic refractive keratectomy,
     476–479, 477*i*, 478*i*
Photodisruption, in laser therapy, 454, 454*i*
Photomicroscopy, specular, 34–35, 35*i*
Photorefractive keratectomy, 440*t*,
     451–452, 452*i*
     for astigmatism, 476–479, 477*i*, 478*i*
     excimer laser for, 470–474
     for hyperopia, 452, 452*i*
     for myopia, 470–474
Phototherapeutic keratectomy, excimer
     laser, 405
     for recurrent corneal erosions, 100
Photothermal laser–tissue interaction, 454
Phthirus pubis (crab louse), ocular
     infection caused by, 130, 130*i*, 160

Propionibacterium
  acnes
    as normal ocular flora, 112, 113*t*
    ocular infection caused by,
      124–125, 125*i*
  propionicus, ocular infection caused
    by, 125
Prostaglandins, 187*t*
Protease inhibitors, 45
Proteases, microbial, in ocular
  infections, 114
Protein AP, 322
Protein metabolism, disorders of, 322–325
Proteoglycans, scleral, 13
Proteus, ocular infection caused by, 122
  keratitis, 171*t*
Protozoa, ocular infection caused
  by, 128–130
  agents for treatment of, 45
Proximal illumination, for slit-lamp
  biomicroscopy, 17
Pseudocryptophthalmos, 266
Pseudoepitheliomatous hyperplasia, 237
Pseudoguttatae, inflammatory, 30
Pseudo–Hurler polydystrophy, 318
Pseudohyphae, 126
Pseudomembrane, conjunctival, 21*t*, 23*t*
Pseudomonas
  aeruginosa, 122, 122*i*
    keratitis caused by, 170, 170*i*, 171*t*
  cepacia, 122
  fluorescens, 122
  ocular infection caused by, 122, 122*i*
    clinical presentation of, 170, 170*i*
    pathogenesis of, 170
Pseudopemphigoid, 204, 213
Psychotropic agents, tear production
  affected by, 83*t*
Pterygium, 339–341, 340*i*
  excision of, 394–396, 395*i*
Ptosis, steroid-induced, after
  photorefractive keratectomy, 472
Punctal occlusion, for dry eye, 86–88, 87*i*
Punctal plugs, for dry eye, 86, 87*i*
Punctate epithelial erosions
  conjunctival, 21*t*
  corneal, 22*t*, 27, 28*i*, 29*t*
    in vernal conjunctivitis, 195

Punctate epithelial keratitis, 22*t*, 27,
    28–29*i*, 29*t*
  measles virus causing, 119, 155
Punctate epithelial keratopathy, 27, 28–29*i*
  exposure causing, 93–94
  microsporidial, 169
  staphylococcal blepharoconjunctivitis
    and, 157, 158*i*
Punctate staining patterns (fluorescein),
    19, 20*i*
Purine bases, 283
Pustule, of eyelid, 21*t*
Pyogenic granuloma, 250, 251
Pyrimidine bases, 283

Racquet flaps (single pedicle flaps), 402
Radial incisions, biomechanics of cornea
  affected by, 449
Radial keratotomy, 439*t*, 457–462, 457*i*
  biomechanics of cornea affected
    by, 449–450
  complications of, 460–461
  corneal topography after, 459
  efficacy and predictability of, 459
  future developments in, 461
  ocular surgery after, 461
  preoperative evaluation for, 457
  refraction after, 459
    stability of, 459
  surgical techniques for, 458
  variables affecting outcome of, 458–459
  visual acuity after, 459
  wound healing and, 453
Radiation. *See* Ionizing radiation;
    Ultraviolet light
Radius of curvature, of cornea, 11
  instantaneous (tangential power), 37,
    444, 444*i*
Rapid plasma reagin (RPR) test, 126
Reactive hyperplasia (lymphoid
  hyperplasia), 252, 253*i*
Rebleeding, after traumatic hyphema,
    364–366, 365*i*, 366*i*
Recessive trait, 285
Recipient eye, preparation of for
  penetrating keratoplasty, 416
Red blood cells (erythrocytes), cytologic
  identification of, 65
Red eye. *See* Inflammation (ocular)

Refraction
    after automated lamellar keratoplasty, 463
        stability of, 463
    after intracorneal lens/ring placement, 465
        stability of, 465
    after keratomileusis, 462
        stability of, 462
    after laser in situ keratomileusis,
        474–475
        stability of, 475
    law of (Snell's law), 442–443
    after photoastigmatic refractive
        keratectomy, 476
        stability of, 476
    after photorefractive keratectomy,
        stability of, 471–472
    after radial keratotomy, 460
        stability of, 460
Refractive index, of cornea, 11
Refractive keratectomy, photoastigmatic,
    476–479, 477i, 478i
Refractive power, of cornea, 442–443
Refractive surgery. See Keratorefractive
    surgery
Reis-Bücklers dystrophy, 293, 294i
    gene linkage of, 289t
Reiter syndrome, 210–211
Rejection, transplant, 412
    after lamellar keratoplasty, 432
    after penetrating keratoplasty, 426–428
Relaxing incision, for corneal astigmatism
    after penetrating keratoplasty,
        424–425
Rendu-Osler-Weber disease (hereditary
    hemorrhagic telangiectasia), 78–79
Replication, as virulence factor, 114
Restriction endonucleases, 288
Restriction fragment length polymorphisms
    (RFLP), 288
Rete ridges, 227, 228i
Retinitis, cytomegalovirus, in HIV
    infection/AIDS, 118
Retinoids, in dry eye syndromes, 90–91
Retinoscopy, 36
Retrocorneal membrane (posterior
    collagenous layer), 32
Retroillumination, for slit-lamp
    biomicroscopy, 17–18
    recurrent corneal erosions seen with, 97

Retroviruses, ocular infection caused
    by, 119–120
    agents for treatment of, 45
Reverse transcriptase inhibitors, 45
RFLP. See Restriction fragment length
    polymorphisms
Rheumatoid arthritis
    human leukocyte antigen (HLA)
        association and, 184t
    peripheral ulcerative keratitis and,
        214, 215i
Rheumatoid factor, testing for, 180t
Rhinophyma, in rosacea, 74
Rhinoviruses, ocular infection caused
    by, 119
Rhizopus, ocular infection caused by, 128
Ribonucleic acid. See RNA
Richner-Hanhart syndrome, 321
Rickettsia, ocular infection caused by, 121
Rieger anomaly/syndrome. See
    Axenfeld-Rieger syndrome
Riley-Day syndrome (familial
    dysautonomia), 92
Rimexolone, 41t
Ring of Schwalbe, displaced (posterior
    embryotoxon), 272, 273i
    in Axenfeld-Rieger syndrome, 272
Risk factors, in ocular infection, 115–116
Ritonavir, 45
Rizzutti's sign, in keratoconus, 306, 307i
RK. See Radial keratotomy
RNA, 284
    messenger, 284
    transfer, 284
RNA viruses, ocular infection caused
    by, 119–120
Rosacea, 73–75, 74i, 75i
Rose bengal staining
    as diagnostic method, 19
    in tear film evaluation, 59, 80, 81i
Rotational corneal autograft, 429–430
Rotational flap, for wound closure after
    pterygium excision, 395i, 396
Rothmund-Thomson syndrome, 329t
Route of infection, 114–115
RPR (rapid plasma reagin) test, 126
Rubeola virus (measles virus), ocular
    infection caused by, 119, 155

Stevens-Johnson syndrome (erythema multiforme major), 201–204, 202t
  human leukocyte antigen (HLA) association and, 184t
  limbal stem-cell dysfunction and, 107
  mucous membrane grafting for, 403
Stings, insect, ocular infection caused by, 131
Stocker's line, 340, 340i, 348t
STR. *See* Short tandem repeats
Streptococcus
  anginosus, 124
  keratitis caused by, 171t
  mitis, 124
  mutans, 124
  ocular infection caused by, 124
  pneumoniae (pneumococcus), 124
    acute purulent conjunctivitis caused by, 162
    keratitis caused by, 171t
  pyogenes, 124
  salivarius, 124
  sanguis, 124
  viridans, 124
Streptolysin, in ocular infections, 114
Streptomycin, 44
Stress model, corneal, 448, 448i
Striate keratopathy, intraocular surgery causing, 384
Striate melanokeratosis, 244
Stroma, corneal, 12–13. *See also under Stromal*
  inflammation of, 27–30, 30i. *See also* Stromal keratitis
    in systemic infections, 180
    varicella-zoster virus causing, 153
  wound healing of, 353–354
Stromal degenerations
  age-related (involutional) changes and, 342–343
  peripheral cornea and, 343–344
  postinflammatory changes and, 344–346
Stromal dystrophies, 293–301, 294t
  congenital hereditary, 276
Stromal edema, 32
Stromal graft rejection, isolated, 427
Stromal keratitis
  acute, scleritis and, 222
  Epstein-Barr virus causing, 154, 155i
  herpes simplex virus causing, 146–149

  in herpes zoster ophthalmicus, 153
  measles virus causing, 119, 155
  microsporidial, 179
  mumps virus causing, 119
  necrotizing, herpes simplex virus causing, 147, 148i
  non-necrotizing, herpes simplex virus causing, 146–147, 147i
  nonsuppurative, 22t, 29, 29t, 30i
  suppurative, 22t, 29, 29t, 30i
  varicella-zoster virus causing, 150–154
Stromal opacification, herpetic keratitis and, 149
Stromal scarring, herpetic keratitis and, 149
Stye (external hordeolum), 73
  in staphylococcal blepharoconjunctivitis, 160
Subconjunctival hemorrhage, 78–79
  causes of, 78t
Subepithelial corneal degenerations, 341–342
Subepithelial graft rejection, 426–427, 427i
Subepithelial infiltrate, 22t
Substantia propria, 11
  immunologic and inflammatory cells in, 183t
Sulfacetamide, 43t
  for chlamydial conjunctivitis, in neonate, 165
  with corticosteroids, 42t
Sulfatase deficiency, multiple, 316–317
Sulfisoxazole, 43t
Sulfonamides, 44
Superficial punctate keratitis of Thygeson, 208–209, 208i
Superior limbic keratoconjunctivitis, 95–97, 96i
Suppressor T cells. *See also* CD8+ T lymphocytes
  in external eye, 183t, 184
Supratarsal corticosteroid injections, for vernal keratoconjunctivitis, 197
Suprofen, 41t
Surface agents, ocular, 40
Surface irregularity, herpetic keratitis and, 149
Surgery. *See also specific procedure*
  anterior segment trauma caused by, 383–385
  for bacterial keratitis, 175–176

for corneal and anterior segment
disease, principles of, 46–50
for dry eye, 86–88, 87*i*
ocular surface, 389–391, 392–408
Surgical fluids, for corneal and anterior
segment surgery, 48
Surgical instruments, for corneal and
anterior segment surgery, 48, 49*t*
Surgical knots, for corneal and anterior
segment surgery, 46*i*
Surgical needles, for corneal and anterior
segment surgery, 46–47, 47*i*, 47*t*
Sutures
compression, for corneal astigmatism
after penetrating keratoplasty, 425
for corneal and anterior segment
surgery, 47, 48*i*
for penetrating keratoplasty, 416–418,
417*i*, 418*i*, 419*i*
postoperative problems related to,
422, 422*i*, 423*i*
Swelling pressure, 13
Symblepharon
in ocular cicatricial pemphigoid,
205, 205*i*
in Stevens-Johnson syndrome, 203, 203*i*
Sympathetic ophthalmia, enucleation for
corneoscleral laceration and,
375–376
Syphilis, 125
endemic (bejel), 125
interstitial keratitis caused by,
209–210, 211*i*
intrauterine, corneal anomalies
and, 278
tests for, 126
Systemic drug therapy, 39

T lymphocytes
in external eye, 183*t*, 184
in HIV infection/AIDS, 119
subsets of, 184
Tacrolimus, 43
Taenia solium, ocular infection caused
by, 130
Tangential incisions, biomechanics of
cornea affected by, 449, 449*i*
Tangential power (instantaneous radius of
curvature), 37, 444, 444*i*
Tangier disease, 315–316

Tarsal conjunctiva, 10
Tarsal muscle, inferior, involutional eyelid
changes and, 94
Tarsorrhaphy, 393–394
for exposure keratopathy, 93, 94
lateral, 393
medial, with canthoplasty, 393–394
for neurotrophic keratopathy, 93
Tarsus, 9, 10*i*
Tattoo, corneal, 348*t*, 408
Tay-Sachs disease (GM_2 gangliosidosis), 316
Tear–air interface. *See* Air–tear surface
Tear breakup time, 19, 56, 59
in meibomian gland dysfunction, 69
Tear–cornea interface, refraction at, 11
Tear deficiency states, 79–88. *See also
specific type*
rose bengal in evaluation of, 19
Tear film, 53–56
defective, 79–88. *See also specific type*
in defense mechanisms of outer eye, 111
evaluation of, 59–61
fluorescein for evaluation of, 19
function of, 53–56
immunoglobulins in, 184
Tear film osmolarity, 61
Tear substitutes. *See* Lubricants;
Tears, artificial
Tearing (epiphora), in ocular
inflammation, 21*t*
Tears
artificial. *See also* Lubricants
for dry eye, 8/85, 85*t*
for hay fever and perennial allergic
conjunctivitis, 194
for Stevens-Johnson syndrome, 202
composition of, assays of, 61
production of, tests of, 60, 60*i*
Telangiectasia, hereditary hemorrhagic
(Rendu-Osler-Weber disease), 78–79
Temperature, anterior segment injury
caused by, 356
TEN. *See* Toxic epidermal necrolysis
Teratogens, congenital corneal anomalies
and, 264–265
Terminal bulbs, 144, 144*i*
Tetracyclines, 43*t*, 44
for chlamydial conjunctivitis, 168
for meibomian gland dysfunction, 70–71
for persistent corneal defects, 101

for rosacea, 75
for trachoma, 166
Tetrahydrozoline, 41*t*
Th1 cells, 184
Th2 cells, 184
Thermal burns
anterior segment, 356
conjunctival autograft for, 397
Thermocauterization, for superior limbic
keratoconjunctivitis, 97
Thermokeratoplasty, 452, 453*i*, 479
for keratoconus, 308
Thiel-Behnke dystrophy, 293
gene linkage of, 289*t*
Thimerosal, allergic reactions to, 104, 105*i*
Thygeson superficial punctate keratitis,
208–209, 208*i*
Tight junctions, in corneal epithelium, 11
Tissue adhesives, cyanoacrylate, therapy
with, 394, 406–407
Tobramycin, 43*t*, 44
for bacterial keratitis, 173, 174, 174*t*
with corticosteroids, 42*t*
Tonometry, applanation, fluorescein for, 19
Topical anesthetics, abuse of,
conjunctivitis caused by, 103, 103*i*
Topical medications, 39. *See also* Eyedrops
Topography, corneal, 444–447, 448*t*
after automated lamellar keratoplasty, 463
indications for, 446–447, 447*i*
after intracorneal lens/ring placement, 465
after keratomileusis, 462
after laser in situ keratomileusis, 474–475
limitations of, 447, 448*t*
measurement of, 36–38
after photoastigmatic refractive
keratectomy, 476
after photorefractive keratectomy, 471
after radial keratotomy, 460
Toxic conjunctivitis, contact lens solutions
causing, 104
Toxic epidermal necrolysis, 201–204, 202*t*
Toxic medication reaction (toxic
conjunctivitis/keratoconjunctivitis),
212–213, 362
Toxic ulcerative keratopathy, 100
Toxocara, ocular infection caused by, 130
canis, 130
Toxoplasma gondii, ocular infection
caused by, 129

Trachoma, 165–166, 166*i*, 167*i*
Trait, 285
Transcription, in RNA formation, 284
Transdifferentiation, conjunctival, 57,
106, 390
Transfer RNA (tRNA), 284
Transitional zone, 437
Transplant rejection, 412
after lamellar keratoplasty, 432
after penetrating keratoplasty, 426–428
Transplantation. *See also specific type*
amniotic membrane, 389*t*, 390–391
conjunctival, 309*t*, 396–397
corneal, 411–413, 414–433. *See also*
Keratoplasty, penetrating
clinical approach to, 414–433
donor selection and, 412–413
eye banking and, 412–413
immunobiology of, 411
histocompatibility antigens and, 411
immune privilege and, 411–412
immunobiology of, 411–412
limbal, 397–400, 398–399*i*
mucous membrane, 389*t*, 390–391,
403–404
Transthyretin gene, mutation in, amyloid
deposits and, 323*t*, 324
Transverse keratotomy, 439–440*t*, 467–469
Traumatic hyphema, 364–368, 364*i*, 365*i*
medical management of, 366–367
rebleeding after, 364–366, 365*i*, 366*i*
sickle cell complications of, 367–368
surgery for, 367
Traumatic iritis, 363
Traumatic miosis, 363
Traumatic mydriasis, 363
Treacher Collins syndrome, 329*t*
Treponema, ocular infection caused
by, 125–126
pallidum, 125, 126
endemicum, 125
Triamcinolone, for chalazion, 72
Trichiasis, 102
Trifluridine, 43*t*
for herpetic dendritic and geographic
epithelial keratitis, 146
Trimethoprim, 43*t*
tRNA. *See* Transfer RNA
Trophic ulcers, herpetic keratitis and, 149

ILLUSTRATIONS

The authors submitted the following figures for this revision. (Illustrations that were reproduced from other sources or submitted by contributors not on the committee are credited in the captions.)

Andrew J. W. Huang, MD: Fig V-12, V-13

Carolyn M. Parrish, MD: Fig VII-1, VIII-10

John E. Sutphin, Jr, MD: Fig XIV-4, XXV-6

Kirk R. Wilhelmus, MD: Fig II-7, II-11, II-14, VI-16, VIII-28, X-8, XII-7, XII-13, XII-15, XII-17, XVIII-3